DEPRESSION

The Evolution of Powerlessness

Paul Gilbert

Mental Health Unit, Pastures Hospital, Derby and University of Leicester, UK

Routledge
Taylor & Francis Group
LONDON AND NEW YORK

First published 1992 Routledge

2 Park Square, Milton Park, Abingdon, Oxon OX14 4RN
711 Third Avenue, New York, NY 10017, USA

Routledge is an imprint of the Taylor & Francis Group, an informa business

First issued in hardback 2016

Transferred to Digital Printing 2009

British Library Cataloguing in Publication Data

Gilbert, Paul
Depression.
I. Title
616.8527

ISBN 978-0-86377-221-4 (pbk)
ISBN 978-1-138-15679-1 (hbk)

Cover design by Joyce Chester

Publisher's Note
The publisher has gone to great lengths to ensure the quality of this reprint but points out that some imperfections in the original may be apparent.

With love and affection to Jean, Hannah and James
May your archetypes serve you well

The rain to the wind said,
'you push and I'll pelt.'
They so smote the garden bed
that the flowers actually knelt,
and lay lodged – though not dead.
I know how they felt.

Robert Frost

Contents

Acknowledgements

The earlier version of this book, *Depression: From Psychology to Brain State*, was written twelve years ago but took time to find a publisher. Eventually Michael Forster at LEA came to the rescue. When *Depression* went out of print Michael came back to me for a second edition. With a desire to explore depression from an evolutionary perspective, I was hooked. I went back to Michael many times. I wanted to change the title and I wanted to expand the size. With persuasion Michael agreed and I am deeply grateful to him.

As a child I could not read until I was ten and my spelling was something else! I mention this to express my deep gratitude to Paul Dukes of LEA and the copy editor, Irene Tuchfeld. They worked tirelessly and without complaint with a manuscript which, in places, was probably unreadable to anyone else but me. My left brain does, of course, accept full responsibility for any remaining errors.

To my family I owe immense gratitude. Jean was always there as a help and support, took interest in how it was going, lifted my spirits when I felt I could not succeed and helped with references and many other things. Hannah and James would also rescue me with cricket on the lawn, snakes and ladders, got me to become a fan of the Gummi bears and other wonders. This book is dedicated to them, for their recognition, love, and constant mirroring.

When I first opened and dismantled the word processor on which I was to produce this book, I hardly dared switch it on. Cognitive distortion or not, I was sure it would blow up. My good friend Dr Dennis Trent set it up and introduced me to the wonders of word-processing. When I phoned him up with "Oh God Dennis I've just lost another chapter", he would speed across and almost by magic find it hiding somewhere on the hard disc, or take it to his system and try to sort it out. It was always the psychoanalytic chapters that played up—I wonder why? At work many friends and colleagues got used to me wandering around mumbling about reptiles and monkeys. Dr Chris Gillespie was very supportive and challenging and Barry Greatorex and Chris took to the model alerting me to research and ideas. Dr Haru Ghadiali provided many opportunities to discuss the links with archetype theory and envy, read various chapters and encouraged me to complete the project. Dr Hema Ghadiali also provided many opportunities for discussion and read chapters. Over the years various clinical trainees have passed through my room and they were challenging and excited. Special thanks go to Alistair Atherton, Nick Moore, Julie Pehl, and Steve Allen. The MSc trainees at Leicester and Birmingham Universities have also encouraged me and advised me what they would find helpful in a revised edition. Special thanks also go to Joyce Chantrill for her very hard work helping to sort out the diagrams, her unruffled support, and "no problem" attitude.

Some time ago a small group of us got together to explore evolution and ethology theory. This group now consists of Dr John Price, Dr Michael Chance, Dr Peter Trower, Dr Dennis Trent, and more recently Dr Dave Stevens. In one sense this book represents our work rather than mine, with a major input from John Price. Over a number of years they have been constant (hedonic) critics, spent pounds on the phone commenting on various chapters, guiding me away from gross errors. Without them this book would not be as it now is.

Also thanks must go to my friend in Texas, Professor Russ Gardner. Again, over many years we have exchanged letters, debated, and discussed. Thanks, too, to Shirley Reynolds, Dr John Teasdale, and Dr Chris Brewin who, although they may not agree with all that is written here, listened and commented on various ideas, sent papers, and were encouraging. I am sure there are many others I should thank since so many have commented and given their insights.

Last but not least thanks go to the many patients who have shared their depression and have taught me much of what I shall relate. Many have become well, some have not and a few have died. To all of them I owe a debt.

Back in 1975 when I started to research depression I was always interested in the question of why depression is possible as part of human experience. In the intervening years I have been enabled to explore many different theoretical models and, perhaps, slowly some kind of understanding is beginning (although at times I am not so sure). It has been 400 million years since we lived in the sea and yet misery still stalks us. Sadly evolution is not about happiness but social success as we shall discuss. To understand depression, in my view, one cannot ignore this history. This book looks mostly at theory although there is also discussion of therapy issues. Theories are the handmaidens of science, however, and in the end must always bow to evidence. Although I have tried to comply with a scientific approach handmaidens can at times be unintentionally wayward. There is much yet to learn but also much that is known. Also I have tried to show that those of different theoretical persusion must talk to and understand each other to be better attendants to the scientific enterprise.

This book is designed to share with you a journey that explores evolutionary theory and the role that power and a sense of belonging have played in the evolution of mental mechanisms. We will explore various theories of depression and how our theories speak to us about different facets of the depressed mind. I hope you will find it useful. Of course no matter how encompassing a theory, at the end of the day the arbiter of ideas is research evidence. But without a decent theory the search for evidence is poorly directed.

As for me, Christmas comes shortly and the wine rack is stocked.

Paul Gilbert, December 1990.

PART I

TYPES

History, Diagnoses, Epidemiology, and Personality

CHAPTER 1

Introduction: Controversies Old and New

Depression has been labelled the common cold of psychopathology. This comparison is unfortunate, for it conveys the impression of a frequent but mild complaint. In reality some depressions end fatally. Depression is responsible for the majority of suicide deaths; those most vulnerable to suicide are depressed and have lost hope (Minkoff, Bergman, Beck, A.T. & Beck, R., 1973; Wetzel, 1976). In many developed countries suicide is in the top ten most frequent causes of death and in younger, male cohorts, in the top three (see Chapter 3). Less easy to calculate, and only recently a subject of study, are those biological correlates of depression which appear to affect adversely immune system function (Farrant & Perez, 1989) and the capacity to combat physical disorder (e.g., via a cortisol — immune system feedback process). Moreover, depression may well reduce life expectancy in certain physical disorders, e.g., cancer (Whitlock & Siskind, 1979).

Outside these physical and life-threatening aspects, depression significantly affects family life. Depressed children suffer various social and academic developmental difficulties (Kovacs, 1989). Parents who are depressed, or who use various mechanisms to defend against a depression, can have a disturbing influence on their children's development and subsequent vulnerability (Gelfand & Teti, 1990; Gotlib & Lee, 1990) and family relationships (Beach, Sandeen & O'Leary, 1990) For all these and other reasons, depression is not only the most frequent mental health problem, but is among the most serious.

Hence, at the biological level, at the psychological level and at the family level, depression exerts a multitude of effects. Rarely discussed in the literature is depression at a cultural level. This is the role the socio-political structures of society play on individuals' feeling state. Recent documentaries, exploring personal experiences of living in totalitarian regimes, have illuminated how many people are often pessimistic and fearful, suffer poor sleep patterns, and are dysphoric. East Germans have told how they feel increasingly marginalised by integration with West Germany, and express openly many symptoms of depression. In a different context, the fragmentation of the Australian Aborigine culture has left in its wake a rise in depression, pessimism, suicide, and alcoholism. These cultural aspects are difficult to explore from a disease theory point of view, since many would argue that these culturally related depressed states are not 'illnesses'. But to social psychiatrists, psychologists, sociologists, and anthropologists, they are important areas of study and our understanding of them is extremely important. Ring fencing depression in terms of disease–not disease is to court various confusions as we shall see later.

There is reason for both some optimism and caution, however. Since the turn of the century progress has been made on understanding the biological bases of depressed states, and developing new drugs and treatments. The psychological aspects are also better known than at any time previously and our understanding of the social conditions that give rise to depression has also advanced. In the biological, psychological, and sociological sciences, as we shall see, there is no shortage of competing theories with varying degrees of evidence to support them. Thus, although frequent and potentially very serious, depression is often a treatable disorder using one or a combination of interventions. Against this optimism however, we should note that during the eighties it has also become apparent that many who are depressed do not come forward for help or are unrecognised as being depressed. Even if depression is recognised many receive inadequate treatment. We have also found that chronic depression can affect up to 20% of cases, and the longer the follow up the less well cohorts do (at least 50% of patients will relapse). Furthermore, for all our progress, depression may be increasing in both the western (Klerman, 1988) and non-western worlds. Schwab (1989, p.16) claims:

> Concern about sociocultural factors contributing to a "new age of melancholy"... is not limited to the Western world. I have been told by psychiatrists in some of the developing nations that they have observed a drastic increase in depression during the past 20 years. In their World Health Organisation (WHO) report on the collaborative study of the

> assessment of the depressive disorders, Sartorius and his colleagues, [Sartorius et al., 1983] maintain that there are probably 100 million depressives in the world and that the number may be increasing because of deleterious sociocultural effects, demographic changes, psychological factors, the increased number of patients with chronic medical disorders, and the widespread use of medications that have depressive side effects.

While I have great respect for my biological colleagues it is quite untenable to believe that in the majority of these cases we are dealing with a disease and can now drug our way out of trouble. To advance our knowledge further, new ways must be found to develop multidisciplinary and biopsychosocial theories. If not we will end up with an ever-increasing number of theories, useless conflicts over whether depression is a disease or not, polarisation into brainless or mindless positions (Eisenberg, 1986) and to regard individuals as socially decontextualised entities, victims to negative thoughts and/or brain amines. In such a world, debate tends to centre on trivia and not on major points of agreement or disagreement. More serious, prevention becomes a fragmented endeavour with different groups peddling different ideas, many of which fail to deal with our life styles as the problem for many. The importance of understanding the causes of depression as a multilevel phenomenon (genetic threshold, early family life, psychological styles and social context) can hardly be overstated.

In this book we tackle this problem from a biopsychosocial perspective. An endeavour is made to indicate how social and psychological processes influence biological processes by virtue of the evolutionary path we have journeyed. We also give due regard to the possibility that a small percentage of depressives may carry genetic vulnerability. It is hoped this will help counteract the growing fragmentation of approaches and models which are often based on faulty conceptions of mind-body distinctions and naive ideas about the evolution of mental mechanisms.

OUTLINE

Our journey is split into three parts. Part 1 contains four chapters that explore the types of depression. Chapter 1 explores how some of our current controversies are products of ages past, and a brief overview is given to historical and philosophical aspects. This is followed in Chapter 2 by a more detailed look at the issues of classification and types of depression. Chapter 3 explores what we know about epidemiology and long term outcome of depression. Chapter 4 engages the thorny problem of the role of personality in depression.

Part 2 contains chapters that explore the evolved mechanisms of depression, or the evolved basic plan(s) for depression. Chapter 5 outlines current theory on the evolution of mental mechanisms. Chapter 6 explores the central theme of this book that depression evolved from a) ranking behaviour (social dominance-subordination) and is associated with innate algorithms for social comparison (inferior-superior) and what we call involuntary, subordinate, self-perception; and b) ingroup-outgroup behaviour which is also associated with innate algorithms for social comparison but of a same-different form. Hence, depression is viewed as a problem of loss/lack of social power and control. Chapter 7 explores how our need for rank, on the one hand, and sense of being like others, on the other, have evolved into a need for self-esteem, to have a sense of positive value to ourselves and others (called living in the minds of others) and hence our concern with our self-presentation and sense of belonging. Chapter 8 explores the experiences of depression under the concept of 'dread' and examines how the experiences of shame, anger and envy are related to a ranking (social dominance) theory of depression. How these are involved in self-organisation is discussed.

Part 3 explores current psychological and social theories of depression. Chapter 9 examines the work of Freud and object relations theory. Chapter 10 follows the view of depression as a thwarting of (innate) human needs and explores the work of Bowlby and Kohut. Chapter 11 takes us back to the idea of underlying social algorithms and biosocial goals (Gilbert, 1989) from the point of view of archetype theory and mentality theory. Here we consider various themes in depressive thinking (of the empty self, the outsider and the subordinate). Chapter 12 explores aspiration and incentive structure in depression and the role of hopelessness. Chapter 13 explores cognitive therapy and some of the recent developments and controversies of this approach. Chapter 14 explores various behavioural theories. Chapter 15 attempts to bring us back in a kind of circle with discussion of the interpersonal theories, the role of life events, social support, and family structure, raising again the issues of power and social dominance, social control and belonging. In the last chapter I summarise the main themes and issues discussed, explore the complexities for studying multilevel interactions and also the role of patterns of self-organisation. That is the outline; let's begin the journey.

HISTORICAL AND PHILOSOPHICAL INFLUENCES

Person or Disease

Early reports of depression can be found in numerous biblical characters. King Solomon is believed to have suffered from an evil spirit and dark moods from which he eventually killed himself. The book of Job is regarded as the work of a depressive. More recent historical sufferers include various composers (e.g., Gustave Mahler, Tchaikovsky, Sibelius) politicians (e.g., Abraham Lincoln and Winston Churchill) and numerous writers, artists and poets (e.g., Edgar Allen Poe and Thomas Mann).

It is worth reminding ourselves that, unlike many illnesses today, depression has been recognised and described in one form or another for over two millennia. Jackson (1986) gives a marvellous overview of the history of thought on depression. The Greeks, especially Hippocrates, Galen and many others, not only outlined the essential characteristics of depression but also had consistent and well described theories for it. The depressed person was described as gloomy and pessimistic, anxious and prone to hide away or take flight, sleepless and also peevish, irritable and prone to outbursts. For the most part the Hippocratic theory was a psychobiological theory. They worked with the idea that there were four basic temperaments related to four bodily substances, the humours: yellow bile, black bile, phlegm, and blood. Melancholia was believed to be the result of excess black bile. This linkage of mood state to some underlying biological disturbance has been with us ever since.

The second aspect of Greek theory was the idea that certain personalities are more prone to depression than others. Thus, the Greeks believed that a preponderance of the different body humours gave rise to different personality types. Melancholia was noted in people of melancholic (black bile) temperament. This view also is still with us although we have exchanged black bile for the concept of neuroticism.

Third, the Greeks believed that various events including the seasons, diets and life events, which could disturb the black bile, could result in depression. The implications for treatment were in terms of rest and diet, and Hippocrates especially argued for a generally supportive and kindly orientation to the depressed person. Here, the approach was very much the study of the individual, inspired by concern with treatment and care of patients. And that depression was a *quantitative* variation from normal. The Hippocratic approach was, then, *person*-centred. It is odd that the biopsychosocial model should have such a promising, early beginning and yet such a disappointing history. Even today this approach still struggles for recognition and we still have what Eisenberg (1986) has called brainlessness and mindlessness science.

Hippocrates was a physician and was concerned to explain various forms of madness as emanating in bodily processes. However, this view was not uncontested and Plato believed in two types of madness: one the result of bodily processes and one due to outside forces, mostly from the Gods. Hence Plato believed that epilepsy was a gift from the Gods that brought with it the power of revelation. Hippocrates was very opposed to this idea (Zilboorg & Henry, 1941). But in a number of other cultures, madness and depression, particularly, have often been viewed as the result of disturbance of the soul rather than the body. For example, that the soul had been afflicted by evil forces or even stolen in some way. Even Jesus is reported to have cured a case of mental illness by the casting out of devils. You may think that today we no longer adhere to these theories but this is not so. Recently, I had a bipolar patient who had fallen in with a religious group who had tried to exorcise her devils. Needless to say, this caused some problems with re-attribution training. But importantly, this conceptualisation of depression led to various ideas that depression was somehow to do with immoral living and a sign of weakness. Such an orientation, dominated by religious thought, has echoed through the centuries (Zilboorg & Henry, 1941; Jackson, 1986).

Plato left his mark in other ways. The Platonic approach to illness, arose from a particular philosophical orientation, "the doctrine of universals" (Kendell, 1975). Plato was not a physician like Hippocrates and therefore did not personally attempt to heal anyone or to be in close contact with suffering. The Platonic approach suggested that illness was a *qualitative* variation from normal, and concern was very much on the illness or disease itself and less on the individual. Disease was a different thing, that had somehow entered or grown in the body; it was alien and abnormal. Hence, the Platonic approach was a *disease*-centred approach. As Kendell (1975) makes clear, considerable controversy has embellished these (Hippocratic-quantitative versus the Platonic-qualitative) positions. Indeed, the study of diseases in psychiatry is still an area of heated debate (Akiskal & McKinney, 1973a,b; Kräupl Taylor, 1980; Scadding, 1980).

Mind and/or Body

As complex and problematic as the qualitative (disease) versus quantitative (person) debate is, it is not the only philosophical stumbling block in psychiatry. When Descartes formalised the distinction between mind and body (in part to get around the problems of the soul in the brain), it was in the very nature of psychiatry that this was to become a second major arena for debate. In spite of major efforts (Hill, 1981;

Popper & Eccles, 1977), dualism remains a controversy in its own right and continues to plague psychiatric discussion. Indeed, it is only by maintaining a very strict dualistic approach that Szasz (1974,pp.12–13) can argue: "The notion of mental illness derives its main support from such phenomena as syphilis of the brain or delirious conditions—intoxications, for instance—in which persons may manifest certain disorders of thinking and behaviour. Correctly speaking these are diseases of the brain, not the mind".

Dualism lies at the heart of the neurotic-psychotic controversy (Hill, 1968). Moreover, as Engle (1977) suggests, to dissociate mind from body provides the rationale for a mechanistic approach to suffering. The mechanistic approach fits neatly with Platonic disease entities. It must be said though, that the Platonic approach, in spite of its questionable corrupting influence on the sensitivities of the physician, has proved enormously useful, especially for the infectious diseases. Indeed, as Kendell (1975) makes clear, by the turn of this century, so successful was this approach in revealing the secrets of many disorders which had plagued humans for centuries, that psychiatry could hardly resist similar endeavours with a similar philosophy. Hence, by the turn of the century a new age in psychiatry was born out of Platonic successes in physical medicine. Yet psychiatry was to enter this era with the two outstanding controversies (qualitative versus quantitative and mind-body) far from resolved. The mind-body problem stirs up a lot of (often) unprofitable debate and in the extreme leads back again to mindless or brainless theory (Eisenberg, 1986).

These difficulties have been long recognised. Psychiatry has tended to regard mental life as capable of considerable, usually arbitrary, dissection. As Zilboorg and Henry (1941, p.496) point out, psychiatry's view of depression was no exception:

> What formal psychiatry chose to consider as emotions were not emotions at all but verbal and muscular manifestations. Emotions were considered a separate functional department of man's body structure; they were considered subject independently to abnormal variations and were therefore thought to cause "affective psychoses" disturbances of the so called "affective field" or of the "emotional level," which could be considered apart from other faculties such as thinking and imagination. Such a departmentalization of the human personality made it easy to give one's methods of psychological investigation the appearance of scientific work. Each part could be studied separately and "objectively", that is to say, only from the standpoint of what it looks like from the outside and not how it works from the inside.

Clearly, such a departmentalisation of emotion obscures the complexity and diversity of emotional experience, and tends to play down the importance of the interaction between thinking, imagination, behaviour, and biology. Moreover, by viewing emotionality (at least in its pathological forms) as an autonomous system, those theories that emphasise the role of biological dysfunction in depressive disturbance have tended to pay little attention to the role of (social) behaviour and cognition in the etiology, maintenance, or treatment of the disturbance. What we now know about the evolution of mental mechanisms shows this view to be quite untenable (Chapters 5-8).

Social Power

There is of course another issue at stake here and that is power (Turner, 1987). Problem definition defines boundaries and domains of expertise. If psychiatric disorder is defined as a disease of the body then it requires specialist knowledge of biological processes to treat and remove/alter it. Much has now been written on this (Turner, 1987). Drug companies have vested interests in the biological treatments and their activities in the third world have not gone uncriticised.

The reason that this issue is important is that all the classification debates carry hidden agendas of who can do what to whom, how preventative programmes should be organised and how resources and power is allocated. Time is money and money and resources dictate what kind of response a society will offer to those that suffer. In my view, in the vast majority of cases (but not all), depression represents a disturbance of biopsychosocial patterns of living. Such a view invites us to grapple with a complexity that is no respecter of our human, constructed, interdisciplinary boundaries. This approach is possible (e.g., Vasile et al., 1987) though difficult.

In the above sections then we have considered three types of problem: (1) the quantitative-qualitative or person versus disease approach; (2) the mind-body or the mindless versus brainless approach; and (3) the issue of social power as a hidden agenda in response to the first two difficulties. Having noted these we can now explore how the disease theories came to dominate (until recently) our conceptualisations of depression.

THE SEARCH FOR DISEASE ENTITIES IN PSYCHIATRY

If Descartes served one important function, it was to allow the brain to become subject to scientific study without fearing the hand of God or damaging someone's soul. Hence, by the time Emil Kraepelin

(1855-1926) came to study psychiatry it was obvious that the brain was the seat of the emotions, thoughts, and behaviour and that various changes in brain functioning could cause changes in behaviour, emotions, and even personality. Most of this work had come from neurology and the study of brain-damaged patients. Kraepelin was born during the Platonic orientation in medicine. It was an orientation whose interest lay not so much in the patient as in the clinical phenomenon itself. For all Kraepelin's abilities, he reflected the spirit of his age in that his interest in the individual patient was, more often than not, notably absent. As Zilboorg and Henry (1941) put it, Kraepelin was "greatly interested in humanity but comparatively little in man". Kraepelin collected data from a number of sources and by careful analysis attempted to impose an ordered system of classification based on the assumption that mental illness could be categorised in terms of a distinct and finite number of disease entities.

The major distinction Kraepelin put forward for psychosis was in terms of dementia praecox and manic-depressive insanity. Kraepelin argued that manic-depressive insanity runs a cyclic course where the patient suffers from attacks of elation and depression, often with returns to normal in between attacks. The prognosis was considered favourable, in that these patients recovered. Dementia praecox was characterised by symptoms of catatonia and hebephrenia, often accompanied by auditory hallucinations. Prognosis for such patients was not good, since it was thought that dementia praecox would eventually terminate in a state of dementia proper. Diagnosis was by prognosis; if the prognosis was correct then the diagnosis was correct. This, unfortunately, led to a rather deterministic attitude to treatment; if the patient suffered from manic-depressive psychosis, the patient would recover. If, however, they suffered from dementia praecox, the individual would eventually deteriorate into dementia.

Although ideas concerning dementia praecox (or schizophrenia as Bleuler renamed it later) had been forming for over 40 years, and concepts of manic depression even longer, Kraepelin's system did not receive uncontested support. Fifty years earlier Griesinger and also Zeller had scorned any attempt to subdivide mental illness, asserting that although mental illness could have different manifestations it was essentially a unitary phenomenon. Fifty years after Kraepelin, Menninger (1963) offered the same rebuke to the Kraepelinian system. As we will see in Chapter 2, concepts of negative affectivity and the effectiveness of antidepressants for various disorders suggest that these writers may yet be correct in essential ways.

Even in Kraepelin's own day many did not accept the Kraepelinian classification system. Hoche argued that there was no evidence that these "well-formed, self-contained, disease entities" actually existed in any pure form (see Lewis, 1967). Hoche viewed Kraepelin's distinct disease entities as no more than convenient symptom clusters. There also appeared to be factual discrepancies in the Kraepelinian system. Sometime earlier Kahlbaum, who had contributed enormously to the development of dementia praecox being labelled as a disease entity, had reported cycles in catatonia. Three years before Kraepelin published *Lehrbuch* in 1899, Mendel had argued that neurasthenia could also be cyclical in its course. Thus, as Zilboorg and Henry (1941) argue, these facts, among others, had to be overlooked in order to preserve the sense of solidity and correctness in the new nosological system. Consequently, Kraepelin's system, even from the time of its first emergence, showed certain characteristics of artificiality.

From a historical point of view it seems that the acceptance of the Kraepelinian system by psychiatry was a product of the age. First, as mentioned earlier, the concept of dementia praecox had been forming for over 40 years, with notable aid from Kahlbaum. Second, it offered psychiatry a fairly concrete paradigm, which had great potential as an integrating framework. Third, the developments and achievements in general medicine placed considerable pressure on psychiatry to produce similar results. The Kraepelinian system seemed to answer the call on behalf of psychiatry. Fourth, it gave the discipline of psychiatry a good grounding in disease theory and established its own social power base.

In a sense Hippocrates won a great victory with the inauguration of the Kraepelinian system; mental illness was firmly in the hands of medicine. Further it began the rudiments of a scientific approach to psychiatry that moved away from charlatanism and arbitrary opinion; one could begin to debate the evidence (although access to gathering the evidence and having the skills to understand what constituted evidence, by virtue of training, was clearly prescribed to lie within the medical domain). Yet paradoxically, in so doing, it had slipped the principles of Hippocrates and had taken up with Plato. Investigations into mental illness became more centred on the "disease entity" and its characteristics, rather than on the individual patient. Gone was the biopsychosocial model of the early Greeks, and Schule's Hippocratic-style warning to psychiatrists to remember that they were treating sick people, not merely sick brains, went unheeded. As Zilboorg and Henry (1941) put it, "this principle clashed too much with the newly established harmonious relationship between medicine and psychiatry."

One of the obvious consequences of Kraepelin's classification system, which became so dominant in European psychiatry, was that it had a significant effect on the orientation of future research. This orientation was based on the philosophy of discontinuities between disorders.

Depressive illness was significantly affected by this approach. Unfortunately, Kraepelin left many pitfalls for subsequent researchers. First, Kraepelin's category of manic-depressive psychosis was a very inclusive category. Lewis (1967) points out that Hoche, in 1910, seized on this problem in his argument with Kraepelin over the existence of disease entities. Hoche argued that by the time of Kraepelin's eighth edition (1909), Kraepelin had relegated "melancholia" (involutional depression) from a disease to a clinical picture: "and that it no longer mattered whether there was mania or melancholia, occurring once in a life or many times, at regular or irregular intervals, whether late or early with predominance of these or those symptoms, it was still manic-depressive insanity."

However, it was not only the over-inclusiveness of the manic-depressive complex that presented problems for future research. Another major confusion arose from the use of terms and distinctions, such as exogenous/endogenous, neurotic/psychotic, which crept into psychiatry at the turn of the century.

The Establishment of the Exogenous/Endogenous Position

The exogenous/endogenous causal distinction has had a major influence on psychiatry in general, and depression in particular (Lewis, 1971). It was introduced into psychiatry by Mobius in 1893, the concept being borrowed directly from the botanist Caudelle 1813 (see Zilboorg & Henry, 1941). This fact is of more than historic interest, however, since the botanist's exogenous/endogenous distinction rested totally on a physical discrimination. Similarly, the original psychiatric use of the exogenous/endogenous distinction was to discriminate between different "physical causes" of mental illness. Mobius labelled those illnesses considered to be due to degenerative or hereditary factors (i.e., internal causes) as "endogenous disorders". Those illnesses considered to be due to bacterial, chemical, or other toxic agents (i.e., external causes) were labelled as "exogenous disorders". As Beck (1973) points out, such definitions left no room for other causal factors, namely social or psychogenic.

Both Kraepelin and Bonhoeffer accepted Mobius' exogenous/endogenous distinction, although Kraepelin did not accept it as a classification system, since it was based totally on etiological considerations. However, Bonhoeffer developed the distinction further and put forward his own concept of exogenous disorders. To Bonhoeffer (1909), exogenous reactions were also of a totally physical origin. They were "modes of response by the brain to injury" (Lewis, 1971). If no direct relationship between a toxin or injury and mental illness could be found, it was suggested that these toxins and/or injuries had produced intermediary products in the body, and it was these intermediary products which were responsible for the mental illness. Thus, Bonhoeffer not only maintained the exogenous/endogenous discrimination as a purely "physical" distinction, but also allowed for exogenous reactions to be of a psychotic magnitude. In contrast to some modern discriminations, which on occasions have loosely equated exogenous with neurotic and endogenous with psychotic, Bonhoeffer's use of these terms was clear. For Bonhoeffer, exogenous and endogenous distinctions referred to differences in physical etiologies, whereas the term "psychotic" referred to the severity of the illness, although definitions of psychosis remained vague. However, subsequent semantic confusions were to arise in the use of these terms.

At the very time psychiatry was celebrating its strengthened union with medicine, with the delineation of the disease entities dementia praecox and manic-depressive insanity, work was being conducted (notably in France on hysteria) which was to intrude into this neat nosological system and raise a host of thorny philosophical problems. These problems presented many conceptual difficulties for Kraepelin's classifications.

Psychogenesis as a Problem for the Exogenous/Endogenous Dichotomy, and the Platonic Concept of Disease

Through the work of Charcot (1825-1893) and later Freud (1856-1939), the importance of psychological processes as major etiological factors in neurosis became established. But the actual concept of "neurosis" was vague and its relationship to psychosis even vaguer. It appears that at the turn of this century, the only illness considered to be of true psychogenic origin was hysteria. For example, in 1911 Bonhoeffer wrote an important paper entitled "How far should all psychogenic illnesses be regarded as hysterical?" In this paper Bonhoeffer (see Hirsch & Shepherd, 1974, p.54) stated: ". . . many psychiatrists would today assume that an illness must be hysterical if in its origin and development it can be seen to depend to a marked degree on psychological causes".

This statement offers some interesting insight into the current attitude of the day toward the role of psychological factors in mental illness. However, it was not a position which Bonhoeffer himself advocated. In the same paper he put forward the view that psychogenesis could play a major role in the development of other disorders besides hysteria. With regard to depressive illness Bonhoeffer argued (see Hirsch & Shepherd, 1974, p.57):

> There is however, a group of depressive illnesses in which the psychological impetus is of prime importance. We are indebted to Reiss for drawing our attention to this group, which he called "reactive depressions." These depressive states are constitutionally based: they occur in individuals who from youth onwards are inclined to take things badly, whose depressive reaction is generally severe and of more than average duration. Severe psychological upsets can be followed by depressive exacerbations of psychotic intensity which are clearly psychogenic since frequently, although not always, when the psychological cause is removed the depressive exacerbation likewise disappears.

The view that "these depressive states are constitutionally based" may imply that Bonhoeffer believed that "reactivity" was an endogenous predisposition, thus placing reactivity within the concept of endogenous factors. Looking back Bonhoeffer's ideas seem to be the forerunner of what later became considered as depressive personality (Phillips, Gunderson, Hirschfield & Smith, 1990) and/or dysthymia. Bonhoeffer further argued that some forms of epilepsy, paranoia, and mania could also be psychologically determined. Bonhoeffer believed that these illnesses could be ascertained by considering precipitating events. He labelled all such forms of illness as "reactive disorders".

Kraepelin accepted Mobius' and Bonhoeffer's exogenous/endogenous etiological distinction. He further accepted the possibility that psychogenic factors could play a role in certain mental disorders. However, unlike Bonhoeffer, Kraepelin placed psychogenic factors within the concept of exogenous causes, and did not distinguish them from physical exogenous causes, ignoring the concept of reactivity (Lewis, 1971). This destroyed the purely physical characteristics of the original exogenous/endogenous distinction. In so doing, Kraepelin introduced into his own nosological system the old philosophical problem of mind–body dualism.

Prior to the absorption of psychogenesis into the exogenous concept of causality, exogenous illness was regarded as physically determined, e.g., through bacteria, toxin, and/or injury. The inclusion of nonphysical factors within the exogenous concept presented considerable problems since it implied that psychological, nonphysical factors could interact with the (physical) disease process. But this position is essentially incompatible with the Platonic concept of a "disease entity". Indeed it is at this point in history that we see the mind/body and the qualitative/quantitative problems becoming entwined within the same sources of reference. So basically the question was, is neurosis an endogenous susceptiblty as various personality theories now argue, or is it purely an acquired trait, the result of some external events (currently or previously) happening to a person (see Chapter 4)?

Various attempts have been made to save the disease entity concept of mental illness, by separating all illnesses of psychogenic origin from the endogenous (physical) illnesses. Thus, as Fish (1974) points out, Schneider argued that neuroses, psychogenic reactions, personality developments, and abnormal personalities are not illnesses in a sense of there being a morbid process in the nervous system, while the functional psychoses are illnesses in this sense. But this solution still leaves the problem of clearly specifying the dividing line between "physical" mental illness (or morbid process) and "nonphysical" mental illness. The attempts to identify this dividing line have been at the heart of many of the controversies regarding mental illness, especially those concerning a meaningful classification of depression.

MODERN APPROACHES TO CLASSIFICATION

As we noted above, the turn of the century saw the beginning of the application of scientific principles to the problems of mental suffering. Modern approaches, reflect this advance in their attempts to quantify, verify and replicate findings. Modern approaches have focused on the notion of the psychiatric syndrome. A syndrome is a set of symptoms that tend to go together. Unfortunately perhaps, the study of syndromes has not being simply concerned with what symptoms tend to go together but also to include notions of causality.

Ever since the development of the Kraepelinian nosology, much was written about the "exogenous" disorders, with their identifiable external etiological characteristics, but very little appeared concerning the endogenous disorders. This situation was particularly noticeable for depression. The endogenous depressive disorders existed as "hypothetical, intangible, elusive predispositions, constitutional or hereditary forces which could be conjectured but not demonstrated" (Lewis, 1971). Thus, classification in terms of etiology was dubious since endogenous disorders were, by definition, simply those disorders for which no precipitator, or exogenous factor could be found. Consequently, the diagnosis of an endogenous disorder rested on the assumption that if no exogenous event presented itself as the cause of the illness, then the illness must be the product of a morbid disease process in the central nervous system. Partly as a result of this dilemma, various methods have been used to try to identify the natural boundaries between the subtypes (syndromes) of depression. In general three alternative approaches have been used (e.g., see Becker, 1974):

1. The cross-sectional approach which seeks consistent groups of signs and symptoms (syndromes).
2. The longitudinal, natural history approach which examines inter-relationships between various factors such as family history, age of onset, duration, severity, periodicity, and outcome.
3. The treatment-response approach which seeks to identify subgroups by examining different responses to various forms of therapeutic intervention.

In each approach, although primarily in the cross-sectional approach, there has been an effort to find a zone of rarity between disorders (Kendell, 1975). Without this, disorders shade imperceptibly into each other. This effort has not been entirely successful. Kendell and Brockington (1980) used a nonlinear method of analysis in an attempt to show a zone of rarity between affective psychosis and schizophrenia. They found little support for the disease entity view. They concluded that the necessary evidence to distinguish the psychoses into Platonic-like disease entities has not been provided, but rather the evidence favours a dimensional classification. Researchers have not been deterred by negative findings and there remains continued concern about the distinction between neurosis and psychosis on the one hand and endogenous and reactive types on the other.

Furthermore, although various early studies often used etiological terms and distinctions as descriptions of their "classified groups", these studies were not directly concerned with etiological considerations. Rather, as Becker (1974, p.38) pointed out:

> . . . they are chiefly concerned with whether depression is unitary or binary, that is, a single syndrome or two syndromes (endogenous and reactive), and whether the syndrome or syndromes is/are categorical or dimensional, that is, whether they are discrete entities (categorical) or whether they are normally distributed and occur in varying combination with each other or with other syndromes (dimensional).

These disputes are still very much with us, and reflect a failure to solve the Platonic (qualitative, categorical) versus the Hippocratic (quantitative, dimensional) concept of disease, assuming, of course, that a resolution is desirable and possible. At the heart of these disputes remain the fundamental problems of the philosophical orientation to the concept of disease. Eysenck (1970) argued that in the study of depressive illness, each of these two philosophical approaches (Platonic versus Hippocratic) has two basic positions. For the Platonic qualitative concept of a disease entity, depression can be either unitary categorical or binary categorical. For the Hippocratic concept of illness, depression can be either unitary dimensional or binary dimensional. A further complication is the view that some depressions are of the mind while others are the direct result of a primary (morbid process) biochemical dysfunction.

For both the unitary categorical and the binary categorical views, a demonstration of the distinctiveness of depression is required. First, it must be established that depression does not shade imperceptibly from normal unhappiness into depression, with various individuals existing somewhere on this continuum. Nor can the same individual move up and down on this continuum. Categorical means they either have it or they don't. Second, depression as an "entity" must be shown to be different from other "entities," and does not shade imperceptibly into, say, anxiety disorder or schizophrenia. In the mid-1960s and early 1970s Roth and his co-workers from Newcastle suggested that they had obtained evidence for distinguishing neurotic from endogenous depressive disorders (Carney, Roth & Garside, 1965; Kiloh & Garside, 1963) and for distinguishing depressive illness from anxiety states. Their position is basically a binary categorical one. But we now know that there is a high comorbidity between depression an anxiety (see Chapter 2).

There are many difficulties in evaluating some of the early work on classification. Major differences in procedure and data gathering have not lent themselves to a consistency of approach or evidence, and it is not surprising, therefore, that evidence is often unclear or contradictory. Moreover, in spite of the errors and questionable assumptions of factor analysis, Kendell (1968, 1975, 1976) argues that factor analysis tends to favour a dimensional, rather than a categorical classification system. He suggests that a dimensional approach more accurately forecasts treatment and outcome than the traditional categorical (disease entity) position. Eysenck (1970) agrees with Kendell but argues that two dimensions, neurotic and psychotic, are required if substantial information is not to be lost. Kendell (1976) rejoins this by suggesting that the same argument can be made for any number of dimensions. The number of dimensions really depends on the purpose for which the classification is designed.

Another problem is the type of symptom to be included. Fatigue (loss of energy) and weight loss are common symptoms of depression but are also rather common in many other disorders including physical disorders. On the other hand may factors that might be helpful in classification, like anger control, hostility, shame, and envy are usually left out. But depression is a psychic state and it makes little sense to focus on symptoms that are highly generalised and common, at the expense of symptoms that are clearly related to psychic processes and influenced by mood state. Hence, perhaps one of the reasons that the classification of depression has difficulty is that it explores too narrow a range of symptoms.

RECENT PERSPECTIVES ON CLASSIFICATION

A plethora of approaches and nosologies has grown up around the depressive disorders. Here we briefly examine some of these.

Statistical

The lack of clear biological markers for major depression and its sub-types has meant that the statistical approach has been very appealing. An often used technique is factor analysis. This involves assessing a range of symptoms and then subjecting them to a statistical procedure that will group them according to how symptoms correlate with each other. During the seventies this procedure provided some support for the neurotic/psychotic distinction and also the neurotic/endogenous distinction (e.g., see Fowles & Gersh, 1979a,b; Kendell, 1976; Mendels & Cochrane, 1968; Nelson & Charney, 1981).

Cluster analysis, as explored by Paykel (1971), suggested four subgroups of depression: (a) psychotic; (b) anxious depression; (c) hostile depression; (d) depression associated with personality disorder (see also Depue & Monroe 1978a). Recently (see Chapter 2) Pilkonis and Frank (1988) found that it was avoidant personality disorder (a form of chronic and severe social anxiety leading to high avoidance of social situations) that was most over represented in hospitalised depressives. In a replication study of their 1971 study, Paykel and Henderson (1977) found only three clusters replicated; the hostile depressives failed to fall out as a separate cluster. On the other hand Overall and Zisook (1980) suggested that (a) anxious; (b) hostile and (c) agitated and retarded depressives do form meaningful subgroups. Cooke (1980a) used a more complex statistical analysis to investigate depressive subtypes in a normal population. He found the subgroupings of: (a) vegetative; (b) anxious; and (c) cognitive; with a fourth consisting of the more classical endogenous symptoms. Cooke suggests that people can experience differing levels of each syndrome, that they are not mutually exclusive, and that a dimensional rather than categorical approach best fits the data.

A Hierarchical Model

The hierarchical classification of depression arises from the work of Foulds (1973) and Foulds and Bedford (1975, 1976). According to this model (which applies to the large spectrum of psychiatric disorders), symptoms can be arranged with regard to the disturbances in personal functioning. The hierarchy consists of four classes of symptoms: (a) dysthymic states—anxiety, depression, and elation; (b) neurotic symptoms—phobic conversion, dissociative, compulsive, and ruminative; (c) integrated delusions—delusions of contrition, grandeur, and/or persecution; (d) delusions of disintegration—primarily of the schizophrenias. Patients with symptoms in higher classes may have symptoms of lower classes, but the reverse does not hold true.

Foulds and Bedford (1976) suggest distinctions of depression along the dimensions of (a) depression versus not depression; (b) psychopathological versus not psychopathological; and (c) psychotic versus neurotic.

This classification is of interest for a number of reasons. It allows for psychotic depressives having neurotic symptoms. In this sense it bears some similarity to Klein's (1974, see further) ideas of the existence of embedded or core symptoms in certain disorders. It allows for the possibility that patients may shift between neurosis and psychosis (Akiskal, Bitar, Puzantian, Rosenthal & Walker, 1978) or indeed, show instability of diagnosis over time (Kendell, 1974). There is some support for this system (e.g., Bagshaw, 1977; Morey, 1985), but it has not attracted much research. Moreover, Surtees and Kendell (1979) failed to demonstrate that psychotics exhibit significant neurotic symptoms as the model predicts.

The Theoretical Approach

Partly in response to the confusion surrounding the statistical approaches some researchers have adopted the idea of a hierarchical approach but in a different way to that of the Fould's model. For example in an influencial paper Klein (1974) suggested that endogenous patients had a primary dysfunction in the pleasure or reward areas of the brain. This made them unresponsive to any rewarding events/stimuli and accounted for the inner deadness and flatness of affect. Hence an individual with endogenous symptoms has a set of key or core symptoms (related to low activity in the reward areas) that are not shared with other groups. However, these may be embedded in host of secondary, non-specific, common stress symptoms (see Chapter 2, Table 2.5). Willner (1984) offers an interesting discussion of this theory. There is now growing agreement that the core of depression is associated with low positive affect, low exploration and low energy (Clark & Watson 1991; see Barlow, 1991, plus peer commentary for a comprehensive discussion of the relation between types of anxiety and depression).

We shall be exploring other theoretical approaches later. But the idea to leave you with is that what you search for depends on your theory and basic orientation. If you believe in autonomus diseases you will look for them. If you believe in psychosocial dysfunctions (cognitions or early life difficulties) then you will look for these. And humans being what they are, each will find evidence to support their theory. The fact that in science we are supposed to try to disprove our theories rather than prove them is an ideal maybe but not the reality. Our human minds simply did not evolve to try to disprove things. Of course exactly the same criticism must be levelled at the theories of power and belonging to be explored later. At the end of the day it comes down to the interpretation of evidence, as much as the evidence itself, and this depends on our internal working models and basic beliefs.

CULTURE

It would be incorrect to believe that in other cultures and in other times people have been ignorant of psychiatric disorder or have not attempted to classify it. It is arrogant to believe that only western science has been concerned with or able to come up with meaningful distinctions. We have already noted that the Hippocratic system had clear ideas about depression. In other cultures too psychiatric classification has been important (Ellenberger, 1970). For example in India, there are ancient systems of classification going back to the Sushruta Samhita written in Sanskrit verse and believed to have been formulated about a hundred years before Hippocrates (Haldipur, 1989). Like Hippocrates, there is the same concern with body humours as causes of illness. It is an interesting, although unanswerable point, whether these classifications represented different boundaries drawn around similar symptoms or whether, in the centuries past, these symptoms/syndromes actually existed in the forms suggested. Given the demise of paralysis as a form of hysteria in the last hundred years, it is an intriguing possibility that in fact syndromes have changed as a result of cultural change.

However, it is primarily in the West that we have developed the notion of platonic-like disease entities. The platonic approach to illness rests on the assumption of universal forms. If depression is in any sense something universal (or a disease) then it should show up in various cultures in more or less the same way. There are enormous problems on this score. First, most cultures have their own definitions for marking what is abnormal to the social functioning of an individual. Furthermore, the cause of an abnormality, so defined, may have various explanations. An experience of loss of energy and wish to die for example may, in the West, be regarded as evidence of underlying biological abnormality but in another culture as loss of the soul (Ellenberger, 1970). Biological change might be taken as evidence for loss of the soul.

Many of these problems reflect the fact that in human evolution the biological bases of behaviour remain but have become 'open' to the central importance of social interaction (Hinde, 1987, 1989). The importance of symbolic representation of the self (Barkow 1975, 1980; Itzkoff, 1990), the socio-historical changes that have taken place in the western world in self-construction (Baumeister, 1986), and the social context of self-definitions (Littlewood, 1990) all speak to the importance of the construction of meaning of internal subjective experience. The way a person constructs and imputes meaning for a change in state will have an effect on the final expression of such a change (Littlewood, 1990) as well as on how an individual may set about coping with such changes. Cultural constraints on certain kinds of activity (e.g., freedom to pursue individual goals) or expectations to achieve, may place different burdens on different personalities in different contexts.

A key issue is presentation. It is now generally agreed that in non-western cultures depressive-like states tend to present with more somatic complaints (Marsella, 1980; Jenkins, Kleinman & Good, 1991). If one were to have crude notions of biological depression and biological symptoms then the implications is that non-western depressions are more biological—an obviously untenable position. In many cultures guilt is notable by its absence and this is a major challenge to those who argued for the dimension of personal blame as a cause of depression (e.g., Abramson, Seligman & Teasdale, 1978, although see Abramson, Metalsky & Alloy, 1989). Murphy (1978) has pointed out that guilt was also absent from western clinical descriptions of depression until the sixteenth century. He suggests that guilt and self-blame are more likely to arise in cultures that emphasise individual differences, self-control, predictability and personal responsibility for pain and pleasure. These cultures separate mind and body and demote the importance of social context and relationships in the causation of distress.

It is in fact paradoxical that despite the medicalisation of depressive states, still in our culture most have a real dread of being diagnosed or being seen as depressed, for it carries the stigma of being inferior, weak or inadequate (Endler, 1990). Many patients seem very keen to find some other explanation for their change of state (e.g., virus). In any event the psychological presentation of depression is very variable across cultures and the boundaries and symptoms that make up a particular classification of disorder in one culture may be different to those in another. Nevertheless cross-cultural comparisons by Sartorius, Jablensky, Gulbinat and Ernberg (1980) show that there are important similarities in depression that outweigh cultural variation. In their view, anxiety and tension, dysphoric mood, loss of energy and pleasure, difficulties concentrating and feelings of low self-worth constitute core depressive symptoms and are relatively culturally invariant. Also many have noted that Hippocrates' depiction of melancholia would be recognised today as depression. So the debates continue becoming more complex but also enriching our understanding of depression and other conditions (Littlewood, 1990; Jenkins et al., 1991). Slowly we are losing our child-like wish for simplicity, and either–or answers, and coming to recognise the complexity of depressed states. The problem here is that this means that different disciplines will need to work more closely together with mutual respect. But then we run into the old problem of social power.

SUMMARY

1. Depression has been noted for many thousands of years. During this time the theories of cause have varied from disturbances in body humours, to metaphysical causes or even the result of evil infestations and moral weakness.

2. In this century, the debates surround three major areas of concern: (a) Is depression a dimensional variation from normal or something alien, abnormal; a disease with its own autonomous action? (b) Can we study the biology of depression separately from psychological and social processes (mindless science) or can we study psychological aspects of depression with no regard to the biological basis of suffering and brain processes (brainless science)? (c) Can we ignore that, whatever approach we take, there are important implications for the social power for the advancer of any particular view? Knowledge and theory can lead to action and action is power.

3. Classification is concerned with the depiction of boundaries and dimensions. Specifically the questions are: (a) Is depression an illness? Depending on how this question is answered a number of subsequent questions follow. (b) If depression is an illness is it best understood as a qualitative (categorical) or quantitative (dimensional) variation from normal; i.e., what is the nature of the distinction (or overlap) between

normal states of unhappiness, reactions to loss or stress, demoralisation and fed-upness and major depression? (c) Is there more than one type of depression and if so, is it meaningful to regard these sub-classifications as being quantitatively or qualitatively distinct from each other? Finally, (d) what is the degree of overlap between some of these sub-classifications and other psychiatric states, e.g., schizophrenia and anxiety states.

Any boundary requires what has been called a "zone of symptom rarity" to be apparent. That is, there have to be symptom clusters that are comparatively rare at the boundary (Kendell 1975; 1988). As yet there is doubt about the presence of any symptom boundaries in psychiatry. However it is more common now to think in terms of a few key symptoms that discriminate between one disorder and another.

4. The approaches to classification discussed here are in terms of phenomenology and statistically, meaningful differences between individuals: (a) cross-sectional studies; (b) longitudinal studies and outcome; (c) treatment response studies.

5. Classification studies may be informed by theoretical rather than pure empiricism. Classification may focus on only one domain e.g., biological or psychological.

6. Classification and meaningful nosologies found in one culture may not translate to other cultures, indicating that depression is not one thing or entity but is culturally variant and quite unlike other diseases like small pox for example. On the other hand cross-cultural work does show some consistency and depression has been recognised for over two thousand years, so some "core" aspect must be present.

CONCLUDING COMMENTS

This chapter has outlined some of the historical debates and controversies surrounding the classification of depression. It is clear that although progress is being made, there is still considerable confusion and debate. Blumenthal (1971) points out that heterogeneity of depression resides at a number of levels, e.g., symptom presentation, treatment response, and etiology (see Chapter 16). Keller and Shapiro (1982) have made the important observation that acute episodes of depression may arise against a background of chronic depression, labelled "double depression". Weissman and Klerman (1977b) also raised the issue of the relationship between acute and chronic depression (see Chapter 3). There are notable gender differences in prevalence and presentation of depression (Weissman & Klerman, 1977a; Nolen-Hoeksema, 1987). Furthermore, various disorders may share common biological mechanisms (e.g., Horrobin & Manku, 1980;

Hudson & Pope, 1990), while the assumption that similar disturbances in neurochemical processes will give rise to similar psychological changes is in doubt (Mendels & Frazer, 1974).

In spite of these many difficulties, the pursuit of meaningful classifications of depression promises to throw up important sources of data. However, to approach the problem from a psychological point of view, the classification issues are puzzling. As Beck (1967; Beck, Rush, Shaw & Emery, 1979) suggests the cognitive themes of the depressive are remarkably similar regardless of subtype. It would also seem that whether depressed patients are anxious, retarded, hypochondriacal, or hysterical, psychological therapies are relatively effective (Weissman, 1979; Blackburn & Davidson 1990), provided the patient is able to engage in a therapeutic process (Blackburn, 1989). This is not to say that there is no attempt to discover which therapies are most effective for which patients. Rather it would seem that for the unipolar depressives at least (who make up the vast majority of cases), distinctions as they exist at present do not seem particularly helpful to the psychotherapist. Understandably, psychotherapists tend to put forward their own systems of classifications (e.g., Blatt, Quinlan, Chevron, McDonald & Zuroff, 1982; Beck, 1983) based on psychological mechanisms. These, at present, do not fit neatly with the more medically orientated nosologies. Hence, as Kendell (1975) suggests, for the majority of cases, classification usefulness depends upon the use to which it is to be put. Data that might guide physical treatment decisions may not always be useful for psychological treatment decisions.

As we go to the next chapter to look at modern approaches to classification and diagnosis in more detail, we can do no better than to end with Kendell's (1988, p.374) summary of the state of the art.

> We have learned how to make reliable diagnoses, but we still have no adequate criterion of their validity, and the achievement focuses on the failure. We draw the boundaries between one syndrome and another, and between illness and normality, in widely differing places and using a variety of different criteria and we have no adequate means of deciding which is right, or even which is preferable for a given purpose. The main reasons for this state of affairs are now well understood. Our ignorance of etiology forces us to define most disorders by their symptoms, and syndromes merge insensibly into one another, and into "normal distress", with no obvious natural boundaries or "points of rarity" to separate them. Many syndromes are disconcertingly unstable over time. The presence of any given symptom tends to increase the likelihood that several others will also be present, or will develop subsequently, and as a result multiple diagnoses can only be avoided by the adoption of

arbitrary hierarchies. Treatment response is too nonspecific to be a useful criterion and "need for treatment" is too obviously subjective and at the mercy of cultural expectations. A further problem, one that is rarely mentioned or discussed, is that we have never succeeded in defining what we mean by mental disorder, which implies that we have failed to established prior agreement on the essential characteristics on that which we are trying to identify.

CHAPTER 2

Depression: Types and Distinctions

The last chapter explored historical and philosophical difficulties inherent in the classification of depression. It is essential however, that we can have some shared understanding of what we mean when we use the term depression. Although depressions vary greatly, honing down these differences has proved rather difficult. This chapter explores some of these difficulties. A further discussion of measurement issues can be found in Appendix A.

TYPES OF DEPRESSION

The fact that depressed patients vary enormously is apparent to all trainees within the first six months of training. Anyone coming to study depression and trying to make sense of the differences can be easily overwhelmed by the different terms and descriptions given to depression. Table 2.1 gives an indication of some of the more common terms one might meet in the literature (see also Gold, 1990).

To complicate matters, formal diagnostic systems only refer to some of these distinctions. The Diagnostic and Statistical Manual (DSM) is the American system (from the American Psychiatric Association, 1987) for the identification and classification of psychiatric disorder. The third edition (DSM-111) was revised in 1987 (DSM-111-R). The DSM provide criteria for the diagnosis of:

TABLE 2.1
Ways of Classifying Depression

Distinction	*Schema*
Neurotic–psychotic	This distinction is an old one but in general is a classification that notes severity. The presence of delusional thinking, which may be either mood-congruent or non-congruent, triggers the diagnosis of psychotic.
Exogenous (reactive)–Endogenous	Exogenous has sometimes been used to describe precipitated disorder (e.g. life events), endogenous being unprecipitated. At other times reactivity has been used to denote patients who can react to events even though depressed. More recently it is the pattern and type of symptoms that trigger the diagnosis endogenous.
Unipolar–Bipolar	This distinction is applied to cyclic variation of mood; bipolar illness involves swings into both depression and at other times (hypo)mania.
Primary–Secondary	Secondary depressions are those that arise in relation to other physical or psychiatric disorders. A primary disorder is "pure" depression.
Agitated–Retarded	This distinction is based on a differentiation of a number of psychobiological and psychomotor differences.
Type A–Type B	This distinction arose from the idea that different depressions might respond to different drugs–i.e. Type A to noradrengeric drugs (e.g. imipramine); Type B to serotonergic drugs (e.g. amitriptyline).

NOTE: the first four distinctions are still very current ways of classifying depression but the last two have not fared so well over time. Nevertheless I believe they are still interesting and merit further research.

1. Major depression: major depressive disorder (single epsiode or recurrent); major depression melancholic type.
2. Bipolar disorder; mixed; depressed; seasonal pattern; cyclothymia.
3. Dysthymia (depressive neurosis).
4. Depressive disorder not otherwise specified.

The European System (devised by the World Health Organisation) uses a system called the International Classification of Diseases which is now in its ninth edition (ICD-9, WHO, 1978)). In 1992 the ICD-10 is due. Farmer and McGuffin (1989) and Cook and Winokur (1989) have given very useful overviews of these two systems and their relationship. Although not all the changes from the DSM-111 to the DSM-111-R are necessarily an advantage (Goldstein & Anthony, 1989) in general the ICD-10 will move closer to the DSM, especially in regard to a multi-axial system (see Mezzich, 1988; Cooper, 1988 for what this up-dated version is likely to look like).

Paykel (1989) outlines the current proposed ICD-10 classification of depression. This system has one division for mania and a number for depression. These are:

1. Bipolar affective disorder: Current episode: manic, hypomanic, depressed, or mixed.
2. Depressive episode: Mild, (a) without somatic symptoms (b) with somatic symptoms. Moderate, (a) without somatic symptoms (b) with somatic symptoms. Severe, without psychotic symptoms or with psychotic symptoms. Psychotic symptoms are divided into mood congruent/incongruent.
3. Recurrent depressive disorder: Current episode of depressive disorder.
4. Persistent Affective disorder: (a) cyclothymia (b) dysthymia.
5. Other mood (affective) disorders: specified/unspecified.

As Paykel points out this new system is something of a 'mixed bag'. It moves closer to the DSM system, but since about 50% of depressives will have subsequent episodes, Paykel sees little point in separating out the recurrent types. Also it may not have handled the endogenous psychotic division particularly well. These debates continue and the above may not be the final form of the ICD-10. Since little work has been possible using the ICD-10 we shall concentrate on findings using the DSM-111-R and other recognised criteria.

Major Depression

The DSM-111-R category of Major Depression represents a superordinate class. Hence, within major depression are a number sub-classifications. Cases can be described as (a) in partial or complete remission; (b) mild, moderate or severe; c) with melancholia (the American equivalent to endogenous) and (d) with psychotic features. Psychotic features may be sub-divided into mood congruent psychotic (e.g., delusions of guilt, poverty, disease) and mood incongruent psychotic features (e.g., persecutory delusions, thought insertion). As Farmer and McGuffin (1989) suggests, British psychiatrists might see the last sub-group as closer to schizophrenia.

As for each of the depressive disorders noted above, the diagnostician selects a number of symptoms from a larger menu. For major depression there is a list of nine possible symptoms of which the patient should have at least five. These are given in Table 2.2

This shopping list approach has been criticised since it is possible for two individuals to qualify for the diagnosis even though they may have

TABLE 2.2
DSM-111-R Criteria for Major Depressive Episode

A

At least five of the following symptoms have been present during the same two-week period and represent a change from previous functioning; at least one of the symptoms is either (1) depressed mood, or (2) loss of interest or pleasure. (Do not include symptoms that at are clearly due to a physical condition, mood-incongruent delusions of hallucinations, incoherence, or marked loosening of associations.)

1. depressed mood (or can be irritable mood in children and adolescents) most of the day, nearly every day, as indicated by subjective account or observation by others
2. markedly diminished interest or pleasure in all, or almost all, activities most of the day, nearly every day (as indicated by either subjective account or observation by others of apathy most of the time)
3. significant weight loss or weight gain when not dieting (e.g., more than 5% of body weight in a month), or decrease or increase in appetite nearly every day (in children, consider failure to make expected weight gains)
4. insomnia or hypersomnia nearly every day
5. psychomotor agitation or retardation nearly every day (observable by others, not merely subjective feelings of restlessness or being slowed down)
6. fatigue or loss of energy nearly every day
7. feelings of worthlessness or excessive or inappropriate guilt (which may be delusional) nearly ever day (not merely self-reproach or guilt about being sick)
8. diminished ability to think or concentrate, or indecisiveness, nearly every day (either by subjective account or as observed by others)
9. recurrent thoughts of death (not just fear of dying), recurrent suicidal ideation without a specific plan,or a suicide attempt or a specific plan for committing suicide

B

1. It cannot be established that an organic factor initiated or maintained the disturbance
2. The disturbance is not a normal reaction to the death of a loved one (Uncomplicated Bereavement)

   NOTE: Morbid preoccupation with worthlessness, suicidal ideation, marked functional impairment or psychomotor retardation, or prolonged duration suggest bereavement complicated by Major Depression.

C At no time during the disturbance have there been delusions of hallucinations for as long as two weeks in the absence of prominent mood symptoms (i.e., before the mood symptoms developed or after they have remitted).

D Not superimposed on schizophrenia, Schizophreniform Disorder, Delusional Disorder, or Psychotic Disorders NOS.

very few symptoms in common. The DSM was been heavily influenced by the research criteria of Spitzer and his colleagues (e.g., Spitzer, Endicott, & Robins, 1975) and hence in the literature you will often see this as the criteria for research. Although there are a number of symptoms that touch on hopelessness (e.g., loss of pleasure), interestingly, hopelessness is not included as a symptom of major depression.

The Unipolar–Bipolar Distinction

This distinction has a rather old pedigree and certainly was not original to Kraepelin although many associate the delineation of manic depression with him. Falret in 1854 for example used the term "folie circulaire" for bipolar illness (see Sedler, 1983). However, it was the work of Leonhard (1959) and Perris (1966) and the advent of lithium that were responsible for the unipolar–bipolar distinction evolving into its current significance. Cohen and Dunner (1989) provide an up to data review of bipolar illness. This classification, to some extent, avoids the controversies engendered by mind–body and qualitative–quantitative issues.

Differentiation of the bipolar disorders has been suggested. Bipolar I patients are those with a positive family history of bipolar illness and who have required hospitalization for both mania and depression. Bipolar II patients have a positive family history of bipolar illness, but have only been hospitalized for depression. Bipolar III patients also have a positive family history for bipolar illness, but have only experienced one depressive episode. These more complex distinctions have yet to be proven (Depue & Monroe, 1978b; Cohen & Dunner, 1989).

One of the difficulties with this system is that the unipolar depressions remain a very mixed and heterogeneous group. Unipolar depression may in practice be little more than a diagnosis of depression in the absence of a bipolar component. Hence, a number of problems still surround this system (Depue & Monroe, 1978b, 1979; Kendell, 1976), including the use of drugs like lithium, which have been found effective for some of the schizophrenias (Hirschowitz, Casper, Garver, & Chang, 1980) and recurrent unipolar depression.

Psychotic Depression

The role of psychotic symptoms in depression is obviously important. As we have seen, in both the DSM-111-R and ICD-10, psychotic symptoms may be sub-divided into mood congruent psychotic (e.g., delusions of guilt, poverty, disease) and mood-incongruent psychotic features (e.g., persecutory delusions, thought insertion). The presence of mood-incongruent symptoms sometimes gives rise to the diagnosis schizo-affective disorder (e.g., Katona, 1989). However, Winokur (1984) argues that there is no reason to believe that mood-incongruent psychotic symptoms are meaningfully different from mood-congruent symptoms in a person with a clear depressive episode. He presents evidence against schizo-affective disorder being an illness distinct from affective illness.

Perhaps one of the most fascinating hypotheses is that susceptibility to psychotic thinking is independent of susceptibility to depression. The idea here is that schizotyptal thinking and experiences are distributed throughout the population (possibly related to inter-hemisphere functioning). Claridge (1985; 1987) has articulated this interesting and important idea. Hence, Winokur (1984, p.241) suggests:

> If there is a predisposition to psychosis, why could not this predisposition manifest itself whenever there was a brain perturbation that was due to any psychiatric illness, including affective disorder, schizophrenia, alcoholism, or organic brain disease.

At the present time we need more research in this area, but consider the following; it is known that depression itself is associated with changes in inter-hemispheric activity (Mandell, 1979; Tucker, 1981; Tucker, Stenslie, Roth, & Shearer, 1981). Could it be that changes in inter-hemisphere activity associated with depression interacts with variation in inter-hemisphere function that may exist independently of the depression? In other words, there is individual variation in the way the hemispheres operate in the population at large and these interact with the changes associated with depression, producing in some psychotic symptoms when depressed.

Such theorising is speculative (although see Claridge, 1987, for evidence to support it). But it means that psychoticism is not simply severe depression (although in one sense the disorder is severe). Secondly reactive psychotic depression is a possibility as is accepted in Swedish classifications. In any event many endogenous depressives are not psychotic and, hence, endogenous depression is certainly not equivalent to psychotic depression.

Primary and Secondary Depression

Primary depression is not preceded by any other psychiatric or physical disorder. Primary depression may be either unipolar or bipolar, the unipolar depressions being further subdivided into "pure depressive disease" and "depressive spectrum disease". Secondary depression is preceded by, and may accompany, other psychiatric disorders (e.g., anxiety neurosis, alcoholism, personality disorder, etc.) or a physical disorder (Robins, Munoz, Martin, & Gentry, 1972). This distinction has the advantage of being accompanied by useful research diagnostic criteria (Feighner et al., 1972). As neat as this nosology appears, it is not without its difficulties (Akiskal et al., 1978; Kendell, 1976).

Endogenous/Melancholic Depression

Within the heterogenous profile of depression it has always been assumed that endogenous depression was likely to be closest to a disease entity. Consequently, the investigation of endogenous/melancholic depression and its distinction from other sub-types have been a main focus for studies of symptom variation. While the neurotic depressions are often regarded as milder states of heterogenous nature and course, it has been assumed that endogenous depression is somehow one thing or (core) entity and that careful description associated with a variety of statistical and other techniques will illuminate it. Various studies cast on this Platonic view (Cooke, 1980a; Young, Sheftner, Klerman, Andreasen & Hirschfeld, 1986).

An early set of criteria for identifying endogenous depression was developed by the Newcastle group (Carney, Roth, & Garside, 1965) and

TABLE 2.3
Criteria for Endogenous Depression

The Newcastle Scale for Endogenous Depression	
No adequate psychogenesis (+2)	Weight loss (+2)
Depressive psychomotor activity (+2)	Nihilistic Delusions (+2)
Adequate personality (+1)	Distinct mood quality (+1)
Previous episode (+1)	Guilt (+1)
Anxiety (-1)	Blame others (-1)
Score > 6 Endogenous depression	
(From Carney, 1989)	
Research Diagnostic Criteria for Endogenous Depression	
Group A	*Group B*
Distinct quality of mood	Self-reproach or excessive guilt
Autonomy of mood	Terminal or middle insomnia
Mood worse a.m.	Psychomotor agitation or retardation
Pervasive loss of interest or pleasure	Poor appetite
	Weight loss
	Decreased sex drive, loss of interest or pleasure
Criteria = at least 6 symptoms with 2 or more from group A	
(From Andreasen, 1975)	

there is also Spitzer, Endicott & Robins (1975) research criteria. These are given in Table 2.3.

The Newcastle scale assigns various weights to different symptoms due to the idea that these symptoms were associated with good outcome. Carney (1989) has recently reviewed the data in support of this instrument. You will note, however, that the Newcastle scale retains the idea of lack of psychogenesis as a key symptom unlike other instruments. It also includes the idea of personality. But, as Katschnig and Nutzinger (1988) point out, there are no clear guidelines for making these judgements and variation in these judgements result in a significant number of individuals crossing the neurotic/endogenous divide.

Since the advent of the Newcastle scale, other classifications have appeared. The most well known being the DSM-111-R criteria for melancholia which is given in Table 2.4.

Unlike the Newcastle endogenous depression scale, symptoms of melancholia (DSM-111-R) are not given weights. Thus, the idea of a hierarchy of symptoms (i.e. some symptoms are more key or core) is not found here. In general the DSM-111-R and the Newcastle criteria are regarded as more "restrictive" than Spitzer's and this may be important when it comes to biological research (Zimmerman, Coryell, Pfohl, & Stangl, 1986; Zimmerman, Coryell, & Black, 1990; and see Free & Oei, 1989, for a discussion).

TABLE 2.4
DSM-111-R Criteria for Melancholia

The presence of at least five of the following:

1. Loss of interest or pleasure in all, or almost all activities.
2. Lack of reactivity to usually pleasurable stimuli (does not feel much better even temporarily, when something good happens).
3. Depression regularly worse in the morning.
4. Early morning awaking (at least two hours before usual time).
5. Psychomotor retardation or agitation (not merely subjective complaints).
6. Significant anorexia or weight loss (e.g., more than 5% of body weight in a month).
7. No significant personality disturbance before first major depressive episode.
8. One or more previous major depressives episodes followed by complete, or nearly complete recovery.
9. Previous good response to specific and adequate somatic antidepressant therapy, e.g., tricyclics, ECT MAOI, lithium.

In a large recent study (N=512) using complex statistical analyses, Grove et al. (1987) derived yet another cluster of symptoms that they labelled nuclear depression. Nuclear depression had some overlap with endogenous depression, but also some differences. Interestingly, they found that these nuclear depressives were more neurotic (as measured by personality scales) than the non-nuclear group. Further, nuclear patients given ECT, functioned worse than non-nuclear depressives with less frequent recovery (although outcome data needs to be considered in the long term (Angst, 1988, and see next chapter). Both the personality data and outcome data are opposite to that predicted by the original endogenous theorists.

Exactly which symptoms are "core" endogenous symptoms remains controversial. Davidson, Turnball, Strickland, & Belya (1984) compared symptoms across five scales for measuring endogenous/melancholic depression. They found that many overlap, but that also each are different in certain ways. Combining the concept of embedded symptoms (Klein, 1974) with those of endogeneity gives rise to a symptom list as outlined in Table 2.5. Since we are going to discuss neurotic symptoms shortly, Table 2.5 presents the endogenous symptoms along with other depressive and so-called stress/neurotic symptoms for comparison purposes.

I would emphasise here, that there is nothing hard and fast about these symptoms and others can be suggested (e.g., Nelson & Charney, 1981; Whybrow, Akiskal, & McKinney, 1984; Andreasen, 1989). Sleep disturbance, especially early morning waking is a debatable core endogenous symptom (as many students with finals coming up will tell you) although it may be important in conjunction with other symptoms. Waking up during the night is also a common stress symptom and reflects hyperarousal. Other patients sleep heavily and feel unrested in the morning. However, the top six symptoms outlined in Table 2.5 rarely occur in stress reactions. Hence, the notion of embedded symptoms remains an interesting one and leads to the notion of a hierarchy of disorder (for a further discussion see Willner, 1984). Symptoms that may be involved in endogenous depression such as significant social withdrawal require further research.

In general different measures of endogenous depression have poor concordance (Free & Oei, 1989) and the so-called core symptoms may represent little more than a severity dimension or individual differences to the same process. The so-called core symptoms may also reflect differences in coping behaviour with those who tend to withdraw (e.g., due to shame?) more likely to develop endogenomorphic symptoms (Gilbert, 1988a). Those who put their hope in others and are seeking support show a more neurotic picture. These individuals might show

TABLE 2.5
Possible Core Symptoms of Endogenous Depression and Neurotic Stress Symptoms

	Core symptoms
1.	Pervasive loss of pleasure (anhedonia)
2.	Non-reactivity in mood
3.	Distinct quality of mood (dead inside; beyond tears; flatness)
4.	Excessive guilt (may be of psychotic magnitude)
5.	Major psychomotor change (agitation or retardation)
6.	Reduced vegetative activity
	Non-specific (Common Stress) symptoms
1.	Diurnal variation *
2.	Early morning waking*
3.	Loss of weight*
4.	Difficulty staying asleep*
5.	Difficulty falling asleep
6.	Suicidal thoughts
7.	Anxiety (of various forms)
8.	Difficulty concentrating (but not retarded or slowed thinking)
9.	Ruminations, worry on problems and intrusive thoughts
10.	Hypochondriasis
11.	Self-pity
12.	Irritability
13.	Tearfulness
14.	Low mood
15.	Mood instablity (quick to anger or feel tearful)
16.	Loss of sexual interest
17.	Easily fatigued

(* These symptoms are often included as core endegenous symptoms, see Zimmerman et al., 1990)

more endogeous symptoms if they lose hope that others can help them. This distinction may explain why the endogenous patient is more likely than the neurotic, to have paranoid ideas. In other words there is a basic mistrust of others or an over-investment in self-control (see Chapters 5–8). Nevertheless, the concept of endogenous depression remains an important research area.

Neurotic Depression

Many have noted that neurotic depression appears to be a heterogenous disorder that is best conceptualised dimensionally (e.g., Kendell, 1976).

The typical symptoms are noted in Table 2.5. It arises from reaction to life events and premorbid personality. There is rather less work in the area of sub-classifying neurotic depression (as opposed to distinguishing it from endogenous depression) and the general impression has been that this is a milder or less serious disorder than psychotic and endogenous depression. The problem here is how you define serious since as we shall see later, recent work suggests that neurotic or non-endogenous depression can have quite poor long-term outcome (Lee & Murray, 1988; Kiloh, Andrews, & Neilson, 1988). In a long-term follow-up Kiloh et al. (1988, p.756) found that compared to endogenous depressives, neurotics tended to be "younger, had shorter index admissions, and were less likely to be readmitted to hospital. In the longer term however they were equally likely to experience further episodes and to commit suicide."

A recent study by Parker, Blignault, & Manicavasagar (1988) looked more closely at neurotic depression. They attempted to study a pure group of neurotic depressives (N=91) by excluding endogenous types although the exact way this was done is unclear. They then explored a variety of symptoms generated from the Beck Depression Inventory and Zung rating scales. A principal component analysis of these clinical symptoms generated four factors; negative cognition (with low self-esteem, guilt, self-criticism, and lowered mood); lack of drive (with loss of libido, anergia, emptiness, anhedonia); anxiety (insomnia, crying, tachycardia, hypochondria) and arousal (appetite loss, weight loss, tiredness, mood worse in the morning). These factors seem close to those suggested as being core symptoms of depression from cross-cultural studies (e.g., Sartorius, et al., 1980; see Chapter 1, this volume). It is clear therefore that endogenous symptoms should not be confused with issues of casuality (Akiskal et al. 1978; see Chapters 3 and 16).

Apart from suggesting major dimensions of neurotic depression, this study is interesting because they were able to explore symptom profiles to a specific life event: break-up of an intimate relationship. Interestingly, they found that depression associated with this life event tended to have a more endogenous profile (e.g., insomnia and weight loss) but was associated with good outcome. They discuss their findings in terms of what is known about the phasic reactions to bereavement. They make the point that often the first phase of bereavement reactions involve symptoms (e.g., weight loss, appetite loss, insomnia) that some researchers might regard as endogenous. They also make the point that there may be differences in neurotic depression arising from loss of an intimate relationship and other types of neurotic depression. In the latter cases the depression is coloured by premorbid personality.

The Comorbidity of Depression and Anxiety

In regard to the relationship of anxiety to depression, Mullaney (1989) has outlined eight hypotheses: (1) anxiety and depression are interwoven and inseparable; (2) anxiety and depression represent distinct disorders; (3) although distinct both in dimensional and categorical terms they can remain difficult to separate; (4) anxiety is part of depressive disorder; (5) anxiety and depression are symptomatically distinct but are not mutually exclusive; (6) they are hierarchically related with depressive symptoms higher up the disfunction hierarchy; hence (7) depression and anxiety generally occur together but depression can manifest as a distinct entity and, (8) depression and anxiety neurosis are indistinguishable and there is little therapeutic point in separating them. All these positions have some evidence to support them.

In a recent study of neurosis in the community, using sophisticated statistical techniques, Goldberg, Bridges, Duncan-Jones, and Grayson, (1987) found that depression and anxiety symptoms are highly correlated and underpin most neurotic conditions. Barlow, Di Nardo, Vermilyea, Vermilyea and Blanchard (1986) have shown that many anxious patients meet a number of DSM criteria at the same time and not just other anxiety classifications. In their study of anxiety cases, depression was often found to reach diagnostic criterion levels. Combining major depression and cyclothymia as a single diagnostic group, 39% of the agoraphobics, 35% of the panic disorders and 19% of the social phobics met the criteria for depression as outlined in the DSM. Although the numbers were small, 4 of 6 obsessional compulsive disordered people also met criteria for major depression.

Sanderson, Beck, and Beck (1990) found that in a large sample (N=260) using structured interviews, over 66% of patients had at least one additional diagnosis. The most common for dysthymia were: anxiety disorder 47.6%; social phobia 27% and generalised anxiety disorder 22.2%. For major depression the figures were: anxiety disorder 41.6%; social phobia 15.2%, and generalised anxiety disorder 20.3%. Exploration of the order of onset suggests that for the vast majority the depressive disorder began first. This contradicts earlier observations that depressives rarely develop other disorders.

In regard to the unipolar bipolar distinction, Murray and Blackburn (1974) found that both unipolar and bipolar depressed patients were as anxious as chronically anxious neurotics. It is my impression that the anxiety of bipolar patients is usually social anxiety rather than separation anxiety (e.g., fears of being alone). This requires validation but may be important from an etiological point of view.

Beck, Emery, and Greenberg (1985) distinguish between anxious and depressed individuals according to their cognitive style. Depressive negative cognitions tend to be more global and restrictive, and more negative about the future. Self is seen as defeated or having lost. The anxious patient is more hopeful and less global in their cognitive style. It is unclear what the evidence of comorbidity has for this view. Kendell (1974) found that a large percentage of people classified as anxious types were often re-diagnosed as depressed at subsequent episodes.

Patients can become more anxious as they improve and prepare to go home from hospital or back to work. In some cases of suicide, it seems to me that it is the return of fear (rather than motivation per se) when having to face the world again that may trigger suicide. As one patient said to me: "While I am here (in hospital) I can shut out the world but the thought of having to face people again fills me with terror. Then I think of suicide."

You may recall that Grove et al. (1987) found their nuclear depressed group to be more neurotic than the non-nuclear group. In the next chapter we will note that because neuroticism often correlates with anxiety scales at 0.7 or above their finding is paramount to saying the nuclear group were also the more anxious. The exact nature of the relationship of anxious symptoms to depressed symptoms continues to stimulate debate and research (Kendall & Watson, 1989; Barlow, 1991).

Negative Affectivity

The study of the relationship between anxiety and depression has proceeded during the eighties and there is growing agreement that most depressed patients are also anxious (e.g., Watson & Clark, 1984; Kendall & Watson, 1989; Clark & Watson, 1991). Watson and Clark (1984) introduced a very important concept called negative affectivity. This concept posits that various negative affects are commonly associated in a general way. Individuals prone to negative affectivity tend to experience more general discomfort and less general well being, are more introspective with negative self-attention and tend to dwell on the negative side of things. Negative affectivity occurs in many psychiatric conditions.

More recently, Watson and Clark (1988) and Clark and Watson (1991) have shown that while negative affectivity is related to depression, anxiety and various other psychiatric conditions, *the lack of positive affectivity is more specific to depression*. Gilbert (1980) found, using a psychophysiological design (GSR), that depressed patients were not more sensitive to failure events than anxious controls, but were much less sensitive (reactive) to success events (solving anagram problems).

For Watson and Clark (1988) and Clark and Watson (1991), positive affectivity appears to be a measure of general energy and engagement in the world, joy and pleasure. This research is important since it suggests that the dimensions of negative affectivity and positive affectivity are not necessarily on a single dimension and need to be considered separately. It maybe that each are independently subject to genetic influence.

This means that depression may arise from either high arousal in punishment areas of the brain, low activity in reward areas or some combination (Gilbert, 1984). Since antidepressants have effects in both the reward and punishment areas (due to the nature of common, neurotransmitter pathways) it is difficult to separate their relative effects pharmacologically. How these concepts of negative and positive affectivity will help to illuminate the endogenous–neurotic question remains to be seen. The interested reader can find further debate of these issues in the excellent recent book by Kendall and Watson (1989).

The older concepts of a general neurotic syndrome have waxed and waned. After great enthusiasm for subclassifying neurotic depressive conditions we are probably returning to a general recognition that, in these conditions at least, there are underlying common traits or factors at work (e.g., Andrews, Stewart, Morris-Yates, Holt, & Henderson, 1990; Barlow, 1991, plus peer commentary). Research on drugs (e.g., MAOIs) show a broad spectrum of effects and research on therapy suggests common elements that are helpful (e.g., Frank, 1982).

Dysthymia and Dysthymic States

In the latter years of the eighties dysthymic disorders have stimulated increasing research (e.g., Burton & Akiskal, 1990). The DSM-111 category of depressive neurosis has become dysthymia in the DSM-111-R. This is however, regarded as distinct from mild major depression. Dysthymia (or depressive neurosis) includes depressed mood for most days for at least two years, plus two of the following: (1) poor appetite or overeating; (2) insomnia or hyposomnia; (3) low energy or fatigue; (4) low self-esteem; (5) poor concentration or difficulty making decisions and (6) feelings of hopelessness. Akiskal (1990) adds the criteria of: insidious onset with origin often in childhood or adolescence; persistent or intermittent course; concurrent "character" pathology; ambulatory disorder compatible with "stable" social functioning.

The concept of dysthymic disorder and the demotion of the concept of neurotic has not gone unchallenged (e.g., Cook & Winokur, 1989). Goldberg and Bridges (1990, p.104) call it, "a new plastic box for some rather old wine". The idea that there are cycles in neurasthenia has been with us for some centuries (see Chapter 1). Akiskal (1988; 1990) and his colleagues (Akiskal, Hirschfeld, & Yerevanian, 1983) suggest three forms of cyclical disorder. These are: (a) hyperthymic disorder, where the individual cycles in and out of hypomanic episodes many of whom may not present for treatment; (b) cyclothymic disorder, where the individual cycles into both hypomania and depression; (c) subaffective dysthymic disorder where the cycle is only into depression, although tricyclic antidepressants may trigger hypomania.

Akiskal proposes that heredity and developmental factors give rise to biologically coded personality traits which result in predispositions to over-react to everyday life and stress—i.e., increased sensitivity to various life events. These traits persist with remission of affective episodes. This is a very similar view of neurotic conditions advanced by neuro-behaviourists (e.g., Gray, 1971) and not far from Watson and Clark's (1984; 1988) concepts of negative affectivity. Personality then, according to Akiskal (1988, p.131), "represents the intermediary stage between remote (e.g., hereditary and developmental) and proximate (e.g., precipitating) causative factors in the origin of full-blown mood disorders".

Vulnerability in the limbic (and probably sub-limbic) system may arise from family pedigrees, early experience of loss/separation and inadequate parenting. Meyersberger and Post (1979) outline the mechanisms of the latter possibilities very clearly. Once laid in, this vulnerability may be activated by one or a number of events, e.g., disabling physical illness; drug treatment affecting the CNS; use of steroid contraceptives; subclinical hypothyroidism; life events particularly in the presence of low support (à la Brown & Harris, 1978a). Especially relevant for bipolar episodes are: use or abuse of catecholaminergic drugs; sleep deprivation; premenstrual phase, the postpartum period; and seasonal photoperiodic change.

Cyclothymia. The cyclothymic temperament is marked by episodes of erratic behaviour—e.g., promiscuity, changes of residence or job, brief religious/cult affiliations followed by disillusion; and episodic drug use (stimulants and sedatives). Patients often talk in terms of their highs (typically lasting a few days) when they may have energy and creative spurts, sleep less and feel confident, and their lows when they become "slothful", lose confidence and self-esteem, withdraw socially and feel guilty, irritable, and nervous. Akiskal suggests their "tempestuous" life styles often create interpersonal havoc.

In his view (1988, p.133) these patients are often given personality disorder diagnoses such as borderline, passive-aggressive, histrionic, or antisocial. However he suggests that: "Only with an in-depth phenomenologic study and prospective follow up did it become clear that their personality maladjustments reflected underlying phasic affective dysregulation". So in Akiskal's view there is an underlying affective instability which gives rise to a "tempestuous" life style and this life style is instrumental in bringing about the life events which exasperate the mood disorder (e.g., broken relationships, loss of job, etc). However, Gunderson and Elliott (1985, see next chapter) suggest that this is only one (Hypothesis 1) of at least four hypotheses of the link between affective disturbance and personality disorder.

Sub-affective Dysthymia. These are sometimes also called characterologic depressives if they have suffered depression since their adolescence. They represent low-grade depression involving low self-esteem and self-critical attitudes, passivity, pessimism and interpersonal dependency which appears to follow rather than precede a well-defined depressive episode from which there is incomplete recovery.

Early and incomplete recovery from affective disturbance seems to set the personality in a particular track which has secondary consequences in terms of relationships and social learning. Hence again in some of these patients Akiskal is considering "personality as a sub-affective expression of mood disorders".

Akiskal has also identified two forms of characterologic depressives according to treatment responsiveness:

1. Those who respond to various treatments (e.g., drug and social skills) when not depressed have a shortened REM latency characteristic of primary depressive states, and often have a family history of affective disorder (especially bipolar).
2. Those who do not respond to usual treatments, have normal REM latency, more personality disorder, history of alcoholism, and higher rates of early loss.

In general Akiskal has raised important points in regard to the possibility of underlying affective dysregulation in personality features associated with depression and also the importance of internal cyclic mechanisms. Especially important are the recent findings that tricyclic antidepressants for some of these cycling states (whatever their origin may be) may run the risk of actually speeding up the cycle. In other words, some may have shorter episodes but the time lag to the next episode is reduced. This is a most important finding and requiring more research. Akiskal also gives an important discussion on the different forms of prevention that might be considered with these people. For a more critical appraisal see Gunderson and Elliott (1985).

Depressive Personality. The concept of depressive personality has a very long history and can be traced back to the early Greeks. More recently, Phillips, Gunderson, Hirschfeld, and Smith (1990) have given an overview of what they call depressive personality. They point out that the assumption that Axis I disorders are somehow biological and Axis II are psychological is to court confusion. Akiskal is also making a similar case for considering some personality dimensions in terms of affect regulation (Watson & Clark, 1984; 1988). For some individuals personality characteristics may be secondary to the affective tone set by limbic structures. This is an important idea especially when we come to consider other personality measures such as neuroticism. However, whether this view proves theoretically superior to the older concepts of punishment sensitivity as a dimension of neuroticism (e.g., Gray, 1971) remains to be seen.

SEASONAL AFFECTIVE DISORDER (SAD)

Another form of cyclic depression has recently become more clearly identified during the eighties. This is seasonal affective disorder (SAD). Mammals evolved in a world of changing seasons. With these seasons a number of internal regulator cycles have evolved, e.g., migration, hibernation, and breeding cycles. The most researched seasonally related disorder studied so far has been depression (Kripke, Risch, & Janowsky, 1983a,b; Rosenthal et al., 1984; Lewy et al., 1985; Wehr et al., 1985; 1986; Kasper & Rosenthal, 1989). As these researchers suggest, many biological functions seem entrained to light/dark cyclic variation. Of special interest has been the hormone melatonin. 5-HT is a precursor of melatonin. Melatonin appears to be concentrated in the hypothalamus and midbrain and may modify neurotransmitter inputs for the hypothalamic control of various hormones (Gilmore, 1981). This pineal hormone increases during dark hours and decreases during exposure to light. Melatonin (among other hormones) is believed to play a role in jet lag symptoms. There is also a seasonal variation to melatonin, being higher in the winter months and lower in the summer months. The pathway that is believed to operate in this mechanism is the retinohypothalmic tract. Melatonin plays an important regulatory role in oscillating mechanisms (biological clocks). Rosenthal et al. (1984) and Kasper & Rosenthal (1989) give excellent overviews of the issues.

Rosenthal et al. (1984) note Kraepelin's observations that some patients exhibit clear excitement during the spring period only to lapse into depressive states during the autumn (the Greeks also observed this). Their own research (Rosenthal et al., 1984, p.73) suggests that "a few single women reported inability to keep a boyfriend in the winter but no difficulty in finding another one during the following summer". Such observations might be expected if these seasonally triggered changes are co-ordinated with (primitive) reproductive social behaviours (Gilbert, 1989).

The typical symptoms of SAD are characterised by: hypersomnia, carbohydrate craving and overeating, mood and energic variation, decreased activity, anxiety and irritability (see Rosenthal et al., 1984, table 2, p.73, and Kasper & Rosenthal, 1989, table 12.2, p. 345). The epidemiology of SAD is unclear. Some reports suggest prevalence could be as high as 5% of the population. Kasper and Rosenthal (1989) quote an in press study by Terman which found that about 25% of a population in New York city complained of symptoms resembling SAD but to a milder degree. Eastwood, Whitton, Krammer and Peter (1985) studied affective cycles in depressed and non-depressed subjects and found that cycles in affective symptoms are universal, those with affective disorders varied in the amplitude of their cycles rather than in the kind of cycle. Kasper and Rosenthal (1989) have so far found that the majority of sufferers are women (83%). The majority (81%) met research criteria for bipolar II and only a minority (12%) for unipolar disorder.

Importantly, from a clinical point of view, there is the growing evidence that sufferers of this condition can be helped by changing their exposure to bright light intensity (Rosenthal et al., 1984; Wehr, Sack, Parry, & Rosenthal, 1986; Kasper & Rosenthal, 1989). However, the effectiveness of light treatment may not be tied to seasonal affective disorder. Depressives (especially of the bipolar form) may benefit (Kripke et al., 1983a,b). Melatonin sensitivity to light may be high in this group (Lewy et al., 1985). I have recently come across two cases of probable SAD but where attitudinal (chronic low self-esteem) problems produced another set of dips superimposed on the seasonal variation. They claimed to have been helped by light therapy. It was only because I had seen these patients over two years that we picked up the two sources of mood difficulties. There is no a priori reason why SAD patients cannot also suffer neurotic type difficulties; both can coexist or interact.

We have only begun to explore the role of light as a therapy for some patients and how it works (Wehr et al., 1986). We do not yet know whether those who benefit will be many in number or few; and whether only depression or other disorders may also be helped. I have had one bulimic patient who showed clear worsening of her cravings seasonally, which were completely cured if she went on holiday to a southern country, but not if she stayed in Britain or went further north. It may be that, in some cases, there is an internal oscillating process which interacts with psychological and social vulnerability. For example, some patients may be more easily able to cope with certain life events in the summer months, but less able if these occur at a critical period, i.e. in winter or autumn. At present, the interaction between life events (e.g., break-up of a marriage during a winter depression), type of event, and season of exposure is still being researched.

POSTNATAL DEPRESSION

It has long been considered that the period after giving birth is a time of increased psychiatric risk (e.g., Marce, 1858). However there is now doubt whether postnatal women are at any more risk of depression that control groups (O'Hara & Zeboski, 1988). Recent television programmes have brought a major public awareness of this distressing condition which many complain was unrecognised by their physician. Cox, Connor, and Kendall (1982) found that 13 of 101 women interviewed had marked depressive illness, the majority of which had gone untreated despite visits from health visitors and GP awareness of the patient's state.

The distinctions of the affective disturbances of childbirth are (a) maternity blues; (b) postnatal depression; and (c) puerperal psychosis. Around 50-60% of women suffer what is known as the maternity blues. Symptoms include bursting into tears for no reason, various anxieties (such as inability to cope), fatigue, sleep difficulties, and poor appetite. Negative affect tends to peak at around the fifth day (Kendell, MacKenzie, West, McGuire & Cox, 1984). Most of these conditions require kindness, support, and understanding, and not psychiatric intervention.

Recent studies however confirm Pitt's (1968) finding that 10–15% suffer more serious depressive disorder or what he called "atypical depression". Symptoms include: various anxieties, tearfulness, confusion, inappropriate obsessional thoughts, irritability, fatigue, insomnia, guilt (often about fatigue and feelings), fears of harming or someone else harming the baby, and loss of interest in sex. Some women report personality changes (e.g., becoming irritable and angry with family), which itself becomes a source for depression and reduced self-esteem. The disorder often arises after leaving hospital (e.g., after the third week) but the exact timing is variable and in some it may be months later. Many studies suggest that postnatal depression is not short-lived and can continue for months, or even years (O'Hara & Zekoski, 1988). It should also be mentioned that I have seen a couple of young depressives who seemed to get a lot better after having a baby. How long they stayed well I do not know but in one case she came to see me a year latter and was doing well, feeling that she had matured. Much may depend on role change and we should not assume that changes are all bad. Puerperal psychosis however is comparatively rare, 1–2 per 1000 and it is likely that the majority are affective illnesses (Platz & Kendell, 1988). These cases require inpatient treatment.

Measurement

There is some concern over whether standard depression measuring instruments (e.g., the Beck Depression Inventory) are appropriate for postnatal depression and some (e.g., Cox, Holder, & Sagovsky, 1987) have devised special screening measures (see also O'Hara & Zekoski, 1988, for a discussion). Cox et al. (1987) point out that self-report scales are not alternatives for proper clinical assessment. Some postnatal depressions may not conform to standard descriptions. For example, a person I knew well, developed intense anxiety and agitation in the dark, with various ideas that someone or thing may break into the house and harm both her and her daughter. The daily onset was clearly marked to the loss of daylight. There was also dysphoric mood (due in part to the fear of the return of agitation each night) and secondary agoraphobia especially at night. I saw this as a break-through of a primitive (possibly prepared) archetypal fear, although there was a history of a rather dominating mother. When it remitted it was sudden. Just one night three months later the anxiety failed to come and never came back, even after a subsequent birth.

Aetiology

The suggested causes of postnatal depression vary from those who emphasise psychosocial factors to those who stress the role of hormones (see Kumar & Brockington, 1988, for detailed reviews). Dalton (1985) for example advocates the use of progesterone as the treatment of choice because there are large hormonal changes (e.g., progesterone and prolactin). Prolactin is believed to give the woman sense of good health in the latter stages of pregnancy. In some cultures eating the placenta (which is high in progesterone) is advocated and this is common in many animal species.

Birth is a time of major changes in biological state and life style. There is a vast number of potential sources of vulnerability to depression such as: biological changes; change in social roles (Oatley & Boulton, 1985); degree of self-complexity (Linville, 1985; those who have less complex and differentiated self-structures are believed to be more vulnerable to depression). The gender and temperament of the infant may also play a role. Many of the life-style factors that appear important in non-postnatal depression are also believed to play a role in depression after childbirth. These include marital relationships, current and previous parental relationships, life events, and the availability and use of supportive relationships (O'Hara, 1986). O'Hara and Zekoski (1988, p.48) in their review of the data conclude:

> What might be suggested from all of the research on etiological factors is that women at "risk" by virtue of past personal or family history of psychopathology and poor social support (particularly from spouse) who experience a high level of negative life events in conjunction with childbirth are likely to experience a postpartum depression.

Cox (1988) has provided a fascinating discussion of cultural practices to childbirth and how these might relate to vulnerability. Rates do seem to vary with cultural practices. It is, he suggests, important to recognise the role changes that have taken place in western society and that there is little in the way of helping women reintegrate themselves into their social roles following childbirth. Indeed it is not uncommon to find women becoming more isolated in the home following childbirth. It also seems to me that in industrial nations the emphasis on production of goods and services acts to demote care-giving roles of all forms (Gilbert, 1989). Cultural attitudes to child-rearing (e.g., the proximity of mother and baby after birth and in the subsequent years) vary greatly (Boulton, 1983; Weisner, 1986). There has also been a cultural myth of the happy carefree mother which fosters unrealistic expectations and denies the difficulties.

Personality

The use of standard measuring instruments have not been particularly useful in identifying at-risk women. Kumar and Robson (1984) did not find any differences in neuroticism between depressed and non-depressed postnatal women. However, Raphael-Leff (1986) suggested it is useful to consider the basic orientation to mothering, to understand the interaction of (post) birth events, personality and depression. She argues that "facilitator" mothers (those who are keen on natural birth and making the baby the focus of their life, etc.) tend to get depressed by separations and inability to perform the role of mother. Regulators mothers (those who prefer working and career and want the baby to fit their own life style) tend to get depressed by enforced togetherness and the loss of independent functioning. Becoming a mother may be seen as a loss of role and status. This approach is rather more inspired and specific than those using standard personality scales like neuroticism. Others consider the preparedness to be a mother as important, suggesting that those vulnerable to depression may not have come to terms with being a mother and may have a critical and dominant mother (Arieti & Bemporad 1980b).

Effects

It is known that postnatal depression is often not a transient condition and can linger on for years. Cox, Rooney, Thomas, & Wrate, (1984) found that postnatal depression was accurately recalled at three years follow-up and that at least half the depressed mothers had not recovered after one year. In clinical practice it is not uncommon to find women with agoraphobia or other problems who date the origin of the problem to a postnatal depressed episode. Increasing evidence points to serious effects of growing up with a depressed mother (Gordon et al., 1989; Gotlib & Lee, 1990; Gelfand & Teti, 1990)

Wrate, Rooney, Thomas, & Cox, (1985) found that at three years many of the children of postnatally depressed mothers showed some behavioural disturbance and postnatal depression may have a deleterious effect on a child's cognitive development (Cogill, Caplan, Alexandra, Robson & Kumar, 1986; Gotlib & Lee, 1990; Gelfand & Teti, 1990). A useful review of the negative effects of maternal depression on infant development is given by Melhuish, Gambles, & Kumar, (1988). Murray (1988) describes her own ethologically based research and explores particularly the nonverbal relationships of baby and depressed mother. The infant suffers because of the lack of interest and reactivity of the mother and this can have effects on the security of attachment, shared affect, concentration, and language development. Generally speaking a depressed and unresponsive mother may have negative effects on the development of a child's internal defence and safety system (see page 292). As outlined elsewhere (Gilbert, 1989) it is the safety system which facilitates open explorative behaviour. Untreated postnatal depression can have serious effects on family life.

There is a growing recognition for the need to increase general and clinical awareness of postnatal complications. In all the antenatal classes Jean and I attended not one raised the issue of postnatal depression or considered the relationship changes that were bound to occur and how these could be dealt with. All of this shows perhaps, the over medicalisation of childbirth.

DEPRESSION IN CHILDREN

There is general agreement that the classification of childhood disorders is not as developed as it is for adult disorders and only a relatively small section of the DSM is concerned with them. There was, until recently, considerable debate as to whether children could suffer from depression and if so, how did it relate to adult forms? Kovacs (1989) points out that criteria that require developed self-constructs, e.g., self as worthless or guilt, are likely to be difficult to use with children because they may not have developed clear self-concepts. Also children may find it difficult to introspect or give clear accounts of their feeling state. So diagnosis is an issue. Izard and Blumberg (1985) suggest that children who are depressed may be more aggressive, as does the DSM-111-R. As in adult depression, the issue of comorbidity with anxiety arises and affective disorders in childhood are associated with anxiety conditions leading again to the idea of general negative affectivity (for a very full review see Finch, Jr, Lipovsky, & Casat, 1989).

Nevertheless, despite these concerns, recent reviews of depression in childhood (Kovacs, 1989) and adolescence (Parry-Jones, 1989) draw attention to their importance. Community surveys suggest a prevalence of about 2–5% for major depression and dysthymia (Kovacs, 1989). Until the teenage years the gender ratio is about equal but by adolescence the ratio changes to 4:1 with girls suffering the highest rates (Parry-Jones, 1989). How far child abuse elevates these ratios is unknown. Prevalence for major depression in adolescence may be about 4.7%, and 3.3% for dysthymia, and depression may constitute up to 25% of psychiatric referrals (Parry-Jones, 1989). These results remain tentative since they are based on DSM criteria and further research will address the issue of whether the rates are higher using more specifically designed identification measures. A particular problem in the movement into adolescence is the rise of risk from suicide (for a full review see Pfeffer, 1989).

Depressed children (often) do not simply grow out of it, nor should depression be seen as part of normal development. An episode can last for 9 months or longer, and it can have serious, adverse effects over the long term and into adulthood. Depressed children are more likely than controls to develop an adult psychopathology. Depression in children can have adverse effects on development and attainment. There is evidence that positive affect facilitates creative problem- solving (Isen, Daubman, & Nowicki, 1987; Isen, 1990) and explorative behaviour, so it is not surprising that these would be effected by depressed states. Depressed children are less attractive as playmates and may have greater difficulties with peer relationships. Residues of social impairment can remain long after an episode has receded. Depressed children can have an adverse effect in a family (Kovacs, 1989). Hammen, Adrian, and Hiroto (1988) in a follow-up study of 8–16-year-olds found that initial symptoms and life stress predicted depression at follow-up. Attributional style was a poor predictor.

This, all too brief, section draws attention to the issues of childhood depression. Kovacs (1989) discusses many of the salient issues in current research and how the old chestnut of endogenous depression again appears in childhood depressions. For obvious reasons the family are often involved in therapy but Parry-Jones (1989) also suggests some cautions when it comes to older adolescents.

RECENT APPROACHES TO CLASSIFICATION AND UNDERSTANDING TYPES

The phenomenological approach to symptom classification is fraught with problems (e.g., Blumenthal, 1971; Kendell, 1988) although it is understandable why researchers are attracted to it. In Kendell's (1975; 1988) view, questions must be raised when we accept our phenomenological classifications as indicating more than just a useful conceptualisation for treatment and research. It is not surprising therefore that researchers have constantly sought to back up accepted phenomenological distinctions with exploration of other forms of evidence. Further on we look briefly at these other forms of evidence. The most obvious first question is, do our classifications and sub-classifications help with predictions of treatment response?

Treatment Studies

Drugs. There have been numerous attempts to classify depression via treatment response (e.g., Rao & Coppen, 1979; Raskin et al., 1970; Raskin & Crook, 1976). Generally the more severe the depression, especially if psychotic, the greater the indication for physical therapy. However, in a comparison of chlorpromazine, imipramine and placebo, Raskin & Crook (1976) make the point that the active treatment affects symptoms, and not patient types. (See Fowles & Gersh, 1979a, for a discussion of Raskin & Crook's findings). A major review of the effectiveness of antidepressant drugs in various psychiatric conditions by Hudson & Pope (1990) suggests that there may be a family of disorders that share common (or at least salient) elements and who show some response to antidepressant medications. The disorders (eight in all) they outline cover a very wide range, including hyperactivity, obsessive–compulsive disorder, panic disorder, eating disorders, as well as depression. Social anxiety has also been shown to respond to MAOIs so this would also have to be included. It is difficult to know what to make of these findings, but they may suggest that our current linkage of phenomenology with biology is very poor. It might also support the idea that monoamines are involved with a general defensive system function (Gilbert, 1989) and/or negative affectivity (Finch, Jr, et al., 1989).

Free & Oei (1989) have reviewed much of the evidence on treatment and classification and suggest that treatment is not a useful criteria for classification, supporting other findings that drugs affect symptoms, not patient types. There is little evidence that neurotic depressives do badly (in the short term at least) with drugs and indeed most studies find that they do fairly well at least for the acute episode. There are questions of the choice of drug—e.g., tricyclics versus MAOIs; the latter may be preferred where anxiety dominates the clinical picture (Stewart et al., 1989). However, we will not explore this further here. Also, it remains a possibility that some patients may have their cycles speeded up by antidepressant drugs (Akiskal, 1988). The use of lithium remains as a central drug for bipolar and recurrent cyclic depression (Rosenbaum, 1989), but it is not used as a major antidepressant but rather a mood stabiliser. It is unlikely that it has much to offer in regard to classification as such and has been suggested for various problems including recurring severe headaches.

Other physical treatments involve relatively non-invasive procedures, such as exercise for mild to moderate depression (I know of no study that has explored exercise in major depression). Exercise is believed to increase central turn-over of biogenic amines (de Coverly Veale, 1987; Simons, McGrowan & Epstein, 1985). More invasive treatments are extroplexsy, or ECT. As Fink (1989) points out however there is still much to learn about how this treatment works and we are still uncertain whether it has much to offer apart from symptomatic improvement. It is not recommended for dysthymia. Generally ECT has not helped the classification debates over and above recognition that some patients do not respond to drugs (although arguments exist about whether non-responders have been given an adequate dose or correct combinations). However, as Hay and Hay (1990) point out, ECT is probably the most effective treatment when hallucinations, delusions, psychomotor retardation and suicidal ideation dominate the clinical picture.

Psychological Interventions. If the path into and out of depression is multifaceted then what do psychological treatment studies tell us about the endogenous–neurotic debates or the idea that some forms of depression represent a disease entity? The evidence on psychotherapy for endogenous patients as far as I am aware is not available. In other words there is no treatment study that has taken a group of endogenous patients and treated them with psychotherapy only. The second issue is that just as it would not be helpful to use any psychotropic medication for depression so also to understand whether a psychological approach works, one should first study a therapy that claims specific benefits for depression. Probably the two contenders here are cognitive therapy (Beck et al., 1979) and interpersonal therapy (Klerman, Weissman, Rounsaville, & Chevron, 1984). In an early study Blackburn, Bishop, Glen, Walley, and Christie, (1981) did not find that the presence of endogenous symptoms mitigated against improvement with cognitive therapy, but the numbers were very small. (For a review of cognitive therapy treatment studies see Blackburn & Davidson 1990; Williams, 1989; Hollon, Shelton & Loosen, 1991.)

In an important study (Elkin et al., 1989) of major depression comparing four treatments, cognitive therapy, interpersonal therapy, anti-depressants with clinical management, and placebo and clinical management, it was found that both psychotherapies where not significantly different from imipramine, and that the psychotherapies had closely comparable effects. However, controlling for severity imipramine came out best and placebo plus clinical management did poorly (clinical management plus placebo did surprisingly well for the less ill group). There was some evidence that interpersonal therapy also did well in the severer group but less evidence for cognitive therapy. Hence it looks as if severity is an important factor in treatment responsiveness. Whether this involves a melancholic/non-melancholic distinction is however unknown. Another interesting finding was how well the less severe depressives did with placebo and supportive management. In a subsequent analysis Imber et al. (1990) failed to find any convincing mode-specific effects of each treatment (although cognitive therapy seemed better for reducing "need for approval"). They see this as further evidence for Frank's (1982) basic idea that various psychotherapies help because of certain common elements that they all share. At the time of going to press we are awaiting follow-up data to see if one therapy is better at preventing relapse or a new episode.

Free & Oei (1989) have given an excellent review of biological and psychological treatment studies and find that there is little evidence to support the idea of two types of depression which respond differentially to drugs or psychological therapy. However, high endorsement of dysfunctional attitudes (Peselow, Robins, Block, Barouche & Fieve, 1990) and marital problems (Gotlib & Colby, 1987) are associated with poor outcome regardless of treatment. In most studies, however, the psychological (mainly cognitive and interpersonal) treatment effects are good, around 70% response rate. Further, the addition of cognitive therapy to medication seems to have a significant effect on relapse rates, suggesting that cognitive therapy may influence the course of major depression (Free & Oei, 1989). This would not be expected if it were an "autonomous disease". In regard to interpersonal therapy in major depression, Frank, Kupfer, and Perel (1989) found that interpersonal therapy (only once a month) was the only predictor of length of interval to a relapse, i.e., the patients receiving it stayed well longer. They say they were surprised by this result. Drug therapy did not predict well intervals. Miller, Norman, and Keitner, (1989) found that cognitive therapy or social skills therapy when added to standard hospital treatment (e.g., drugs) gave significant benefit to the prevention of relapse (at one year).

As Beckham (1990) points out, in an important review of psychotherapy for depression, we are at something of a crossroads. No less than for drugs, we remain unclear of how it works and much depends on the theories we hold. Nevertheless, there is a growing recognition that psychosocial therapy matters a lot (see Chapter 15). Where attention is now focused is in exploring in more detail those who don't respond, and attempts to identify those patients who remain vulnerable to relapse regardless of remission at the end of an acute episode, and regardless of which treatment is given (e.g., Rush et al., 1986; Giles, Jarrett, Roffwarg, & Rush, 1987; Akiskal, 1988; Scott, 1988; Teasdale, 1988).

Summary. Taken as a whole these data cast serious doubt on the therapeutic assumptions that lay behind the endogenous–neurotic distinction. Nevertheless, cognitive therapy is not a cure-all and Blackburn (1989) has recently indicated that patients who have delusional beliefs, who lack insight or attribute their illness to a physical condition, who are too severely depressed to establish a rapport, and have had chronic depression of many years, do poorly with cognitive therapy. What emerges then is severity, insight, and chronicity as indicators of response to cognitive therapy. As with the dexmathesone suppression test, severity may be a more important factor than depressive type (Arana, Baldessarini, & Ornsteen, 1985).

Genes for Depression?

If you approach the phenomenology of depression with the preconceived idea (or hypothesis) that somewhere in the confusion of symptom variation lies a disease entity (and that this disease is not acquired, say, as a result of negative parenting on the maturing nervous system) then it makes sense to consider the possibility of genetic loadings for depression. One way of exploring the idea that some symptoms of depression represent a core disease which have a significant genetic loading is with family studies.

Weissman et al. (1986) found that symptom patterns (including endogenous, delusional, melancholic or autonomous) in the index patient did not predict major depression in relatives. Rather, age of onset, major depression with anxiety or secondary alcoholism were independently related to increased risk in relatives. Andreasen et al. (1986; see also Andreasen, 1989) examined 2,942 first degree relatives of 566 individuals diagnosed as having unipolar depression. They were interested in whether endogenous depressives had higher rates of familial affective illness than those with non-endogenous disorder. They used four different criteria of endogenous (Newcastle; RDC; DSM-111-R for Melancholia; and the Yale autonomous depression criteria). Contrary to their expectations they did not find that "first-degree relatives of patients with endogenous depression have a higher rate of affective illness" (p. 246); and this was regardless of the diagnostic criteria used. Moreover the rates of endogenous depression where quite different depending on the criteria used (the Newcastle scale being the most restrictive). Hence the idea of family loading for endogenous depression (which has often been an important assumption) was not found. However they where not able to test the idea that endogenous depressives tend to have relatives who are endogenously depressed, when depressed (i.e. the breed true argument).

In general then, for specifically endogenous depression, the evidence for genetic loadings is rather poor. Andreasen et al. (1986) fall for the usual mind-body fallacy that lurks in all these debates when they argue that endogenous depression may still be biological but not genetically based. All depressions are in some sense biological and the important question is, in what sense?

What is also unanswered by a lot of research of families is the specificity problem, that is, what is inherited? Is it a general sensitivity to psychiatric disturbance—for example, neuroticism or emotional instability, a predisposition to negative affectivity or defence system functioning (e.g., see Torgersen, 1990)? How far does the expression of type of illness depend on many factors, such as developmental and psychosocial (Reiss, Plomin & Hetherington, 1991)? In reality genetic questions require adoption studies, since anything else can't really rule out the possibility of the effects of growing up with disturbed families. Wender et al. (1986) have conducted such a study looking at psychiatric disturbance in the biological relatives of adopted individuals who have affective disorder. They found an eight-fold increase in rates of unipolar depression in these biological relatives of adoptees. They also found much higher suicide rates (a fifteen-fold increase in suicide among biological relatives). As they point out, since low 5-HT has been associated with suicide and impulsiveness, it is possible that some genetic effect on an internal biological 5-HT control mechanism is involved. But 5-HT is probably involved in many psychiatric disorders.

Genetic studies are becoming increasingly complex as our understanding of depression complexifies. Two recent reviews are helpful in articulating the main issues (McGuffin & Katz, 1989; Merikangas, Spence, & Kupfer, 1989). Both reviews on the genetics of depression come down strongly in favour of an inherited vulnerability especially for bipolar disorder. The degree to which life events are necessary to light up a genetic vulnerability is an important question however. Even bipolar disorder seems to be influenced by life events (Ellicott, Hammen, Gitlin, Brown & Jamison, 1990). McGuffin and Katz (1989) and Bebbington, Katz, McGuffin, Sturt and Wing (1989) suggest that there appears to be a tendency for those vulnerable to depression to have (or at least report) higher rates of life events (see Chapter 15).

One thing is clear; the road from gene to pathology is complex and not linear (Merikangas et al., 1989). There may be any number of different genetic influences increasing risk of depression; e.g., some may be related to traits for dominance and need for achievement while others may relate to attachment concerns or sensitivity to attachment failure. In this scheme vulnerability is dimensional and relates to *thresholds*; that is, some individuals may need very negative life experience to fall into depression while others may succumb with less severe events (McGuffin, Katz & Rutherford, 1991). A protective factor for one person may not be protective for another (Reynolds & Gilbert, 1991, and Chapter 15). Coping behaviour itself may be genetically influenced (Kendler, Kessler, Heath & Neale, 1991). It seems to me that in our culture, negative life events—e.g., major increases in mortgage rates that increase stress and divorce in families, losing one's job, being passed over for promotion, having to compete and needing a lot of luck to succeed, the increased importance of the demonstration of competency and positive self-presentation, and so on (e.g., Lasch, 1985; Klerman, 1988)—are all falling on us in a far greater density than they might in stable hunter gather societies (Glantz & Pearce, 1989). Under this kind of environmental influence we may be pushing our biological tolerance to the limit. Just as in heart disease there may well be a genetic component but this only begins to show up under the great distortion of life styles (e.g., diet and exercise, as shown by cross-cultural studies) from which we evolved, so the same may be true for depression. Klerman (1988) has argued that the increased incidence of depression in postwar cohorts cannot be explained by simple gene arguments.

Life Events

We shall be looking at life events more closely in Chapter 15. However, we should mention here that there is now evidence that life events are not predictive of type of depression. Certainly precipitated endogenous depression does occur (Akiskal et al., 1978). Hence there is very little evidence for the view that endogenous depression is not associated with life events (Brugha & Conroy, 1985; Grove et al., 1987; Paykel & Dowlatshahi, 1988). Also in one recent study of 400 working-class women with children, Brown, Adler and Bifulco (1988) found that 60% of remissions of chronic depression were due to positive (fresh start) life events.

Biology

McAllister and Price (1990, p.361) in a review of depression following brain injury, point out that "depression is almost certainly the most common behavioural concomitant of disorders afflicting the nervous system". However, depression, as a result of brain injury does not map neatly onto the endogenous–neurotic divide. Depression is known to be associated with a host of side effects from certain drugs; it may arise from various hormone changes (e.g., at the menopause, and hormone replacement therapy is growing in use), is associated with thyroid dysfunction (Calloway, 1989), can be a complication in viral infections, and has a variety of different neurotransmitter changes (Healy & Paykel, 1989). Depression and stress also affect the immune system (Farrant & Perez, 1989). In all these cases the researchers find important interactions between life stress, coping, and personality. Individual differences are important. There has been no consistent evidence that one kind of biological variable can be extracted as specifically related to a specific type of pure depressive disease.

In general then, there is no outstanding biological marker that differentiates depressive types, although, as in much of this area of research there are teasing possibilities and conflicting findings. For example, Braddock (1986) found that the Newcastle scale was one of the better predictors of the response to the dexamethasone suppression test (DST) of cortisol (see also Carney, 1989). However, DST non-suppression seems related to a dimension of severity (Arana, Baldessarini, & Ornsteen, 1985) and the issue of whether endogenous symptoms are a reflection of severity remains unresolved. Recently Zimmerman, Coryell, and Black (1990) pointed out that some of the inconsistency of findings using biological markers like the DST may relate to how diagnostic criteria are used.

Another area of interest is sleep architecture (e.g. Sitaram, Nurnberger, Gershon, & Gillin, 1982) which may be associated with acetylcholine sensitivity (Gilbert, 1984). Debus & Rush (1990) review the evidence and suggest than indicators of sleep architecture may help to separate out depressive types along the classical endogenous–non-endogenous divide although again these findings are confounded by issues of severity (REM sleep is shifted forward in time in depressives). To date however sleep variables do not seem to discriminate bipolar from unipolar. In conjunction with other measures (like the DST), Debus and Rush believe that sleep architecture may help in the prediction of treatment response and relapse. This fascinating area is likely to grow over the next few years and it will be interesting to see if these promising results do eventually collapse into an issue of severity or can be used to distinguish types. It would be interesting if this work could be associated with ranking theory (see Chapters 5–8) because ranking theory suggests possible differences between defeat depression and the more chronic submissive forms. The former (putting it crudely) involves older, reptilian patterns of defeat.

It would in fact be very surprising if there were not biological differences between people who are depressed. However, it is likely to be in patterns of biological change rather than single response systems (Gilbert, 1984; 1989). When these differences are more clearly understood, debate will continue as to their etiological significance and most theorists now speak in terms of "*threshold*" rather than some autonomous internal disease. It is almost certain that some carry a biological sensitivity to various forms of depression but never manifest the disorder and researchers are obviously interested in this. Hence, one can predict that over the next decade greater research will be directed to those who might be vulnerable but stay well. We also know that once an episode has occurred a patient is at greater risk from subsequent episodes; almost as if once the pathway has been opened up somehow, or a depressive brain state organisation has been switched on for a certain period, it is more easily recruited again. (It's always easier second time around and this seems as true for crystal formation as it is for biological systems.) On the other hand, we know that social factors play an important role in relapse and subsequent episodes (see Chapter 15).

SUMMARY

As Kendell (1988) makes clear, although we can make reliable diagnoses it remains uncertain how much more we can say about depression. Clearly severity stands out as the single most important aspect for treatment considerations, but how genes, psychological style, life events, and culture all interact to produce an individual's symptom profile at any point in time (and these profiles are often highly unstable) remains mysterious.

1. Classification remains a fascinating area for research with a long history of ideas. But it has only been in the the last thirty years or so that scientific techniques have been systematically applied.
2. The main classification systems are the American DSM and the European ICD which have recently moved closer together. The unipolar–bipolar distinction seems to be one of the most important distinctions.
3. The role of psychotic symptoms remains of interest but the meaning of the difference between mood congruent and mood incongruent is unknown.
4. The separation of the endogenous subgroup from other types continues to claim interest often with the assumption that it represents some "core" depressive disease whereas neurotic depressions are a mixture of personality and life events. The evidence that supports this distinction is at best mixed. The assumption that endogenous symptoms are biologcial and neurotic symptoms are somehow psychological is simply wrong and is grossly confusing. Treatment issues seem more related to degree of severity, cyclicity, and the role of supportive environments.
5. Evidence has now built up that depressives often have other Axis I conditions, of which the most common is anxiety. In many cases the depression predates subsequent disorders. However anxiety and depression present across a wide spectrum of disorders. Recent ideas of "negative affectivity" and defence system function (Gilbert, 1989) have been suggested to explain such findings.
6. The role of personality and the meaning of personality traits (i.e., whether they reflect underlying affect control

modulators) has given rise to various concepts of dysthymia and cyclothymia. The implications are that recovery may be limited in those who have some kind of underlying instability in affect systems, which have become part of the personality structure.

7. Postnatal depression has received more research interest this decade and it has become an essential public health concern. Further training is necessary to alert clinicians to its prevalence and long-term effects on the growing child.
8. Research into depression early in life and late in life has also developed in this decade. Much evidence now suggests that depression in childhood does exist. Further longitudinal work is needed to explore the distinction from adult types and its long-term course.
9. Efforts to distinguish depressive types according to treatment response have not been successful; treatments affect symptoms rather than patient types. However, severity, delusions, retardation, and lack of insight may mitigate against psychological treatments at least in the acute state.
10. The biologic distinction of types remains an elusive but important research area. There are no clear biological distinctions between types although it is likely that in time differences in "patterns of biological functioning" will emerge. Severity accounts for much of the variance in these studies.

CONCLUDING COMMENTS

It has be noted that every new statistical approach tends to produce slightly different results and groupings. Not surprisingly then many new adjectives have become increasing peppered in the literature, e.g., autonomous depression and nuclear depression. If not in written then certainly in spoken discourse (e.g., in ward rounds) some use terms like clinical depression, biological depression and even worse "real" depression. These terms are sometimes used so idiosyncratically that they are meaningless. Also we have the continuing tendency to speak of "biological symptoms" or "biological features". Again such views reflect serious mind–body confusions of dualism. For example, in many cultures depression presents with a greater degree of somatic complaints and fewer psychological symptoms such as guilt. Are we to assume therefore that such depressions are more biological? When is a belief (in say personal inferiority and low self-esteem) a biological feature and when not? How can drugs sometimes produce increases in self-esteem? It is not mind versus body but rather variations in biopsychosocial patterns that distnguish patients.

By now the reader is perhaps more familiar with the complexity that faces us in understanding depression. To my mind the platonic disease approach to depression is fraught with problems and can be as much a hinderance as a help. This is not because syndromes do not exist, nor because genetic and biological studies are unimportant; indeed there is clear evidence of biological variation between people. In fact I doubt that anyone would be surprised at the findings that humans vary genetically, we are not all exact copies. Hence, it would seem to me perfectly reasonable to suppose that there may be a dimension of variability in the capacity to shift brain state in one direction or another. What is less clear to me is whether we can march from here to the proposition that depression is a specifically inherited disease.

The problem with the disease approach is that it tends to be theoretically impoverished and simplistic in the social-psychological domain. If depression is somehow a disease then there is little point in looking at its phylogenetic evolution and considering how depression may have played a role in group living. That is, it would not be seen to have any functional utility; it's an abnormality. Ethological theorists (see Chapters 5–8) on the other hand believe that the capacity to be depressed probably exists in most people, that this brain state possibility within the population was positively selected for rather than against, and that what we should be studying is thresholds for the activation of this state. At the end of the day phenomenological and statistical approaches can only investigate expression or phenotype. The degree to which one can move from phenotypic expression to a theory of genotype or disease entity is fraught with difficulty (see Chisholm, 1988 for a general discussion of the complexity of phenotype/genotype relationships in regard to evolution theory and Merikangas, Spence, & Kupfer 1989, for a discussion in regard to depression). What we need it seems to me is a greater preparation to work psychobiologically, encapsulating the human mind, body, and spirit, an example well set by Vasile et al. (1987). They note, however, that it is difficult to get clinicians to appreciate this.

If I would want this book to achieve one aim it would be to help this dialogue along. Depression is often a state of intense suffering for self and family members and sometimes leads to loss of life. Future generations require of us a preparedness to tackle the complexities of the disorder and not hide behind professional fences.

CHAPTER 3

Epidemiology, Relapse, and Long-term Outcome

> The basic facts regarding rates of depression are easily summarized. About 1 per 1000 of the general population are admitted to hospital annually with depression; about 3 per 1000 are referred to psychiatrists, of whom two are treated as out-patients. However, around 3 percent of the general population are treated in this country by general practioners and an equal number probably consult and are not recognised. The prevalence rate in the general population is about 5 percent although estimates vary considerably. Depression is therefore a kind of iceberg of which only the tip sticks up to reach the psychiatrist. The frequencies of the disorder will depend very much on how one defines it and where one studies it. (Paykel, 1989, p.3)

Increasingly large numbers of depressed people are referred to psychologists, social workers and community nurses without recourse to psychiatry. This has serious training implications. Furthermore, if education of the rates and diagnosis of depression increase and the shame or stigma is reduced then more people may come forward for help. It is vital that we can work cooperatively across disciplines. A good model is given by Vasile et al. (1987).

EPIDEMIOLOGY: SOME ISSUES

Epidemiologists use various terms to describe their statistics. Point or period prevalence refers to the proportion of the population suffering the disorder at any point in time; incidence refers to the number of new cases over a set time period; morbid or life-time risk refers to an individual's risk for the disorder over his/her life time. Risk factor refers to a factor that increases risk or vulnerability of developing the disorder (see Williams & Poling, 1989, and Brown, 1991, for a clear discussion).

Epidemiology depends very much on the criteria one uses to diagnose individuals and how the diagnosis is made (e.g., by interview or the use of self-report scales). There remains considerable controversy over this (Kendell, 1988). As criteria loosen the rates of depression in the community rise steadily, sometimes dramatically. Self-report measures, which some believe tap general demoralisation and stress, can give prevalence as high as 40% and above.

Depression and Stress

The new area of stress research is of concern. In the first place, stress is sometimes used to refer to external events, sometimes a subjective state (one is suffering from stress) and at other times a coping style (see Hobfoll, 1989, for a good review). A stressful event can include just about any type of event from loss of job, shortage of resources, interpersonal conflict and so on. Much of the careful work conducted by Brown and his colleagues (see Chapter 15) on understanding precise relationships of life events with depression and self-esteem is blurred and lost on stress concepts. Psychologists frequently talk about stress reactions. It does not matter if the patient suffers from depression, anxiety, worry or irritability, is autocratic or submissive, is hypochondriacal or suffers suicidal feelings, has alcoholic problems or uses tranquillisers, suffers physical disorder such as hypertension or ulcers, has one episode or many episodes, has good outcome or poor outcome; these variables can all be related to the stress concept. Where stress shades into neurosis, personality disorder, or other psychiatric conditions is very unclear. Having decided that stress is somehow one thing we then devise stress packages, to help people manage their stress. These include a bit of relaxation training, thought monitoring and so forth. There is hardly any evidence on who benefits, or on long-term effects. Although I have serious worries about current phenomenological classifications of psychiatric conditions and concepts of disease, the concept of stress is equally worrying. Stress somehow makes mental disorder more acceptable. It is less alarmist than mental or emotional disorder. We feel better if we diagnose someone as suffering stress rather than major depressive disorder or dysthymia.[1]

Stress remains a useful and important concept however, provided we remain clear of its meaning and limitations and separate its meaning in regard to cause, affective state, and response. The treatment implications are salient concerns.

DEPRESSION

In 1981 Boyd and Weissman (p.1044) outlined what was currently known of epidemiology using agreed criteria: (1) The point prevalence of depressive symptoms ranges between 9% and 20%. (2) The life-time risk of bipolar depression is less than 1%. The annual incidence of bipolar disorder is 0.009% to 0.015% for men and 0.007% to 0.03% for women. (3) Using the new diagnostic techniques in industrial nations, the point prevalence of nonbipolar depression is 3% for men and 4% to 9% for women. The life-time risk of nonbipolar depression is 8% to 12% for men and 20% to 26% for women, and the annual incidence of nonbipolar depression is 8% for women.

The last figure is provisional since it was based on one study, but for the other statistics various studies show consistency. Hence around one fifth of women and one tenth of men were believed to suffer depression at some point in their lives. Unfortunately, this was ten years ago and if anything things look worse now.

To take bipolar illness, the above review suggests a ratio of 10–20:1. However so much depends on the type of population studied and the criteria used that estimates in fact vary widely. Also it is known that over time a large percentage of patients may switch from unipolar to bipolar. In a major review Angst (1988) presented evidence for ratios of 8:1 down to 1:1, and that bipolars are likely to suffer about twice the number of episodes as unipolars. Bipolar illness has an earlier age of onset than unipolar illness, but whether bipolar illness starts with (hypo)mania or depression has no prognostic value (Angst, 1988).

The epidemiological relationship between anxiety and depression suggests that various anxiety conditions coexist with depression (for a review see Williams & Poling, 1989; see Chapter 2). Also in using questionnaires or even objective measures it is not entirely clear if patients scoring at a mild level on many symptoms are the same as patients scoring highly on only a few (Shapiro, 1989).

Brown and Harris (1978a) using the Present State Examination (PSE) with a group of working-class women, found that 36% met criteria for either definite or probable caseness. Amenson and Lewinsohn (1981) found that 48% of males and 62% of females reported a prior episode of depression and, of the 998 individuals in the sample, 38% indicated that they had sought various forms of treatment for episodes. Recently, Bebbington et al. (1989) raised a number of important methodological questions to this research area. For example using the PSE, in the working-class area of Camberwell, they found that under one set of assumptions, risk of a minor episode of depression was 46% for men and 72% for women. Changing the method reduced this to 16% and 30% respectively. Thus, as these researchers point out the risk of minor affective disorder is extremely high, and with these kinds of statistics we should also look at resilience.[2]

In 1980 the American Institute of Mental Health set up an epidemiological catchment area community survey (ECA). Each area has about 200,000 individuals. Yale received the first grant and others (e.g., John Hopkins, in Baltimore, and others) soon followed. As expressed by Weissman (1985), the aim was to study and provide information on: "1) the prevalence and incidence of specific psychiatric disorders in the community; and 2) for newly developed mental disorders (i.e. incidence cases), the concomitant factors associated with or causative of the disorder."

Weissman (1985) has reviewed the not inconsiderable achievements of the ECA studies. In common with work on negative affectivity (Watson & Clark, 1984; 1988) major depression and anxiety conditions are heterogenous. Panic disorder and major depression may have an underlying common diathesis. Risk is positively related to family history and children of depressed parents are more at risk from separation anxiety. Of course none of these findings necessarily indicates how risk is conveyed (see Chapter 2) but some role for genetic sensitivity remains a possibility.

The issue of shame (see Chapter 8) complicates this area of research. For example we are unsure of the levels of psychopathology in organisations. Hence, another complication is that people must be prepared to reveal symptoms if asked so that they can be diagnosed as a case. It is not clear that individuals are always prepared to reveal depressive symptoms (e.g., Bucholz & Dinwiddie, 1989).

Gender

It is currently believed that women suffer depression in a ratio of 2 or 3:1 compared to men. Various hypotheses have been put forward for these differences, including biological differences and how females and males cope with dysphoric affect (Nolen-Hoeksema, 1987). However, one recent study has cast doubt on the idea that the higher prevalence of female depression is related to something about being female. Wilhelm and Parker (1989) followed a group of teachers for five years and found no gender differences in depressive episodes. Since there were no role differences in this cohort (and also no clear gender differences in personality as measured by the masculinity–femininity scale) they suggest that gender variation may relate to role differences. Hence social factors may be a key issue, accounting for gender variation. Of course there may be particular individual aspects that are related to choosing a profession of teaching which may interact with vulnerability. (For a further discussion see Harris, Surtees & Bancroft, 1991.)

Summary

How we move from epidemiological work to considerations of other factors such as vulnerability factors, risk or natural course is complex. Williams and Poling (1989) point to the Berksonian fallacy (or clinical illusion) in which one can make inappropriate generalisations from a sub-sample (e.g., hospitalised depressives) to the population at large. The vast majority of depressives in the population are not recognised by medical agencies, do not present for treatment, and may not even recognise themselves as suffering from a diagnosable psychiatric condition, or even if they do are too ashamed to seek help. Whether we can draw inferences about cause and course of depression from the minority of cases that come to our attention is doubtful. This is why large random community surveys, with socially-skilled trained interviewers who can spot issues of shame, are so important.

In view of the very high rates of depression noted above we might also remember the comments made by Schwab (1989; see Chapter 1) that world wide there could be as many as 100 million depressives. At this level I do not think there is much doubt that we have an epidemic of misery and suffering.

RELAPSE

Recent reviews and long term follow-up studies suggest that the chances of relapse from major depression are high. Belsher and Costello (1988) have given an excellent review of factors effecting relapse and discussion of the considerable methodological problems in this area of research. In their conclusion (p.94) they suggest:

> (a) relapse is frequent after unipolar depression has been successfully treated—within 2 years of recovery, around 50% of patients relapse; (b) although the cumulative probability of relapse increases with time, the longer patients stay well, the less likely they are to relapse in the future;

(c) recent environmental stress increases the likelihood of relapse; (d) the absence of social support from family members increases the risk of relapse; (e) a history of depressive episodes increases the probability of relapse; (f) persistent neuroendocrine dysregulation after recovery from depression increases the probability of relapse; (g) maintenance doses of amitriptyline or lithium decrease the probability of relapse; and (h) research has failed to demonstrate significant associations between relapse and gender, marital status, or socioeconomic status.

In regard to drugs, it should be pointed out that while drugs do reduce relapse rates compared to placebo, nevertheless significant numbers of patients on drugs relapse (Belsher & Costello, 1988). In a three-year follow up study comparing lithium with amitriptyline Glen, Johnson, & Shepherd (1984) divided patients into two groups. Group I were those with more than one episode in the five years before the index episode and group II were those with only one episode within the same five years. It was found that 69% of patients in group I with severe recurrent depression relapsed and 61% of patients in group II relapsed. Both groups included people on placebo. When only the drug-treated patients were compared relapse was 42% for lithium and 57% for amitriptyline. However studies vary greatly and worse figures have also been reported for drugs (Belsher & Costello, 1988). Of course a central issue here is compliance with medication.

In regard to psychological factors Teasdale (1988) has suggested a cognitive model of vulnerability to relapse. The first aspect is the tendency to evaluate life events in more extreme terms producing intense rather than mild depression. The second aspect involves depression producing a vicious cycle of negative construing and more depression. A host of factors such as biological and social can feed this cycle. Hooley and Teasdale (1989) explored the predictive validity of expressed emotion, marital satisfaction, and perceived criticism of spouse. All factors were associated with relapse at nine months but perceived spouse criticism was the best predictor. This finding supports Price's (1988) ethological and social ranking model of depression, which suggests that a high rate of "put downs" increase risk to depression and relapse. Frank, Kupfer and Perel, (1989) found that in a group of unipolar depressives pharmacological treatments failed to predict time to recurrence, although interpersonal therapy did.

Cognitive therapy shows some promising indications that either alone or in combination with drugs it has a significant effect on relapse, especially if associated with booster sessions (Free & Oei, 1989). We still await the long-term (e.g., five to ten years) follow-up studies but if these prove to bear the promise hoped for then this is a major contribution.

LONG-TERM FOLLOW-UP

I would like to discuss one study in detail because I think it highlights the difficulty with our classification system. In one of the most informative studies of the 1970s, Akiskal et al. (1978) used a longitudinal approach to investigate the heterogeneity of neurotic depression. Using a standard psychiatric diagnostic procedure (DSM II), these authors argued that neurotic (non-psychotic) depression was the only appropriate diagnosis for each of the 100 cases studied. Patients with other diagnoses, e.g., manic-depressive illness; anxiety, obsessional and phobic neuroses, and organic brain damage, were excluded.

In 22% of cases depression appeared to be clearly related to situational events, but for the other 78% situational events tended to act as a trigger mechanism for the depressive episode. On the question of reactivity of neurotic depression Akiskal et al. (1978, p.759) argue that: "... neurotic depression was viewed as a functional illness, representing a psychological, understandable reaction to adverse environmental contingencies in both vulnerable and non-vulnerable personalities."

At the index episode, symptoms were generally mild, i.e., a clear absence of psychoses (as required by selection criteria) plus a relative absence of major vegetative disturbances (e.g., sleep, appetite, and libido) and psychomotor (retardation and agitation) disturbance. Symptomatology presented largely on the subjective (psychological) level, with few clinical signs of endogenous depression. In 90% of cases other symptoms of non-affective neuroses were evident, e.g., obsessional, anxiety, and phobic symptoms; 24% of cases showed a characterological difficulty, designated as a life-long tendency to overreact to normative stress. The overall impression then is of a very mixed group of individuals and symptoms.

Akiskal et al. (1978) present many important points for consideration, only some of which can be summarised here. Their findings include:

1. Of the 100 patients studied, 36% went on to develop depressions with an endogenous profile of symptoms. Given the authors' initial exclusion criteria and the mild, reactive nature of the neurotic depressed state at the indexed episode, they are led to agree with others (e.g., Klein, 1974) that the endogenous concept of depression should be divorced from considerations of severity or cause. In their view mild, non-psychotic, endogenomorphic depressions, which may be either precipitated or not, do indeed exist.

2. These researchers were unable to demonstrate a relationship between a neurotic episode and a subsequent psychotic one, i.e., some patients having been diagnosed as neurotically depressed had subsequent episodes of psychotic depression, or moved into a depression of psychotic depth via a neurotic depression. These researchers do not mention the possibility that specific life events, e.g., childbirth, may play some role in these transitions. Clinical observations suggest, however, that women who suffer a psychotic puerperal episode can be left with a neurosis which may take longer to clear. In any event Akiskal et al. (1978) believe that their data support a hierarchical conceptualisation of illness as advocated by Foulds (1973) and Foulds and Bedford (1976). This evidence seriously undermines the idea that neurotic and psychotic depression are qualitatively separate or are different diseases. The neurotic–psychotic distinction may hold little validity for predicting the course of an individual's illness over time, or for the development of a meaningful nosology. A further interesting point not discussed by these researchers is that a treatment not effective at one time in the subject's history (i.e., neurotic depressive condition) may become effective at a later point (psychotic depressive condition). Furthermore, the person may (or may not) make a complete recovery with physical treatment when psychotic, but the same treatment may be less effective when neurotic symptoms dominate presentation. This seems one of the puzzling but important questions for both the classification and treatment-response studies. It would, however, seem to echo Raskin and Crook's (1976) findings that drugs affect symptoms, not people or illness types.
3. The view that neurotic depression is equivalent to secondary depression (Winokur, 1973) was found to be true for only 50% of cases. Moreover, one-fifth of those studied went on to develop bipolar illness, which also casts doubt on the view that neurotic depression is a subgroup of unipolar depression. Nevertheless these researchers still believe that a primary–secondary distinction has some usefulness for depressions that arise in the course of some other non-affective disorder.
4. The presence of a characterological disorder significantly affected outcome. Akiskal et al. (1978) suggest that these patients may overlap with Paykel and co-workers' clusters of hostile and personality disorder patients (see Chapter 1). Akiskal et al. (1978, p.764) point out that:

> ... a patient may suffer from a pure primary affective illness or primary affective illness in the context of severe characterological disorder (in which instance it will have poor prognosis). Conversely, a patient may suffer from a character disorder (such as hysteria, sociopathy, or related disorders) with concomitant alcohol and drug abuse as well as depressive symptoms.

In later work Akiskal et al. (1980) and Akiskal (1988; 1990) have suggested that characterological depressions may be subdivided into "sub-affective dysthymias" and "character spectrum disorders." These have been discussed in Chapter 2.

There is mixed evidence as to which depressed population does best in the long term. In the original endogenous–neurotic debate it was argued that with proper treatment endogenous types had good outcome. Grove et al. (1987) however found that their nuclear depressives did less well, but their results are complicated because (as measured by personality scales) the nuclear group were more neurotic.

Recent Findings on Long-Term Outcome

Recent evidence has revealed clearly that the longer the time over which recovery is measured, the worst the outcome. Angst (1988) and Belsher and Costello (1988) point out that recovery is not well defined and ranges on a dimension, from symptom-free to mild or moderate symptoms, making studies difficult to compare. Angst (1988) found that recovery rates were comparable for both unipolar and bipolar depression. He also found little evidence that outpatients had better or worse outcome than inpatients. This is a surprising finding since patients come into hospital for a variety of reasons apart from objective symptomatology.

Lee and Murray (1988) found that although psychotic patients may "race ahead" showing good recovery in the short term, in the long term (e.g., ten to twenty years) they actually do much worse. This study followed up 89 consecutive admission with primary depression as diagnosed by R.E. Kendell between 1965 and 1966). He also allocated them a position on a neurotic psychotic continuum. Of these 89, a change in diagnosis was common: 12 had episodes of schizo-affective disorder, 10 become bipolar, 7 developed alcoholism, 3 developed schizophrenia, 3 developed chronic paranoid psychosis, 3 became bulimic, (these three had leucotomies leaving them with marked defects), 9 died "unnaturally" and a further 9 developed malignant disease. They take this latter finding to argue against the idea that modern treatment has eliminated the risk of unnatural death.

Lee and Murray (1988) also agree with Bebbington that complicated cases must be included in outcome data, for not to do so gives an over optimistic picture of long-term outcome. They also point out that follow-up needs to be very careful. Over half of the 19 disabled patients were not in contact with psychiatric services. It may be that with recurrent episodes people become disheartened or ashamed (e.g., patients have said to me "I didn't like to go back to my doctor because I am sure he/she would think, 'Oh no not you again' "). Since a lot of patients coming to psychological services complain about the lack of time to talk to their psychiatrists, or that their psychiatrist appears only interested in monitoring drugs, we do not know whether co-ordinated counselling or psychotherapy would increase contact.

Kiloh, Andrews and Neilson (1988) followed up 133 patients from an original group of 145, who had been admitted to hospital during the period 1966-70. Kiloh was one of the leading researchers advocating the neurotic–endogenous distinction in the 1960s and 1970s and therefore their work allows careful consideration of outcome with respect to these distinctions. The endogenous group did slightly better than the psychotic group of the Lee and Murray (1988, p.756) study and no patient was re-diagnosed as suffering from schizophrenia. They found that 7% had committed suicide, 12% had remained incapacitated by depression, with only 20% remaining continuously well. In their discussion they say:

> We have always advocated the value of distinguishing between endogenous and neurotic depression. In the present study, patients with neurotic depression spent less time in hospital during the index admission and were less likely to be readmitted, yet at follow-up they were just as likely to have died from, or remained incapacitated by, their depression as patients with endogenous depression. We would see these data as supporting a different course for each illness; that is an episodically severe course for endogenous depression and a more chronic course for neurotic depression. But over the years there was no difference in overall severity, and both varieties of depression appear to produce the same amount of despair and disability.

Chronic Depression

As we have mentioned above (e.g., Belsher & Costello, 1988) one of the difficulties in comparing studies is that recovery can be defined in various ways and therefore it is not always clear whether patients in follow up cohorts have fully recovered or not. Keller et al. (1984; 1986) followed up a cohort of patients with major depression. Of these 64%

had recovered at six months, rising to 74% by one year but only to 79% at two years. In other words 21% remained unwell at two years.

Scott (1988) has given an important review of chronic depression (see also Angst, 1988). Scott points out that chronic depression has sometimes been used interchangeably with the concepts of characterological depression or treatment-resistant depression but argues that this is unjustified for a number of reasons. In her view chronic depression has many forms and can arise for many reasons. For example, only about a third of depressives come forward for treatment and even of these some are given inadequate treatments. Furthermore, many years may have elapsed between onset and seeking help, by which time many changes may have occurred in the family and other social relationships.

Scott (1988) suggests the following classification:

Chronic major depression: This is usually of late onset and develops from an unresolved episode of major depression, which can be either unipolar or bipolar. In these patients there appears to be little evidence of pre-existing minor depressive difficulties.

Chronic secondary major depression: This appears as an unremitting episode of major depression associated with physical ill-health or some other non-affective condition.

Characterological or chronic mild depression: This is sometimes referred to as dsythymic disorder. This appears to be a rather heterogeneous, ill-defined group with early onset of symptoms (e.g., Akiskal, 1990) and where symptoms have either distorted or become woven into the personality.

Double depression: These patients suffered an acute episode of major depression which is superimposed or arises out of a neurotic or minor chronic disorder. On recovery from the major episode the individual returns to a premorbid level of minor depression. Prognosis is poor with frequent returns of more severe episodes.

Scott explores a number of factors that may be associated with chronic depression and the reader should note that factors affecting chronicity are often similar to those predicting relapse. Females appear more at risk to developing chronic conditions. Life events such as loss of employment, dependency on family, lack of intimate relationships or marital discord either preceding or following depression can affect outcome. These kinds of factors are known to affect onset (see Chapter 15) and it is no surprise that they should affect chronicity if they remain unresolved. On the other hand early loss of a parent and having three or more children under fourteen did not seem related to chronicity.

Personality may well be important in a subgroup although the extent to which personality is distorted by a depression also warrants consideration. Also the degree to which personality influences vulnerability via its effects on such traits as sociability and capacity for forming and maintaining intimate relationships needs to be considered as the effects of personality on chronicity may be indirect (see Chapter 4). IQ may be a factor for some. A possibility of family loading exists, with one study cited by Scott (1988) finding that 40% to 50% of chronic depressives had family histories. This is not necessarily evidence of genetic transmission but could be accounted for by the social influence of depression in families. Postnatal depression for example is now known to affect a child's development (see Chapter 2).

In Scott's view symptoms provide no clear evidence for predicting chronicity. Some psychotic symptoms may be associated with chronicity but these may relate to schizo-affective illness. The role of SAD in chronicity has not yet been properly addressed.

SUICIDE

One of the most serious complications of depression is suicide. In Britain, between 4,500 and 5,000 people commit suicide each year. This figure may be higher and much depends on choice of death (e.g., car accidents are not recorded as suicide and other suicides may be given open verdicts). Males more often than females kill themselves while females are more prone to suicide attempts (e.g., overdosing, often with prescribed drugs). Some 80,000–100,000 may attempt suicide each year.

Given better detection and treatment for depression one might expect suicide to be falling, but many researchers have found that suicide is increasing. Let us first look at some American statistics. (Shneidman, 1989, p.5):

> ... during the eleven-year period, 1970 to 1980, 272,322 suicides were recorded in the United States. The suicide rate is about 12 per 100,000 population—it was 12.4 in 1984 (National Center for Health Statistics, 1986). Except for those over 65, it ranks as one of the ten leading causes of death in all age groups. Suicide rates gradually rise during adolescence, increase sharply in early adulthood, and parallel advancing age up to the 75 to 84 age bracket when they reach a rate of 22.0 suicides per 100,000 (in 1984). Male suicides outnumber female suicides by a ratio of three to one (3.4:1 1984). More whites than nonwhites commit suicide (27,002 versus 2,284, respectively, in 1984). Suicide is more prevalent among the single, widowed, separated, and divorced. The commonest method is firearms.

These figures may represent the fact that there are more whites than nonwhites in the country and choice of method may reflect the ease of access of firearms. As Hyman and Arana (1989, p.178) point out, evidence also suggests that in some age groups suicide is increasing faster than in others.

> Since 1970 there has been a large percentage increase in rates for males between the ages of 15 and 34. During the period 1970-1980 suicide for white males increased 60 percent within the 15- to 19-year-old group and 44 percent in the 20- to 24-year-old group. Thus, although older white males are still at the highest risk, the risk appears to be increasing rapidly among younger white males.

Two recent studies, on this side of the Atlantic, have shown complex but similar trends in suicide. Crombie (1990) noted that suicide in Scotland was below that of England and Wales through most of this century, but in the last decade Scotland's rates have increased at a faster pace, with young males' rates being particularly important. In Britain as a whole, some falls in suicide in previous decades may be attributed to the phasing out of coal gas, but death by hanging and drugs is now increasing.

Kelleher and Daly (1990, p.536) explored suicide rates in Ireland. Looking at the patterns of changes in rates against a backdrop of social changes they say:

> Suicide no longer occurs mainly in the elderly. The suicide rate among Irish males under the age of 35 years increased over 300% from 1970-1985. This appears to be part of an international trend. Increased rates in men between the ages of 24 and 44 years have been reported from a number of countries ... there has been a great increase in the suicide rates of the two largest cities. In the past, the urban suicide rate was always considerably lower than the rural rate in Ireland, and in the 1960s the suicide rates of Dublin and Cork were actually lower than the aggregate urban rates. From the mid-1970s however, the suicide rate of these two cities, particularly Cork city, rose to a level well above the national average.

There are many factors responsible for these effects. But as Kelleher and Daly (1990) point out, poverty is not one of them since this has lessened in Ireland, at least as measured by GNP. However, as will be pointed out shortly (Chapters 6–8) much may depend on the social comparative evaluations a person makes, and culture to some extent imposes these. Also, these rates can be set against a rising tide of various psychiatric problems (e.g., alcoholism) and other social disturbances such as crime, all of which may point to the change in patterns of social behaviour and cultural values.[3]

In regard to primary depression Slater and Depue (1981, p.282) found that:

> ... the occurrence of serious suicide attempts in primary depressives is strongly associated with an increased rate of independent events in the year preceding the attempts and that a particularly high density of events between episodic onset and the attempt may further enhance the probability of an attempt.

Furthermore, the significance of events was that they tended to represent a loss of an important, confidant relationship. Thus, social and relationship factors are important in suicide and attempted suicide. However, there are other factors that are related to suicide. These include: history of attempts, alcoholism, recent bereavement, living alone, chronic and/or terminal illness, and personality disorder. The assessment of suicide risk is complex and relates to many factors, not just depression (see Hawton, 1987, and Hawton & Catalan, 1987, for a comprehensive overview), but depression is a major factor.

In general then, suicide seems to be yet another indicator of the growing mental health difficulties that are slowly increasing in the western world. Our responses tend to be piecemeal, individually focused (Murphy, 1978) with implicit self-blame (patients need to learn how to cope with stress better) and miss a main source of disturbance—patterns of social relationship and sense of belonging.

Depression on the increase?

Suicide appears to be on the increase; what about depression? A number of authors have suggested that we are entering an age of increased depression (e.g., Schwab, 1970; 1989; Klerman, 1988). Klerman (1988) documents several trends in the research literature: increased prevalence in the "baby boom", post World War II generation; an earlier age of onset; an apparent decrease in depression in cohorts born before 1920; increased evidence of family aggregation, suggestive but not conclusive of a genetic transmission for certain types of depression; increased risk in females across cohorts.

Among the explanations for these changes, Klerman (1988) outlines both biological and psychosocial possibilities. Biological causes could include: changes in nutrition; virus or some unknown environmental toxin. In regard to the latter, it may be the effects of ionisation in air produced by living near pylons. In regard to psychosocial factors, he outlines: urbanisation (which is known to be highly correlated with crimes and murder rates); demographic factors; changes in family structure and attachment patterns; an increased role of women in the work force and increasing social anomy.

A major complication in research is the alarming increase in drug problems and high growing suicide rates in these people, especially in parts of America. We do not as yet know whether these rates reflect an increase in underlying depressive problems, though this is almost certainly likely. Shaw, Steer, Beck, and Schut (1979) found that the factor structure of Beck Depression Inventory responses for heroin addicts was similar to non-addicted depressed patients. This takes us back to the difficulties illuminated by Kendell (1988) and noted in Chapter 1 concerning the arbitrary nature of the boundaries we draw around conditions. If we start to include drug addiction and alcoholism as secondary disorders to depression (i.e., they are forms of self-medication for underlying depressive problems) then our rates of depression will soar. And since these are also increasing then problems of depression are probably increasing at a faster rate than we currently estimate.

SUMMARY

1. Evidence suggests that where we put the boundary between illness and not-illness determines the rates of depression. We can move from 5% as a conservative estimate to over 30% based on the work of Brown and his colleagues. Some studies suggested higher rates for less severe disorders in some sections of the community. Life-time risk can be 20% or higher with women at the highest risk. Debate surrounds the question as to whether those who self-medicate for depression or dysthymia (e.g., become substance abusers) should or should not be included in figures of depression prevalence and incidence.
2. Stress is a problematic and confusing concept that shades boundaries and fails to acknowledge the often serious emotional disturbance that is involved or is hidden until some event lights it up.
3. The longer cohorts are followed the worse they do. About 50% of depressives will relapse although debate surrounds the issue of relapse versus new episode. Various diagnostic groups do not seem to do better in the long term: endogenous patients and neurotic patients are equally prone to suicide, have

subsequent episodes and various poor outcomes in terms of functioning.

4. The longer the follow-up the more often it is found that depression changes it form. A first episode of unipolar or neurotic depression may subsequently present as bipolar or endogenous at subsequent episodes.
5. Up to 20% of depressives have chronic disturbance. These acute episodes may wax and wane but there remains an underlying chronic disorder. Various forms of chronic depression have been outlined.
6. Suicide, as a complication of depression, is on the increase throughout to western world especially in the younger male age group. The change in social behaviour and economic cultural values seems to be an important factor.
7. Depression is also on the increase but again clear facts are obscured by increases in rates of substance abuse and other disorders.

CONCLUDING COMMENTS

Whether one is an organic psychiatrist or a more social evolutionary theorist like myself, we would all agree that depression is one of the most serious mental health problems that face us. The rates are so high that there is little chance of us doing a great deal at an individual level except help those who present for treatment and try to ensure they are treated adequately (in my view with a biopsychosocial model). All would agree that we need better prevention, educational and social policies. We need to de-stigmatise depression and not hide it under a stress concept, which in my view increases the chances of failed detection and inadequate treatment. At this level our differences on whether depression is a disease or not are trivial since evidence shows that even those who suffer from the (so-called) milder forms are at risk from suicide, may have deleterious effects on their family, fail to achieve life goals and live life in some misery.

We are a long way from reaching our ideals and much more research is necessary (as usual) in all the domains of the biology, psychology, and sociology of affective disorder.

NOTES

1. Can you imagine going to managers and saying that you have in your organisation; A% with major depressive disorder, B% who suffer dysthymia, C% with achohol problems, D% who have suffered childhood abuse, E% who

are violent at home, F% who are the recipients of violence and abuse, and so forth. Furthermore, K% are so emotionally disturbed, aggressive and fearful of losing their jobs that their autocratic styles are seriously affecting others below them in the hierarchy. This is not (as some of my colleagues suggest) alarmist but realistic.

Two recent events alerted me to this problem. First, in discussing a psychological report on stress in the health service, going to the region, two managers objected to the term emotional disorder. They argued that people in their organistion did not suffer emotional disorder (apparently only patients suffer from this). Their view of emotional disorder was naive to say the least and also conveyed the idea that stress could be dealt with simply. The second event was when I was asked to do some stress work with nursing staff. I gave the usual package but subsequently I was approached on an individual level. Out came a history of abuse, major family and financial worries, long-lived low self-esteem and so on. All psychologists that get involved with staff will tell similar stories, so why are we colluding in this smoke screen? It was a testament to their resilience that some of these people were coping at all. And if I had approached them as an outside researcher they would have denied problems (they told me). I found both events sobering and worrying.

2. I personally do not like the term minor depression because it takes us back to the common cold idea. Are the people we call minor depressives less at risk from suicide or marital discord, detrimental influences on children or other serious complications? Also in today's climate of fighting for resources as we are, is it a useful term? Our managers throw around terms like "walking worried" to denote all kinds of psychlogical problems. Our use of terms must take account of political realities.
3. Ranking theory would suggest that it is social differences, social inequality, and wide variations between individuals that influences depression. When social differences are divisive, social comparison shows individuals that they are less able, have less opportunities and less resources than others they see around them. Thus economic policies that produce wide variations (the haves, the have-nots and the have-lots) are not neutral in regard to health in general and mental health in particular. Media and observation can set our aspiration levels which economic reality makes inaccessible to many (see Gilbert, 1989, p.342-348).

CHAPTER 4

Personality, Personality Disorder, and Depression

The idea that proneness to depression and personality may be related is traceable to the Greeks. The physicians Hippocrates, Empoedocles, and Galen believed that there were four basic elements (water, fire, air, and earth) four qualities (heat, cold, dry, and damp) four body humours (blood, phlegm, yellow bile, and black bile) and, according to the preponderance of various body humours, four personality types (sanguine, phlegmatic, choleric, and melancholic). Consequently, depression was seen in terms of a dimensional variation of premorbid personality. This view has been with us ever since. You may recall from Chapter 1, Bonhoeffer (1911) noted individuals who from "youth onwards are inclined to take things badly, whose depressive reactions are generally severe and of more than average duration". These reactions were regarded as being constitutionally based (i.e., partly endogenous). And so the notion of depressive personality has been with us a long time and continues to stimulate debate (Phillips, Gunderson, Hirschfeld, & Smith, 1990).

BACKGROUND ISSUES

The search for personality types and dimensions remains a key area of psychology with many specialist journals devoted to it. Variation is seen to arise from inheritance, acquired biological variation (e.g., Meyersburg & Post, 1979) social learning, and social interaction.

Various terms such as temperament, character, and personality have evolved to describe these variations and have often been used interchangeably. However, nowadays temperament tends to be reserved as a description for possible inherited biological differences (Akiskal, Hirschfeld & Yerevanian, 1983; Rutter, 1987a). Included here are arousability and autonomic reactivity, degree of internal inhibition and activity level (Kagan, 1984), and sociability. Impulsiveness may also be a temperament (MacDonald, 1988; Zuckerman, 1989). A main characteristic of temperaments is that they are stable over a long period although their expression may alter with development.

In the large Minnesota studies of twins reared apart and together (Tellegen, Lykken, Bouchard, Wilcox, & Rich, 1988) there is accumulating evidence that about 50% of personality variation may be inherited. Depending on the model used, these researchers found rates of inheritance varied from 0.39 to 0.58. However, models are complex and caution should be used in translating such findings to genes on the one hand, and to theories of psychopathology on the other. In regard to the latter issue, twins obviously share the same womb environment as they develop and this environment can have major effects (Hofer, 1981). Consequently, a variety of factors that influence the environment of the womb will affect both twins; factors such as various drugs, alcohol or cigarette smoking; various hormones (e.g., progesterone is believed to effect the relative development of the two hemispheres); stress or shocks to the mother that produce biological changes in the womb; effects of a poor nutrient environment and low birth weight. In short any perinatal factor that influences CNS development will be shared by twins and these factors influence personality (Blackwood, 1988) and possible susceptibility to psychopathology. Also of course in comparing monozygotic and dizygotic there is the issue of sex differences. In the Tellegen et al. (1988) study the age of separation varied from birth to 4.5 years with a mean of 0.2. These variables need careful control. We do not know how the very earliest relations with caregivers influence subsequent relational style. (For further discussion of the gene-environment issues, see *American Psychologist*, Feb. 1989 Special issue: *Children and their development*; and Reiss et al., 1991).

But whatever the source of temperament differences between individuals, temperament characteristics do matter in regard to later development (Rutter, 1987a; MacDonald, 1988). For one thing they influence how others (e.g., parents) will react to the child and the kinds of interactive styles that develop. These in turn influence subsequent development. In other words the baby is not a passive recipient of external (social) events but is also a shaper of its social environment. In Anna Freud's words "babies are born themselves". Second, different children may require (and have preferences for) different types of rearing environment (see Stevens, 1982, for a discussion of how different children may prefer different caregivers). Hence poor outcome seems related to a "poor fit" of the child's temperament with the demands made by parents and teachers (Wolff, 1988).

Personality has been conceptualised in numerous ways (Ewen, 1988; Liebert & Spielger, 1990). Some traits maybe more important than others. Recently, Buss (1988), following an evolutionary perspective, has described basic personality domains: activity, fearfulness, impulsivity, sociability, nurturance, aggressiveness, and dominance. The search for basic domains of personality continues and Buss' work gives a good overview (see also Buss, 1991). But it must be remembered that in any one person who has a modicum of development we can only measure the outcome of complex dispositions and (socially adapted) maturity of those traits.

In a sense personality is the hybrid of temperament in interaction. As Sroufe and Fleeson (1986) point out, a child does not move through life with a set of temperamental characteristics in one bag and acquired characteristics in another. Rather the child moves forward with a set of organised feelings, attitudes, expectations, internal models of self and others, and behavioural repertoires; everything is in the same bag. To put it another way, innate temperament and social learning do not operate like a lego model (one stacked on top of, or next to, another) but rather are mixed together as in a cake mix (Tyson, 1986). In our later discussions of self-organisation we will refer back to this basic issue. As Hinde (1989) points out, the tendency to divide behaviour into innate and acquired should have been abandoned years ago. Any observable social behaviour represents what each person brings to a relationship and the style of the interaction itself (see Chapter 16 for his model). Furthermore, the manner by which such combinations of temperament and social experience shape subsequent vulnerability to psychopathology is complex (Sroufe & Rutter, 1984). Recent work on cooperation and aggressive individualism, which might be regarded as basic personality characteristics, has shown that these social dispositions are shaped by the social environment (Eisenberg & Mussen, 1989). In this chapter we have not the space to engage the details of the biological substrate of personality, but the interested reader is referred to Gray (1971); MacDonald (1988); Zuckerman (1989).

PERSONALITY AND DEPRESSION

Suffice to say that it is patterns of internal organisation that give rise to personality. Given this, we can explore some research on personality in relation to depression. Frank, Kupfer, Jacob, and Jarrett (1987, p.14) have suggested four possible types of relationship between personality and depression: "1) certain personality features predispose an individual to affective illness; 2) personality modifies affective illness; 3) personality disturbance represents a complication of affective illness; 4) personality pathology represents an attenuated expression of affective illness". To complicate matters any one of these links may hold for some cases but not for others: e.g., for some link 1 may exist, for others link 4. Also trying to explore such linkages as if they were mutually exclusive is fraught with problems.

Neuroticism

Neuroticism is an old favourite in personality theory. It is associated with a variety of negative affects (Watson & Clark, 1984; 1988) and psychiatric conditions, including unipolar depression (Akiskal et al., 1983). However what exactly is neuroticism? Eysenck and Eysenck (1975) defined the neurotic personality as moody, anxious, over emotional, and frequently depressed. Although neuroticism has been considered distinct from trait anxiety the fact that they correlate at 0.70 or above, and the kinds of question appearing on the scale (e.g., do you suffer from "nerves") raise serious doubt to this view (Eysenck, 1988). It should also be noted that the Eysenck Personality Questionnaire (EPQ) has a number of clear mood questions (e.g., does your mood often go up and down? do you ever feel just miserable for no reason? do you often "feel fed-up"? have you ever wished you were dead?).

In a recent study of outpatients and day patients (N=75; Gilbert & Reynolds, 1990) neuroticism correlated at 0.56 with BDI. Controlling for social dependency left a significant correlation of 0.40. Clarke and Hemsley (1985) in a study of students found that depressive self-statements (e.g., on loss and failure) actually correlated more highly with trait anxiety and neuroticism than did anxious cognitions. Teasdale and Dent (1987) found that those selected for elevated neuroticism scores and depressed individuals shared a common disposition to attend to negative information and endorse negative attitudes. Low grade susceptibility to anxiety, depression, and neuroticism run together then (Watson & Clark, 1984; Barlow, 1991), and to advance our understanding of why this is the case we need to consider psychobiological aspects of the affect control systems. Various theories exist (Eysenck, 1967) including the idea that neuroticism derives from limbic system tone (Gray, 1971), sensitivity to punishment, or heightened defence system information processing (Gilbert, 1989).

A central question is: To what extent does neurotic personality (measuring, as it may, low grade chronic negative moods) predict depression? Hirschfeld et al. (1989) investigated personality characteristics in a group of individuals at risk from depression due to family history. In a six-year follow-up study, they compared those individuals who had an onset of major depression during the six years (N=29) with those who remained depression free (N=370). Measures of emotional strength and resiliency distinguished the onset from the no-onset cases. The measure of emotional strength was derived from a number of self-report scales including the MPI neuroticism scale. Low emotional strength is depicted by the person who is "likely to be emotionally labile, over-reactive, hypersensitive, passive and self-doubting" (p.346). However, it appeared that age was a significant factor in that for younger subjects (17–30) the predictive value of neuroticism did not occur. In fact they found that the effect of neuroticism was three times greater for the forty-year-old subject than the twenty-year-old. As they say, "the lack of any predictive value of the personality features among the younger age group is startling" (p.348). Indeed it is and goes against a long history of beliefs to the contrary. Clearly this work needs replicating. [1]

Although depression is associated with neuroticism, so are a variety of psychiatric conditions. Hence, its relationship to major depression is not straightforward (see Note 1). It is certainly not a specific predictor and most neurotic individuals do not develop major depression. You may also recall from Chapter 2 that Grove et al. (1987) found that their group of nuclear depressives (closely associated with endogenous depression) were actually more neurotic than non-nuclear depressives.

At the end of their study Hirschfeld et al. (1989, p.350) ponder the extent to which premorbid personality measures are really premorbid. They say:

> This raises a difficult question of what premorbid personality really means. Since sub-syndromal states are likely to be long lasting, how can these states be separated conceptually and operationally from abnormalities of personality? Do individuals have abnormal personality features(personality disorders perhaps) or do they have chronic (sub-syndromal) affective states? Does it make any difference? At this point we have no answer to these vexing problems.

Comment. We are left with the question: How conceptually distinct are measures such as neuroticism from measures of low grade affective dysthymias? Are they the same thing? If they are then it is not too surprising that a scale designed to measure moodiness and "frequently depressed" should correlate with depression. The main issues for research are: (1) the degree of mood-state variability in this aspect of personality; (2) whether it forms in the wake of an affective disturbance or before, and whether neuroticism that forms following a depressive episode is more or less pathogenic than neuroticism which predates an episode; (3) the degree to which some "neuroticism" scores represent incomplete recovery from a depressive episode; (4) the degree to which early life history sets the affective brain regulation system's "operating tone"; (5) the degree to which life events are necessary to push the person from affective instability into a major depression; and (6) further work on the role of positive affectivity as a distinct vulnerability factor for depression (Watson & Clark, 1988; Clark & Watson, 1991).

If, as seems likely, neuroticism (or sub-syndromal dysthymia?) represents some properties of the limbic system, then these biological variables in relationship to factors that are known to effect limbic system activity such as social relationship history (e.g., Reite & Field, 1985) and life events need further research.

Introversion

Introversion–extraversion is believed to represent a distinct dimension of personality (Gray, 1971; Eysenck & Eysenck, 1975; MacDonald, 1988). However, it is important to be aware that different scales measure slightly different things. Morris (1979, p.41) points out that extraversion is associated with a number of traits that tend to covary "but this tendency should not be over overestimated." These traits include:

1. Social activity: the amount of energy expended and the intensity of one's activities in social contexts, time spent in social encounters, talkativeness.
2. Social facility: social and interpersonal skill, leadership qualities, dominance, conversation skill.
3. Risk taking and adventuresomeness: spontaneity and flexibility in social behaviour, contrasted with social inhibition and restraint.
4. Preference for action and objectivity in contrast to reflectiveness, introspection, and abstract-intellectual pursuits.

Morris (1979) reviews some of the evidence which suggests a link between introversion and depression. Given this definition, extraversion would be expected to relate to positive affectivity (Watson & Clark, 1988) and this seems to be the case (Argyle, 1987). Emmons and Diener (1986) looked at two separate factors of extraversion; sociability and impulsiveness in regard to life satisfaction and positive and negative affect. Sociability was associated with positive affect and life satisfaction whereas impulsiveness was associated with negative affect.

Many researchers have found a relationship between introversion and unipolar depression (e.g., Akiskal et al., 1983; Hirschfeld et al., 1983a; Hirschfeld, Klerman, Clayton & Keller, 1983b) during both the depressed phase and on recovery. Especially important seems to be reduced sociability. Using an ethological approach Pedersen et al. (1988) found that as patients recovered from depression they increased their verbal communications with more than one person. This suggests perhaps that as a person becomes depressed their ability to communicate with more than one (or a limited number of others) is reduced. It has also been found that under stress non-human primates increase the amount of time they spend with a preferred ally and reduce the amount of time they spend in general social activities (Gilbert, 1989). In so far as depression can increase hostility, this also may generally reduce sociability or its rewarding qualities (see Chapter 8).

Some individuals may have difficulty in relating to others because they see themselves as different from others (Brewin & Furnham, 1986) and fear scorn or censure (see Chapter 8). Thus, social anxiety may account for at least a part of social avoidance and low sociability. Introversion may result from previous or early trauma and though individuals may wish to be more sociable they are fearful of being so. Also, as with neuroticism, it is unclear how much introversion may be the result of an incomplete recovery from a depressive episode. Another possibility is lack of social skills. These aspects may be different from the introvert who has a genuine preference for solitude. Indeed in our study of 75 neurotic and personality disordered patients (Gilbert & Reynolds, 1990) we found that introversion had a nonsignificant, negative correlation with a measure of preference for solitude ($r= -0.04$; P 0.36). Hence we are left wondering how much introversion in depression is social fear based, or whether there are people who are not socially fearful but simply prefer their own company. Add to this the view of Gray (1971) that introversion is related to sensitivity to punishment, and the concept becomes more complex. How much is introversion social avoidance? Is it this avoidance that accounts for its link with depression?

Davidson, Zisook, Giller, and Helms (1989) explored the issue of "interpersonal sensitivity" in depression. They relate this concept to a person's sensitivity to personal deficit in comparison to others. Their findings are extremely relevant to ideas, to be developed later, that depressive patterns evolved from sexual selection and ranking behaviour (see Chapters 6 and 7). Their measure of interpersonal sensitivity explores a number of related concerns: feeling inferior to others, feeling others are unfriendly and do not understand one, feeling shy or uneasy with the opposite sex, sensitivity to criticism and put-down. High scorers, compared to low(er) scorers on interpersonal sensitivity, had an earlier age of onset, more chronicity, and more severe depression, as measured by the Hamilton rating scale. These patients were also more retarded, had higher guilt and suicidality and were more paranoid. Greater impairment of work and interests was also noted. They suggest that MAOIs may help these patients. These symptoms fit very well with a ranking theory of depression (Chapters 5–8) and are important findings since clearly interpersonal sensitivity does not seem to be related to only mild or moderate depressions.

Hirschfeld et al. (1989) used a composite of five scales to measure introversion–extroversion in their study of onset of depression in vulnerable people, described above. However their onset cases included both unipolars and bipolars. They failed to find introversion to be a significant predictor of depression, although one of their scales, "thoughtfulness" did significantly differ in the 31 to 41 age group (this trait has been related to negative affectivity (Watson & Clark, 1984). However, it is believed that it is only unipolars that tend to be more introverted and less sociable (Akiskal et al., 1983) whereas the premorbid personality of bipolars tends to be more sociable work/ achievement orientated and extroverted and more like that of normals on recovery (MacVane, Lange Brown, & Zayat, 1978). Matussek and Feil (1983) found that endogenous depressives also tended to be more achievement orientated. By combining unipolars and bipolars Hirschfeld et al. (1989) may have cancelled out any effect for unipolars and introversion.

The other issue that needs consideration is specificity. In other words, of the traits that are frequently associated with depression, how specific to depression are they? In a recent comparison of major depression with panic disorder Reich, Noyes, Hirschfeld, Coryell and O'Gorman (1987) found that the differences in personality between these two groups (as measured for traits of emotional strength; interpersonal dependency; extraversion–introversion, and various others) were far from significantly different, although both were different from controls. In comparison of unipolar, bipolar, and anxious patients, Murray and Blackburn (1974) found that on recovery the unipolars where not different from anxious patients but the bipolars varied from both, indicating again perhaps of the importance of the unipolar–bipolar distinction.

When it comes to introversion the factor that appears most important is sociability and this presumably must be influenced by how comfortable people feel in relation to others. In our study (Gilbert & Reynolds, 1990) an unreported finding was a significant correlation of neuroticism and introversion ($r = 0.33$, $P < 0.002$) in 75 neurotic patients.

Overview

Research suggests a number of things about these two well researched personality traits: (1) neuroticism is a nonspecific personality variable and is associated with a variety of negative affects and a variety of psychiatric disorders. Emotional instability in general may be conceptualised as a measure of sub-syndromal dysthymia or negative affectivity; (2) both introversion and neuroticism are state sensitive (i.e., as mood state worsens individuals tend to become more neurotic and introverted/less sociable); (3) unipolars seem more similar to other neurotic groups especially anxiety groups in regard to personality; (4) the unipolar–bipolar distinction is important in regard to these personality variables; the trait of extraversion (associated as it is with positive affectivity) may mean that individual variation here leads to a more bipolar pattern; (5) the extent to which it is the interpersonal sensitivity of introversion that carries risk of psychopathology is yet to be fully established; (6) the degree to which introverts tend to be more socially submissive is unresearched, but is an important area for the social (dominance ranking) theories of depressions that will be developed later.

DEPENDENCY AND ACHIEVEMENT

It has long been considered that social dependency, on the one hand, and excessive achievement and anakastic personality, on the other, give rise to depressive vulnerability. Most of these formulations have been derived from psychoanalytic theory (Chodoff, 1972). Macdiarmid (1989) has recently reviewed the history of psychoanalytic thought which has long recognised that individuals may vary as to whether they primarily (emotionally) invest in forming relationships or are individualistic in the pursuit of goals. There is no shortage of recent research that supports this distinction, at least for social dependency and unipolar disorder (Nietzel & Harris, 1990). However, interpersonal dependency shows a strong mood-state effect (Hirschfeld et al., 1983a,b). Also the concept of social dependency is often confused with the needs to maintain status/rank (see Chapters 6 and 7) on the one hand and need for nurturance on the other. Hirschfeld's Interpersonal Dependency Scale, which is used in most of his studies, has three factors (emotional reliance on another person; lack of social self-confidence; and assertion of autonomy) that account for about 50% of the variance in studies (Nietzel & Harris, 1990). It is not obvious how these factors, especially the last two, relate to dependency, since dependency continues to be seen in terms of oral needs and needs for nurturance. It may be that the above traits are more obviously seen as a solution for low self-esteem and subordinate self-evaluation (Gilbert & Trent, submitted for publication). In ranking theory there is a fundamental difference between needs for oral dependency and nurturance and needs for protection in social situations.

Sociotropy and Autonomy

Beck (1983) also proposed that both the vulnerability to depression and the type of symptoms a patient expresses may be related to variation in the dimensions of personality called sociotropy and autonomy. Sociotropy (or social dependency) relates to social needs; for example, needing others for safety or help, fear of social isolation, fear of rejection, approval dependence and so on. It was predicted that socially dependent people would be more likely to become depressed by interpersonal disruptions and that their symptoms would be more like those of neurotic depression. Autonomy relates to individualistic needs: for example need for achievement—judges worth by success or failure; prefers his/her own judgements—likes to be in control. It was predicted that these individuals would be more likely to become depressed following failure and achievement-blocking events and that their pattern of symptoms would be of a more endogenous form.

Beck et al. (1983) developed a sixty item scale to measure these two dimensions. A factor analysis produced three factors for sociotropy (fear of disapproval; abandonment/separation fears; need to please others); and three factors for autonomy (individualistic/autonomous action; mobility/freedom from others' control; preference for solitude). Recent evidence suggests that sociotropy may mediate the reaction to both interpersonal and autonomous life events, but Beck's measure of autonomy does not exert any effect (Robins & Block, 1988; Robins, Block, & Peselow, 1989). In regard to symptom variation the relation between sociotropy and neurotic-type symptoms did seem to be supported but the relationship between autonomy and endogenous symptoms was not (Robins et al., 1989). If anything autonomy seems related to a certain resilience to depression (Gilbert & Trent, submitted for publication). One explanation for these findings is that the autonomy measure does not really measure the construct as described by Beck (Robins, personal communication). A modified version of the scales to better measure the theoretical constructs has actually yielded more positive results (Robins & Luten, 1991).

Another reason may be that it is social competitiveness and rank sensitivity that carries the risk of depression (Gilbert, 1988a). Or as Arieti and Bemporad (1980a,b; see Chapter 12, this volume) suggest achievement strivings that carry risk of depression are those that are being pursued to gain social approval and exert social control. For the genuinely autonomous person there may be no such hidden agenda. This distinction echoes McClelland, Atkinson, Clark, & Lowell's (1953) distinction of value achievers and need achievers. The high-need achiever is the individual whose behaviour is determined by internal standards. Such individuals prefer moderate risks and are relatively independent of social or authoritarian influences. Value achievers, on the other hand, overtly avow to high standards, but these may be unrelated to actual performance and are significantly influenced and guided by social approval and expectations of social approval. McClelland et al. (1953, p.419) speculated that value achievers develop in response to: "... authoritarian pressure from parents to be ambitious and the resultant motive which has originated in external sources shows itself as a fear of being unsuccessful". This is a fundamental distinction, as pointed out previously (Gilbert, 1984).

This points up possible links between high (ideal) standard setting—value achievement motivation—and consequences for styles of attribution in failure situations. High achievers tend to blame themselves for failure while low achievers blame external factors (Weiner, 1972). This may be a form of defensive exclusion, i.e., one has learnt to blame oneself rather than the parents for imposing high standards (Gilbert 1984; Driscoll, 1989; Gut, 1989; Chapter 10 this volume). These subtle but important distinctions are not obvious in Beck's concept of autonomy. Certainly, in my view (Gilbert, 1984; Gilbert & Trent submitted for publication), approval needs share a complex relationship between attachment on the one hand and achievement striving on the other and cannot be separated as Beck suggests. Fear of disapproval may arise from child–parent relationships, since child–parent relationships are also rank (social dominance) relationships (Hartup, 1989), but they can lead to achievement striving, needs to gain social control, and not just attachment/nurturance needs.

Another possibility is that the symptoms associated with autonomy may need to be re-examined. Parker et al. (1988), for example, found that endogenous type symptoms could arise from loss of an intimate bond and they point out that bereavement can also be associated with short-term endogenous symptoms. Matussek and Feil (1983) found exactly the reverse of Beck's predictions for unipolar depressives but some support for his views with bipolar endogenous patients. Non-endogenous depressives were aggressive and over-autonomous while the unipolar endogenous depressives lacked autonomy. However, bipolar endogenous depressives were more aggressive and had a hypomanic drive towards achievement and were more obsessional. Hence the unipolar–bipolar distinction once again comes out as an important variant.

In a study of 75 outpatients and day patients Gilbert and Reynolds (1990) found that all the sociotropic factors share a significant positive relationship with depression, the highest being fear of disapproval ($r=0.48$, $P > 0.000$). A similar pattern was found for neuroticism, the highest being with fear of disapproval ($r=0.49$, $P > 0.000$). Fear of disapproval also shared a small but significantly positive relationship with introversion ($r= 0.3$, $P > 0.005$). However, only the autonomous factor, mobility/freedom from control, showed a weak relationship to depression ($r= 0.22$, $P > 0.032$) whereas the factor individual autonomous action showed a weak relationship to psychoticism ($r= 0.25$, $P > 0.02$) and extraversion ($r= 0.21$, $P > 0.035$).

Blackburn, Roxborough, Muir, Glabus and Blackwood (1990) while exploring physiological aspects of depression also found that both sociotropy and autonomy tended to return to normal levels in recovered depressives (cross-sectional data), suggesting a degree of mood-state variability. Given the important role that need for approval and fear of disapproval seems to play in depression it is of some interest that Imber et al. (1990) found that cognitive therapy was rather better at reducing this than other therapies. We await follow-up data to see if this lowering of need for approval has relapse prevention effects. Ranking theory (Chapters 5–8) predicts that it would.

Anaclitic and Self-criticism Depressions

Blatt and his colleagues (Blatt, 1974; Blatt, Quinlan, Chevron, McDonald, & Zuroff, 1982) have developed similar concepts to the above but their approach is derived from psychoanalytic theory. Their two dimensions are labelled anaclitic (dependency) and self-criticism. Blatt et al., (1982) regard anaclitic vulnerability as an earlier form of vulnerability linked to the frustration of oral needs and infant dependency. The individual has deep fears of being abandoned and of their own weakness and vulnerability. When depressed, these fears become prominent giving rise to feelings of weakness and helplessness and the seeking of others for protection, care, and support. The more these needs are frustrated the greater the depression.

A developmentally later self-critical, depressive, vulnerability arises at the individuation stage. This is similar to Bibring's (1953) ego analytic theory (see Chapter 12). Blatt views self-critical types as marked by self-rebuke for failing to live up to internalised standards. They are prone to excessive feelings of inferiority and worthlessness. Hence, whereas the disturbance of the anaclitic is from self–other relationships, it is the evaluations of the self and achievement goals that are the source of suffering in the self-critical types.

Blatt et al. (1982) have designed the depressive experience questionnaire to measure their constructs (they also fail to distinguish value achievers from need achievers). From a review of clinical records they suggest that self-critical types suffer from:

> social isolation, intense and self-critical involvement with work, professional and/or academic striving, feelings of worthlessness and failure, a history of very critical or idealised parent, obsessive and paranoid features, anxiety and agitation, acting out (sex, alcohol and aggression), fear of loss of control, childhood history of enuresis and bowel difficulties and feelings of being a social failure. Members of this group made serious and violent suicide attempts and most often were diagnosed as "depressed with psychotic features". (P. 120)

They note a history of critical and idealised parenting, suggesting that this is value achievement (see page 89) that is involved in these depressions. The relationship between Beck's and Blatt's concepts is very close. At the time of going to press Moore and Blackburn (in preparation) investigated these scales in 21 depressed patients. They found that Blatt's measure of dependency and Beck's measure of sociotropy were significantly correlated. However, Blatt's measure of self-criticism did not correlate significantly with Beck's measure of autonomy. Furthermore, the correlations of these scales with different measures of depression was complex and showed different patterns. It is inappropriate to explore here in detail the research that explores the overlap of these various constructs but the interested reader is referred to Nietzel and Harris (1990) for an overview.

Dominant Other, Dominant Goal

Like Beck, Arieti and Bemporad (1980a,b) suggest there are different basic dispositions to interpersonal and achievement goals that convey vulnerability to depression. The dominant other type are excessively reliant on others to provide sources of meaning and self-esteem. They strike what is called a "bargain relationship" with others in which they forego independent gratification in return for the continual support and nurturance from a dominant other to maintain self-confidence.

The dominant (or lofty) goal individuals are highly achievement orientated. Unlike Beck's approach however, Arieti and Bemporad, see this seeking after achievement as full of surplus meaning; behind this striving is a desire to be valued and appreciated by others. Achievement then is a goal designed to produce interpersonal pay-offs. We shall look at this theory in more detail in Chapter 12 .

Existential Pursuits

The existential psychotherapist (Yalom, 1980) suggests very similar vulnerabilities to those outlined above, although these are not linked specifically to depression. The pursuit of the ultimate rescuer is an individual who looks to others to provide sources of meaning and gratification and also salvation and/or protection. In therapy they can be demanding and clingy or passive and dependent. In distinction is the pursuit of specialness. As the term implies these individuals are seen to demand special attention or admiration, can dominate others (especially in group therapy). Yalom (1980) links this type with narcissistic vulnerability and its associated problems of rage and shame sensitivity.

Yalom's (1980) book is an excellent introduction to existential psychotherapy and therapists of all persuasions will find much that is useful and resonates with the personal. Perhaps because of the similarity of the concepts (at least those related here) it has not stimulated much research.

INTERPERSONAL THEORIES

It is surprising that, although much of the theorising centres on interpersonal traits, the interpersonal theories of personality have been consistently ignored by those interested in dependency and autonomy. For this reason I would like to spend time with it here. In 1957 Leary published his book, Interpersonal Diagnosis of Personality. Leary did not derive his model from ethological or biological work, but he does acknowledge the influence of Jung and other analysts, notably Sullivan and Karen Horney. Leary used statistical procedures to derive two orthogonal constructs labelled dominance–submission and love–hate. The love–hate dimension may also be labelled in different ways such as linking–distancing. These orthogonal dimensions produce what is called a circumplex model as illustrated in Fig.4.1.

The reason for using a circumplex model relates to the pattern of correlations obtained whereby ratings of different behavioural traits are highly correlated to their immediate neighbours, but with movement around the circle the degree of correlation falls. In this system, the model

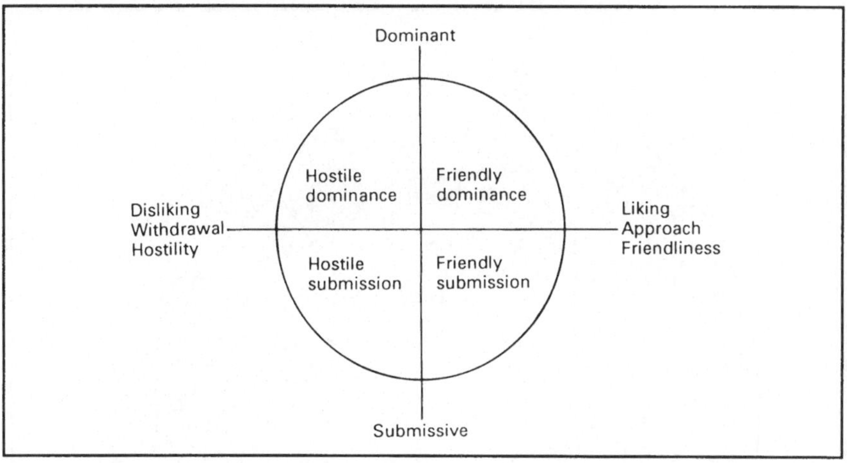

FIG. 4.1. Circumplex model of status and solidarity in interpersonal behaviour (From Crook 1980; reproduced with kind permission of Oxford University Press).

suggests four basic classes of behaviour: friendly dominance, friendly submission, hostile submission and hostile dominance. These in turn can be subdivided into eight further categories and have been labelled as: managerial-autocratic, responsive-hypernormal and so on, as represented by the outer circle in Fig.4.2.

Fig.4.2 is taken from Carson (1969), who extended Leary's work. Looking from the perimeter inwards, the second circle suggests the types of behaviour associated with the various subdivisions. The circle nearest the centre suggests the least extreme versions of these classes of behaviour. As a result, the model has built into it a strength of arousal component measured via the radius of the circle. The central circle suggests the complementary behaviour that is provoked in others.

Much of Leary's theory relates to the idea of interaction between social others. Duke and Nowicki (1982) have examined the degrees of complementarity in the sender's and respondent's behaviour. For example, in the love–hate affiliative dimension friendliness in one gives rise to friendliness in the other, hostility in one gives rise to hostility in the other. However, in the dominance–submission dimension the reaction of the individual at whom the behaviour is targeted gives rise to the opposite (submissiveness elicits dominance in the other). Anti-complementarity and non-complementarity also exist between sender and respondent. (For a detailed discussion of these issues and redeveloped interpersonal circle, see Kiesler, 1983; Orford, 1986; Birtchnell, 1990).

An important aspect of this system is the concept of interpersonal adjustment. In later chapters we will explore in detail issues of

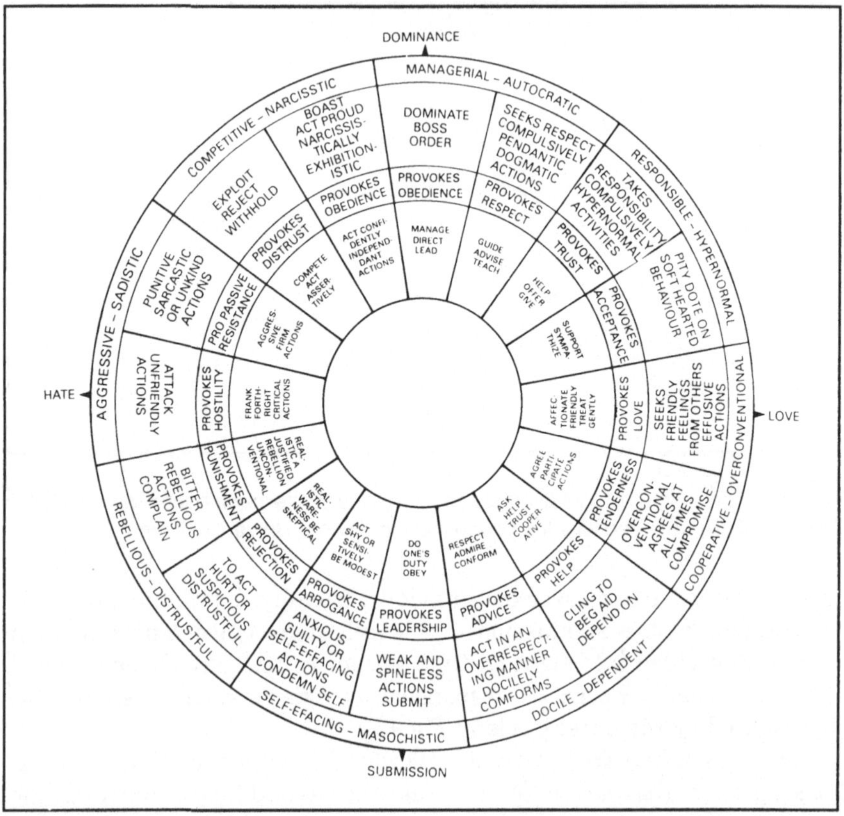

FIG. 4.2. The circumplex model of Fig. 4.1 divided into 16 behaviour categories. Circle segments define qualitative contrasts in behaviour and distance from centre suggests strengths. In the outer ring the 16 categories have been reduced to 8 names defining overall dispositional traits; the first word indicates the less extreme form of the type (from Crook 1980, reproduced with kind permission of Oxford University Press).

dominance and submission and therefore this approach has special appeal to the evolutionary theory discussed later. The description of these personality patterns of adjustment has clear overlaps with the notion of self-organisation, also discussed later. For these reasons the outlines of the Leary system of personality as "patterns of adjustment", is given in Appendix B.

Developments of the Interpersonal Model

Carson (1969, p.113, quoting Foa) maintains that each of these personality styles, represented in different personality acts, "is an attempt to establish the emotional relationship of the actor towards himself and towards the other, as well as to establish the social relationship of the self and the other with respect to a larger reference group ... Each behaviour serves the purpose of giving or denying love and status to the self and to the other." Carson suggests therefore, that dominance–submission and love–hate present three dimensions: (1) acceptance vs rejection; (2) self vs other; and (3) emotional vs social. Thus, for example, the cooperative behavioural style offers love to both self and other, but is rejecting of hostile, status-seeking, competitive responses in both self and other. The masochist denies status to the self but amplifies it in the other. The different styles have implications to both self and other in the three domains noted above. These may also be seen as role enactment patterns.

As Carson (1969) points out, social context may recruit these various patterns to a greater or lesser degree. The same style may not be seen in all contexts. An autocrat at work may be quite loving and docile at home. A cooperative individual may be quite loving of the world at large (e.g., religious) but rather neglectful of his close relationships or deliberately avoid aspects of intimacy (e.g., as in celibacy). Hence, both in terms of the relationship between these different personality types and the degree to which they are expressed, they should be regarded as dimensional rather than categorical.

Some Recent Developments

Leary was of the view that high self-esteem related to the ability to coordinate the complex repertoire of social displays in context appropriate ways, i.e., an individual can nurture and trust when appropriate, distrust when appropriate, submit, follow or lead when appropriate, and so on. The knowledge that one can enact these roles provides some security for self-esteem. In social learning theory, this ability to respond according to context might be called self-efficacy (Bandura, 1977). In this sense, it is like a sports person who can play all the shots and is therefore able to treat each one on its merit. This is in contrast to the player who has a limited repertoire and must continually navigate himself into a position that enables him to play his limited range (sometimes quite awkwardly). Furthermore, this is close to Jung's concept of individuation, i.e., the individual who has articulated and mastered and blended the full keyboard or range of their human archetypal nature (see Chapter 11).

In a recent new approach to personality, Paulhus and Martin (1987) provide some evidence for this view. They found that self-esteem does indeed relate to mixed capabilities. For example, high self-esteem people who are capable of being nurturant are also capable of being hostile. Hence, high self-esteem individuals are not fixed in any one interpersonal style. These authors also highlight important distinctions relating personality to social behaviour. These are: (1) ability; related to knowledge and degree of skill for enacting certain social behaviours; (2) capability; related to the ease of enacting particular social repertoires; and (3) traits; relating to index-typical behaviour. In their view, capability, i.e., the ease by which certain social repertoires are expressed, may be important to self-esteem. Capability may be significantly influenced by anxiety. Anxiety will not only lower the probability of attempting the behaviour, but will also disrupt the performance if it is attempted. In this regard, anxiety does not affect the ability, since individuals may know what to do, but it does affect capability; i.e., there is a distinction between knowing what to do and actually being able to do it. A similar case can be made for depression.

In regard to the disruptive effects of anxiety, however, it may be that any strongly aroused emotion, be it anger, anxiety or even sympathy, may disrupt performance. Moreover, individuals may inhibit certain classes of behaviour for all kinds of reasons, e.g., fear of becoming too angry or anxious (losing control), catastrophising the counter-response (i.e., fear of being overwhelmed), moral beliefs related to self-esteem, and so on.

The interpersonal approach has generated much research and many ideas, although its impact on psychotherapeutic practice has been disappointingly limited. In this theory, depression proneness is related to the dominance–submissive dimension, rather than the love–hate or attachment dimension. This fits with an evolutionary theory (Chapters 6 & 7), which argues that perception of social power is a crucial variable in depression. Also important is the distinction of hostile and docile submission. Although depression may be linked with subordinacy, this can often result in increases in hostility (see Chapter 8).

Many of these ideas have been expanded and well articulated in a classic paper by Kiesler (1983). J.Andrews (1989) explores how the interpersonal circle can be used to explain people's different cognitive models of the world and also variation in therapeutic style (e.g., some styles are more hostile and autocratic than others). The interested reader is also referred to the work of Horowitz and Vitkus (1986) who have articulated some important ideas on the value of using interpersonal theories to study both pathological behaviour and psychotherapeutic processes.

Birtchnell (1990) gives an overview of current thinking in this area and offers a new conceptual schema for the approach. In his view the dominance–submission dimension should be labelled upperness (for those seen of higher rank) and lowerness (for those seen as lower in rank). Love–hate is relabelled as closeness–distance. The reason for this is that love–hate are affects whereas dominance–submission refer to interpersonal relationships. Birtchnell argues that at present the Leary system confounds affects and relationship. In his system the two dimensions are proximity and power, both of which refer to relationship and are spatial concepts. Hence affects (e.g., love, hate, anxiety, depression) maybe related to any position on his interpersonal system. In other words, one may feel depressed from too much closeness (closeness that is being forced on one from another), or too much distance. Preference for distance from others need not relate to hate. The central dimension seems to be one of social control. That is if one can control the various interpersonal possibilities then negative affects are less likely. Thus, perceived control may be a third dimension. This system is depicted in Fig. 4.3.

Birtchnell (personal communication) agrees, however, that depression is often associated with the position of lowerness. Also this model helps us understand that entrapment (uncontrollable closeness) may relate to negative affect. Hence it fits with theories to be discussed

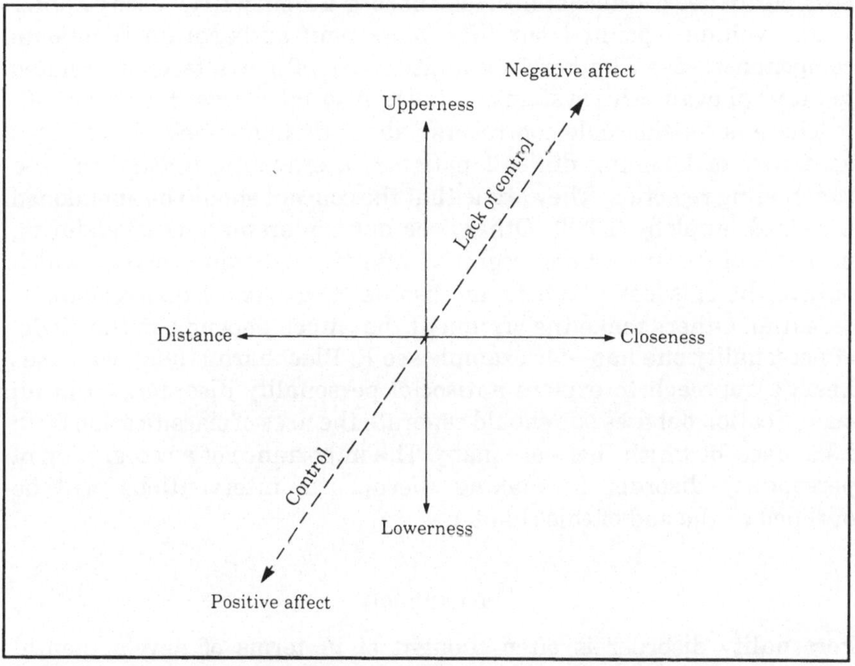

FIG. 4.3. Relationship between interpersonal spacing, control, and affect (in three dimensions) (Adapted from, and in consultation with J. Birtchnell, 1990).

later (Chapter 6–8) that depression is associated with involuntary, subordinate self-perception. Certainly depression is not simply, or always, the result of a lack of closeness. Birtchnell (personal communication) also points to adaptive and maladaptive social distance. In other words we can be adaptively close or clingy, adaptively distant or avoidant. etc.

PERSONALITY DISORDER

The study of personality traits brings us to one of the most thorny areas in research: the relationship between personality disorder and affective illness (for a comprehensive review see Farmer & Nelson-Gray, 1990). In Akiskal's (1988; 1990) view it is mood disregulation that accounts for both proneness to depression and various behavioural characteristics of personality disorder. Personality disorders, then, are not seen as variations of normal traits (e.g., neuroticism, introversion, sociotropy, etc.) but rather as various mixtures of symptoms, behavioural traits and emotional experiences which are abnormal. Like so much thinking in this area, affect is not placed in a social or evolutionary context, so it is possible to theorise about affect (as Zilboorg & Henry 1941—see Chapter 1 this volume—pointed out fifty years ago) as separate functional components. (See Chapter 5 for a discussion of how affects are related to internal evaluative systems for judging social success.)

There is considerable controversy about this approach. Some see it as a way of labelling difficult patients, therapeutic pessimism, and sanctioning rejection. They argue that the concept should be abandoned (Lewis & Appleby, 1988). Others see our understanding of enduring patterns of symptoms and cognitive-affective-behaviour styles, which outlive the episodes of functional disorder (e.g., Axis 1 depression), as essential. Others make the argument that much depends on the model of personality one has—for example see R. Blackburn (1988), who uses Leary's approach to explore antisocial personality disorder. As in all classification debates one should separate the uses of classification from its abuses, of which there are many. The importance of a recognition of personality disorder in making therapeutic interventions will be outlined at the end of this chapter.

Development

Personality disorder is often thought of in terms of developmental difficulties. The patient may be blocked, stuck, has failed to develop or has distorted development in key areas of emotive, cognitive, and social awareness and competencies (e.g., Kegan, 1982; Lane & Schwartz, 1987;

Rutter, 1987a,b; Beck, Freeman and associates, 1990). For example, borderline personality disorders are noted for their rage, inability to articulate, discriminate and control feeling states, and a chronic sense of emptiness. While narcissists are noted for their lack of empathy, their exploitiveness, and their omnipotent fantasies. However, because (for example) self-mutilation (which borderlines are prone to) is not a hallmark of early life it must be concluded that, at least in part, these problems represent not just blocked development but distorted development. Be this as it may, it is certainly the case that their difficulties show up early and age of onset and a history of developmental difficulties are a key to their diagnosis. Rutter (1987a) has pointed out that the hallmarks of personality disorder are:

1. Onset of problems in early childhood or adolescence.
2. Long standing and persistence over time without marked remission.
3. Abnormalities and difficulties in functioning seem to constitute a basic aspect of that individual's usual functioning.

Hence symptoms and behaviours associated with personality disorder may be more or less constant and not just thrown up in the presence of an episode. The problem with such a view is that a depressive episode or life event stress may trigger a number of symptoms that appear to be like those of personality disorder. Many of the symptoms of personality disorder have no equivalent in Axis I classification and therefore how one should code symptoms of envy, shame, rage, dependency, impulsiveness, lack of empathy, etc., which may well be the result of depression, is not known.

Types

To explore the issues that arise in the literature a brief outline of personality disorders is given. At the present time there are two basic systems of classification; the DSM (the American system) and the ICD (the European system). These have rather different nosologies for personality disorders. The ICD-9 includes the forms of: Paranoid; Affective (which includes concepts like cycloid, cyclothymic, and depressive); Schizoid; Explosive; Anankastic (basically obsessional); Hysterical; Asthenic (which is also inadequate, passive and/or dependent); Sociopathic/antisocial; plus various others such as passive aggressive, immature, and eccentric.

The DSM-111-R divides the personality disorders into three groupings. In group A there are: Paranoid; Schizoid, and Schizotypal.

Some believe that this group may have underlying biological similarities to psychoticism (see Claridge, 1985; 1987 for an interesting discussion of schizotypal traits as a normal variant in the population). In group B there are: Antisocial; Borderline; Histrionic; and Narcissistic. In general these are regarded as disorders of affect instability or as some have called them 'dramatic'; individuals who are subject to them are easily triggered into extreme affective or behavioural responses. In group C there are: Avoidant (a form of extreme and generalised social phobia leading to excessive avoidance of social interaction); Dependent; Obsessive Compulsive; and Passive Aggressive. These are basically fear-dominated personalities. Finally there is a group for Unspecified.

Whether or not any of these categories will stand the test of time remains to be seen. Furthermore, Morey (1988) has pointed out that the revised DSM-III-R represents a substantial divergence from the DSM-111 and has produced considerable overlap among the personality disorders. Also, the way personality is assessed is important since informants (e.g., friends and spouses) tend to depict the patient's normal personality differently from the patient (Zimmerman, Pfohl, Coryell, Stangl, & Corenthal, 1988). As with Axis 1 affective disorders there is some concern over the DSM shopping list approach to diagnosis (e.g., having to have five from a list of nine symptoms).

Nevertheless clinicians would benefit from having a working knowledge of these syndromes since personality disorder is one of the reasons that various therapies, both drug and psychosocial, can come unstuck (Beck et al., 1990). The interested reader is directed to Millon and Klerman's (1986) edited volume which contains may interesting papers arguing for and against these systems of classification. Millon himself has articulated a set of ideas about the psychological functioning of these individuals. The chapter on personality disorder by Rosenham and Seligman (1984) also provides a useful introduction to the area and gives short case histories for each form of the DSM types.

Pilkonis and Frank (1988) explored the types and rates of personality disorder in 119 treatment-responsive recurrent depressed patients. Using a battery of self-report and objective ratings they found that 48% showed some personality problems. These broke down into 30.4% with avoidant features, 18.6% compulsive, and 15.7% dependent (hence the majority fell into the fearful anxious cluster C). They also argue that their results support Bowlby's (1977a) view that distorted patterns of attachment underline those personality styles that are vulnerable to depression. However, it is unclear how strict their diagnosis was and they talk in terms of features rather than full syndromes. In fact full syndromes as depicted by DSM may be rare and most show mixed patterns, i.e., a bit of this and a bit of that (Zimmerman & Coryell, 1989).

Nevertheless, Pilkonis and Frank's work is an interesting exploration of the degree to which the range of personality disorders are represented in depressed populations.

Borderline Personality Disorder

Borderline personality disorder can be diagnosed by DSM-111-R with five types of symptom selected from: (1) unstable interpersonal relations often involving idealisation or devaluation of others; (2) at least two areas of impulsive behaviour (sex, spending, eating, driving, shoplifting, substance abuse, etc.); (3) marked instability of mood (depression, anxiety, anger) but rarely lasting more than hours; (4) inappropriate feelings or expression of anger and temper (e.g., fights); (5) recurrent suicidal threats or gestures, or self-mutilating behaviour; (6) persistent and marked identity disturbance (e.g., in self-image, sexual orientation, choice of friends, etc.) (7) chronic feelings of emptiness or boredom; (8) frantic efforts to avoid abandonment.

Although not included in the DSM it is believed that, under stress, borderlines can have psychotic episodes although only a small minority may go on to develop schizophrenia (unlike schizotypals). Stone (1989) points out that the term borderline has been used in at least four different ways: (1) a borderline between treatable and untreatable with psychoanalytic therapy; (2) a borderline between neurosis and psychosis; (3) an imprecise region of psychic functioning according to defenses; (4) a term of despair for narcissistic patients that don't respond to analytic therapy.

The borderline category has had a very mixed history and does not appear at all in the ICD-9, although there may be overlap with explosive and hysterical personality disorder. There are a number of changes in the ICD-10, which includes the category, impulsive personality disorder (Mezzich, 1988). Tarnopolsky and Berelowitz (1987) have provided an important review of the evolution of the concept of borderline, the different ways of assessing it—e.g., family and drug studies—and its validity as a concept and working diagnostic category. On the whole they believe it remains a useful category. According to these authors one unpublished study by Gunderson found that as many as four-fifths of inpatients with personality disorder could be diagnosed as borderline (Gunderson has developed his own research instrument for diagnosis). Although other studies report lower figures, borderlines make up a high percentage of inpatients with personality disorders.

Tarnopolsky and Berelowitz (1987) review the evidence of the relationship between borderline personality disorder and depression. In regard to the specificity of borderline to depression they say: "The majority of borderlines do not develop affective illness; a variable number display affective symptoms at follow up but probably no more than other personality disorders" (p.729). Farmer and Nelson-Gray (1990) reach a similar conclusion. As in all such findings, much depends on how a diagnosis of depression is made since in my experience borderlines (like other personality disorders) can frequently score highly on self-report measures of depression (e.g., the BDI). Hence, clear criteria for diagnosing depression is essential.

Gunderson and Elliott (1985) have also presented a comprehensive overview of the relationship of borderline personality disorder and depression. From their review of the data they outlined four possible forms of association. However, it is likely that their hypotheses may apply to other forms of personality disorder:

I. Affective disorder underpins borderline personality disorder, and impulsive drug use and sexual activities are efforts to alleviate chronic depression. Hence mood regulation is a central preoccupation of borderlines. However, Gunderson and Elliott (1985) find little support for this view, e.g., the lack of efficacy of drug treatment for the majority of borderlines. Indeed tricyclics like amitriptyline may make them worse (Tarnoposky & Berelowitz, 1987) but they may fare better with monoamine oxidase inhibitors. Also, non-affective symptoms such as impulsiveness and chronic interpersonal difficulties discriminate unipolar depressed from borderlines.

II. Borderline personality disorder itself can give rise to affective disorder. In this view impulsiveness and poor social relational styles give rise, secondarily, to poor mood regulation and depression proneness.

III. Personality disorder and affective disorder are qualitatively distinct (as suggested by DSM-111-R). Any apparent correlations between them arise from the relative prevalence in the population of these two disorders. However studies show that the two disorders coexist more frequently than would be predicted.

Gunderson and Elliott (1985) find some supporting evidence for each of the above although as outlined there is also negative evidence. Hence they argue that both disorders can be diagnosed from signs and symptoms that have a variety of sources. This leads them to a fourth hypothesis, namely:

> Hypothesis IV suggests that the observed concurrence of affective and borderline symptoms result from their heterogeneity. For either

> disorder, individuals may start with a biophysiological vulnerability that increases risk of being psychologically impaired in early development. Such early traumas may create vulnerability to either or both disorders, but the actual presentation varies as a function of later physiological and psychological reactions to environment and temperament. The key to overlap and dissimilarities between these two disorders, then, may be a constellation of innate and external factors that are inconsequential individually but combine to shape depression, chronic dysphoria, or borderline behaviour—alone or in any possible combination. (P.286)

Theories and therapies of borderlines are primarily psychoanalytic (for a review see Aronson, 1989) but recently an interesting model has been put forward by Melges and Swartz (1989). They suggest that borderlines have problems in interpersonal distance. If they start to get too close to others they fear domination and being controlled. If they are too distanced however, they fear abandonment. It is at these times they may show depressive features. The idea then is of intense instability in these interpersonal components. Melges and Swartz (1989) note preliminary evidence that in their family background the father tends to be absent and under-involved, while mother tends to be over-involved, intrusive, and negative.

However, recent work on borderline patients has shown a very high incidence of sexual abuse (Ogata et al., 1990; see Chapter 10 this volume). Thus Gunderson and Elliott's view that external factors may be cumulative and inconsequential separately is not borne out by the evidence on child abuse and borderline symptoms. Needless to say these findings have enormous implications for therapy and detection. Given a history of abuse it is hardly surprising that borderline patients may have problems with interpersonal distance.[2]

Narcissistic Personality Disorder

The DSM-111-R again goes for five out of nine as a way of making this diagnosis. Included here are: (1) has marked feeling of rage/shame to criticism; (2) is exploitative of others; (3) has sense of specialness or grandiosity, exaggerates achievements, etc.; (4) believes his/her problems are unique; (5) engages in fantasies of success, ideal love, beauty etc; (6) has an unreasonable sense of entitlement; (7) needs constant attention and admiration from others; (8) lacks capacity for empathy or feelings for others; (9) is preoccupied with envy.

There is an old saying that some people don't understand, while others don't understand that they don't understand. The narcissist is like the latter and the main characteristic that Freud outlined was intense egocentricity, making it difficult for them to form a meaningful therapeutic relationship. Recently, there has been interest in how this group of traits relate to others—e.g., to borderline—and what has been called malignant narcissism. Malignant narcissism overlaps with anti-social personality disorder (see Kernberg, 1989). Stone (1989) has suggested that females are more likely to be diagnosed as borderline while the full narcissistic picture occurs far more commonly in men. The more aggressive and malignant the narcissistic disturbance the more likely the patient is to be male.

The relationship of narcissistic personality disorder to depression is extremely complicated, not least because the term narcissism or narcissistic vulnerability has been used in so many different ways. Whereas borderline, anti-social, and paranoid (for example) are not regarded as having any normal developmental components the same is not true of narcissism. Hence, the omnipotent, idealising egocentric and exhibitionist stage of childhood development has sometimes been called narcissistic (e.g., Kohut, 1971; 1977). This has led to discussion in the literature of the relation between healthy and unhealthy narcissism (for a review see Gottschalk, 1988). To complicate the picture further, some talk in terms of narcissistic injury or narcissistic vulnerability by which they mean traumas to the experience of the self (e.g., shame). Yet another complication is that there are many different theories suggesting how (so-called) normal narcissism gets distorted into a pathological personality development (see Russell, 1985; Adler, 1986).

Research using the narcissistic personality inventory (NPI) suggests a positive relationship between Eysenck's dimensions of extraversion and psychoticism (Emmons, 1984; 1987). A factor analysis of the NPI generated four separate factors: exploitativeness/entitlement; leadership/authority; superiority/arrogance; and self-absorption/self-admiration. Emmons (1987) suggests that it is exploitativeness/entitlement that loads on pathological narcissism and that this is associated "with neuroticism, social anxiety and interpersonal styles of aggressive/sadistic and rebellious distrustfulness".

Gilbert (1989) argued that the social mentality that dominates the narcissistic style is social competitiveness rather than cooperativeness or social affiliation. Moral awareness and recognition of the rights and needs of others are notably absent. The vulnerability to depression is commonly thought to arise from shame or a build-up of defeats that activate powerful feelings of inferiority. This may be the same reason that Type A personalities get depressed (V. Price, 1982; Gilbert, 1989). Hence this vulnerability is very similar to that outlined by Bibring (1953) but in the case of narcissistic personality disorder it is associated with egocentricity and a significant lack of empathy. In my experience these individuals can be difficult to engage in therapy. There may be little capacity for self-reflection or ability to recognise that they must change rather than the world around them.

I also believe that these patients should be distinguished from the straightforward shame-prone personality, or those carrying narcissistic injuries (with whom in my view they are often confused). The shame-prone personality crops up in many disguises in depression but not all these lack the empathy of the true narcissist. I am not sure why the lack of empathy and exploitativeness makes such a difference to psychotherapy outcome but in my experience it does and therapists should be mindful of this. It probably relates to lack of insight. One should also make a distinction between dependency and the more arrogant exploitativeness of the narcissistic personality disorder. In regard to psychotherapy the interested reader might consult (Adler, 1986; Kahn, 1985).

As we shall discuss later (see Chapter 8) shame proneness and an underlying sense of inferiority and low self-esteem are very much related to depression, not least because they tend to be associated with marked social withdrawal, fear or distrustfulness. Hence I find it helpful to keep in mind Emmons' (1986) findings of exploitativeness as the key symptom of narcissistic personality rather than shame proneness or fantasies of beauty or success. Indeed fantasies of success and belief in one's own ability can be very energising (e.g., Christ?), but this does not mean that such a person lacks empathy or is exploitive. In my view, it is shame proneness, especially when associated with a sense of inferiority, fear of others' scorn and consequent withdrawal/concealment that often carries risk of depression (see Chapter 8). Indeed, it is shame rather than exploitativeness that most writers are speaking of when they talk of narcissistic problems in depression (Mollon & Parry, 1984). Perhaps this is why Pilkonis and Frank (1988) found that avoidant personality disorder was the most over-represented in the depressed population and not narcissistic personality disorder.

As noted elsewhere (Gilbert, 1989) there are different theories as to its development. Some stress the lack of a positive admiring early relationship (e.g., Kohut, 1977) while others stress the more Adlerian idea of the spoilt child syndrome. Again much may depend on which aspect of narcissism one is focused on. Another aspect that one might consider is intense sibling rivalry. I have, over the years seen patients who appear to have shame-prone problems with a sense of inferiority, who can become angry and act out, are envious and also if not hypomanic then at least highly energetic from time to time, although it rarely lasts. In nearly all of these cases there was some kind of intense sibling rivalry sometimes associated with the idea that the parents preferred siblings. In my view sibling relationships have been ignored in this area.

Dependent Personality Disorder

As we have already seen from our earlier discussion in this chapter interpersonal dependency crops up in most theories of vulnerability to unipolar depression. The outlines of dependent personality are very similar to Beck's concept of sociotropy and Blatt et al.'s (1982) concept of anaclitic, Arieti and Bemporad's (1980) concept of dominant other, and Yalom's view of pursuit of the ultimate rescuer. For this reason I will give less time to it here. For the diagnosis of dependent personality disorder (which is also present in the ICD-10) the DSM-111-R uses the five out of nine system. Included are: (1) needs excessive advice/ reassurance to make everyday decisions; (2) allows others to make important decisions (e.g., place of abode, job); (3) agrees with others even if they believe others are wrong, for fear of rejection; (4) has difficulty initiating or doing things; 5) volunteers to do unpleasant things to win approval; (6) feels uncomfortable and avoids being alone; (7) feels devastated when close relationships end; (8) preoccupied with fears of abandonment; (9) is easily hurt by criticism.

In effect the dimensions that are presented here are intense sensitivity to aloneness (loneliness), submissiveness and need for approval. As with all the DSM criteria these kinds of problems are quite common in other disorders and may also be state (depression) sensitive. Hence, they may, as Akiskal (1988; 1990) suggests actually represent chronic, mild, depressive states of long duration. In everyday practice sometimes these folk are given the appalling label "inadequate personality". This seems to be in part an angry response to their (at times) annoying clinginess, and "tell me what I should do" style. They are well described on the interpersonal circle.

Birtchnell (1988a, p.121) has recently reviewed the issue of dependency. He takes the view that dependency is failed development in: becoming securely separate; acquiring an adequate level of self-worth; feeling accepted and welcome in a world of adults. All these Jung might have called "failures in individuation".

The problem in all these kinds of theories is the linking of phenomenology with casual theories. The concern is that the person might be held responsible for these development failures when in fact this is almost certainly not the case. Dependent personality is more likely to arise as an issue in women and the reasons for this are probably social rather than purely psychological. Women who marry or become pregnant early in life (perhaps to escape an intolerable home situation) may not have had the opportunity to individuate. Lacking a career they become dependent (economically and in other ways, as noted by Birtchnell, 1988a) on a spouse and/or may make poor choices of spouses. They may model dependent behaviours from mother and cultural attitudes to the dominance of men. Marriage may be fear dominated and we may be at risk of missing the social context of these behaviours (e.g., Hinde, 1989).

The other problem is that dependency in men may spring from a different path. Need for approval for example is common to a number of personality disorders. However men may be able to use power and threat more effectively to cover their real fears of loss of a supporting (sexually) available wife. Bird, Martin, and Schulman (1983) found that a number of high status men could suffer an ego collapse with loss of a wife's support. In fact all of Birtchnell's development failures could also be applied to narcissistic disorder but the narcissist has very different ways of dealing with them.

Comment

My own view on personality disorder is one of ambivalence. One of the main reasons that I see an understanding of personality to be important is because in today's climate we hear a lot about short-term treatments for depression which for some people are very helpful. However, in my clinical work many patients I see probably have personality difficulties (since it is common for GPs and other agencies to refer patients that have not responded to drugs and are regarded as difficult). It is unreasonable to expect rapid change. Thankfully this is now being recognised (e.g., Beck et al., 1990). Indeed, Frank et al. (1987) have shown that patients with personality difficulties tend to respond more slowly regardless of treatment used. In a heterogenous group of patients in private therapy, Persons, Burns, and Perloff (1988) found that those who dropped out of cognitive therapy had personality disorders, non-endogenous symptoms and high initial BDI scores. These authors quote previous findings that those with personality problems tend to experience less emotional improvement over the early stages of cognitive therapy compared to those without personality disorder.

Psychological work with these people is often about development not simply re education. This has economic and resource implications not to mention training. I have seen some therapists become despondent when patients don't seem to work so neatly as the textbooks suggest and more often than not when one explores the history the reasons are obvious. As a rule of thumb with personality disorders the pace is much slower and the relationship with the therapist crucial. Also you cannot avoid working with historical data.

Second, I think that an understanding of personality brings attention to a number of difficulties that are not dealt with within functional disorder discription and certainly are not best viewed as diseases. It is most important for clinicians to be aware of the great complexity that may confront them in their clinical work in depression, and the very intense struggles some people have to change. So maybe we should ask why do the personality disorders have such difficulty changing?

A PSYCHOLOGICAL APPROACH TO PERSONALITY DISORDERS

There is a very different approach to personality disorder which is based not on classification of symptoms but a careful understanding of psychological abilities (Beck et al., 1990). This approach arises from concerns with treatment rather than developing neat nosologies. Here the concern is not to understand the type of disorder or even the symptoms but to understand how the person construes their interpersonal world. The two aims of this approach are to process and to understand content. Leaving aside the issue of diagnosis, there has recently has been some awareness of why these individuals are difficult to treat with short-term therapies.

1. No clear focus: Personality disorders may present with no specific problem area or a mass of interconnected difficulties. When one tries to work with one area it slips away into another or else the patient feels hopeless and overwhelmed.
2. Rigidity: These patients may have very rigid ways of construing the world and flexibility does not come easy to them. Black and white thinking is typical (Beck et al., 1990). For example, 'people are either for you or against you; love you or hate you.' Millon (1986) particularly has written on the subject of the rigidity of their internal construing.
3. Avoidance: These patients may avoid or refuse point blank to look at themselves or their internal construing. Often this is the result of extensive shame, or rage–shame spirals (see Chapter 8) and needs careful handling. There can be long silences and painful "don't knows". Revealing what is really going on inside is painful and difficult and they are easily inhibited in revealing thoughts and feeling or past traumas such as abuse. Powerful transference feelings can distort active engagement (e.g., feeling let down or being very distrustful). One patient recently refused to talk about anything that might make her cry because of intense shame of being seen to cry. It was six months before, gradually, enough trust had been built by to begin the painful work on those things she felt so ashamed about.

4. Long-term interpersonal difficulties: This is a hall mark of personality disorders and can make it difficult to form a therapeutic relationship, especially one that can instil any kind of hope. Few will stay in therapy unless there seems some kind of possibility to change and finding ways to help. These patients may never have had a relationship that was trustworthy, may perhaps be victims of abuse or neglect, and hence, there can be deep suspiciousness of others especially in allowing any degree of vulnerability to be worked with. On the other hand other types are only too ready to hand over all responsibility to the therapist and become demanding and clingy doing very little work themselves.

5. Self/Role complexity: Individuals can judge themselves in a multitude of different roles such as parent, academic, gardener, friend, artist, singer in the bath, and so on. Linville (1985) suggests that self-complexity is related to proneness to depression in that those who have few self-defining constructs/roles, and in whom these constructs are highly interdependent, are likely to experience extreme shifts of mood in association with negative events. A simple description is putting all one's eggs in the same basket. A lack of self-complexity results in global thinking (black/white & either/thinking) and a tendency to catastrophise. These individuals may also have rather limited and restricted constructs for judging others.

In therapy helping patients to complexify their self-constructs is important. Ideas like "if I fail at X I am a total failure as a person", are common. Extreme affective reactions maybe a result of this lack of complexity. Although depression itself can result in a loss of self-complexity (Beck, Rush, Shaw, & Emery, 1979) in non-personality disordered folk it is a transient effect of mood state. Consequently, therapy tends to be easier to the extent that one is able to reactivate a previously developed complex and differentiated self-system (stored in long-term memory). In personality-disordered individuals, however, this self-complexity is not available to be reinstated and has to be developed, sometimes almost from scratch. Not surprisingly therapy can take time.

Also, for some, incentives can be in serious conflict, e.g., to be independent and free from control and domination by others yet also to be anxiously attached, clingy, and fearful of abandonment/separation. This can produce massive oscillations as movement towards one incentive produces fear of loosing another (see Melges & Swartz, 1989). Beck et al. (1990) also draw a distinction between conditional self-beliefs and unconditional self-beliefs. Unconditional beliefs are "I am bad regardless. There is nothing I can do to redeem myself. I am bad through and through." The same way of thinking can be directed at others: "They are bad through and through."

Personality disorders often have high levels of dysfunctional attitudes and high levels of dysfunctional attitudes may predict poor outcome to various therapies (Peselow et al., 1990).

6. Affect complexity: Like self-complexity, affect complexity relates to the ability to differentiate emotional experience. Lane and Schwartz (1987) suggest that emotional development goes through a set of stages that may parallel Piaget's cognitive stages. The stages they suggest are awareness of: (1) bodily sensations; (2) the body in action; (3) individual feelings; (4) blends of feelings; (5) blends of blends of feelings. At the lowest level, the baby is only aware of experiences in body sensations and these are generally crudely differentiated in some pleasure–pain dimension. Subsequently, comes the awareness of feelings derived from actions. Later come the more differentiated affects of sadness, anger, anxiety, joy, etc. Later the capacity to experience blends of these feelings and the capacity to cope with ambivalence. Later still comes blends of blends of feelings.

In therapies that focus on affect (e.g., gestalt), the therapist enables the patient to focus on body states and body feelings, e.g., "Your jaw looks tight when you say that. Can you focus on that and tell me what that is associated with that tightness?" Safran and Segal (1990) note how this can help to bring about further processing of internally generated, emotional arousal (e.g., unrecognised anger, sadness, fear, etc.).

Lane and Schwartz (1987) suggest that those who are vulnerable to personality problems (e.g., dysthymia) may have poorly articulated emotional schema for decoding complex emotional states. As a result, their emotional life tends be less well differentiated than those without these problems and subject to extremes. Lane and Schwartz, and also Sommers (1981) point out that affect complexity is not independent of cognitive complexity. For example, Sommers suggests that an individual's "emotional range" is related to their cognitive complexity and role-taking. She notes that:

> A person who is capable of shifting viewpoints and of considering a situation from its multiple perspectives is essentially likely to rapidly alter his or her initial evaluations and to transform the corresponding emotions. To respond with more emotions may thus require particular cognitive endeavours: to recognise the privileged character of one's own viewpoint and to search for further information by which to evaluate a situation. Conversely, a relative inability to shift perspectives may impede emotional changes. Characteristic cognitive acts, such as intense focus on one aspect of an event may function as a barrier blocking the inflow of new information necessary for the process of reappraisal and or the transformation of emotion. (P. 559)

In essence then, both self-complexity and affect complexity relate to the range and variability an individual has in the way they are able to make sense of both internal sources of information (e.g., affective arousal) and external sources of information (e.g., other people's behaviour). These are not independent abilities and their constriction leads to more extreme cognitive judgements and affective responses.

7. Egocentricity: The above leads on to the issue of egocentricity and the capacity to shift view points, to recognise that there is more than one view of any situation and that other people may take different and equally valid views (Liotti, in press). Depressed patients who are highly egocentric are often difficult to help.

8. Emotional Lability: Extreme sensitivity to minor triggers which can recruit anger, anxiety or depressed mood are typical of those with emotional lability. These patients are also interpersonally sensitive (see Davidson et al., 1989; see also pages 85 and 201). This is not quite the same as neuroticism. It is well represented in borderline patients.

9. The good–bad self paradox: It took me some time to work this one out but it works something like this: "I know I am bad because I was abused, had an abortion or whatever. However I must be a little bit good because I feel guilty and am paying for it. If I didn't feel bad about myself then I would really be a completely wicked person." Trying to help someone give up the guilt and self-dislike becomes difficult because they may see it as taking the only decent thing about them away. Their bad feelings about themselves are actually a source of positive self-construction. Another variant of this can be: "My bad screwed-up life is a testament to what others have done to me. In this sense it becomes a way of remaining vengeful. I cannot forgive." Use of the advantages–disadvantages technique (Beck et al., 1979) or the two chairs (Greenberg, 1979) can be helpful here. Unresolved anger is common (see also Fitzgibbons, 1986). Yet another variant is in anorexia. Anorexia patients are often fairly competitive with other women, take pride in their control and size. The only positive thing about them may be their control over their eating and weight. Sometimes it is difficult to change these without first developing more positive self-constructs. No patient will move towards health if they see it as taking away their positive self identity (however fragile) or if they think it will make them worse in some way, or they will lose their self indentity.

The above nine points are by no means the only way of thinking about the special problems the personality-disordered patient brings—for example, Beck et al. (1990) outline how different attributes may be over or underdeveloped in different personality disorders. Other workers have used Piaget's concepts and focus on the issue of emergent patterns (e.g., Kegan, 1982). Some understanding of these complexities in treatment are essential if therapy is not to come to grief. Later we shall consider innate needs (Chapter 10) and basic archetypes and themes (Chapter 11).

SUMMARY

1. Interest in the relationship between enduring personality traits and depression has been with us for many centuries. However it has only been in the last forty years that these have been systematically studied. This research has shown us that the role of personality in depression is complex.
2. There is growing evidence that a sizable proportion of those vulnerable to depression have personality styles that reflect lability in affect control systems, although there remains debate on how these traits should be operationalised.
3. Traits of emotional dependency, interpersonal sensitivity, need for approval, inhibited or intense achievement striving as a (secret) way to achieve approval and status, have long been regarded as carrying vulnerability to depression. Social dependency and negative interpersonal events seem especially problematic. Considerable concern exists on the issue of the specificity of these traits to depression however (e.g., Nietzel & Harris, 1990).
4. Few theories of the role of personality in depression come at the problem with any kind of comprehensive theory of personality, or of the basic archetypal core structures. A promising approach that may help this is that of the interpersonal theorist (e.g., Leary, 1957), and evolution theory.
5. The role of personality disorder is controversial but some insight into personality difficulties is essential to understand the complications in presentation and treatment. However, where traits like social dependency and lack of self-assertion become a matter of personality disorder is anyone's guess. Borderline, narcissistic, avoidant, and dependent personalities are all noted for their extreme sensitivity on these traits.
6. Looking at personality difficulty from a developmental point of view suggests that affect lability and fear may relate to underdeveloped functions of self (cognitive and affective complexity). This can lead to rigidity, avoidance, and egocentricity. In psychological therapy these problems need careful consideration. It is difficult to teach someone how to run if they are having difficulty walking.

CONCLUDING COMMENTS

In any therapy of depression the therapist must have some insight into what a patient is capable of doing in therapy. It is one thing to take a highly articulated therapy like cognitive therapy (Beck et al., 1979) which uses very restrictive exclusion criteria for patient selection (Safran & Segal, 1990) but quite another to apply such techniques to unselected inpatients and outpatients, as is becoming increasingly common. In our hospitals we are only slowly changing from a highly medicalised, drug-based treatment approach, and while it is understandable that nurses, occupational therapists, psychologists and others are desperately searching around for more psychosocial approaches, the training implications are serious and not fully recognised. With the evidence that up to 50% of patients on acute wards have personality/developmental problems, and 20% of depressions are chronic, where do we stand in terms of awareness of the length of possible treatment?

The pressure to get results is riddled throughout our treatment establishments. In my experience this causes intense stress for various kinds of therapists. Older members of the nursing and medical profession can undermine efforts seeing some patients as "just wasters". Some psychologists, who should know better, refuse to even contemplate the idea of personality disorder since this seems to offend their liberal ideas of not labelling people. Personality disorder in depression is a very serious complication. It may be that we have not the skills or resources to help these patients, but then we should be honest about this.

But let us not be pessimistic either. Our understanding of therapy is moving ahead at a great pace. Drug treatments that may help to soothe the patient while they are attempting to change are being researched. Also just as Kohut (1977) gave analysts "permission" to be empathic (Eagle, 1987) so new developments in cognitive therapy (e.g., Freeman, Simon, Beutler, & Arkowitz, 1989; Beck et al., 1990) are giving "permission" to some therapists to slow down and think of the issue of development and therapeutic relationship (of course many therapists always did think of these things). It may turn out that we need to change radically the way we conduct therapy and may find that self-help groups, outward-bound courses (Gilbert, 1989) and other kinds of social experience that facilitate a sense of belonging and self-worth are more effective than our individual therapies. All this awaits research in the future. We all have our personal hunches about what might be helpful for patients whose depression in part relates to personality, but we don't really know and still await long-term outcome studies.

NOTES

1. There are a number of possible hypotheses that may account for these findings—one being the small number of cases involved. Another may be that depression itself can have a destabilising effect on personality (Akiskal, 1988; 1990). Since few previous studies have looked at personality before first onset this remains to be investigated. To account for the age differences, one possibility is that neuroticism over time may (a) influence the selection of spouses/partners, and/or (b) the effect of neuroticism may lead to poor social relationships and it is through the poor quality of social relationships over time that vulnerability builds up. The hypothesis here would be that if the neurotic or anxious individual is lucky enough to find a supportive and tolerant partner then they may be protected, but if their relationships are marked by conflicts (perhaps as a result of their personality and cognitive style, poor selection of partner or just the usual marital problems) then depression is more likely.
2. At the time of going to press Gunderson and Phillips (1991) have published a new, major review of the relation between borderline personality disorder and depression. Their general conclusion is that their relationship and overlap is "surprisingly weak".

PART II

CONCEPTS

The Evolution of Mental Mechanisms and the Needs for Power, Belonging, and Self-value

CHAPTER 5

The Evolution of Mental Mechanisms

Many psychopathologists are often ambivalent about evolutionary theory. When it comes to exploring similarities in general biological structures between us and other animals, for some, this is almost a no-go area. However, gene-biological structures represent units of stored knowledge laid down over millions of years; they are our internal libraries that make biological life possible. The structure of our bodily form (two eyes, four limbs, the timing of sexual maturity, etc) and the potentialities of our socio-emotional lives are stored in our genes. When this knowledge is lost (i.e., words on the pages of our library books are missed out or misspelt) malformation often occurs. On the other hand, mental suffering is rarely the result of genetic error. Rather it is the activation of certain types of potential within us. Even those that suggest a genetic linkage with certain forms of suffering should not automatically posit disease or malformation. The evolution of mental mechanisms is not concerned with happiness or feeling good. For example, anxiety may feel bad but it evolved to regulate how danger is responded to. In certain kinds of environment those who have higher thresholds for anxiety and are cautious may survive better than those who have low thresholds. If we by-pass the biological we are ignoring a source of knowledge, or what Jung called the archetypal (Chapter 11). If we need at least a modicum of love, respect, and freedom from fear in order to prosper and flourish then we need these things by virtue of having become a certain kind of species (Chapter 10).

Another problem that some people have is with the whole concept of innateness. Some believe it is largely irrelevant because social life plays such an overriding role on our mental states and psychological functioning. In this volume however, we shall argue that while this is true, it is true precisely because we are a certain kind of species. Our concern is to outline the biological infrastructures on which our mental life depends. This is not reductionist but rather highlights three central issues. First, humans have various basic needs (to be loved, respected, have a sense of value to others, relate positively to ingroups and less positively to outgroups, all of which signal social success). Second, an evolutionary approach argues against the fragmentation and artificial divisions of behaviour, affect, and cognition and in terms of coassembled modular processes (Gilbert, 1989). The fragmented approach to mental life has dominated psychiatric thinking for centuries as noted by Zilboorg and Henry (1941; see Chapter 1 this volume), making illness formulations of dysphoric states more likely and locating the error in the person. This has allowed us to define mental suffering via affects (depression, anxiety, etc.) when in fact affect is only one aspect of dysfunction and the source of depression may lie in the environment. Third, an evolutionary approach suggests that many forms of mental suffering are not diseases in any recognisable sense, rather they represent the activation of internal potential, or earlier adapted solutions to social living. Social anxiety, for example, is fundamental to certain types of group living and it has taken major adaptations in late primate evolution to enable social activity to become predominantly hedonic.

Innateness of psychological functioning is concerned with the idea of a given potential, a possibility, not a fixed action plan. Within us are possibilities that evolved many millions of years ago together with possibilities that are of much later origin. We seem to have little trouble with these ideas when it comes to language or attachment behaviour and yet when we consider preparation for other dispositions problems begin and people worry about over-biologising. I hope to show that this worry is unfounded. This chapter attempts to outline the background that will allow us to approach our theories of depression from an evolutionary perspective. We will see how the brain is a modular system that is concerned with social success and not rationality. It cannot be easily split into artificial components of thinking, feeling, and behaving. A superb review of an evolutionary approach to personality, which bears centrally on the approach taken here, can be found in Buss (1991).

EVOLUTION: A KEY TO OUR WAY OF BEING

The evolutionary approach starts with the not surprising idea that humans evolved from primate stock some 5 or less million years ago. The primate line in turn evolved from previous evolved species reaching back to the stem reptiles who first appear some 250 million years ago (MacLean, 1977; 1985; Bailey, 1987). Most vertebrates have four limbs, heart and lungs and so forth. The basic design of the nervous system, with the spinal cord along the dorsal surface and computer and sensory organs (eyes, ears, olfaction, and mouth, etc.) in the head find their beginnings in changes occurring in the sea some 400 million years ago. The avenues of this phylogenetic history remain with us and we can refer to this as a conservation of form or basic plan(s). The human embryo goes through a brief period when gills form and then disappear. As Gardner (1988) points out, evolution allows species to transform but yet maintain certain general designs or basic plans (e.g., such as four limbs, pairs of sensory organs, etc. See Lorenz, 1987, for some fascinating examples). Unfortunately, having to adapt to previous structures is not always helpful. A very common example is the human skeleton. We have so many back problems because the "basic plan" of the spinal column evolved in the sea and is retained, although it is not well suited for upright locomotion on land. The development of the child before birth is limited by the basic female anatomy. So having to accommodate to earlier "basic plans" in our biology is not without costs. This is true of brain mechanisms also. Various levels of brain structure have their origins at different phylogenetic times.

The Brain

The basic architecture of the brain is represented in Fig. 5.1.

As selective pressure produced increasingly complex adaptations, what was being laid down in gene-neural structures were strategies for successful adaption to the environment operated via affective and behaviour repertoires (Nesse, 1990). Certain basic plans (Gardner, 1988), strategies (Wenegrat, 1984), and biosocial goals (Gilbert, 1989) were highly conserved in the gene-neural structures because of their influence on the reproduction of individuals and were passed on. Amongst these was the innate predisposition to care for the young (and the need to be cared for during infancy), to compete for resources with other conspecifics (members of the same species) to cooperate with and help others. Along this varied and dimly understood journey the behavioural–emotive potentials for much that we now see in

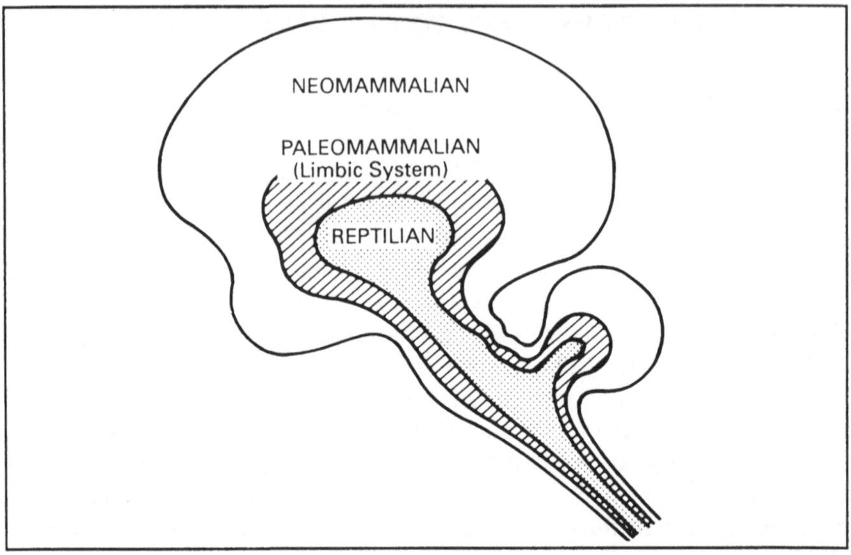

FIG. 5.1. Components of the human brain. The forebrain evolves and expands along lines of three basic formations that anatomically and biochemically reflect ancestral commonalities with reptiles, early mammals and late mammals (from MacLean 1985).

social behaviour, the sources of our sense of fulfilment and depression arose from, and found expression in, evolution.

r-K Selection

The species-typic breeding strategies have been classified in terms of r-K strategies. Chisholm (1988) suggests this idea is traceable back to Dobzhansky in 1950. It suggests that the environmental carrying capacity selects for different types of reproduction strategy. r-strategies involve coming into breeding cycles early and the production of high numbers of offspring. Usually only a very small percentage of offspring survive into adulthood to reproduce. K-strategies however, are evolved in situations of keen intraspecies competition and where reproductive success is determined by the efficient reproduction at replacement levels (a kind of quality versus quantity distinction). Chisholm (1988) has provided a useful table of these distinctions (see Table 5.1).

There is much debate in the literature regarding the contexts of these strategies. Ideas exist that males tend to be more r than females, for example. However, what is now fairly well accepted is that

TABLE 5.1
General Characteristics of r and K Selected Species

r-selected	*K-selected*
Variable or uncertain environment	More constant environment
Dispersal after birth	Occupation of same niche
High mortality before breeding	Low(er) mortality
Little intraspecific competition	Keen intraspecific competition
Many offspring	Few offspring
Low parental investment	High parental investment
Short birth intervals	Long birth intervals
Rapid development	Slow development
Early reproduction	Delayed reproduction
Short life span	Long life span
Little social behaviour	Complex social behaviour
Little play	More play
Inflexible behavioural repertoires	Flexible behaviour repertoires

Adapted from Chisholm (1988)

K-selection necessitates the evolution of a number of mental mechanisms that allow the animal to perform in line with their selected reproduction strategies. K-strategies produce animals that are required to learn about their social and non-social environments in order to exploit them successfully. Hence they are biologically disposed to attach themselves to care-givers and postpone breeding until adult enough to act as care-givers to their own offspring, invest in them (i.e., making offspring survival and prosperity a central preoccupation for at least some part of their adult lives). Further, K-selection requires that conspecifics become more aware of, and capable of, influencing the actions of those with whom they will share their breeding environment. Play (MacLean, 1985) may be one arena where this occurs (i.e., in play animals are learning about others and practising certain interactional skills). Indeed K-strategies require that individuals are able to manipulate others profitably, e.g., able to elicit support from others in their child-rearing, resource acquisition strategies, and so on (Charlesworth, 1988).

Genotype and Phenotype

One of the most important aspects of K-selection is the genotype–phenotype interaction (Chisholm, 1988; MacDonald, 1988). K-strategies, on the whole, give rise to neural mechanisms that are more flexible and with "open behavioural repertoires". This allows for enormous variety in phenotypic expression (via modification of behaviour through learning) of the genotype. This flexibility reduces the control of "fixed action patterns" and allows novel behaviour in new situations. Genes share complex relations with behaviour however. Some traits are influenced by many genes (called polygenic) and a single gene may influence a variety of traits (called pleiotropic). Although genotype constrains, to some degree, the variability allowed by phenotype, the greater the flexibility for learning the more variable phenotypes will be (MacDonald, 1988; Buss, 1991). As Chisholm (1988) argues, life history is essential to understanding the phenotype–genotype linkage. Furthermore, the environmental contribution to development influences biological substrates (Meyersburg & Post, 1979; Hofer, 1981). That is, environments that provide poor quality in nourishment/ diet, or social factors (e.g., availability of caring others/mother) result in major disturbances in the maturation of the nervous system.

MacDonald (1988) points out that our flexibility and dependence on input (learning) is a double-edged sword for it becomes possible that environments can have either helpful or pathological effects. Although the very long periods of dependency that a child has on its parents or care-giving individuals allows the child to learn an enormous amount about the social life of which the child will become a part, it carries a great potential cost. If the environment turns out to be punitive in some way, or fails to provide what is needed, then serious disturbance can result. McGuire and Troisi (1987) have suggested how environments lacking in certain social characteristics, such as care and respect for others, can have serious pathological effects. Furthermore, pathological effects occurring early in life can have an enormous influence on subsequent development (Rohner, 1986; Bowlby, 1988; MacDonald, 1988; Gilbert, 1989). It is as if the basic plans of humans require and anticipate a certain type of environment for the nervous system to mature in a certain way. The emergence of the person is a dialectical process between genetic endowment and self in interaction.

THE SOCIOBIOLOGICAL REVOLUTION

Sociobiology is a development of basic Darwinian principals of selection which have the effect of transforming species over time. Darwin argued for three basic forms of selection: natural, intersexual, and intrasexual. Natural selection favours the inheritance of traits that confer advantage in the struggle with the physical environment (e.g., body fat in cold climates; ability to camouflage against predators, etc.). Intrasexual selection favours the inheritance of traits that will confer advantage in social competition with members of the same sex (e.g., strength, antlers, threat displays, etc.). Intersexual selection favours the inheritance of traits that attracts desirable mates (e.g., plumage, courtship displays).

However, sociobiologists with a particular interest in insect life (Wilson, 1975) point out that personal, individual reproductive history is not the whole story. In many insects (ants and bees) members toil for the benefit of the colony/hive without personally reproducing (workers are sterile). Also individual reproductive theory fails to address questions such as the evolution of altruism (Dawkins, 1976). Indeed, it has been the obvious importance of apparent altruism which has been a main concern of sociobiologists.

Kin Altruism

In 1964 Hamilton put forward a mathematical theory for kin altruism which suggested that in some situations, self-sacrificing altruism had the effect of increasing the chances of survival of related members who carried shared genes. In other words behavioural characteristics can evolve that may be detrimental to an individual animal expressing them (e.g., self-sacrifice) but are of benefit to genetically related members. Consequently, it was proposed that it is genes that are selected for rather than individuals. However, to call genes selfish, as Dawkins (1976) has, is to play loose with language and convey an impression that genes have motives which they obviously can't have. It has clouded the whole area with emotive terms that are meaningless. All kin selection really points to is a possible mechanism derived from probability theory. Kin altruism is likely (as part of K-strategies) to increase the probability of genetic representation in succeeding generations. In fact at the individual level this means that on the whole, K-selected individuals will be less selfish and more concerned about relatives than r-strategists. Indeed Dawkins (1976) makes this point.[1]

This approach to selection is called inclusive fitness. At its simplest it suggests evolution operates via increasing the representation of genetic material in the next generation (Wilson, 1975; Dawkins, 1976; Crook, 1980). Wenegrat (1984, p.17) puts it this way:

> Accounting for genetic material in other than direct descendants acknowledges the fact that particular behavioural traits may affect not only the individual's reproductive history, but the reproductive history of those companions who share his or her genes. For this reason, inclusive fitness can be used to account for evolution of behavioural traits whose reproductive benefits are reaped by kin, rather than just by the individuals who actually manifest them.

The shift to considering gene replication as the mechanism underlying the evolutionary process has been fascinating. Over the last decade or so sociobiologists have been concerned with exploring behavioural traits in terms of whether they carry a potential for increasing chances of genetic representation (i.e., inclusive fitness). Hence sociobiologists have been interested in mathematical modelling of behavioural traits in populations to estimate their fitness. Among these traits are: preference for sisters' offspring, rates of parental investment in offspring and spacing, incest taboo, moral behaviour, and deception, to name a few. But remember as powerful a theory as sociobiology is, at its heart it is a statistical theory and is concerned with probabilities not absolutes.

However, arranging things such that one's relatives may benefit is hardly altrusim and is usually called nepotism. So again the sociobiologists use of language leaves much to be desired. Furthermore, many human parents do not give (invest in) their children what they need to survive and prosper, thus rendering them lacking in self-confidence, vulnerable to early suicide, unable to maintain long-term relationships, or making poor choices of partners, and so forth. The interaction between socio-cultural success and biological-reproductive success is extremely complex.

Reciprocal Altruism

Using the same basic formula of genetic representation and probability theory, Trivers (1971; 1985) presented another aspect of selective influence. Reciprocal altruism relates to the evolution of helping (non-related) others. Helping others will have evolved (been selected for) where the donor is able to benefit from the donation in terms of subsequent help from the recipient. However, help given is on a cost benefit analysis such that the cost (in terms of the probability of advancing gene replication) does not exceed the benefits. Some theorists have been extremely critical of this idea (Richards, 1987). But in America there is growing interest in seeking explanations of psychopathology in terms of reciprocal altruism (Glantz & Pearce, 1989; Nesse, 1990). The hypotheses here are that people can become disturbed when they feel they are giving more than they receive, receiving more than they can repay, or that they can damage relationships because they are exploitative and don't recognise that they will stir others' anger/withdrawal by failure to reciprocate.

In humans, helping behaviour is under the influence of complex cognitive emotional mechanisms—e.g., empathy, sympathy or the concern with feeling guilty for not helping (Eisenberg, 1986; Eisenberg

& Mussen, 1989). Furthermore, receiving may increase the attractiveness of the donor in the eyes of the receiver (Hill, 1984) This idea of attractiveness as a ranking issue will be discussed more fully in Chapter 7. Indeed, it may be that reciprocal support of self-esteem by the formation of alliances and cooperation and the preparedness to bestow status on talented members of a group has had a major effect on human evolution. In any event it is important to recognise that in social psychology ideas of reciprocal altruism have been around a long time under a different term (e.g., equity; see Brown, 1986). Crook (1980) has utilised reciprocal altruism to present a model of the evolution of guilt and friendship (Gilbert, 1989). Guilt acts as an internal alerting mechanism that one has transgressed the boundaries of reciprocal relationships and is acting exploitively or has failed to care/protect others—i.e., has allowed or caused injury.

Response Rules

An important concept in sociobiology is the notion of response rules (Wenegrat, 1984), sometimes also called epigenetic rules. Response rules are the species-typic psychobiological response patterns that can be recruited to certain environmental stimuli. For example, salivate if hungry when cues signalling food are present; increase arousal, freeze or run like hell, to unexpected noises or movement in the bushes. Do Z if A happens; do Y if B happens. In one sense unconditioned responses (e.g., salivation) are examples of response rules. They are part of an innate preparation for action. In another sense response rules can also be preparations for learning. For example, we know that it is easier to classically condition certain responses to certain stimuli but some associations are more difficult to learn. Rescorla (1988) has argued that we should view classical conditioning as the way animals acquire information about their environment. As he points out many clinical psychologists, who are keen on classical conditioning theory, actually don't understand it.

Response rules can be represented in a sequence of hierarchical decisions. Wenegrat conveys this idea by using the example of driving: stop if lights are red, drive on if green. However a higher rule is "drive if too far to walk." A yet higher rule might be "learn to drive if you want to get about". Response rules also cluster into social strategies. For example, "dominate others if you can, otherwise submit and wait your chance" (Hinde, 1987); or "select certain types of mating partner with certain characteristics" (Buss, 1989); or "invest in a child until a certain time, then turn attention to reproduction again." Response rules are another example of basic plans.

Sociobiological Controversies

Consider the fact that chimpanzees share about 99% of our genes, as Jane Goodall frequently tells us on her various documentary programmes, and are more like humans than other monkeys. Genetic variation then, between humans and chimpanzees, is very very small. Consider how much less it is between individuals of the same species (Eibl-Eibesfeldt, 1989). Thus if we are to consider genetic influences on behaviour it is important to keep this fact in mind. Further, many genes are modifiers (Day, 1990; Gardner, personal communication) that function to make small changes in more basic systems (e.g., attachment behaviour, dominance and ranking behaviour, and mate selection). For this reason ethologists and psychologists are interested in cross species comparisons, to study archetypal social behaviour (e.g., attachment behaviour, dominance and ranking behaviour, tactics of mate selection). This leads us to consider what Gardner (1988) has called basic plans, which are encoded in gene-neural structures and which can be observed in a variety of species. These gene neural structures provide the general rules that have been adaptive over the long term (again, e.g., attachment behaviour, dominance and ranking behaviour, and tactics of mate selection).

The issue of self-interest is a favourite of the sociobiologists. But self-interest can be analysed at the genetic level, the group level (we tend to support those we identify with), the social level (creating a positive self-presentation), the personal level (following one's own goals and plans), and the level of reinforcement (following the pursuit of pleasure and the avoidance of pain). The sociobiologists often use these different levels interchangeably, but one does not necessarily produce the other. Considerable confusion not to say false moral superiority is claimed by those who see human behaviour as guided (only) by self-interest. Do they mean we do things that are positively reinforcing (but how would they deal with smoking)? Do they mean following one's own goals? But what about when this conflicts with genetic interest? The language of self-interest can only be used in a psychological sense for beings that have some notion of self. All other forms are simply the enactment of underlying species, typic programmes that (for statistical reasons) may at one time have led to inclusive fitness and become established in the gene pool. [1]

Once there is a high degree of flexibility, (i.e., enormous variation can occur as a result of learning) and neuronal plasticity, then humans become more shaped and shaping of their social networks/ environments, than they are simple enactors of biological programmes. Learning changes biological structures and neuronal patterning (Hofer,

1981; Gilbert, 1989) with profound effects on the subsequent organisation of the CNS. Consequently, we find that many of our basic human behaviours require input to mature and be utilised proficiently. A child that does not receive adequate caring from his/her parents is more likely to develop various forms of psychopathology and become a poor parent themselves than a child that has been loved. If this person becomes highly promiscuous, does this mean they are reverting to r-selection tactics or are we seeing dysfunction of K-selection tactics, a searching for love, or a malformation of attachment systems, and so forth?

The debates surrounding the mechanisms and dynamics of evolution remain controversial (Wilson, 1975; Dawkins, 1976; Crook, 1980; Jantsch, 1980; Plotkin & Odling-Smee, 1981; Rose, Lewontin, & Kamin, 1984; Wenegrat, 1984; Fox, 1986; Schwartz, 1986; Vining, 1986; Richards, 1987; MacDonald, 1988; Eibl-Eibesfeldt, 1989; Itzkoff, 1990). Fox (1986) makes the point that individuals are motivated to acquire mates, copulate, seek dominance, care for children and so on. If all goes well inclusive fitness may follow, but gene representation in the next generation is the result rather than a cause of behaviour. This is obviously correct when we hold onto the fact that in regard to the question of ultimate causation we are talking of selective influence and probability estimates. In humans with culture there are great complications in the relations between symbolic thought processes and various strategies of inclusive fitness—i.e., the relations between cultural and biological fitness (Jantsch, 1980; Hill 1984; Rose et al., 1984; Schwartz, 1986; Vining, 1986; Itzkoff, 1990). Some individuals may be so concerned to gain socio-cultural advance (e.g., follow a career or make money) that they forego any interest in leaving replicators of their genes after them.

Behaviour is controlled by proximate mechanisms (genes, hormones, motivational states, cues in the environment, and so forth—that is, things that can exert their influence at a point in time, or now). In humans, neural structures must be genetically laid down otherwise humans could not be born as potential humans. But the plasticity of these neural structures, where plasticity (phenotype variability) itself was a K-selected strategy, means that variation in expression of behaviour is determined by life history (Chisholm 1988; Macdonald, 1988) and current social context (Hinde, 1987; Buss, 1991). So understanding gene-behaviour relations without careful analysis of phenotype is problematic and reduces the predictive power of sociobiology. Some (e.g., Itzkoff, 1990) go so far as to suggest that symbolic thought allows for such variation of phenotype via the exercise of intelligence that the linkage with inclusive fitness theory is considerably weakened. Yet another problem is that inclusive fitness theory assumes a gradual unfolding process of selection when in fact changes in species are often rapid and explosive following a period of stability. This is certainly true in the evolution of humans (Itzkoff, 1990).

PSYCHOBIOLOGICAL RESPONSE ROUTINES AND PATTERN GENERATION

It is important to note that although response rules relate to certain types of calculation, they execute their instructions via changing biological state (e.g., affect and motivations; Nesse, 1990); hence my use of the term psychobiological response pattern (Gilbert, 1984; 1988a,b; 1989). In general we seek out certain types of mate because they affect us via sexual attraction; we care for offspring because we love them. A psychobiological response pattern is an innate, pattern generating option. We can think of it as a preparedness within the system to organise itself (to coassemble affects, cognitions, and action tendencies) in certain ways (Gilbert, 1989). For example, most are aware of the fight/flight system. In flight there is arousal which recruits various aspects of: the cardiac system (heart beats faster), changes in blood flow, changes in blood clotting, changes in gastric-intestinal activity, changes in oxygen to the muscles, changes in the release of various neurotransmitters and hormones, changes in attention, and so on. The patterning and coordinating of various psychobiological processes is in part the result of experience but also comes as part of an innate organisational competency (e.g., anger or sexual behaviour work more or less in species-typic way—similar patterns of arousal, action tendencies, and so forth). Hence, we are thinking of systemic changes (see also Iran-Nejad & Ontony, 1984). We also now know that there are various forms of feedback that occur in these systemic changes. Continual activation of the flight pattern will lead to exhaustion and possibly, in the extreme, death. Or to give a more specific example, changes in cortisol may have a modulating effect on central neural activity (e.g., the hippocampus has receptors for cortisol).

An example of a psychobiological response pattern that changes in a set sequence is protest–despair (Bowlby, 1969; 1973; Gilbert, 1988b) When an infant is separated from its attachment object the first response is usually protest, an active calling to and searching for the lost attachment object. If this is unsuccessful it is followed subsequently by despair, which is a (relatively) non-reactive or a "closed down state". Again this patterning and sequencing is innately available, observable in many primates, but changes with maturation and experience (Hofer, 1984; Kagan, 1984). Another example is from the learned helplessness paradigm (Seligman, 1975). The first response to uncontrollable trauma is often (though not always) to become fearful and to struggle to find an escape. If this is not successful the system changes to a state of helpless passivity. Genetic differences may influence how quickly the first response lasts, the form of later responses, and so on.

The problem with sociobiology, as applied to psychopathology, is that (paradoxically) it is not very biological or psychological, but statistical. The way response rules are actually organised and "run" in the CNS has received scant attention. However, this idea of *"pattern generation" as a property of innate potential* is a crucial factor for understanding psychopathology. Under certain kinds of stress, elements of the psychic system may become organised in such a way that we say the person is ill, or dysfunctional. Various patterns can be recruited within us that are against our conscious wishes (e.g., when giving a prestigious talk I may find it difficult to get out of the toilet).

Our fear of various stimuli may diminish with repeated exposure without harm. Thus learning and experience not only give us flexibility of response but change the organisational properties of psychobiological systems. Many patterns of potential internal organisation are developmentally influenced, giving rise to phenotypic variation as discussed above. How we come to understand the world and respond to it, our sense of self and empathy for others are properties of psychic organisation. These require certain types of internal integration of abilities, affects, and competencies. Here we are thinking of the recipe model of personality rather than the lego model (see Chapter 4). However, our dependency on the environment means that some forms of potential self-organisation may never become developed. Very negative experiences with our parents may result in failure of the attachment system to mature and become organised within us. We become unable to reach our evolved potential of becoming loving partners and parents. Our potential to become organised into the pattern of a loved, lovable, and loving self does mature within.

At this point we leave our discussion of innate organisational potentials, but will refer back to it throughout the rest of the book. To understand psychopathology it is helpful to keep in mind this aspect since it lies behind new notions of self-organisation (e.g., Greenberg, Elliott, & Foerster, 1990), mentality theory and archetype theory (Gilbert, 1989, and Chapter 11 this volume). Further, depression is a potential brain state organisation which has as part of its pattern, behavioural, affective, cognitive, and biological aspects. This pattern may be switched on via genes, abnormal rearing patterns, maladaptive cognitions, thwarting life events, and so forth. The patterns may vary according to a host of factors but there are certain characteristics of the pattern that must remain, otherwise depression would be so infinitely variable that it could not be recognised. Depression is then, a potential internal organisational pattern. The reasons for the evolution of this pattern, and its maintenance in our gene-neural structures, is the subject of our next two chapters.

THE SELF-DEFENSE–PROTECT SYSTEM

Stumuli have two important properties. They cue arousal or dampen it, and they are sources of information. Memory affects both arousal to stimuli and the meaning given to stumuli. Both arousal and meaning cue responses. Psychobiological response patterns differ according to whether they (a) are defensive and self-protective or (b) arise from safety and are concerned with exploring the environment for positive reinforcers and resources—i.e., an early decision in extracting the meaning of stimuli and priming type of response is "safe–not safe". The self-defense–protect system, operating under conditions of threat, has a menu of possible responses options for responding to various threat events.

Types of Threat. Threats can be divided into non-social and social. Non-social threats are things like predators, and these often activate the defensive system via sensory input (e.g., visual shapes, smells, sounds in the bushes, etc.). Height cues and falling cues can also be non-social threats. Some theorists see these as triggering the alarm reaction (Marks, 1987). Social threats relate to threats coming from conspecifics (members of the same species or group). Here threats come from others who may attempt to take resources, such as pushing an animal out of a territory. In primates social threats are mostly (dominance) rank related. In humans we may speak of threats to status, self-presentation, or self-esteem. In this situation the person acts to defend something that he/she has and in this sense (like most defensive responses) they are protective.

Also the withdrawal of safety cues can activate the defense–protect system. For example, removal of the mother can shift the psychobiological pattern of the child to defense and involves seeking and calling to the parent and signalling distress.

Types of Response. The types of response are either active/ excitatory or go, or inhibitory/stop. Go/stop options, however, are not mutually exclusive and both options can be primed. For example, a person may feel both urged to flee yet also feel inhibited from doing so. Examples of excitatory-go responses to non-social threats involve psychomotor discharge and include: fight, flight, escape, and active avoidance. Examples of inhibitory-stop responses include: freeze, faint (demobilisation), or camouflage (Beck et al., 1985; Marks, 1987). To social threatening events the active/excitatory options may be: fight or counter aggression to protect status or elicit subordinate compliant responses from conspecifics; flight/withdraw, or submit/yield. This menu of options is dependent on the type of stimuli. For example, no chimpanzee has ever been seen to submit to a baboon even though they may fear them.

In psychotherapy when the self-defense–protect system is aroused one may see various efforts to avoid harm. These can range from submissive concealing (as in shame) through to anger to repel possible attack or force compliance. The defense–protect system is designed to shut down open exploration and attend to self defense. In therapy, internal exploration may also be blocked and this inhibits work on further emotional processing (Greenberg & Safran, 1987). For example, internal cues signalling anger may be blocked because anger is perceived to be threatening in some way. A climate of safety is needed to reduce this blocking/avoidance and facilitate an internal climate for exploration.

THE SAFETY SYSTEM

When animals feel relatively safe and secure in their environment, the activity is focused on exploration, seeking resources or resting. The most obvious cues that activate the safety system are those that signal an absence of threat. Under these conditions the explorative and resource acquisitions menu of options may be primed, including such behaviours as seeking food, nest building, finding a mate or interacting with friends and lovers, and so on. The response options here are go/no-go and there is no inhibitory component to the safety system. Rather it operates on a gradient of arousal (Gilbert, 1989) related to *positive affectivity*. Inhibition always comes for the defense system.

The defense and safety systems are not mutually exclusive concerns (e.g., the excitement of parachuting). However, the degree of social control determines the levels of arousal that can be tolerated before self-protect action switches in and blocks exploration. Under conditions of safety the attention is focused on acting in, and learning about, the environment in order to obtain positive reinforcement, acquire knowledge/ skills, or mastery, etc.

In highly social animals like humans the safety system operates when individuals feel comfortable with others; as when acting with friends and attachment objects. The presence and behaviours (e.g., smiles, winks, etc.) of others can have the effect of calming and reducing defensive arousal and activating the positive reward areas of the brain, making interaction pleasurable. In these situations the social environment is not a focus of threat (which it might be without these signals being present). However the rather elaborate social safety system evolved later than the defense system. To see how safety signals are necessary in order to avoid automatic activation of the defense system consider this simple example. You are about to meet a new boss. As you walk in his/her nonverbal behaviour is friendly, he/she smiles at you and we say "puts you at your easy". Suppose these cues are not present however. He/she does not smile or shake your hand but in a neutral voice asks you to take a seat. Under these conditions you are likely to be more self-defensive and protective, feel anxious or uneasy. Will you have to defend your self-presentation? Of course you may not want the job or you may feel more dominant than your boss, i.e., you feel in control and in that situation you may be more prepared to be aggressive if he/she gives you any trouble. In any event the relationship will proceed differently if both individuals adhere to a safety signal interaction. In essence these nonverbal safety signals follow rules and are important in interpersonal behaviour. They are innate and vary little cross-culturally (Argyle, 1984).

A sense of relative safety promotes open exploration of the environment (Gilbert, 1989). As another example, imagine the child who feels safe with its parent. In the presence of the parent the child will show a natural inquisitiveness and exploration, tries things out and so forth. The child who does not feel safe/secure with its parent, however, will need to direct a certain amount of its activity to watching for threat cues emanating from the parent (or separation from the parent). Further, because the parent cannot be relied on to provide a safe environment if things go wrong, the child needs to be extremely cautious in its explorative and resource gathering behaviour.

Perhaps the biggest problem is on the issue of how individuals try to create the climate of safety that will allow them to explore and gather, or have access to resources. Some try to create safety by making friends, some form dependency relationships with real people or God, whereas others feel safety is only assured by knocking out or dominating potential opponents, or investing in their own efforts (see Charlesworth, 1988, for a fascinating discussion of the tactics of resource gathering). Response rules can vary from person to person, situation to situation, and time to time as a reflection of the context and state of individuals. Each individual has a slightly different set of preferences for each response in their internal menus. Some are cooperative while others are more competitive (Eisenberg & Mussen, 1989; Gilbert, 1989).

I have properly laboured the point, but basically the defensive–protect response menus tend to be stereotyped, automatic, involuntary, and non-exploratory, while the safety system menu of responses tends to be exploratory and more open. The internal climate (defense or safe) also has major effects on the integration of personality attributes and possiblities.

Integration and Segregation of Internal Traits and Abilities

The safety system allows for the openness to, and exploration of, the environment. This is helpful in that it enables the child to be exposed to, and integrate various inputs. Moreover, it may also be presumed that it facilitates a more integrating orientation to internal psychic propensities, facilitating intelligence and creative thinking (e,g., Isen, Daubman, & Nowicki, 1987; Isen, 1990) and personality development. Insight into oneself and empathy for others depend on an openness to the self and other. The non-defensive personality tends also to be an open personality (Hampden-Turner, 1970) able to explore and integrate information. They also tend to be more giving of positive reinforcement to others. This links with self-esteem, but what is interesting here is that self-esteem in turn seems to be related to a personality who is able to exercise traits over various domains.

Recent evidence suggests that it is the integration of various elements of internal possibilities (for love, empathy, self-assertion, caring of others, leadership, and so forth) that is associated with self-esteem (Paulhus & Martin, 1987). If some of these are defensively blocked then one becomes more defensive in certain areas and self-esteem more vulnerable (e.g., like a one-club golfer). Certain aspects maybe less likely to mature in a highly defensive oriented person and are not integrated into self-organisational patterns.

Internally, the balance between the safety system and self-defense system is moderated via internal models of self. For example, an internal model of self as inferior, shifts the balance to self-defense–protect operations. This will increase vigilance to threat and also increase self-focusing to ensure that the self is not sending signals that might provoke punishments/aggressions/put-downs from others (see Chapters 7 and 8). Attention is therefore constrained, an openness to experience and free exploration (and initiative taking) is lost. The affect system shifts towards greater negative affectivity.[2] Another way to think of this is that high levels of defensive arousal produce regressive (and disintegrating) alterations in self-organisation (Horowitz & Zilberg, 1983).

AFFECTS

Affects are essential components of the self-defense and safety systems. As reviewed elsewhere (Gilbert, 1989) affects provide the energy for responding, planning, and anticipating, they give us our sense of urgency and impetus; affects provide information of internal state; affects can often be related to social signals and are important for nonverbal communicative behaviour; affects give us our sense of values and affects keep us on track of important incentives and biologically relevant (biosocial) goals. As Nesse (1990) points out, happiness and positive affect are often associated with finding a lover, having children, gaining status, being admired, acquiring resources, forming friendships and alliances, becoming an ingroup member, and so forth. Negative affects tend to be associated with failing to find a lover, failing to gain respect and status, failing to form alliances and friendships, being an outsider, and losing resources. In primates, social success is an important vehicle to reproductive success and consequently positive affects are often associated with social success. Affects, then, inform us that we are tracking biologically relevant goals. This is why our sense of self-value (see Chapter 7) influences our affective lives, and why both are linked to our social lives.

To return to the issue of response rules, then, we can suggest that all humans have inherited a set of response rules and a menu of options of response and affects for dealing with particular environmental events. At birth these are no more than possibilities but are shaped and developed through life. Anxiety and depression represent the activation of internal options (psychobiological response patterns and states) that have their roots in the gene-neural architecture of early (non-human) brain designs. When and if they are activated is rarely the result of disease. Moreover, since negative affects have been so important to conveying information about threat and (lack of) social success an illness model may be inappropriate for understanding them.

Once we recognise that depression and anxiety are innate potentials and not the result of malfunctioning "organs" (at least in the majority of cases) then our conceptualisation of depression changes. To give one example, in agressive groups, primates at the bottom of the hierarchy are tense and anxious and this is self-protective and adaptive. Evolution is unconcerned with individual happiness and our expectation that humans should be happy is a human construct. If we wish to reduce depression then we will need to look at both historical factors (e.g., early rearing patterns) and sociocultural influences which have brought about the depressive pattern of organisation in an individual.

ETHOLOGY

Ethologists have been critical of sociobiology for its rigidity and failure to accommodate the fact that both ontogeny and culture (or social climate of interactions and values) exert a significant influence on behaviour in their own right. Also the idea that the gene rather than the individual or even group is the selective unit has been disputed (Eibl-Eibesfeldt, 1989). Others have argued that the sociobiologists tend to look for evidence to support their theories (e.g., incest taboo) and discount as aberrant the evidence that contradicts it. Ethologists approach the issue of the evolved basis of behaviour from a different perspective.

Tinbergen (1963) suggested that ethology is concerned with four basic but related questions: (1) *the study of causation*, meaning the exploration of psychobiological mechanisms underlying behaviour; (2) *the study of function*, that is the survival value of any given behaviour: its fitness; (3) *the study of ontogeny*, that is development over the life cycle; (4) *the study of phylogeny*, that is the study of the transformation of behaviour over evolutionary time (see also Hinde, 1982; Eibl-Eibesfeldt, 1989).

While the sociobiologists have put forward a statistical theory for ultimate causation, called inclusive fitness theory (as the way of understanding behaviour traits, and how they may have become laid down in gene-neural structures over millions of years), ethologists have been interested in how individuals expressing certain behavioural traits actually function in the natural environment and how the environment reacts to them. This leads us to the behavioural argument of the importance of the social milieu as the dispenser of rewards and punishments and that individuals above all else must accommodate themselves to this fact. Furthermore, ethologists make the point that unless you study behaviour in the natural environment, you have no way of classifying response rules and you may not even know what an animal is capable of. For example, we now know that chimpanzees hunt other monkeys in a well organised way, with division of activities, (e.g., trackers, blockers, and capturers, etc.). This was simply not known before they were observed in their natural environment and is a very recent discovery (Boesch, 1990). Artificial conditions (e.g., cages and zoos) may produce consistencies in behaviours, but these consistencies may none the less be pathological and rarely seen in the natural habitat.

Hence, ethology is concerned with the proximate mechanisms of behaviour. In this regard they view the social context as far more important than the imperative to pass on genes since it is the social environment that calls forth and acts on the developing nervous system, exploiting what plasticity there is. Since animals do not know they are attempting to maximise their genes, behavioural analysis requires understanding of social dynamics. Ethologists, then, highlight the interactional nature of behaviour rather than some internally controlled robotic-like organisms that are busy ferreting out the best manner to leave genes after them. There is relatively little disagreement about the role of inclusive fitness as an ultimate explanation but there is disagreement in terms of understanding ontogeny, the function of behaviour and the importance of social context as shaping behaviour.

THE PSYCHOLOGICAL PERSPECTIVE

Whereas the sociobiologist is interested in mathematically modelling social behaviour from the point of view of inclusive fitness theory and the ethologist is interested in the interactional aspects, the psychologist is interested in trying to get inside the head as it were, and consider how the person is actually doing all those things that the evolutionist suggests they are supposed to be doing. Hence the psychologist is interested in things like: how do people learn, how do people make attributions, what are the dimensions of attributions, how do people construe and evaluate themselves; what are self-schema, self-esteem, self-organisation and self-identity and how are they arrived at; how do people reason; how does memory and language work and so forth. Furthermore, psychologists are interested in how these may be changed. Is it possible to change attributional style, teach assertive behaviour and via psychological or psychosocial interventions bring about a change in that person's internal organisation that reduces suffering, reduces vulnerability, and moves the person on in their maturation process? At the end of the day, although social context is undoubtedly a source of suffering it is individual minds that suffer; it is an experience of being; an internal organisation pattern; it is a way of knowing or being in touch with archetypal states.

The psychological psychopathologist needs to have feet in both the camps of biology and sociology. Without this there is the risk of developing not only a brainless or mindless science (Eisenberg, 1986) but also a highly socially decontextualised one. Nowhere is this problem more noticeable than in the current cognitive notions that it is not things in themselves that disturb us but the view we take of them. This is simply not true. While it may be a useful model for helping people take control and exert choice over their lives and give up negative self-evaluations, from a biological point of view it fails to acknowledge basic needs (Chapter 10). People prosper in certain environments (those that provide access to a degree of social success; see the above discussion on affects) and not others and on the average these environments are pretty similar across cultures (Rohner, 1986; MacDonald, 1988). Supportive caring environments with low levels of social threat and which provide a sense of belonging and worth tend to produce happier individuals than environments in which social structures are fragmented and disorganised, cannot provide a sense of belonging and where relationships are marked by suspiciousness and hostility (see MacDonald's, 1988, comparison of the Gussi and Kung!). If adults are not loved or respected or are subjected to abuse, harassment or are marginalised in their main roles, they may become depressed or aggressive (Chapter 15). The cognitive model is important when we begin to recognise that humans evolved to require certain types of input, and have certain internal mentalities (evaluative systems) for making sense out of the world and orienting themselves to it.Thus people can become trapped in styles of evaluation that produce suffering but, by means of education and a switching to alternative ways of evaluating self and others, they can move out of distressed states (Chapters 7, 8, and 13).

The psychologist's contribution to an understanding of mental suffering is to furnish insight into the socio-typic internal cognitive affective system of individuals. In the rest of this chapter we will explore the internal psychological mechanisms that facilitate meaning-making in the social world (Gilbert, 1989) or, to put it another way, the psychological proximate mechanisms of human behaviour.

RESPONSE RULES AND MEANING-MAKING SYSTEMS: BIOSOCIAL GOALS AND SOCIAL MENTALITIES

Biosocial Goals

We believe that K-selection has given rise to a host of response rules and social strategies that are primarily to do with conspecific interaction (Crook, 1980; Wenegrat, 1984; Gardner, 1988). We have also discussed the idea that these strategies have a degree of plasticity to them which allow for history of reward and punishment to be carried forward in time exerting their impact on the expression of phenotype (Chisholm,1988; MacDonald, 1988). Another way of thinking about K-selection is that K-selection gives rise to biosocial goals (Gilbert, 1989) or motivational systems (McClelland, 1985). These goals are important to achieve social success and, as we have argued, social success in primates is linked to reproductive success. The brain is not a passive responder to the environment but is actively searching, processing, encoding and selecting responses in the pursuance of goals. These goals are not arbitrary but are the products of K-selection. Gilbert (1989) outlined three basic social goals: *Attachment* (which relates to care-giving and care-receiving), *alliance formation* (which relates to cooperation) and *ranking* (which relates to competing), but various blends are possible (see also Buss, 1991).

What many of the psychoanalysts (e.g., Freud and Jung) and the behaviourists have in common is the assumption that humans are goal directed and future orientated. What an evolutionary approach tells us is that the general nature of these goals will be products of K-selection. As Jung suggested, there are archetypal themes to human life; to elicit care from care-givers, to develop relationships with peers and become a group member with a sense of belonging; to find a mate, to care for offspring, to strive for recognition, respect, and status; to make sense of life and to come to terms with death. We may wish to debate the exact number or content of our biosocial goals but what is generally accepted is that each species has species-typic goals that it must achieve to be able to function within its social domain and prosper.

Mentalities

If there are different (K-selected) biosocial goals that act as internal guiding mechanisms, then are there also internal processing modules for organising information as to how far that goal has been achieved, and what needs to be done to achieve it? Could different goals use different processing mentalities to make these calculations? The answer is probably, yes. There is now much evidence that human mental functioning is made up of individual sub-units or modules. Ornstein (1986, p.9) tells us:

> The long progression in our self-understanding has been from a simple and usually 'intellectual' view to the view that the mind is a mixed structure, for it contains a complex set of 'talents', 'modules' and 'policies' within ... All of these general components of the mind can act independently of each other, they may well have different priorities.
>
> The discovery of increased complexity and differentiation has occurred in many different areas of research...: in the study of brain function and localisation; in the conceptions of the nature of intelligence; in personality testing; and the theories of the general characteristics of the mind.

Neurological work has demonstrated very clearly that the brain is a modual structure with a high degree of functional specificity

(Gazzaniga, 1989). There is also evidence in support of: Specialised forms of modular processing systems (Fodor, 1985); specialised social intelligences (Gardner, 1985); specific communication propensities (Gardner, 1988); archetypes (Jung, 1964; Wenegrate, 1984); biosocial goals (Gilbert, 1989); reasoning modules (Cosmides, 1989) and interacting cognitive subsystems (Barnard & Teasdale,1991). All these data point to a basic modular system of mind. In a fascinating paper Power and Brewin (in press) have reviewed some of the new areas of cognitive science, which is exploring modular, unconscious processing. Such modular processes tend to work in parallel, are relatively inflexible and task focused (see also Chapter 13). As we go through this book we will speak often of self-organisational patterns. This concept is concerned with the internal organisation of these modual processing systems. Via their organisation we come to "experience and know ourselves." One thing seems clear, these modual systems did not evolve for rational reasoning, but to advance social success. On the latter point Cosmides (1989, p.193) says:

> ... thus, the realization that the human mind evolved to accomplish adaptive ends indicates that natural selection would have produced special-purpose, domain specific, mental algorithms—including rules of inference—for solving important and recurrent adaptive problems (such as learning a language; ...). It is advantageous to reason adaptively, instead of logically, when this allows one to draw conclusions that are likely to be true, but cannot be inferred by strict adherence to the propositional calculus. Adaptive algorithms would be selected to contain expectations about specific domains that have proven reliable over a species' evolutionary history. These expectations would differ from domain to domain. Consequently, if natural selection had shaped how humans reason, reasoning about different domains would be governed by different, content-dependent cognitive processes.

Biosocial goals (Gilbert, 1989) have the potential to create a nucleus of meaning around social interaction. These were labelled: *care eliciting, care giving, cooperating, and competing.* A mentality provides the necessary internal structure(s) to be able to construe relationships in certain ways; it is a core potential for the construction of meaning. A mentality is a complex assembly of affective couplings, action tendencies, and cognitive and attentional structures (see Gilbert, 1989, pp.26-27). A rough conceptualisation of the these different goals is given in Table 5.2.

For example, the cooperative goal recruits styles of reasoning and evaluations of social situations in terms of mutual gain, sense of belonging, and moral interaction. The competitive goal recruits styles

TABLE 5.2
Core Social Mentalities

	Self as	*Other as*
Care Eliciting	Needing inputs from other(s): care, protection, safety, reassurance.	Source of: care, nurturance, protection, safety, reassurance.
Care Giving	Provider of: care, protection, safety, nurturance.	Recipient of: care, protection, safety, nurturance.
Cooperation	Of value to other, sharing, appreciating, contributing, affiliative.	Valuing, contribution sharing, appreciating, affiliative.
Competition	Contestant, inferior-superior.	Contestant, inferior-superior.

of reasoning about where one's place is, in a social hierarchy. The care-giving goal recruits styles of reasoning and evaluation that are concerned with help giving. Care eliciting recruits styles of reasoning and evaluation that are concerned with inputs from others. These basic orientations to social life provide the bases for our repetitive human themes of social interaction as told by the novelist and enacted in myth and ritual (Chapter 11). Hence the need for love, a sense of belonging and purpose make life meaningful and are associated with positive affect. While rejection, a loss of social place and marginalisation can make life seem meaningless and are associated with negative affect.

The fact that humans are able to "make sense" of certain kinds of interaction (e.g., as infants we are soothed by the comfort of being held, Montagu, 1986) implies that there is a basic preparation for the construction of social meaning along the various dimensions mentioned above. However, this preparation is only in terms of possibilities and not eventualities. How the social environment, from the cradle to the grave, acts and reinforces the development of these mentalities will influence much that finally becomes part of our self-understanding and self-organisation. Certain parts of our potential will be developed and become part of self-awareness. Other aspects may lie dormant unless circumstances arise that show us different aspects of our potential. We may never know what lies within unless the environment pulls on this aspect of our potential.[3] Learning in early life is crucial because throughout evolution for any individual life the context of life was, until recently, (usually) stable. Only with humans do we find massive variations of context over an individual life.

It would be inappropriate to go into details of the mentalities here and the interested reader is referred to Gilbert (1989). MacDonald (personal communication) has asked the very important question of how biosocial goals relate to personality theory of traits (e.g., Buss, 1988; Macdonald, 1988). Biosocial goals are K-selected goals that will increase the likelihood of acquiring resources and becoming socially successful. Thwarting of these goals activates negative affects for reasons noted above. Individual variation occurs by different individuals being predisposed to follow slightly different mixtures of strategies (Buss, 1991).

One major variation is the degree to which an individual is motivated to invest in self, or individualistic strategies, or the degree to which the focus is on eliciting investment/help/support from others. This basic distinction has a long history in psychological theorising (Macdiarmid, 1989). Another distinction relates to basic affiliative mechanisms of love–hate (Leary, 1957). MacDonald (1988) has explored in detail how different traits might relate to various r–K strategies. At the present time the relationships between the concepts of mentalities, meaning-making, internal systems, and basic human traits are under intense discussion and research, and no final resolution and integration of these ideas is yet possible.

DEPRESSION

In the above we have outlined some of the basic concepts that will be used to explore the evolutionary basis of depression. Also the above aspects will act as a backdrop for the many theories to be discussed in subsequent chapters.

Depression and Biosocial Goals

Any biosocial goal can become central to self-organisation and become the most important route to social success. Furthermore, in adults at least, different goals may be *invested with self-value*. The affects of social success depend on moving towards this biosocial goal. Hence some individuals become competitive and the roles they enact with others are concerned with rising up the hierarchy, getting on, taking the initiative, accumulating resources, and so forth. They feel good about themselves when they are achieving success, gaining status and recognition for talent. At times they may use fight-aggressiveness to overcome reluctance in others and feel good if people obey them.

Other individuals follow more the biosocial goal of care eliciting. Self-worth and value come from perceiving that others care for them and are available for help. Yet others become care-givers and seek out roles that allow them to look after others, care for them, and have a sense of being needed and important. While some individuals do not wish to be cared for but seek affiliative opportunities to cooperate with others and become appreciated members of a group or network. Of course these biosocial goals are not in any sense mutually exclusive, so it is probably better to think of their pattern of organisation within an individual (see Chapter 11 on the nature of social themes).

Compensation. A failure to achieve one goal may be compensated for by pursuing another, since each goal will have social success pay-offs. For example, someone might, as a result of parental failure to nurture care eliciting, turn to competitiveness so that others can be kept under control or become admirers. Or an individual whose basic autonomy and individuation is blocked might turn to care eliciting, trying to elicit from others what they are unable to do for themselves. However, as we see in Chapter 10, compensation goals that are blocked may lead to the re-emergence of the feelings associated with the goal that was originally blocked. For example, a competitive individual who fails may experience again feelings of not being loved or wanted early in life or only being loved if they are successful. In another typical case, a patient lived to please parents and act as a care-giver to them. She was known amongst her friends for being very caring. What was blocked and being compensated for was autonomy. As she passed through therapy she found her energy coming on when she started to rebel and become more competitive, assertive, and irresponsible. She felt she was in touch again with a child-like enthusiasm. When she no longer acted like the timid caring person, needing to please others as she had been, some of her friends were shocked and made various comments and jokes to force her back into her old self-identity.

Segregation, Integration, and Depression

We suggested above that when the self-defense–protect system is activated, this shifts the mental system towards a more automatic and less integrated system. Thus, as Beck et al. (1979) point out, depressed people are more "primitive" in their thinking, more global and absolutistic, less flexible and less integrated. Positive affectivity, creativity, and exploration are lost. At times however finding a way out of depression can result in creative works (e.g., the mildly depressed novelist) but usually depression does not result in creativity. Hence depression tends to have a segregating effect on mental mechanisms (that is, we become less flexible, integrative, and open). In this sense depression can act to encapsulate a particular sytle of experiencing (see also Gilbert, 1989).

In the next three chapters we shall explore depression from an evolutionary prespective. The arguments that have been outlined here help us keep in mind that depression has some in-built pattern; it is a potential brain state organisaticn and any of us are potential suffers. It will have great phenotypic variability from person to person but still there will be commonalities; an experience of misery, low levels of explorative behaviour, loss of energy, negative self-organisations and perceptions of inferiority, and poor assertiveness.

SUMMARY

1. The gene-neural structures of mind represent stored knowledge and can be understood as accumulated knowledge units from previous adaptations and selections.
2. The morphological structure of the human CNS emerged from the reptilian period and was added to as new adaptations took place leading to the triune structure of the human brain.
3. The selective process that has had greatest effect on changes in brain function and structure has been K-selection. With K-selection came the need for new social dispositions and competencies. Consequently, many of the response rules and strategies that are coded in human gene-neural structures are those designed to engage in species-typic social behaviour. Species-typic social behaviours arose from response rules serving inclusive fitness.
4. A consequence of K-selection was to allow for increasing variation between genotype and phenotype in the enactment of social response rules, i.e., learning and flexibility of responses associated with the positive rewards and punishments as occurs in the social environment.
5. The degree to which individuals experience safety or threat has an effect on the internal biological (e.g., levels of cortisol) environment and this affects the primed menu of options for responding to the environment. During maturation, development that takes place in an internal (biological) environment of defensiveness can skew development towards defensiveness. Alternatively, development that takes place where the internal biological environment has low levels of defensive arousal is more likely to lead to a confident and relaxed individual who is more likely to develop greater flexibility in the pursuit of biosocial goals.
6. Ethological approaches suggest that behaviour should be viewed with respect to four issues: (1) the study of causation,

meaning the exploration of psychobiological mechanisms underlying behaviour; (2) the study of function, that is the survival value of any given behaviour, its fitness; (3) the study of ontogeny, that is development over the life cycle; (4) the study of phylogeny, that is the study of the transformation of behaviour over evolutionary time.
7. K-selection has given rise to a number of biosocial goals that are important to follow if an individual is to prosper in their species-typic social environment; these are care eliciting, care giving, cooperating and competing. There are innate internal algorithms that help track these goals. Affects also help us to track and pursue these biologically relevant goals.
8. The social environment can block, amplify, and modify these goals. Depression and other primitive responses can arise when the central biologically relevant goals are blocked, (e.g., loss of respect, status or value, failure to find friends and allies, loss of control over resources, and so forth).

CONCLUDING COMMENTS

For too long the human sciences have sought to avoid and ignore the biological realities of life. Only now, as the planet dies, are we gaining awareness that our abuse of our own living space and our insistence that we can make up our own rules is a dangerous illusion. Similarly, we are now slowly recognising that, while it is true we have much freedom in how we conduct ourselves, this freedom is not absolute. The human race is a species of animal, extraordinarily complex, but one which was not created anew overnight. Maybe we never did get over the shock that Darwin confronted us with. In our search for meaning that goes beyond the self and reaches out towards the transpersonal we may forget that this search itself is sometimes because our own lives have become so empty of the things that we evolved to require from our fellows.

The irony is that following an evolutionary and psychobiological approach suggests that the long-term solutions to our suffering (for the many but not all) do not lie with changing our biology, swallowing handfuls of tranquillizers or in alcoholic control, but in a coming together to insist on a better social milieu in which to exist and grow; to claim our evolved biological heritage. Whether it be in our architecture (e.g., high rises), in our family units or work and economic environments, we must ask for what purpose have we allowed these to develop in the way that they have. We are in a sense all victims of ignorance, of system building that has no other motive than its own efficiency. Only slowly may we realise that efficiency, as the sole criteria of a social-economic system, is not necessarily biological or socially sensible.

Humans are clever in that they can understand systems and think systemically, i.e., discover that the relationship between events follow rules, even if these rules cannot be directly observed (e.g., gravity). In the non-social sciences the researcher simply studies the system and does not make up rules to suit themselves. In the human sciences however, it is our values that influence systems. If you believe that economic happiness comes from material resources, then bravo unbridled competition! Yet material resources are only marginally related to happiness (Argyle, 1987) and suicide is increasing in Ireland and world-wide despite increases in national GNP (Chapter 3). As we move into the next century, and as an ex-economist, my greatest fear is that economic values will gradually dominate sociocultural values more than now and the social costs will be disastrous. Social and human scientists must come together, stop fighting over whether these are true sciences or not, be extremely cautious of disease theories in mental health, yet also be more aware of the biological realities and needs of humans, and require economists to develop systems that serve people rather than the other way around.

An evolutionary, biopsychosocial approach to suffering attempts to find a harmony that resonates with the biological and archetypal. It does not assume that we are free to construct ourselves in any way we choose. Rather we are constrained by virtue of being an evolved and fascinating animal.

NOTES

1. The fact that altruism (or nepotism) evolved because it may increase the probability of getting one's own genes in the gene pool is an important concept, but we cannot go from here to a concept of selfish individuals. If Dawkins had called his book "replicators" or some other such non-emotive term then there would probably be less confusion and hostility to the concepts than there has been, and certainly it would have been less easy for right wing politicians to high jack. If genes were really so selfish and concerned with their own survival then it is doubtful that they would be carried in animals that significantly threaten not only their own survival but every gene carrying member on the planet.
2. Humans also like to act directly on their biological state. When defensively aroused some eat to comfort self or slim, others drink or take drugs, others withdraw, others throw themselves into some task that distracts and allows a certain fantasy or hope of success leading to a better internal feeling. Indeed much of our behaviour is aimed at attempting to control our biological state, to create within us the pleasurable and hopeful and reduce the painful.

3. Perhaps war is the most graphic example. The home-loving boy who finds himself blowing someone's head off may be haunted by recognition of potential that only a disturbed environment could call forth. Or take the competent female who is confident and able until she finds a man whom she falls for sexually (he is exciting). Only gradually does she find that his dominance behaviour is now turned on her and calling forth from (activating within) her a depressive pattern of yielding.

CHAPTER 6

The Evolution of Social Power and its Role in Depression

> Micropolitics, like all politics, has to do with the creation and negotiation of hierarchy: getting and keeping power, rank and standing, or what I call "social place" ... In everyday, face-to-face encounters and relationships, we constantly monitor the shifting micropolitical balance. We want to know where we stand, relative to others, at a given moment. And we want to have a say in negotiating our standing.—Clark (1990, p. 305)

INTRODUCTION

This chapter explores the theory that depression is about not being able to control one's social place. Stated briefly, depression is associated with unfavourable changes in one's relative social place, or (having a perception of) occupying a low social place. From an evolutionary point of view the questions are: (1) why is social standing and rank so important to humans?; (2) what are the psychobiological correlates of rank position?; and (3) how might the evolved mechanisms and state patterns associated with rank be related to depression?

Karen Horney (1885–1952, see Ewen, 1988) suggested that people have three basic interpersonal options: they can either move towards each other, away from each other, or against each other. To these I would add two others: (1) the ability to make others move away and/or inhibit their actions (e.g., as in threatening) and (2) the ability to attract others to move towards one (e.g., in courtship). Brought down to basics then there is an attract-repel/inhibit dimension (or as Gardner, 1988, suggests, link or space) to conspecific relating. These are tactics of social control.

Origins of Social Power in Depression

Sexual selection necessitates adaptations to two basic problems of social control: (a) competing with other conspecifics (members of the same species) who are going after the same breeding resources (relating to intrasexual selection); and (b) attracting mates (relating to intersexual selection). As far back as fish we see these two basic behavioural dispositions in action. Mating requires the inhibition of the aggression and flight system and the exhibition of characteristics (e.g., courtship display) that are designed to attract rather than repel. Indeed, so important is the attracting-attractiveness dimension that there evolved multi-colouring in fish and plumage in birds; these evolved even at the expense of anti-predator abilities.

In the last chapter we introduced the ideas of evolved response rules, psychobiological response patterns, social mentalities and the concept of domain specific reasoning and evolved algorithms. Now consider the following. The reasoning of the depressed person is (often but not always) focused on negative data and inferences about the self and the world (Beck et al., 1979); they may judge themselves negatively in comparison to others (Swallow & Kuiper, 1988); attention and memory shift towards the negative (Blaney, 1986) and various psychological abilities are impaired (Miller, 1975); there is loss of energy, reduced positive affect (Clark & Watson, 1991), and the depressed person becomes generally hopeless (Beck, 1976; Abramson, Metalsky, & Alloy, 1989; Alloy, Abramson, Metalsky, & Hartledge, 1988) and pessimistic (Seligman, 1989). Looked at from sexual selection theory, depression results in poor abilities to compete for resources and depressed people are unattractive (e.g., as mates or allies) to others (Coyne, 1976a,b).

Three questions arise therefore: (1) is the depressed person locked into specific reasoning modules, algorithms, and internal organisational patterns that act to inhibit their actions and produce loss of energy to pursue biologically relevant goals? (2) could such a style of reasoning and psychobiological response patterns have evolved, i.e., do they have an innate basis? (3) are rank (social place) evaluations associated with these patterns?

In this chapter we shall answer these questions affirmatively and suggest that the depressed response pattern evolved from ranking behaviour, on the one hand, and algorithms for ingroup–outgroup behaviour, on the other. Specifically, it will be suggested that an important component of depression is involuntary, subordinate self-appraisal or perception (the older term, taken from Alfred Adler and Karen Horney, would be inferiority complex). However, I would stress at the outset that involuntary, subordinate self-perception is not equivalent to low self-esteem. For example, an endogenously depressed lady became ill when new noisy neighbours moved next to her. This was her retirement home with which she had been pleased for some years. No appeals to them or the council did any good and she developed the idea that they had completely ruined her life. She felt "as if my life is controlled by them". Her experience was of powerlessness and entrapment (she could not afford to move). At no time did she accept that she was to blame or there was anything bad about her. Indeed, quite the opposite. The junior doctor's appeal that maybe she could learn to cope with the noise only made her worse. In our theory her depression was centred on involuntary subordinate self-perception; that is a lack of social power and the experience of her life as being dominated by others and that she had been defeated.

One the other other hand self-esteem is, in the majority of cases, linked with involuntary subordinate self-perception (Chapter 7). In this book we shall be concentrating on this linkage.

The potential for involuntary, subordinate self-appraisal and its co-assembled affects and behaviours, evolved (perhaps) precisely to inhibit an animal from challenging for breeding resources in situations that it could not win. The archetypal root of involuntary, subordinate self-appraisal can therefore be considered from the point of view of ranking behaviour and the evolution of reasoning systems (basic algorithms) that make ranking behaviour possible.

There are five central ideas that inform this approach:

1. Social comparison as a basic evaluative (or reasoning) ability (algorithm) for all animals that form ranks and exhibit ingroup–outgroup preferences.
2. The psychobiological response and state patterns that flow in the wake of certain types of social evaluation and social events (those that signal social failure) mirror changes noted in depression.
3. The role of internal inhibitory mechanisms are essential to allow ranks to form and be viable, and subordinates in various primate groups are more inhibited than dominants.

And in the next chapter:

4. Reassurance has evolved as a way to control arousal consequent to rank differences in recent primate and human

evolution. The need for reassurance has become central to the social behaviour of humans.

5. The major shift in how humans rank themselves, via the display of attractiveness and talent rather than aggression and power, underlies many of our tactics to gain and maintain self-esteem.

THE IMPORTANCE AND PREVALENCE OF SOCIAL RANKING

The idea that the human capacity to become depressed evolved from changes of psychobiological state consequent to ranking (dominance) stress is not new (Price, 1972; 1988; 1989; Henry & Stephens, 1977; Henry, 1982; Gardner 1982; 1988; Bergner, 1988). However, Price (personal communication) has pointed out that, whereas there is increasing research into renal disorders, immunological deficiency and cardiac disease, as a consequence of aggression down the hierarchy (and there is growing evidence that being the recipient of "down hierarchy aggression" is associated with various risks of organ failure), psychopathologists have yet to engage in detailed and coherent psychobiological research studies of ranking stress (although see Henry, 1982). If depressive states evolved from defensive responses to rank stress on the one hand, and outgroup fear on the other (as I shall argue) then the first question is, why should animals rank themselves? The short answer to this is that a rank provides a social infrastructure that allows animals to reduce the degree of energy expenditure in competing/fighting where conspecifics are going after the same resources (Barash, 1977). That is, the recognition of rank difference reduces aggressive behaviour and exerts an effect on resource accessibility (Dunbar, 1988). Ranking is above all a means of deciding social control and preferential access to resources. Subordinates occupying a low rank position have little social control over access to breeding resources, are tense and biologically stressed (e.g., Henry & Stephens, 1977; Sapolsky, 1989).

Ranking behaviour is an important dimension of human social life and covers a diverse set of social concepts. It is implied in terms such as social power, dominance, status, respect, prestige, and authority (Clark, 1990; Kemper, 1988, 1990a,b; Kemper & Collins, 1990; Gilbert, 1990). We may speak of the status of individuals, groups, or nations. Objects can also be described as "status symbols" and even abstract ideas (e.g., academic theories) can be ascribed a rank/status. The common thread that runs through this diversity is that there is a natural tendency to understand, think about or construe relationships, between things, people and objects, in terms of some ranked relationship, and these constructions influence our attention and behaviour towards them.

In humans, ranks can arise from the power to move against others but also the ability to attract others and have social attention and status bestowed. Savin-Williams (1979, p.923) explored dominance hierarchies in young adolescents and found that: "The dominance hierarchy appears to foster a reduction in intragroup antagonism, to focus division of labour responsibilities, to distribute any scarce resources, and to provide knowledge of where one's social place is among peers". Female ranks are more related to situation than male ranks and are more flexible. The sociologist Kemper (1988; 1990a,b; Kemper & Collins, 1990) makes a distinction between power hierarchies derived from threat/aggression and status hierarchies derived from positive social behaviours. Arnold Buss (1988) has recently suggested that dominance (which is a rank related trait) has three components: (1) aggression; (2) non-aggressive competition (i.e., competing in a beauty contest, or expression of talent) and (3) initiative taking. Apart from deviant groups, on the whole humans acquire status by the demonstration of positive qualities about the self (e.g., talent, abilities, knowledge, beauty etc.).

However we might think of rank, there are important consequences to gaining and loosing it. Be it academic theories or individuals, those that have a high rank are accorded (usually) more attention and resources than those that have a low rank. Although ranks are properties of relationships (Dunbar, 1988) individuals also form internal schematic representations (or cognitive affective maps) of their position/location in these relationships. Also, Clark (1990) notes how emotions provide internal information about one's relative standing and threats to it. Positive affects are associated with gaining rank (e.g., pride) and negative affects are associated with losing it or not having it (Gilbert, 1990). Furthermore, our affect towards others is related to perceptions of their relative rank, power or status. To some extent this internal representation provides information for the construction of social comparison (Swallow & Kuiper, 1988; Wood, 1989; Suls & Wills, 1991) and self-esteem (Barkow, 1975; 1980). The ways of human ranking are complex however, and often depend on a voluntary bestowing from others (e.g., parents, friends, teachers, bosses) and what we could call audience participation. Also, in humans, rank is often influenced by the roles an individual can perform and their functional utility to others (e.g., medicine, law, mother, friend, etc., Crook, 1986). Considerable training may be undertaken to prove competency to fulfil a role and hence be "worthy" of respect.

The evolution of ranking via attractiveness is the source of our next chapter; here we are primarily concerned with the aggression side of

TABLE 6.1
The Two Ranking Systems Showing Possible Outcomes Associated with a Perception of an Involuntary Inferior-Subordinate Position

COMPETITIVE RANKING[a]
Inferior ↔ Superior
Controller ↔ Controlled

RANKING SYSTEMS
(TACTICS)

POWER AGGRESSION	ATTRACTIVENESS
Cohesion	Talent
Threat	Role competence
Authoritarian	Democratic-authoritative
To be obeyed	To be valued
To be reckoned with	To be chosen

IF SELF IS CONSTRUED AS LOSING/INFERIOR

Shame
Envy
Hostile resentment
Revenge
Depression
Social Anxiety
Defeated
Controlled by others
Involuntary subordinate
Internal attack

[a] The relationship of self-other can be internalised leading to self-attacking or self-valuing

ranking. However, these two chapters are part of the same theme and need to be considered together to convey the complex of changes that have occurred to human ranking dispositions. Table 6.1 is designed to offer an overview of these ideas and concepts, both for this and later chapters. It outlines the two forms of social ranking and depicts the various phenomena and internal experiences that can be associated with involuntary, subordinate self-perception.

INGROUP–OUTGROUP

Our main focus in this chapter is with ingroup ranking behaviour and the affects, behaviour, cognitions, and biological correlates that go with it. However, we should keep in mind that the issue of ingroup–outgroup often lurks here also. The beliefs of inferiority tend to arouse both primitive anxieties of subordinacy and also the persecutory anxieties of being an outsider. We should note that animals come together in groups for various reasons, one of which is predatory pressure (Trivers, 1985). Early humans were not only subject to predatory pressure, but were also subject to hostility from other humanoid groups (Itzkoff, 1990). Having a place in a group was vital for safety and social success (and, as we noted in Chapter 5, in general social success tracks reproductive fitness). Wenegrat (1984, pp.114-115) suggests that:

> The persons comprising a group with which an individual maintains contact will inevitably be those with whom he or she has specific interactions of a sexual, competitive, dependent, or nurturing kind. Nonetheless, it is possible to argue that an individual's relationship to a group as a whole is not determined by the sum of his or her interactions with persons in the group, and that social strategies exist that predispose men and women to perceive social aggregates as unitary bodies. They either seek them out or avoid them, according to previous experience.

The idea that we can relate to a group as if it were a unitary body helps us to understand why ingroup–outgroup evaluations are often strongly associated with a sense of social place and rank. The selection for ingroup–outgroup distinctions possibly arose from kin selection (Wenegrat, 1984). Small hunter-gatherer bands tended to be genetically related. However, whatever the root of such behaviour and discrimination, it seems that humans are particularly sensitive to group membership, and self-identity is related to it (e.g., Brown, 1986; Abrams, Cochrane, Hogg, & Turner, 1990). The social algorithm is probably *same/similar-different*. The degree of "fit" of a member to their group is central to rank and popularity (Wright, Giammarino, & Parad, 1986). This construct system, as we shall see throughout this book, can be strongly aroused in depressed people. Depressed people often see themselves as different from others and are fearful of this difference being revealed. We shall explore the implications of this evolved need to belong and feel similar to others in Chapters 7 & 8.

In our society people can find themselves in groups which they did not select—e.g., in coming to a new job or school, or moving to a new location; others are, as it were, already there and one attempts to relate to them. If they turn out to be unsatisfactory there may be limits on the opportunities to move off to another group. On the other hand we can voluntarily seek out groups with whom to share interests and goals. These can vary from sporting and hobby groups and religious groups to more aggressive groups like the Klu Klux Klan. What attracts us to a particular group reflects our personality. What determines our ability to come and go depends on a variety of factors (fear of loss of support if one leaves, activating the aggression of the group, having alternatives to go to, etc.). And groups exert pressure to belong and conform (e.g., trade unions). Yet again we can join groups for reasons unassociated with the group's activities (e.g., the man/woman joins the tennis club to find a spouse). For the moment, however, we wish to focus on the evolution of mental mechanisms that may underlie ingroup ranking behaviour.

THE ORIGINS OF RANKING: CLUES TO THE EVOLUTION OF DEPRESSION?

If ranking behaviour is a major source of depression then one way of illuminating this is to attempt to trace the themes and tactics of ranking over phylogenetic time. The reader should appreciate, however, that there will be a degree of artificiality about this way of analysing ranking and it runs the risk of glossing over many complexities. For example, we can only study species as they are now and not how they were millions of years ago. On the whole, I think the risk is warranted.

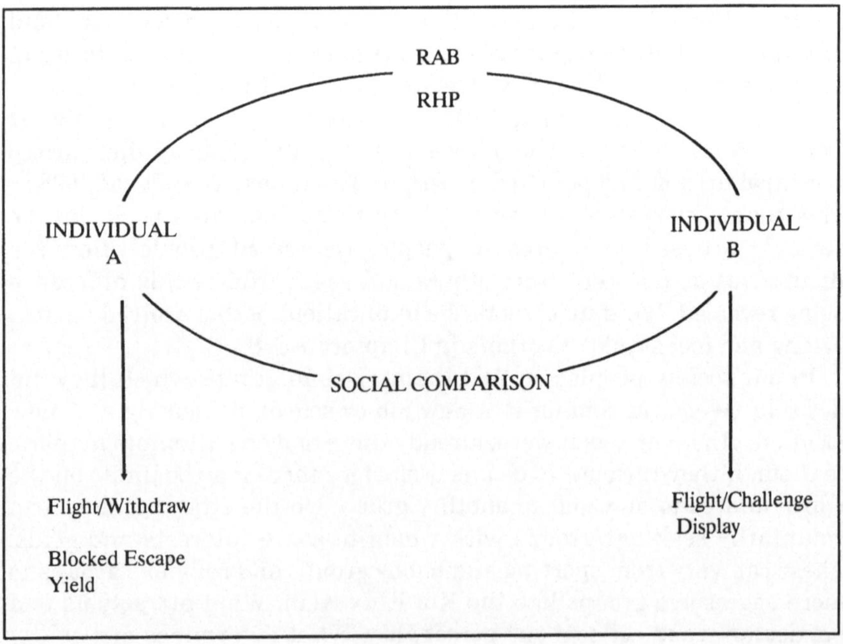

FIG. 6.1. Behaviours in territorial intraspecific competition.

Territorial ranking

The beginnings of our story go back a long way. Both reptiles and birds form ranks which result in ownership of a breeding territory. In many cases the territory owner has the advantage (Archer, 1988; recognition of ownership is important in primates also, Dunbar, 1988). When contests for territory occur there is a particular kind of interactional display. First, the contestants face each other and stand erect, stiff-legged, and/or puff themselves up; they engage in what is called ritualistic agonistic behaviour, RAB (Lorenz, 1981; MacLean, 1977, 1985; Archer, 1988). There may be various head-bobbing and sideways movements. This may be a stand-off situation and still occurs in humans, such as standing erect and meeting eye gaze, especially when there is to be a physical contest (e.g., in boxing, wrestling, and American football perhaps). To maintain eye gaze in such situations is to show a lack of fear. This is a very primitive power signal. The standard "body stiff and erect" postures of armies on display, engage a similar muscular pattern to reptiles (MacLean, 1985).

The display ritual of RAB forms part of what is called "an assessor strategy". Maynard Smith (1982), using game theory, showed that the assessor strategy is evolutionary stable. It allows an individual to work out if the contestant facing them is stronger or weaker and then respond appropriately. In technical terms the animals display to each other their fighting ability, strength or resource holding potential/power, RHP (Parker, 1974; 1984). If an animal evaluates it would lose if it came to a fight (i.e., has unfavourable relative RHP) it is free to take flight relatively uninjured. So it's quite important that the animal gets that judgement of comparative strength correct, not only to avoid getting into (or prolonging) dangerous fights, but also to contest those situations that it could win (and be socially successful in). The animal that evaluates it is stronger than its contestant is free to engage in fight (i.e., is not inhibited or avoidant). This situation is outlined in Fig. 6.1

Now in reality things are a little more complicated (Archer, 1988) but three main points at issue here are: (1) the necessity and evolutionary advantage of the ability to assess the self in relation to the other (mutual evaluation), that is to be able to make an evaluation/calculation of relative or comparative RHP, called social comparison; (2) the ability to move against another or away subsequent to this evaluation; and (3) the very primitive origins of social comparison. There may be various such (internal and external) reasons why an animal cannot move away from an aggressive dominant and we will call this blocked escape and entrapment (discussed shortly and in Chapter 15).

Displays of RHP (and, in humans, self-presentation) allow animals to weigh each other up; that is to evaluate (the strength of) each other. Exactly how they evaluate whether to disengage or fight is unknown since, although each can see the other, they are unable to see themselves. Various cues such as eye angle and body size/shape (Hinde, 1987) enter into this evaluation, but as we shall argue shortly, however the calculation is made, it is to a large degree an internal calculation that is also context dependent (Hinde, 1987; Gilbert, 1989). The fact that animals cannot see themselves but only the other, suggests some kind of internal algorithm(s) for making these calculations which allow self–other matching. These social algorithms can be effected by various events (e.g., past history of success or failure, age, hormonal state, etc.).

This evaluative competency/ability, with its associated fight/flight response options seems to be highly conserved in gene-neural structures (Gardner, 1988). Although the criteria for making social comparisons in humans have become rich and complex (Festinger, 1954; Swallow & Kuiper, 1988; Wood, 1989; Abrams et al., 1990), nevertheless, the biologic linkage between social comparison and ranking behaviour may lie in these primitive breeding strategies.

Blocked Escape

So first comes the evaluation (which does not require a high level cortex) and then the response. In general, the main coping responses in territorial species are fight and flight and birds often have skirmishes at the boundaries of their territory. However, in limited territory or where escape (ability to move away) is not possible (called blocked escape) we see a different pattern. For example, Schjelderup-Ebbe (1935), who coined the term "pecking order", described the consequences of losing dominance in farmyard fowl, where escape to a new territory was not possible. Following defeat the bird's:

> ... behaviour becomes entirely changed. Deeply depressed in spirit, humble with dropping wings and head in the dust, it is—at any rate, directly upon being vanquished—overcome with paralysis, although one cannot detect any physical injury. The bird's resistance now seems broken, and in some cases the effects of the psychological condition are so strong that the bird will sooner or later come to grief. (As quoted by Price & Sloman, 1987)

Schjerlderup-Ebbe (1935) made the point, which others have confirmed, that this "coming to grief" is the result of the animal's change of state and not the result of physical injury. Because this state of defeat often follows loss of rank, Price and Sloman (1987) have called it the *yielding subroutine of ritualistic agonistic behaviour*. MacLean (1985) noted how reptiles that had lost rank, lost their bright colours and died shortly thereafter. The important point is that defeat is not too much of a problem provided the animal can escape. It is only when escape is blocked that the serious changes of state occur. A similar response set to uncontrollable trauma has been found using the learned helplessness paradigm (Seligman, 1975; see pages 174–180 this volume).

These types of finding allow us to zero in on ranking relationships as offering possible clues to the evolved function of depression. For example, did the early programmes for depression evolve to inhibit animals in situations of social competition that they would lose and where escape was impossible? From inclusive fitness theory, might the serious biological changes that result from defeat plus blocked escape act to reduce the numbers of animals occupying and utilising resources in a limited space? (For a similar view of suicide see deCatanzaro, 1980.) If defeated animals die off quickly might this have inclusive fitness benefits—for example by making way for kin? Has this "go down and die" process been modified in subsequent adaptations or is human depression something totally new with very different origins? If depressives reduce their claim and contesting for resources, what does this mean for inclusive fitness?

However, at this point these are only clues. I do not wish to enter into too much speculation and such propositions are difficult to test. At this point I would say that, in ways that are obscure, increased mortality and depression do seem linked. I am not convinced we had an adequate theory of this (although Seligman's, 1975, book was originally named *Helplessness: On depression, development and death*). Nevertheless, if the reptilian brain exerts more control over our behaviour than we would like to admit (e.g., Bailey, 1987) then these findings should be considered when we think about the biological changes that are part of involuntary, subordinate self-appraisal (i.e., sense of inferiority).

GROUP LIVING AND THE STRATEGIES OF INGROUP RANKING

Once the basic plan or archetypal mechanism for group living evolved, then various subsidiary tactics for surviving, competing, and living in close proximity with conspecifics followed. In primates there appear to be two basic forms of group living noted by the typical interactional styles shared by conspecifics (Chance, 1988a,b). These are called the agonic and hedonic modes. In the *agonic mode* (the type for most primates) conspecifics are oriented towards aggression or its inhibition (via submission/appeasement). In the *hedonic mode*, noted primarily in chimpanzees and humans, the orientation is more affectional with high levels of reassurance and reconciliation following agonistic encounters (although this is usually reserved for ingroup members). In this chapter our analysis of depression is primarily on the agonic mode. In the next chapter we will consider changes brought by hedonic life styles.

The Agonic Threat/Aggress-Submit System

In group-living animals there is no home base, nest site or territory to contest. Rather animals remain in close proximity to each other. Escape is now blocked (in part) by internal factors. The reason for this is that to escape/flee the group would reduce breeding chances in the future and increase chances of predation. The breeding strategies of group living require that those who are inferior to the more dominant animals are (often) internally prevented from leaving. If this were not so then we would be back to spaced/territorial structures. However, animals sometimes migrate from one group to another and males or females may leave their group of birth. Species vary in this regard (Dunbar, 1988), but humans also can leave groups they are disgruntled with (Haviland, 1990).

Dunbar (1988) has pointed out that breeding success must be estimated over the lifetime of an animal. Animals that have short life spans and few chances of breeding may function differently from animals that have longer life spans and a number of chances of breeding from year to year. When lifetime chance is calculated it becomes apparent that there are at least two possible strategies: (1) a high-gain/high-risk strategy which means that an animal might do very well, especially when in its prime, but could also do poorly if beaten or weaker than others; (2) low-gain/low-risk that offers moderate success but extends over the breeding lifetime of the individual. There are a number of strategies that might be associated with low-gain/low-risk such as accepting a subordinate position and waiting to take over a harem or waiting/working with allies for help, or being sneaky and opportunistic.

The social comparative competency (evaluation of relative strength and chances of making a successful challenge) has been maintained in primates. They form dominance hierarchies, and evaluation of comparative or relative strength remains an important component of how they behave towards each other and maintain group cohesion. When the control of social behaviour is via threat/aggression the group structure is called agonic, meaning that the behaviours in subordinates are designed to inhibit, limit or terminate ritualistic agonistic behaviour when in close proximity to more dominant or powerful animals (Chance

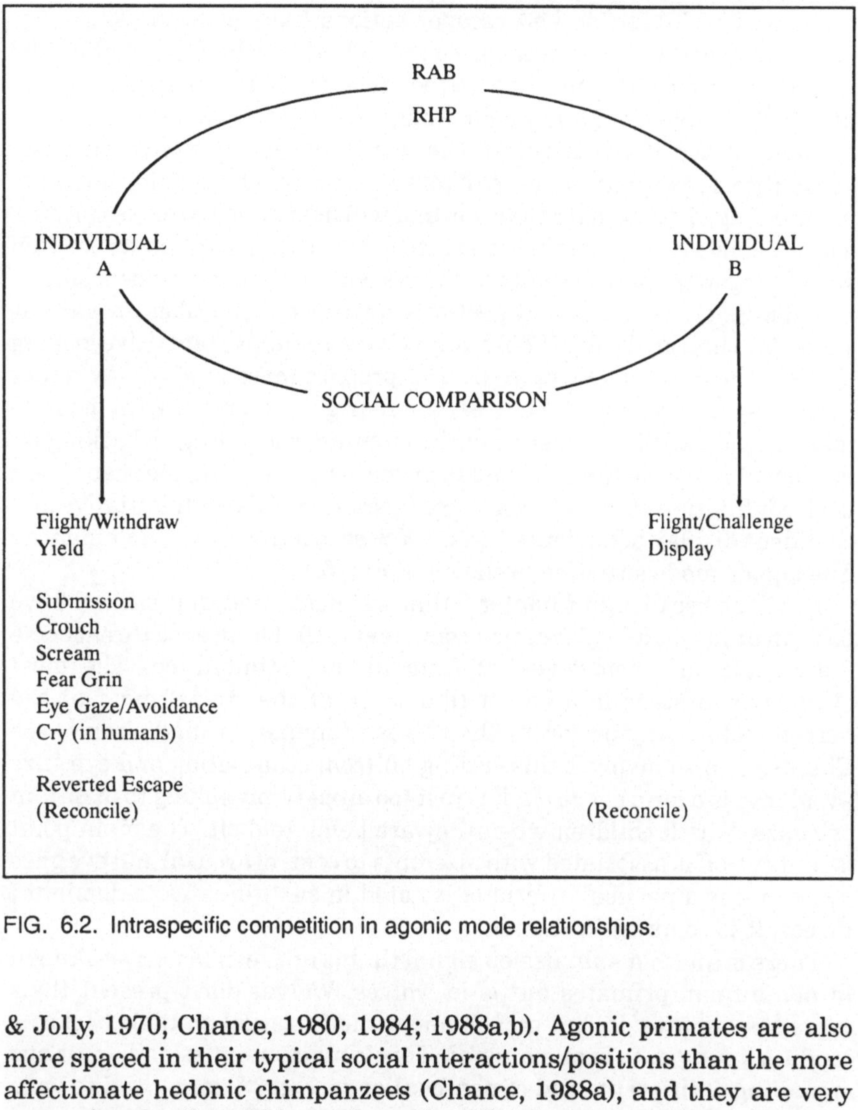

FIG. 6.2. Intraspecific competition in agonic mode relationships.

& Jolly, 1970; Chance, 1980; 1984; 1988a,b). Agonic primates are also more spaced in their typical social interactions/positions than the more affectionate hedonic chimpanzees (Chance, 1988a), and they are very wary of each other. This wariness is called braced readiness (Chance, 1980; 1988a), indicating a high level of self-defensive–protective arousal, facilitating a preparedness to engage in submissive or retreat behaviour should the need arise, or even counter-aggression.

Submission Signals

In group-living animals inhibition and control of RAB is necessary, to avoid constant fighting. Hence, two very important adaptations to the flight and yielding (blocked escape) options have evolved. These are submission and reverted escape. An individual who believes that he/she is weaker than another has to be able to: (a) avoid eliciting an attack/challenge from a more dominant and (b) be able to terminate a possible attack if elicited. In other words there is a nonverbal body vocabulary for expressing an animal's evaluation of itself in relation to another (e.g., I am weaker than you and will not challenge for resources). These signals also convey a high state of arousal. A solution for dealing with living with more dominant others is submission and appeasement.

Submission postures and gestures have been described in various ways (Mitchell & Maple, 1985) but involve screaming, repetitive looking at, then away, or sideways glances, a preparedness to give way under challenge, a lowering of the eyes, the fear grin, crouching the body to make it look smaller rather than threatening, retreating or backing off or "down", lowering the chin, and in primates, presenting the rear. There is also inhibition of initiative and confident display. (Both initiative and confident display behaviours Buss, 1988, sees as aspects of dominance.) The agonic mode situation is shown in Fig. 6.2. [1]

It will be recalled in Chapter 5 that we mentioned that stimuli have both an arousal and information component. Under intense threat some individuals cut themselves off from further stimulation. The most obvious example is in a horror film when at the crucial moment the person looks away or covers their eyes. Submission (and shame, see Chapter 8) also involves this cutting off from stimulation and eye gaze avoidance is a form of cut-off; it is just too anxiety-provoking to maintain eye gaze. Watch children when they are being told off. The main point is that cut-off is associated with attempts to control arousal and eye gaze avoidance is a particular form of it noted in subordinates to dominant threat. It is common in shame.

There is another submission signal that is not seen (as far as I know) in non-human primates but is in wolves. Wolves don't present their rears as primates do, but crouch and sometimes roll on their backs as might a young or juvenile animal. This kind of submission is perhaps signalling a different kind of non-challenge, e.g., "I am a child to your adult" (Price, personal communication, 1990). Also in birds, females may beg food in order to reduce male aggression. Both these are examples of signalling child-like status to inhibit conspecific aggression. Humans can also show tearful behaviour as an act of submission, and tearful behaviour has been identified as a submissive act (Buss & Craik, 1986). Tearful behaviour would only be classified as a submissive act in the context of conflict however. Interestingly, males may be more eager to suppress these signals in order not to be seen as submissive and weak (but again I stress the context is important). Tearfulness can also be elicited as part of an attempt to elicit reassurance behaviour from another. Individuals may burst into tears after being shamed/humiliated by a dominant (e.g., an attack by the boss or parent) which acts both to signal that the attacker is recognised as being stronger in some way, and a need for reassurance. Such signals may also produce guilt in the dominant and efforts at reparation from the dominant or attacker/shamer.

The facial expression of the "fear grin" is also an important submissive signal. On the way to becoming human, the fear grin may have been adapted to the smile and become a signal of no threat—i.e., as a way of avoiding the elicitation of aggressive behaviour and relaxing the other (Hinde, 1987). The smile is often used as a signal of friendship and reassurance and is seen as attractive rather than a mark of inferiority. Most individuals appear less threatening when they smile.

In general then, there are a number of social signals and gestures that can be elicited *involuntarily* to the evaluation of a social event. However, from our current perspective the most important aspect of submission and the awareness of being in an inferior position is the activation of *internal inhibition*. That is, subordinates are less explorative, initiate less (except perhaps grooming others), and are tense. Their psychobiological states are very different compared to more dominant animals (Henry & Stephens, 1977; Henry, 1982; McGuire, 1988) Furthermore, inhibition, resulting from dominance relations within a group, have been put forward as an explanation for the passivity and inhibitedness in some group therapy members, especially those who are depressed (Kennedy & McKenzie, 1986).

Signals of Power

Price (1988) has suggested that signals of social power can be classified in two ways. Signals that are emitted with the purpose of reducing rank/status or maintaining a conspecific in a subordinate position can be called catathetic signals. These involve various signals of threat, put-down or non-recognition of another's attempts to achieve status/respect. Signals that boost status in others are anathetic signals. These can be involuntary, such as submissive signals (a receiver of submission signals from another has their dominance and social power confirmed), or voluntary. Voluntary anathetic signals relate to various forms of respect, morale boosting, appreciation, and adulation.

At a behavioural level catathetic signals relate to signals of punishment and signals of non-reward. Anathetic signals relate to rewards. This links with Gray's (1982) concept of a behavioural inhibition system which monitors the environment for rewards and punishments.

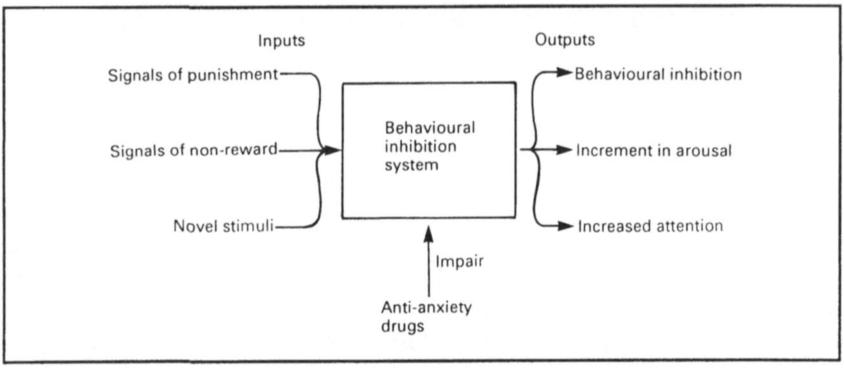

FIG. 6.3. The behavioural inhibition system (Gray 1982).

A major aspect of this model is the role of non-reward in activating the behavioural inhibition system. Two factors are involved here: (1) the amount of rewarding, reassuring or anathetic signals a person needs to overcome any internal defensiveness or inhibition; and (2) the internal models of self (in specific social settings) that in part determine whether reassurance and reward signals are necessary or to what degree and type. In some contexts the lack of anathetic signals acts like catathetic signals (i.e., lack of positive rewards or reassuring social signals activate the inhibition system). The degree and type of social reward/reassuring signals perceived to be needed may arise from internal models of self. If we see ourselves as higher in status/rank that others then inhibition is much less likely, for one evaluates that one could cope with any threat signals from subordinates. Also the more safe we feel in ourselves and the less reassurance we need, the less inhibited and more open we are likely to be.

Our evolutionary theory is not a brainless science but attempts to form links with what we know of basic brain structures (Gilbert, 1989). However we believe that behaviourists have often ignored the social domain and social evolution in particular. They fail to recognise that social success is of prime importance to the evolution of mental mechanisms. Once this is recognised then many of the debates between behaviourists and other types of theorist (e.g., Bowlby 1980; Kohut, 1977) become less competitive and more a matter of focusing on commonalities (see Chapters 10 and 14). The concept of catathetic and anathetic signals only relate to social rewards and punishments. These signals relate to issues of social control, power and belonging, and internal models of self and others. As mentioned previously (Chapter 4), our social signals either offer respect, love, status, reassurance to self or others, or withhold it.

Nonverbal Behaviour

If we are saying that depression is somehow about the activation of basic programmes of submission and/or defeat/yielding then we should be able to note this in nonverbal behaviour. Unfortunately the evidence here is not clear. In regard to nonverbal behaviour it has become apparent that the relationship of mood to nonverbal behaviour is exceedingly complex.

Ellgring (1989) reviewed the literature and reported on an extensive set of experiments with depressed patients exploring eye gaze, speech pattern, facial expression, and gestures. I can only mention some of the conclusions here. The relationship of nonverbal behaviour to mood is complicated by large individual differences and personality factors; nonverbal behaviour is only moderately associated with depth of depression; modes of expression vary from situation to situation and person to person; individual changes are relatively stable for that individual; a variety of facial expressions are observed in depression, not just the sad face for example; at the individual level, gaze and speech change in a state-dependent way. Unfortunately, Ellgring does not control for rank difference in interaction. A depressed unskilled worker who has never been near a hospital may behave quite differently compared (say) to a depressed university professor undergoing the same experiments. One may view the experimenter as very dominant and the other as much less so. This does not change our basic theory since individuals may choose their common social groups with which they compare themselves (Abrams et al., 1990).

The issue of individual variation is highlighted with exemplary cases. For example, exploring four cases of endogenous depression, in one case both eye gaze and speech pattern were closely associated with mood changes. For another, the association was negligible with various changes in mood state occurring despite an abnormal gaze pattern. For the third patient, changes in mood were primarily associated with changes in gaze behaviour while for a fourth changes were primarily associated with changes in speech activity (p.141). Hence, Ellgring (1989, p.169) concludes: "...it cannot be expected that each of the behaviours reacts to mood changes, to a similar degree, for all individuals. Moreover, different expressive functions have to be taken into account. Facial expression can indicate short term negative affects, gaze social reactivity etc." In other words Ellgring brings our attention to the fact that there may be various combinations of affects in the depressive experience—e.g., anger, anxiety, sadness, etc., and that these will influence different aspects of overall nonverbal presentation. Any depression can involve blends of different, negative affects and reduced positive affects (Clark & Watson, 1991; Watson & Clark, 1984).

One other aspect of Ellgring's (1989, p.172) findings should be noted. They compare endogenous and neurotic depression.

> In general endogenous depressed patients showed marked reduction in nonverbal behaviour more frequently during depression and had more marked changes with improvement than neurotic depressed patients. In contrast, neurotic depressed patients more frequently remained stable in their nonverbal behaviour or contrary to expectation it was even reduced with improvement of subjective well being.

The author suggests that this may be because the endogenous patients were treated with drugs and improved more rapidly. However, they also found that in regard to smiling, some neurotic depressives actually came to smile less as they improved and his explanation does not account for this. It is possible that endogenous depression may represent the activation of a more primitive defeat/yielding response (whose phylogenetic origin is reptilian), while neurotic depression is more linked in with the group-living submissive response. This has credence since the smile evolved from the submissive, appeasement fear grin (Hinde, 1987) and the reduction of smiling in some neurotics may represent a reduction of appeasement signalling. Unfortunately, ethological concepts such as submissive signals are hardly discussed in this work.

In general, depression often results in powerful verbal and nonverbal communication patterns. From an evolutionary perspective such communication needs to be considered in terms of the four questions posed by the ethologists: function, survival value, development, and phylogenetic origin (see Chapter 5). These changes in communication change the attractiveness of a person (e.g., as a confidant or friend) and elicit from the social environment responses that may act to maintain depressed behaviour and negative perceptions of the self (e.g., Coyne, 1976a,b).

Verbal behaviour follows different rules to nonverbal behaviour. For one thing a person can contradict what they said: "I didn't mean it that way." A negative message given with a wink changes the whole meaning of the message. Here, of course, lies the basis of the double bind. A person says, "I love you," but their nonverbal behaviour does not conform with loving (i.e., is tense and cold). Many researchers now believe that it is nonverbal behaviour that has the most powerful effect on our emotions. This makes sense from an evolutionary point of view since so much of our phylogenetic history has been concerned with decoding and responding to nonverbal behaviour. This causes considerable difficulty in depression research. Two people may claim to feel equally inferior, but observation shows they behave with others in very different ways. Hence, verbal reports as indicators of some biological state may be extremely unreliable.

Obedience/Conformity

Another human behaviour that relates to perceived rank and submission is obedience to authority. Milgram (1974) demonstrated that individuals can be made to behave in harmful ways (e.g., delivering apparently painful electric shocks) to others and the only factor that seemed to be responsible for such acts was human preparedness to ascribe rank to others (i.e., endow them with authority) and then to obey them (submit to their orders). It would seem that the presence of authority figures acted to inhibit more prosocial moral behaviour (Sabini & Silver, 1982). Hence, again, we see the powerful inhibitory effects that perception of dominance/rank can produce. In Milgram's experiments subjects continued to do what they were asked even though it was clearly distressing to them to do it. Inhibition of moral behaviour in order not to offend a more dominant individual is a very serious issue for humans.

We also know that individuals will change their minds if confronted with others who have different opinions. For example, Asch (1956) found that individuals could be made to change their judgements of the relative length of a line in the face of others who gave a different judgement (these "others" were primed by the experimenter to give the wrong answer). Why would someone change their opinions to conform, and in the face of clear evidence that they are correct and the others are wrong?

Scheff (1988) argues that this is the result of fear of being different and invoking scorn. Exploring this research from the point of view of there being a basic conforming/deference system he notes (p.403, italics added):

> A reaction that occurred both in independent and yielding subjects was the fear that they were suffering from a defect and that the study would disclose this defect: "I felt like a silly *fool* ... A question of being a *misfit* ... they'd think I was queer. It made me seem weak eyed or weak headed, like a black sheep.

In our view this arises from a basic submission system consequent to fear of being perceived as weaker/inferior, and also fear of being seen as different from others. Note how these two types of concern inferior (being a fool) and being different from others (a misfit) arise together. It goes without saying that to be seen as different is usually only a problem if this is associated with inferiority in some way, otherwise a person may take pride in their differences (see Abrams et al., 1990, for a more complex discussion). The exception to this is fear of envy (see Chapter 8). The effects of depression on conformity have not been well studied but Katkin, Sasmor and Tan (1966) found that depressives tend to be highly conformative in their values and attitudes, suggesting perhaps an increased disposition to submissiveness and need to signal ingroup membership. (See also Wenegrat, 1984, for a discussion of the importance of cognitive conformity and group identification.)

Reverted Escape

Submission is concerned with the inhibition of aggression. However, there is a primate adaptation to the sequence of threat–submit interactions that should be noted. A threatened subordinate may actually return to (move towards) the source of the threat (higher ranking individual) and seek reconciliation. This sequence of withdraw and return to the source of threat has been called reverted escape (Chance, 1980; 1984; 1988a). Jane Goodall (1975) has given graphic descriptions of this. Young chimpanzee males that have run into trouble and been hurt by a dominant may return and hound the dominant for stroking and reassurance, even throwing tantrums if they don't get it. It is usual however, for the dominant to gently stroke the younger animal until it becomes calm. Hence, reconciliation has become an important social behaviour following agonistic encounters and acts to reduce the level of tension between individuals. Reverted escape and reconciliation are examples of approach behaviour used in the service to control fear. Religious confession is one example of reverted escape (e.g., going to one's priest in a certain apologetic, submissive way and seeking forgiveness, which offers a sense of relief and continued acceptance from a powerful other, e.g., God). They are designed to solicit certain behaviours from another member of a group and this act of solicitation is crucial to understanding subsequent evolved changes in social and ranking behaviour. Flight and withdrawal however are basically avoidance strategies, to stay away from threat.

Chance (1988a) has suggested that a dominant animal may activate the reverted escape behaviours in subordinates by threatening or biting them and in this way test the "loyalties" of those in his group. Consequently, aggression and threat are used to bind individuals to the dominant and ensure continued attention to him. Human tyrants can punish others, or make "examples" and teach lessons, for similar reasons—to ensure or renew compliance. If these aggressions are unpredictable then this will further raise the arousal in subordinates and increase their attention to the dominant.

Chance (personal communication) also suggested that certain forms of dependency which involve returns to an aggressive other may actually reflect this process of reverted escape. The aggression of the other keeps a person in a very subordinate, inhibited position yet at the same time movement away also increases the attractiveness of the dominant via desires for reconciliation and needs for security. (Some religions know well this mechanism.) This kind of emotional dependency (which I would see as quite distinct from other forms of attachment) bodes ill for women who remain attracted to their abusive husbands. However, it is perhaps more common for women to be forced into a subordinate position by abuse which inhibits their own problem-solving and explorative behaviour. This is reinforced by serious economic and socio-cultural restraints (lack of support from family or friends) and concerns to be able to provide for self and children. This in effect acts as a form of blocked escape.

Explorative Behaviour

In the agonic mode, subordinates are in a state of high arousal (Henry & Stephens, 1977; Sapolsky, 1989), called braced readiness, which, at the same time is a form of inhibitory control (Chance, 1984; 1988a,b). This general blocking of explorative and resource acquiring behaviour is probably the result of the avoidance of risk of eliciting the aggressive attentions of the dominant. This behaviour is very easy to see in humans. For example, think of the committee or group situation where the leader is a rather aggressive-dominant sort of person. At these meetings arousal can be high, but the amount of exploration and free exchange, fun and play is very low. If the dominant is called away or is absent then the whole situation may change. People start bouncing around ideas (exploring), telling jokes, and so on. Hence, the inhibitory effect of aggressive individuals is easy to see. This inhibition is the result (in part at least) of the relationship for, as Gardner (1982) has pointed out, animals that have behaved in a subordinate and inhibited way may completely change their behaviour with removal of the dominant. Such effects are easily seen from a behavioural (operant) point of view (that is, the dominant acts as an aversive stimulus, blocking exploration).

In human depression we may be tapping into a more internal block on exploration flowing from unfavourable models of the self. McGuire (1990) has recently noted that exploratory behaviour is very low in depressives. For example, he observed that if a non-depressed individual has to achieve a number of things (e.g., go to the bank, buy groceries, pay some bills, etc.) then finding a queue at the bank results in a shift to getting the groceries and returning to the bank when the queue may be shorter. The non-depressed switches plans quickly to achieve goals. However, the depressed person, finding the same cue at the bank stays there and is unable to switch plans. This, we would argue, represents a significant block on free, explorative (initiative-taking) behaviour. A different line of research (Isen et al., 1987; Isen, 1990) suggests that positive affect is associated with creative problem-solving, which in our view is associated with low levels of internal inhibition and open explorativeness. McCrea (1987) also found that individuals who are "open to experience" tend to be more creative. Hence, explorativeness, creativity, and flexibility probably relate to low levels of internal inhibition and are negatively associated with high submissiveness or sense of personal defeat. However, it may be that any individual who is rank and power orientated may also be less "open to experience" and less creative than individuals who are less rank or power focused (for a fascinating discussion see Hampden-Turner, 1970). On this issue further research is needed.

The suggestion is that one can be blocked in explorative behaviour from within and without. Low self-esteem, commensurate with negative social comparison (inferiority), tends to reduce explorative behaviour and this is because it has been biologically adaptive (in agonic groups) for subordinates to be inhibited. So if there is some kind of inhibitory mechanism that switches in, and is associated to subordinate status, could such a mechanism influence other general processing systems? Quite possibly.

Energy

Lader (1975) found that, as measured psychophysiologically, the basic state of depression is retardation (see also Barlow, 1991). Agitation, if and when it occurs, is superimposed on this basic retardation. Explorative behaviour requires a certain energy and certainly not psychophysical retardation. One symptom that depressives often complain of is loss of energy and this loss of energy is different to sleepiness. In sleepiness we may be relaxed, have difficulty keeping our eyes open, but sleep is refreshing. In depressive fatigue and loss of energy states we are rarely sleepy, our bodies feel slowed down or heavy with various feelings of tiredness or achiness in muscles, sleep may not be refreshing and is disrupted. Fatigue is a complex state (Kennedy, 1988; Blakely et al., 1991) and its relationship to psychophysiological retardation (Lader, 1975) is unknown. It has effects on attention, information processing, and distractibility and often accompanies certain organic and viral disorders. In one sense sleepiness may tell us that we need to sleep whereas fatigue may tell us that we are in no fit state to compete in life. Hence fatigue is related to exploratory behaviour and many patients tell us that they are unable to explore or carry out tasks for they feel just too tired to do them and can't muster the energy. Loss of energy is also noted in low, positive affect states (Clark & Watson, 1991).

In depression some patients experience acute losses of energy. For example, a patient managed to get out of bed and go to the shops. When she returned she collapsed on the bed and stayed there for some hours. After an argument a patient may say how they felt drained of all their energy. Psychomotor retardation may also be part of depressive fatigue, but agitation is not the opposite of fatigue and agitated patients also complain of loss of energy.

In ranking theory it is possible to suggest that part of the control system for explorative and competitive behaviour involves biological processes that regulate energy. Margaret Thatcher is a good example of someone who seems to need little sleep and is rarely fatigued. She is also known for being highly dominant and autocratic (power is energising). One should stress, however, that fatigue states are complex and here we simply introduce the possible linkage of fatigue, explorative behaviour, and perception of power and social control. Also internal evaluations of one's general energy level can feed into negative self-perceptions, sense of inferiority and incapacity, and predictions about obtaining future goals. Fatigued individuals are often unattractive as friends (see next chapter, they rarely take the initiative), especially if one feels one has to continually boost them up. People often say how "draining" they find a depressed person. Energetic people are attractive, (chronically) fatigued people are not.

Information Processing Capacity

Cohen, Weingartner, Smallberg, Pickar, and Murphey (1982) suggest that the more difficult a task and the greater the level of effort required, the greater the probability of deficits being manifest in depressed individuals. They suggest that in depression there is a general deterioration in the capacity to structure and organise responses. This may be in response to general cognitive efficiency change, and/or general changes in a central motivational system. Whether this is related to fatigue and whether other (non-depression) causes of fatigue produce similar effects is unknown. Weingartner, Cohen, Murphy, Martello, and Gerdt (1981) examined both qualitative and quantitative changes in information processing in depression. Generally, depressed patients exhibit difficulty in structuring inputs for recall, but when provided with structure, learning deficits were not significant. These data may link with the evidence presented earlier (Gilbert, 1984) that disturbance in brain-stem activity may make it difficult to "switch analysers". This, we could argue, is the result of inhibition of explorative behaviour. Problem-solving behaviour requires the ability to switch options around in one's head, "to play" with various possibilities.

If there is high internal inhibition then this capacity may be reduced. The consequence is that the capacity to integrate new information and be creative may also be reduced. It follows that psychotherapy must have an element that reactivates the explorative system, reduces internal inhibition, and allows new forms of information to become integrated. In this way new organisations of information and insight might be possible. At one level therapy is a kind of play (not in the "funny game" sense, but in the relaxed explorative sense).

On the biological side, drugs can significantly affect information processing capacity (Davis, Hollister, Overall, Johnson, & Train, 1976; Warburton, 1979). Henry, Weingartner, and Murphy (1973) and Glass, Uhlenhuth, Hartel, Matuzas, and Fischman, (1981) demonstrated that depression-drug-information-processing interactions are highly complex. Findings suggest that antidepressant drugs may improve brain state efficiency before affecting mood. This area is controversial, however, as a review demonstrates (Thompson & Trimble, 1982). For example, the cognitive functioning of normals given non-MAOI antidepressants tends to deteriorate, while for depressives it improves. Lyons, Rosen, and Dysken (1985) found that antidepressants affected instrumental behaviour and that changes in social behaviour may be secondary to increased levels of general activity.

Memory. Explorative behaviour requires at least some degree of anticipation of good outcome. If one anticipates failure then there may be little point in exploration. It is of interest therefore that memory for positive and negative events may influence explorative behaviour. I know of no research in this area, however. What we do know is that depression has a negative effect on memory. Depression is associated with poorer recall of positive memories compared to negative memories, especially for specific personal memories (Blaney, 1986; Williams & Scott, 1988). It is a possibility that this inhibition in recall of positive information is associated with involuntary, subordinate self-appraisal and the inhibitory mechanisms that evolve to reduce challenge behaviour in subordinates.

Brain State Patterns

So far we have tried to make links between a number of research findings that at present seem unconnected. Ranking theory may be able to show how they are linked together. The suggestion is that the need to form groups meant that some individuals (subordinates) had to be inhibited from challenging for resources in order to: (a) reduce agonism and maintain group cohesion and (b) avoid eliciting fights, or be able to terminate conflicts that they could not win. This is mediated by general inhibitory processes consequent to recognition of low rank. In depression the brain state is such as to ensure reduced challenging and explorative (resource gathering) behaviour. Consequently, its pattern involves reductions in efficient cognitive processing, inhibition of explorative behaviour and creative thinking, distortions in memory, reduced effectiveness of positive reinforcers (they lose their energising properties), and in humans, self-organisation giving rise to perceptions of inferiority, weakness, and inability. Depressed people also send unattractive signals (Coyne, 1976a,b) and in severe cases they lose all interest in their own appearance. This signal of low attractiveness also signals a reduced competency to attract breeding partners; these are signals that one is "out of the running".

Chance (1988a; personal communication) has argued that those who are (or become) orientated to the outside world as if the social structure were agonic in form (i.e., there are more powerful threatening others around who can exert control) attend to, and selectively process information from, the social environment in a self-defensive or harm-avoidance way. Attention and reasoning is not open and free because so much attention is taken up with keeping out of trouble. This is clearly marked in therapy where fear of shame and attack inhibits a person from exploring their own memories, feelings, and cognitions (Mollon & Parry, 1984, and Chapter 8 this volume). This is associated with shut down or shut out self defensive-protective behaviours. With the development of safety, such that the social environment is not seen to be a source of threat, then the attention structure becomes more open. In this state inputs can be integrated by virtue of explorative and curiosity mechanisms, new insights and possibilities arise, growth and integration of mental mechanisms become possible (see Chapter 5). Previous memories, for example, that remained in a state of inhibited processing, can now be re-worked and integrated with new affective responses (Greenberg & Safran, 1987; Safran & Segal, 1990).

In the next sections of this chapter we explore in more detail what might be going on inside the depressed person, especially their internal relationships and patterns of biological state.

THE INTERNAL REFEREE

Greenberg (1979; Greenberg et al., 1990) noted that many theories of psychopathology have drawn attention to a basic split in self-relationships. An individual can become the object for their own self-attacks. The gestalt therapist Perls, for example, suggested that we could be split into topdog–underdog and that the topdog acts like an internal bully. The topdog engages in repetitive hostile put-downs (Greenberg, 1979). In behavioural language this is internal self-punishment. Why has the mind evolved to be able to function thus, since its effects are to reduce exploration and initiative taking, reduce the chances of achieving goals and seem quite non-adaptive?

Earlier we suggested that the ranking dimension of behaviour relies on a certain type of (evolved) algorithm or social reasoning module. If this is true then depressed persons may talk to themselves as if they are subordinate (for a more detailed discussion of how these reasoning models become internalised, and directed at the self, derived from the ideas of George Herbert Mead, see Gilbert, 1989). A clue to the internal mechanisms of the control of the depressed state has been suggested by Price (1988, p. 162):

> Another thing to strike me is that the constraint of giving up is imposed on the yielder from within. The winner does not stand guard over what it is he has won; he assumes that the loser will behave like a loser and not either recontest the issue at a symbolic level or escalate to a level at which death or serious wounds are likely. The instructions of the yielding subroutine are like an internalised referee who says: 'You have lost. Behave like a loser.' The yielding subroutine is a symbolic or ritual equivalent of death or serious physical incapacity, in the same way as the elaborate threat signals of RAB are a symbolic equivalent of hitting and biting. This is consistent with the fact that many depressed people feel incapacitated, some feel dead and others feel like 'losers'.

What Price (1988) has indicated here is the possible presence of an innately available, psychobiological response pattern (no different in principal to the idea of there being an innate anxiety based fight–flight mechanism for dealing with threats) consequent to defeat in a no-escape situation. The importance of an animal going down and staying down has been discussed already. Without some mechanism that powerfully puts a brake on the animal's (breeding and resource acquisition) aspiration level agonism would escalate to points that were maladaptive.

The yielding internal referee is also a reasoning module of sorts in that it changes the self-evaluative process considerably as well as access to positively and negatively toned memory. Now in animals, internal reasoning or evaluative algorithms are obviously not represented in internal language or self-dialogues. However, humans can have (but often do not, Greenberg & Safran, 1987; Brewin, 1988) conscious access to their internal evaluative algorithms and can elaborate them. Interestingly, patients may have difficulty in putting this sense of inferiority into words, but experience it at an affective level. Images can be powerful for helping this articulation. One patient described her inner sense of self as a lump of distorted black plastic. Hence, people can "sense" and "feel" inferior even though in putting it into language they may see it is irrational. However, all humans have an archetype for subordinate functioning; it is not learnt but can of course be developed (and/or emotionally conditioned) to various self-perceptions by life experience. However, the internal referee does not always involve changes in self-perception (remember the lady with the noisy neighbours, page 144) but there is always a sense of defeat and being overpowered in some way. Another example is of someone who construes their state in terms of illness rather than any personal badness or ability.

When the sense of subordinancy is linked to self-evaluation (as it most often is) then the Freudian equivalent would be a hostile super-ego. The "self as subordinate" algorithm can be articulated in self-constructions and self-dialogues as a result (say) of early parenting that was hostile or authoritarian. Indeed, there is now much evidence that those with low self-esteem come from either neglectful or authoritarian families (Coopersmith, 1967; Rohner, 1986) and that depressives see their parents as rather low on warmth (see Chapter 10) and requiring them to submit to the parental wishes (McCraine & Buss, 1984). However subordinate self-perception becomes articulated or activated (be it via genes, learning, and/or current environmental contingencies) the internal dialogue, style of reasoning with and about the self, will be predominately one that inhibits action. Consider the internal dialogue of a depressed, suicidal woman (Firestone, 1986, p.443):

> ... I tell myself things like 'just be quiet. Don't say anything. Don't bother people with what you have to say. Just stop talking. Shut up. Just don't say anything, okay? Just don't bother me okay? I don't want to hear anything from you.'

We see here the extreme negativity of the self and the blocks on outward directed behaviour being operated from within. Usually things are not quite so graphic but people talk of the internal voices, or what Beck (1976) calls automatic, self-evaluative thoughts: "You're a failure, you are all washed up, who would love you? what have you got to offer?

you're pathetic, etc." As Beck says, while this style of reasoning and thinking dominates the person's evaluative life there is little chance that the things necessary to break out from the depression will follow. This is an agonic type mentality, it is an internal representation of agonic dominance relations. The self experiences both the anger of the put-down and the sense of weakness/badness that the attack produces (Greenberg et al., 1990).

So then the theory suggests there is a mentality and associated special reasoning ability, laid into gene-neural structures that evolved from situations of forced subordination and blocked escape. It is an archetypal experience, a way of construing the self and inhibiting action. It has a built-in biological code.

Another key question is the degree to which appraisals of signals acting on one's own sense of inferiority are conscious and go through conscious cognitive mechanisms before they activate submissive or yielding states. Can early memories play a role (see Chapter 10)? On this question the evidence is unclear. One view is that, as for most animals, yielding need not be conscious (although it often is in humans). Indeed in all kinds of states of inhibition a person may consciously hate what their body insists on doing with them. Generally, then, the person does not wish to be depressed but biologically the programme is up and running, the response rule is activated. Furthermore, in nonverbal animals these response rules and algorithms convey their instructions by changing the biological state of the organism (Henry, 1982).

THE BIOLOGY OF INVOLUNTARY SUBORDINATE STATUS AND THE LOSS OF CONTROL

Changes in physical state, as a result of changes in the status hierarchy, have also been noted in reptiles (Maclean, 1985) who may not only lose their colours but may die. In primates, 5-HT appears sensitive to status relationships (Releigh, McGuire, Brammer, & Yuwieler, 1984) as does cortisol (Henry & Stephens, 1977; Leshner, 1978; Gilbert, 1989; McGuire, 1988; Sapolsky, 1989). Androgens are also affected, as are central neurochemical processes (Henry & Stephens, 1977). Subordinate females come into their breeding cycles later than dominants, possibly as a result of the social stress of being in a subordinate position (Bowman, Dilley, & Keverne, 1978; Kevles, 1986). Also physical display characteristics are sensitive to rank position (Price, 1989) and low ranking birds are inhibited from display by the displays of higher ranks (Hinde, 1982). Subordinate animals may be more vulnerable to depression and to certain types of losses (Rasmussen & Reite, 1982).

Learned Helplessness

One question the reader may ask is: "How similar is ranking theory to that of learned helplessness?" This is a central issue. The antecedents of the experimental data on helplessness stretch back some 40 years. In 1948 Mowrer and Viek discovered that if rats were pretreated with inescapable shock they demonstrated subsequent deficits in escape-avoidance learning. Some 20 years later Seligman and his colleagues (Overmier & Seligman, 1967; Seligman & Maier, 1967) studied the effects of inescapable shock on escape-avoidance learning in dogs. In this procedure dogs were placed in a Pavlovian harness and inescapable shocks contingent on a conditioned stimulus (CS) were presented. The original idea was to study the incubation of fear produced by inescapable shock. When the dogs were released from the harness and allowed to learn an appropriate escape response, a majority (though not all) of these animals demonstrated considerable difficulty in learning how to avoid the shock. Instead of actively attempting to avoid the shock, following the presentation of the CS, many of the pretreated dogs passively accepted the shock in a clear state of distress. Seligman found that this passivity was very difficult to extinguish. This apparently unexpected finding led Seligman to postulate that, rather than "no learning" in the inescapable situation, these animals actually learnt that their responses were ineffective in controlling the shock. Subsequent research (Seligman, 1975) points to this being a very reproducible finding in a variety of species.

The idea that learning about the uncontrollability of trauma could have powerful effects on subsequent behaviour led Seligman to suggest that there may be a parallel between such learning and depressive states. Seligman (1975, pp. 53-54) reasoned that:

> When a traumatic event first occurs, it causes a heightened state of emotionality that can loosely be called fear. This state continues until one of two things happens; if the subject learns that he can control the trauma, fear is reduced and may disappear altogether; or if the subject finally learns he cannot control the trauma, fear will decrease and be replaced by depression.

Thus, the central axiom of the learned helplessness theory is controllability. Although the above extract suggests that anxiety is replaced by depression, when a trauma is perceived as uncontrollable, this "replacement" idea does not appear to be crucial to the learned helplessness theory. Rather it is controllability over reinforcers in general that relates to depression. In this way Seligman attempts to provide a solution to the so-called success depressions. (However, in our model, success depression may relate to being promoted out of one's ingroup and not feeling a sense of belonging in the new group situation).

While Seligman has popularised the helplessness view and has pointed up many parallels between learned helplessness states and depressive states (Seligman, 1975, especially p. 106), there are, of course, many other theorists who place special emphasis on perceptions of helplessness (Bibring, 1953; Lazarus, 1966; Beck, 1967; 1976; Melges & Bowlby, 1969, to name but a few). Nevertheless, it is probably fair to suggest that much of the subsequent research on learned helplessness and depression was largely stimulated by Seligman's ideas.

The early work on helplessness has been extensively extended by Anisman and his colleagues (Anisman, 1978; Anisman & Sklar, 1979; Anisman & Zacharko, 1982; Anisman, Suissa, & Sklar, 1980a, Anisman, 1980b) and also Weiss (Weiss, Glazer, & Pohorecky, 1976; Weiss et al., 1979; Weiss & Simson, 1985). Interest has focused on synthesis-utilisation rates of brain amines in specific brain areas as a result of loss of control. There is some evidence to suggest that in uncontrollable stress situations utilisation outruns synthesis, producing monoamine depletion. The processes are complex and may involve a number of mechanisms in the rate limiting steps of catecholamine production (e.g., changes in tyrosine hydroxylase, MAO, presynaptic receptor mechanisms, and so on).

Anisman and his colleagues have shown that various drugs which deplete monoamine stores can produce behavioural coping deficits similar to those associated with inescapable shock. Moreover, MAOI's tend to protect against the development of behavioural deficits associated with inescapable trauma.

Anisman (1978, pp.159-160) has provided an excellent summary of the neurochemical changes associated with stress, and for conciseness and clarity this is reproduced in full. The following observations have been noted:

1. Moderate levels of stress tend not to affect the endogenous level of NE and 5-HT. Given that stress does result in faster disappearance of labelled NE and 5-HT, and since stress after enzyme inhibition results in greater reduction of NE and 5-HT, it is probable that stress increases both synthesis and release of NE and 5-HT.

2. Besides increased synthesis of amines, partial inhibition of MAO occurs, thereby preserving NE and 5-HT. The net effect of the increased synthesis of amines together with the MAO inhibition is that the demands of the organism are met. Indeed, with relatively mild stress, an initial increase of NE and 5-HT levels may be observed.
3. With intense stress, a decline in endogenous levels of NE and 5-HT is seen. Presumably, synthesis does not keep up with utilisation. The effectiveness of NE released apparently is also reduced by increased reuptake of NE under these conditions.
4. With mild stress, DA, ACh, and 5-HT are unaffected. As the stress severity increases, ACh levels rise. While DA has been reported to decrease, the effect of stress on DA is considerably less pronounced than on NE neurons. The differential effects of stress on DA and 5-HT relative to NE might indicate that the former two systems have superior regulatory systems, thereby maintaining balance between synthesis and utilization of the neurochemical. [. . .]
5. Under conditions of stress, activity of anterior pituitary hormones increases, as do levels of plasma corticosterone.
6. Under conditions in which control over the stress is possible, whether this is considered in terms of actual escape/avoidance responding or coping by fighting, NE levels are not found to decline. Moreover, the source of degradation is also varied away from the side of COMT and toward MAO. Additional reports also indicate that with controllable stress neither ACh nor corticosterone levels are affected.
7. The effect of stress on neurochemical activity varies as a function of the excitability of the organism and may vary as a function of the strain involved.
8. After repeated exposure to the stress, neurochemical adaptation may occur, i.e., NE and corticosterone levels, which might otherwise vary, remain constant after exposure to stress over a series of sessions.
9. Stimuli associated with stress may come to elicit neurochemical changes.

Anisman makes it clear that it is the controllability which is crucial for determining the patterns of neurochemical change. The observation is so consistent that its importance cannot be overemphasised. In a human research, Breier et al. (1987) found that in laboratory conditions even a mildly aversive stimulus (uncontrollable noise 100db) activated the hypothalmic–pituitar–adrenal axis. Over recent years researchers have focused on the role that different amine and other biological systems may play in the effects of lack of control (e.g., see Weiss & Simson, 1985; Willner, 1985; Healy & Williams, 1988) and debate continues as to which of the amine and other biological systems are the more important and in what way, drawing distinction between acute helplessness (which may dissipate within days) and more chronic forms. Most now agree that it is the pattern of changes in neurotransmitter pathways that is important to this distinction. However, recall that rank also is a dimension of social control.

Learned Helplessness: A Basic Plan?

Learned helplessness theory has become one of the most important theories of depression for a number of reasons: (1) it is a clear psychobiological theory that outlines a relationship between control and biological change. It therefore indicates that severe biological disturbance can be reactive and not the result of an autonomous disease process; (2) the effects of helplessness have been observed in many species suggesting that it is a highly conserved psychobiological response pattern in evolutionary terms. It is in this sense an archetypal potential; (3) the effects of loss of control on avoidance learning, explorative behaviour, vegetative and appetitive processes are so consistent as to suggest that this is a basic plan and not a random effect of psychobiological disorganisation producing arbitrary effects; (4) it provides a testable theory with clear predictions and has stimulated an enormous amount of research.

In the literature there have been notes that fighting might protect against helplessness and that subordinate animals might succumb more easily to helplessness. For ranking theory these are important observations, but as far as I am aware little has been made of them.

As discussed in Chapter 5 and later in this book, it is helpful to understand depression as a change in internal patterns of organisation. In 1984 an earlier version of this book was called *Depression: From Psychology to Brain State*. The title told the theme. At this time I was concerned to put across this aspect of pattern organisation. As here, I reviewed some of the evidence that biological changes to events (e.g., uncontrollable trauma) produce biological effects that could influence cognitions. Hence, it was possible to have a negative life event/uncontrollable stress–biological change–negative cognitive style relationship. Negative cognitions could modify or maintain the biological state of depression. A rather more sophisticated approach, but with the same idea, has been developed by Healy and Williams (1988) to explain the patterns of symptoms of depression (e.g., vegetative, cognitive affective, behavioural). They focus on circadian rhythms as part of the disrupted pattern in depression. However, the evolutionary implications of disturbance in circadian rhythms is unclear.

Nevertheless, this is a fascinating attempt to explore pattern changes in depression and link them with learned helplessness research. In this chapter we have explored the idea that internal inhibition, triggered by involuntary, subordinate self-perception and/or a sense of entrapment, may block the exploration of coping options necessary to overcome depression. Also, the actions of others (e.g., put-downs, criticism) may maintain involuntary, subordinate self-perception (Hooley & Teasdale, 1989).

Ranking Theory and Learned Helplessness

It is obvious that experimental helplessness does not require negative self-perception. How does ranking theory fit with learned helplessness theory? First, I do not see any major conflict between helplessness theory and ranking theory. Both draw attention to the issue of perceived defeat and controllability of outcomes. Ranking theory, however, addresses the problem of depression from a purely social perspective. Many of the social dimensions of control are ignored by the learned helplessness theory. Second, ranking theory argues in favour of innate social algorithms (social comparisons) that set the internal conditions of inhibition in social interaction and in this sense opens us up to a more complex analysis of helplessness that links it directly with self-esteem (see next chapter). Further, the aspect of internal self-attacking is understandable from ranking theory (see pp.172–173) but is less clear with learned helplessness theory. Third, ranking theory also points out that submissive behaviour and the issue of perceived defeat evolved from social living. Hence, the internal modulators (in everyday life) of helplessness experience are most often related to social evaluations or micropolitics as Clark (1990) calls them. We do not know whether subordinates show disturbances in circadian rhythms, although we do know that they show heightened cortisol functioning which originates in the CNS (e.g., McGuire, 1988; Sapolsky, 1989).

There is much work to do before we really understand how helplessness theory and ranking theory relate to each other. They make different predictions however. These are:

1. Helplessness brought on by non-social events (and perceived to have little impact on long-term social success) would extinguish faster than helplessness brought on by inferiority or social events, especially if the person remains in the presence of others who are seen as (more) dominant.

2. Ranking theory helps us understand why a pattern of response options, especially those of shame, anger control, assertiveness, envy, self-attacking and the social complexities of the depressed person often arise together (see Chapters 8 and 15). All these are potential responses to the perception of low status and being involuntarily subordinate. Helplessness theory has little to say on these issues.
3. Ranking theory makes predictions about the expression of hostility in depression. It suggests that up hierarchy aggression is often inhibited but not down hierarchy aggression. Hence, the depressed person may behave in a more subordinate, inhibited, and anxious way in the presence of those who are seen as potentially stronger or superior but irritability and anger may be expressed in the presence of those seen as inferior. As Price (personal communication) points out it is not unusual to find the depressed man complaining of his depression but his wife and children complaining of his anger. However anger control in depression is complex (see Chapter 8).
4. Ranking theory would predict that the more inferior the negative self-perceptions the more closely post traumatic stress disorder will mirror depressed-like states. For example, aggression will be more inhibited in situations of negative self-evaluations following trauma, whereas in the absence of inferiority beliefs anger may actually be more likely to be expressed (see Riley, Treiber & Woods, 1989).

At this time I will leave the issue of the relationship of ranking theory and helplessness theory as an area for future research and discussion. My main concern has been to direct attention to the potential for a fuller integration of learned helplessness theory and ranking theory.

RANK AND THE ISSUE OF THE OUTSIDER

In the above sections we have explored the evolution of ranking behaviour and the origin of involuntary, subordinate self-perception. However, as we mentioned earlier, this is not the whole story. One of the other characteristics of the depressed person's thinking is that they also see themselves as different from others (see next chapter). How does this perception fit into our story?

Same–different evaluations are very important to group membership (Brown, 1986). For example, Wright et al. (1986) point out that, while aggressive and withdrawn children are often unpopular, in groups of aggressive children, aggression does not lead to unpopularity as often as might be expected. Thus, the degree of "fit" of the child's behaviour to the group norm can be a better predictor of popularity and acceptance. Gardner (1988) has suggested that there is a separate basic plan (or social algorithm) for evaluating and responding to ingroup and outgroup members and making these judgements of "fit". He suggests that a strong sense of being an outgroup member can elicit feelings of paranoia and being subject to persecution from others. And of course outgroups are often persecuted and victimised. Wenegrat (1984) explores the evolutionary influence for selection of this kind of behaviour. There is, therefore, an archetypal fear of outsiders and also of being made an outsider. Many films and other forms of art reflect this basic fear. Furthermore, group membership is an important aspect of self-esteem and self-identity (see Abrams et al., 1990, and Chapter 7 this volume). Another interesting observation is that following loss of rank an animal (e.g., in gorillas) may take up a solitary life. Once someone has involuntarily fallen in rank (been deposed) they can be ejected from groups quite quickly. Group living, therefore, runs parallel with the need to feel part of a group, supported by a group, and hence free from potential persecution. Lone primates often find it difficult to be accepted in a group unless they can make some bid for dominance or attract allies. In humans also non-acceptance can elicit aggression, but submission/ withdrawal/ avoidance is probably more common.

Unfortunately, human history shows that for an outgroup member, submission may not terminate attacks (Itzkoff, 1990) and those identified as different/outsiders can be killed and tortured (sometimes in a terrifying manner, e.g., the holocaust). In the process they are rendered "inferior, scum and vermin". Like subordinates within groups, outsiders are often denied access to resources. The need to belong is, therefore, of great importance for humans to feel safe. (Some personality disorders do not have this social affinity, e.g., schizoids, but nevertheless can have fears of persecution).

It not surprising, therefore, that much of what we do, feel, and think is related to our experience of ourselves as being part of, or becoming an ingroup member and avoidance of being an outsider. The old sociological term was alienation, although this does not convey the fear that can be involved with outgroup membership. But even without fear, outgroup members are unlikely to be socially successful. Thus, if affects track social success or the potential for success (see Chapter 5) it is not surprising that the sense of being different and alone is so common in depression. Self-help groups can help enormously because they provide a reference group, break down the sense of being different and alone (the only one who feels or thinks this), reduce the sense of inferiority, and can send reassurance signals (Wilson, 1989). The problem about this is that some depressives may be too depressed to send such signals, be non-communicative and self-focused, and envious.

At the present time further work needs to be carried out on how (a) the algorithms for "social place estimates" within a group and (b) those for estimating whether one actually belongs to the group are related and are coassembled. While the ranking algorithms provide for the *superior–inferior judgements*, the ingroup–outgroup judgements arise from *same/similar–different* algorithms. Because networks and alliances (which are both family and friendship based) have become so important in humans (see Chapter 7), our internal evaluative algorithms, for making both types of judgement (rank and belonging or "fit") have become linked. In the latter case we tend to orientate ourselves to the group in general, i.e., "them" or "us".

The non-depressed paranoid feels an outsider but not inferior. The depressed paranoid feels both inferior and different from others. By exploring the relative involvement of ingroup ranking evaluations and those of being different or an outsider, we may be able to furnish clues to the distinction between neurotic and endogenous depression (see Appendix C).

VOLUNTARY AND INVOLUNTARY SUBMITTING/YIELDING

There is a major complication to the above story. It is obviously true that most of us most of the time do not reach particularly high status and we are happy playing in the lower ranks; examples may also be subordinating oneself to a leader or religious figure. In some situations we are quite happy to have our behaviour directed by others (Gilbert, 1989). Hence we need to make it clear that the kind of "subordinate self-perception" we are discussing is involuntary; the person would prefer not to be subordinate, or "out of the running". It is also the case that an individual may not fully accept the subordinate status that another person is trying to push them into, in which case more aggressive/resentful behaviour is likely. Indeed, in many depressives we can see complaints about how others treat them and aggressive outbursts may be followed by collapse into more submissive/yielding states. As we shall see in Chapter 8, anger control (as distinct from assertiveness) is actually quite complex in depression.

However, this dimension is rather more complex that this. Suppose you are standing in a queue and a seven foot criminal-looking type pushes in front of you. In one sense you voluntarily don't argue, but since this is a fear-based backing off it is also involuntary and you may be very resentful. Suppose an old lady pushes in front of you, again you may concede (because you would feel guilt at telling old ladies to get to the back of the queue) but not willingly and may feel resentful that they have pulled rank of "old age". However this is not fear based as it clearly is with the seven-footer. Suppose someone puts you down. You may voluntarily agree and self-blame, but how far is this fear based and an effort to maintain support and not escalate conflict? Andrews and Brewin (1990) found that when women were in an abusive relationship they blamed themselves but when they left the relationship they changed to become more partner blaming. In depression, it is common to hear of the accommodating and submissive style which was designed to win love and affection.

Suppose you have a virus and start to feel you have no energy to fight the usual day-to-day hassles. Hence you may start to back down or out of life's arena because you just don't feel up to it. Many depressed people complain about this aspect and say: "If only I felt better I could get on with my life", and many are convinced they are physically ill. This is also involuntary yielding but not necessarily submitting (although the person may come to feel inferior because of their feeling state). The chairman who gives up due to ill health has clearly had to yield but again not willingly and not from fear. Rather his biological state informs him (by reducing his energy) that he is not up to the tasks of the job. If he voluntarily accepts this and comes to terms with it then he may be spared depression. But he if cannot come to terms with it he may become depressed.

Suppose your family have groomed you for high office (e.g. to be a famous brain surgeon) but in your heart you would like to be a painter. Here you would like to back down and give up your status but are constrained from doing so (e.g., don't wish to disobey your parents or feel you must continue to work in medicine). In this sense you cannot voluntarily yield. Eventually our surgeon may get depressed and have to yield.

There was recently a documentary on people who had accidents. Two cases struck my attention; let me mention one. A person had a prestigious job in the film world. He felt unable to get out and in many ways didn't want to, but he was drinking heavily, sleeping badly, had thoughts of suicide (which he didn't fully understand) and had become reckless. Following a bad car accident he was out of action for nine months. During this time he had to slow down and had time to reflect. It occurred to him that he did not want to go back to his old life style. At first he became more depressed but then began to think that maybe he didn't have to go back. As this thought grew in his mind he felt, he said, "a burden lift from my shoulders and for the first time in my life I felt free. I then realised how depressed I had actually been all those years." True to form there was a history of a very ambitious mother in his early life.

The point of this digression is that in humans yielding and giving up is actually very complex. There seems at least three dimensions: voluntary–involuntary, fear-related–not fear-related, and conscious–nonconscious; and therapists need to be sensitive to this. Sometimes a patient needs to stand up for themselves more and not back off, at other times they need to learn how to bow out gracefully without feeling inferior. All the therapist can do is to facilitate a process that does not activate involuntary, subordinate self-evaluation and sense of having been defeated. This is why I think that if patients consistently refuse to down themselves they are less likely to get depressed. If we could be more open to our own needs without self-downing or seeing ourselves as inferior then we would be spared much suffering, as the Rational Emotive therapist Ellis (1977a,b,c) tells us.

These themes will come up in various disguises throughout this book.

SUMMARY

1. Rank is a key social dimension for all social animals. There are specific styles of processing/reasoning (e.g., social comparison and mutual evaluation) that, in animals using ritualised contests, allow them to make estimates of their relative rank and respond accordingly.
2. In territorial animals defeat is rarely a problem unless escape is blocked and then we see major changes of state occurring. The subsequent defeat-blocked escape repertoire may be an early forerunner of later depressive responses in humans (especially endogenous depression?). Defeat can be internal in the sense of a gradual recognition that one is not achieving one's aspirations.
3. A number of defensive and self-protective responses have evolved with group living that are organised around an agonic mode—that is where aggression and its inhibition are central social dispositions.
4. The tactics are basically to dominate those who are weaker and submit to those who are stronger. In these groups it is the subordinates who, to a large degree, are responsible for recognising who are stronger or more powerful, submitting to them, inhibiting their (overt) reproductive behaviour and challenge for resources (explorations). Via their submissions and general states of inhibitedness, tense arousal and

vigilance to the more dominant, they are enabled to control the levels of aggression within the group. Hence, their states of internal inhibition, social anxiety, and wariness, in this context, are not maladaptive. When these relations of dominance recognition, and the threat/submit relationships are not in place, as in overcrowded zoo conditions, the outcome is often fatal for many (Stevens, 1982). But again I should emphasise that these are simplifications.

5. Depression (may have) evolved as a motivational (internal) state to reduce aspiration level and inhibit agonism, it is the "go down stay put" programme. But this programme will have been modified to fit different social environments. Specifically, there may be two archetypal forms: defeat arising from blocks to, or reversals of, up-hierarchy motivation, and high submissiveness directed at other conspecifics.
6. These basic programmes have been extensively modified over evolutionary time but, nevertheless, remain as potential responses to perceptions of defeat, inferiority or low rank, making the individual more fearful of others, more avoidant and/or more compliant. Low mood may be the motivational state that set the (internal) parameters and conditions that would lead to (the speed of) giving up or not challenging.
7. There are biological similarities between low rank, status, and depression and these underlying state variables control the various behaviours discussed above. Learned helplessness appears to share many of the same basic mechanisms of low rank.
8. Ranking theory is a new way to conceptualise depression and in this sense it can, at present, give only crude approximations to underlying mechanisms. This analysis should not be taken too literally but only as marking out an area of study, an approach yet to be developed.

CONCLUDING COMMENTS

We humans like to think that we are created somehow anew. Maybe we have never really come to terms with Darwin's dethronement of us. It is true of course that humans are capable of much more than other animals and we shall address this issue in the next chapter. However, evolution is conservative, a bit of a hoarder; it does not throw things away but rather adapts them to new purposes (Lorenz, 1989, gives some fascinating examples of this). Most of us are aware of the our appendix, for example, that does not do much but can kill you nevertheless. If we take the idea of the triune brain (Chapter 5) seriously then, as Maclean (1977; 1985) and Bailey (1987) point out, these different structures of the brain do not always work smoothly with each other. Second, it is probably incorrect to assume that cognitive evaluative processes only go on in cortex or at some high level. Many brain structures seem to be responsible for specific forms of evaluation (Ornstein, 1986).

In this chapter we have explored the idea that there are primitive "potentials" that exist within the brain that (mostly) are now are maladaptive. Modified versions of the defeat programme may be adaptive to the extent that we give up pursuing the unobtainable. But such adaptive responding requires that the subsequently evolved moderating aspects be working. Hence, a disappointment is not turned into a major defeat. But if, for some reason, these modifications don't work too well then more primitive and crude changes may take place. Furthermore, we may have internal working models of ourselves, built up from previous interactions with others, that actually facilitate their recruitment rather than inhibit them (e.g., being labelled or treated as inferior, or subordinate, by siblings and parents). And more often than not, we may inhabit a social world were we are in reality constantly being subjected to various forms of put-down—in our marriages, at work and in the economic structures of living—that convey a sense of inferiority in more subtle terms.

Only now are psychologists beginning to wake up to the enormous importance of social power, something that philosophers have been concerned with for hundreds of years. And even those who profess to be interested in power usually do not recognise how large a role social power (accommodating oneself to how to get it, and to those who have more of it) has played in the evolution of brain mechanisms. The de-biologising of humans has exacted a high price in my view for we have turned a blind eye to the biological consequences of power exerted over others and ourselves. The rest of this book attempts to move to the human level and to articulate how the problem of power can be understood in terms of attractiveness and how it lurks in much of the depressive experience.

NOTE

1. The sexual dimension in dominance behaviour is very well known in humans also and occurs in slang language (fuck you, up your arse, and other such pleasantries), nonverbal gestures indicating sexual activity (Morris, 1978), and in rituals and objects of threat. An erect phallus is often used as a threat or potency signal in many cultures (Eibl-Eibesfeldt, 1989).

CHAPTER 7

Notes on the Evolution of the Self

> We do not content ourselves with the life we have in ourselves and in our being, we desire to live an imaginary life in the minds of others, and for this purpose we endeavour to shine.—Pascal (1670)

According to Buss (1988) dominance is a basic human trait with three dimensions of expression: (1) aggression over others; (2) non-aggressive competition; e.g., via games, demonstrating talent, ability etc; (3) leadership, that is a preparedness to take the initiative, to make suggestions and step in in a crisis. Buss argues that most animals have the first of these but not the latter two. Evidence is growing that evaluations of dominance are made very rapidly with little in the way of cognitive processing, rely on nonverbal behaviour and arise at the beginning of interpersonal interaction (Kalma, 1991). Buss (1988) links the dominance–submission domain to self-esteem. In this chapter we will explore the idea that our aspirations are often concerned with appearing attractive to others and "courting" others' appreciation, being seen as competent, able, and so on. In other words, we are orientated to social success (see Chapter 5). We will explore the evolutionary changes that have moved from social success via aggression, to social success via affiliation and the demonstration of attractiveness, and the implications for a theory of depression.

THE HEDONIC MODE: HIERARCHY AND NETWORKS

The social group of chimpanzees tends to be relaxed and affectionate. For this reason the social structure has been called hedonic, in contrast to the more (agonic) aggressive and spaced social structures of other non-human primates (Chance & Jolly, 1970; Chance, 1988). Chance and Jolly (1970) noted that much of chimpanzee behaviour cannot be understood as aggressive since, often, it does not result in submission or withdrawal, but rather leads to forms of associative behaviour such as grooming, play, alliance formation, joint exploration, foraging, sexual and mothering behaviour. To put this another way, display often activates approach behaviour of conspecifics, soliciting reassurance and affiliation. The result is a group structure that tends to be relaxed, affectionately based, and where affectional ties are important to an individual's pursuit of goals.

In the hedonic mode reassurance may be given voluntarily to others rather than being dependent on elicitation. The motive for affiliative relationships is much stronger in chimpanzees than in other non-human primates. For example, on returning from foraging chimpanzees may greet and display to each other as a kind of reassurance of good relations (Power, 1988). An important consequence of this hedonic style of interaction is the reduction of inhibition in subordinates–i.e., they are more explorative and relaxed in the presence of others. Although humans have not evolved from chimpanzees, it is likely that humans evolved through a stage similar to chimpanzees (Hinde, 1987). As Jane Goodall has often pointed out, chimpanzees are more similar to humans than they are to other monkeys, sharing about 99% of our genes.

Aggressive interactions still occur and power and threat still play important roles in the acquisition of dominance for chimpanzees (physically inferior animals never become top rankers unless they find tactics to frighten others like rolling tin cans, as Goodall notes). However, the post-agonistic encounters are usually marked by reconciliation, cuddling, and stroking. Indeed, de Waal (1988) has pointed out that previous adversaries, rather than avoid each other, may become allies, through this reconciling process. Hence, we cannot understand the functional meaning of aggression in their social behaviours unless we consider both its antecedents and consequences. The consequences are often to increase rather than decrease affiliative behaviour.[1]

Submission/appeasement may be a way of inhibiting aggression, but reassurance/affiliation and reconciliation are ways of avoiding it (or at least its long-term consequences, e.g., spacing, avoidance) and reducing the tension generated by rank differences. Those of higher rank are not feared in the same way as they are in agonic groups. With its high level of reconciliatory and reassuring behaviour, the hedonic group structure has the effect of reducing the threat that exists within the social environment. This facilitates greater levels of exploration of, and interest in, each other.

Alliances and Networks

An important form of solicitation of positively rewarding responses from others arises from alliance formation. In a number of mammalian groups, alliances or coalitions (Crook, 1980; Wenegrat, 1984; Trivers, 1985; Dunbar, 1988) are important for reproductive success. Reproductive success may be advanced via a preparedness to share with an ally who helps support the indivdual's rank. Females may use males to support their rank. Indeed, in primates who form these kinds of alliances, an individual may fall in a hierarchy with removal of the ally (Crook, 1980).

Chance (1988, personal communication) suggests that what we observe in chimpanzees is less a marked, rigid hierarchy as in the agonic mode (although a hierarchy still exists, it is less obvious) and more a system of friendship networks. These networks are often kin based, especially for females (Kevles, 1986), but by no means always so. They are crucial to the animal's ability to play an active part in social life. Networks form especially for foraging and small numbers of individuals may spend time foraging together. Often tense individuals may link up with more confident individuals (Power, 1988). Individuals may move from one small group to another within the larger group. Also evidence is now mounting that chimpanzees do hunt and work cooperatively with a division of activities, and they share their kill, especially with their allies and associates (Boesch, 1990). The chimpanzee hierarchy is therefore not always obvious and more important to individuals are their networks. Also in times of stress—e.g., when encountering predators chimpanzees come together to hug each other and gain the confidence to attack or harass the predator (Chance, 1980). Over all then, networks are an important evolved social adaption in group-living primates. Networks were also crucial in the hunter–gatherer band (see also Chapter 15).

Networks are also important in ingroup–outgroup evaluations. The formation of a network marks the boundaries of ingroup–outgroup membership, even within a larger group. Help is more likely to be directed to individuals recognised as part of the network compared to those who are not part of the network. Presumably this allows for a more efficient operation of kin and reciprocal altruism (Wenegrat, 1984). In humans, networks often form around shared values and, as we have seen, cognitive conformity is important so as not to be rendered an outsider. This makes sense, because it means that in offering help/support to someone who believes, acts, or feels the same as you, you are not only fighting for similar objectives or values, but also you are more likely to receive reciprocal help in seeking to secure your objectives (because they are shared). This is the basis of cooperation (Gilbert, 1989). Humans can share common goals and outsiders can become those who do not share these goals. In the miners' strike of the early eighties, families were split and fragmented, precisely on the issue of shared goals. An example, perhaps, where kinship networks break down in the face of competing goals.

Alliance formation gives rise to certain types of social reasoning and awareness (Chenery, Seyfarth, & Smuts, 1986) and behaviour-affective patterns. In non-human primates, aggression is less often directed at allies (Trivers, 1985) but it requires a social-cognitive competency to know who your allies are (Chenery et al., 1986). In humans this is developed into the need for friends. In children, networks and friendships modify the nature of competitive hostile relationships; friends are less aggressive and competitive and engage in more positively rewarding behaviour than non-friends (Hartup, 1989). Trivers (1985) notes however, that in non-human primates anger can be directed at an ally if they do not offer support as expected (and as, perhaps, happened in the miners strike). Hence, some degree of coercion can be part of alliance formation.

Networking is related to the trait of sociability (Buss, 1988). There is now much evidence that being able to operate in a supportive network protects against various forms of psychopathology. Children who are poorly socially integrated with their peers are more at risk of mental ill health, or to put it another way, good peer relations are important to mental health (Hartup, 1989; Goodyer, Wright, & Altham, 1989). How do networks function to produce these effects?

Reassurance

We cannot over-emphasise the enormous importance of the evolutionary development of reassurance. It is seen clearly in attachment behaviour, where a threatened or fearful infant may return to the mother and be calmed by her stroking and holding (Bowlby 1969; 1973; 1980; Harlow & Mears, 1979). Reassurance has biological effects, primarily of calming (Gilbert, 1989). Further, we now know that this reassurance enables the child to increase its exploration (see also Chapter 10). In this way the child encounters others and learns how to operate in a network of peers, or cooperative relationships (or what Hartup [1989] has called horizontal relationships—as opposed to the more ranked vertical relationships). Chimpanzees, more than any other non-human primates, express reassurance behaviour to many conspecifics and often. They are in fact well known for their touching, hugging, stroking, and kissing behaviours.

Gilbert (1989) suggested that what has evolved and become amplified in chimpanzees and humans is the operation of a safety system. The safety system is open to cues signalling no threat, reassurance, and help (e.g., smiles, voice tone, hugs, etc.), and when these signals are present in the environment they have the effect of calming (defensive) arousal. They also convey a sense of belonging and acceptance in the network. The safety system allows for the potential to feel calmed by others. The activation of the safety system facilitates exploration via reducing internal inhibition since, as we have also noted, aggression is less likely to members within the network. Our capacity for affiliative networking offers new strategies for the avoidance of the threat–submit repertoires and opens the possibility for various forms of cooperation.

However, as important as the attachment and friendship systems are, they are not the only domain of reassurance giving. For example, we may seek reassurance from people we have no attachment relationship with (e.g., doctors, priests, bosses) and we can seek reassurance for our self-presentations by examining the environment for signs of approval and acceptance. Status plays a part in these relationships in that it is unusual to feel reassured from those we see as lower in rank or less skilled than ourselves (unless of course we want to be reassured of our superiority). Part of the reason that Type As are reluctant to accept help is because of the ranking implications (Gilbert, 1989). [2]

In humans the need for reassurance is elevated to a new symbolic level as we shall discuss below. Humans desire reassurance for their self-presentation and the roles they share with others. Reassurance is given via signals of approval. For example, before going to a party one may ask one's partner, "How do I look?". Before giving a talk one may practice on colleagues, "How does this sound?". In developing our networks much effort may go into ensuring that our self-presentation conforms to the norms of our identified group. Much of our social life involves a certain seeking of confirmation of acceptability, both to confirm our rank and place in a social group, and also to convey a sense of belonging, being like others, an accepted group member. As suggested in the previous chapter the negative consequence of being seen as different (e.g., Scheff, 1988) is that it invokes both fears of inferiority and also fears of being made an outsider.

RANKING AND NETWORKING VIA ATTRACTIVENESS: THE SWITCH TO THE HEDONIC SOCIAL STRUCTURE

It is against these types of social structure (the hedonic mode) that we can begin to consider the role that ranking and networking via attractiveness plays in our social and personal lives. Our need for reassurance of self-presentation is known to be a fundamental human concern (Schlenker, 1987, and as we shall discuss below). In essence, to know that others find us attractive acts like a reassurance signal, relaxing us and orientating us to affiliation rather that to threat–submit. Ranking via attractiveness depends on the ability to elicit positive rewarding responses from others. It is likely that a number of evolutionary adaptations have come together to result in the motivation to create a good impression on others and in this way have rank bestowed. Although we cannot be precise in how ranking by attractiveness came to have such prominence in human social motivation, there is no doubt that it represents a fundamental shift from the agonic mode. One very obvious dimension is in mate choice (Richards, 1987).

Mate Selection. The domain of social control via attractiveness has been important in selective mate choice and in determining reproductive success (Shively, 1985; Trivers, 1985; Richards, 1987; Dunbar, 1988). The importance of soliciting the attentions of a potential mate cannot be over-stated. It is seen in nearly all species from fish to reptiles, birds and mammals, and is the domain of the courtship display.

Buss (1989) has shown that mate choice across human cultures is not based on strength and aggression but on attractiveness of targets and that men and women may have different criteria for evaluating an attractive mate. With the movement for r to K selective strategies, the female becomes more interested in securing a mate who will be able to protect her young and invest in them. To be attractive therefore males should be able to convey the information that they are good protectors, will be reliable mates and also have control over resources. Hence status remains a domain of attractiveness for women's choice of men. Men on the other hand follow a different strategy. Their concern is with spreading their genes, and selecting good (biological) quality mates as may be demonstrated by natural beauty and youth. The fairy tale of Cinderella tells the story well. This may affect the experience of shame (see Chapter 8).

ATTENTION STRUCTURE

Chance (1980; 1984; 1988; Chance & Jolly, 1970) has pointed out that we can understand dominance (ranked) hierarchies in a number of ways; for example who gets access to resources and in what context, who threatens who, and so forth (see also, Buss, 1988; Dunbar, 1988). One way to understand the evolution of ranking and networking via attractiveness is to think of ranked relationships in a different way, that is as an attention structure. As pointed out in the last chapter, be it objects, theories, people or groups, those that have rank are accorded more attention than those who do not. They are also more desirable to have in one's network. Consequently, attention elicitation and attention control are important components of ranking behaviour. Attention can be studied even when animals are not in direct conflict.

Chance argued and has shown that a dominance hierarchy is also an attention hierarchy, i.e., who pays attention to whom, when, where, etc. And this is an important parameter for understanding subsequent changes to ranking and how humans evaluate their relative status. Networks can also be studied via attentional patterns. Those that are well integrated into a network will elicit and receive more attention than those who are not well integrated. As Buss (1988) points out, this attention is socially reinforcing. But it is more than this; positive attention also reduces defensive arousal, while positive attention from high ranking figures, especially if they show appreciation of (our) efforts, is mood elevating.

Eibl-Eibesfeldt (1989) has reviewed the evidence for attention ranking structures which supports this approach. He concluded that high ranking children in various cultures show off more (are more self-referencing, which Kohut [1977] would call exhibitionist), are more affiliative and helpful to others, and are attended to more. They also tend to be more protective of lower ranking children who may defer to them. High ranking children still use threats (and more often than subordinates) but this is not the main tactic to gain rank (see also Hold-Cavell & Borsutzky, 1986). Indeed, aggressive children may be unpopular, at least in groups of affiliative children (Wright et al., 1986). Lower ranking children are more inhibited in their displays to others (show off less), are less self-referencing, are less explorative, initiate less, and are attended to less. It might be argued which came first, inhibition or rank. This can be resolved by considering what happens when high ranks move out of a group. In this situation a new child takes over and displays and becomes the centre of attention. The same is true of primates (Gardner, 1982). Hence, in most cases the inhibition is a result of the interaction between the subject and the presence of others.

Attention structure is a crucial idea for understanding subsequent phylogenetic changes to human ranking and networking behaviour. Surely one of the most important changes that has taken place in human ranking behaviour is the shift from asymmetries derived from power and threat to asymmetries of attractiveness (Kemper, 1988; 1990; Kemper & Collins, 1990). In our contests of beauty (note that we use the term beauty contest), in our examination rooms and in sports, in our art and literature, and in our race to win Nobel prizes, to be recognised and valued by others, what is being competed for here is positive attention, admiration, and prestige (Barkow 1975; 1980). That is, there is a desire to express ourselves with the aim of gaining recognition of having made a positive contribution and/or of having talents/attributes; that is, we are valued (Gilbert, 1984). We have institutionalised this by setting up various arenas that allow people to show us what they can do.

SOCIAL INVESTMENT

The sociobiological view of child–parent relationship has been framed in terms of investment (Trivers, 1985). With K-selection the parent is motivated to invest in the child and the child is motivated to elicit investment. Social attention can also be considered as a type of tactic for elicitation of investment. For example, by being seen as talented, others may be persuaded to invest in us, bestow resources, form friendly relations, become mates, allow us to join the ingroup, and so forth. A multitude of possibilities to gain social attention are therefore allowed; from friendship and altruism, to beauty and talent. These are tactics which give rise to socio-cultural fitness (Hill, 1984).

To put this at a more general level, there has been a complexification in the social reward areas of the brain (MacDonald, 1988) such that humans are motivated to show off, develop their talents, and share with others to gain approval and admiration. This is designed to bring social success (which at some point in our history was related to reproductive success). The common theme in our need for social attention (or what Kohut, 1977, has called mirroring; see Chapter 10) is that it is aimed at eliciting a voluntary bestowing of attention/resources from others and when this is forthcoming the inner experience is approval, acceptance, pride, admiration, and so on. No other animal as far as we know is motivated to work for years on projects, with the hope that one day they will find acceptance/admiration in the eyes of others. We want to be appreciated (to use Williams James' term). And when this is not forthcoming we may switch to more coercive tactics or become depressed—a scenario beautifully expressed in Arthur Miller's play, *Death of a Salesman*. Thus we attempt *to elicit others' investment in us*.

Social Attention-holding Power (SAHP) and the Evolution of "Self-presentation"

Gilbert (1989) has suggested that over evolutionary time the RHP system (gaining attention and exerting social control via threat/aggression) has been added to and to some degree modified (but not replaced) by the need to present self as attractive to others. The social signals that others display are less, "I am stronger than you" but rather, "pay attention to, or select/invest in me and I will be useful to you" (Buss, 1988). These signals are designed to elicit positive, voluntary bestowing of status from others on the one hand and a sense of belonging on the other. Both have resource implications. High ranks are likely to have resources bestowed on them (e.g., research monies) and allies are likely to share resources. Technically this was called social attention- holding potential/power SAHP (Gilbert, 1989). Favourable estimates of one's SAHP arise from the ability to control others' attention in a favourable way; unfavourable estimates of SAHP arise when we believe that we have little to interest others or are viewed negatively. Estimates of favourable and unfavourable SAHP seem to function in a similar way to estimates of favourable and unfavourable RHP in other animals; that is, favourable estimates facilitate open display and exploration (confidence), unfavourable estimates are associated with inhibition, withdrawal, and lack of confidence. I suggest that our internal estimates of SAHP signal the degree of social success we enjoy and hence are related to our attractiveness and power to elicit investment from others. As the cognitive therapists point out, however, (Beck et al., 1979) these estimates may be faulty.

This shift from (but not replacement of) aggression, as a way to control others, via attractiveness, has taken place against a background of changes in r-K selection—e.g., mate selection/choice and intersexual strategies, affiliative behaviour, reconciliation and reassurance giving, evolution of attachment and alliance (friendship) formation, the importance of joint exploration of the environment and the sharing of food and knowledge. Indeed, the sharing of knowledge/information and the evolution of language are part of an explosion of social behaviours that allow individuals to control the attention of others and alter their cognitive (meaning-making) schema. Our lives can be changed by arguments and discourses. All of these modifications and changes call forth the need to be able to evaluate what will be attractive to conspecifics, for without this (assuming we do not try to coerce) we will not be attended to. Hence, the motive to gain positive attention from others has become a powerful proximate mechanism as it is associated with access to resources on the one hand, and is reassuring and calming on the other.

Is this a new idea? Well, actually no it isn't. Consider what Pascal wrote in 1670, quoted at the beginning of this chapter. Scheff (1988, p.398) also notes a similar idea suggested by Cooley in 1922:

> Many people of balanced mind and congenial activity scarcely know that they care about what others think of them, and will deny, perhaps with indignation, that such care is an important factor in what they are and do. But this is illusion. If failure or disgrace arrives, if one suddenly finds that the faces of men show coldness and contempt instead of the kindness and deference that he is used to, he will perceive from shock, the fear, the sense of being outcast and helpless, that he was living in the minds of others without knowing it, just as we daily walk the solid ground without thinking of how it bears us up.

Cooley apparently believed that this "looking glass effect" had three aspects (see again Scheff, 1988, p.398):

> A self-ideal of this sort seems to have three principle elements: the imagination of our appearance to the other person; the imagination of his judgement of that appearance; and some sort of self feeling, such as pride or mortification.

It seems then that we have known for a long time that we try to *live in the minds of others.* To create a good impression is associated with pride, which is probably rank related, in that similar experiences come from winning contests, passing examinations, and so on. With pride we say a person "walks tall" indicating confidence and taking on the postures of a dominant animal. If our success is demoted in value ("anyone can do that") then pride may turn to disappointment or resentment.

Taking the Initiative

Buss (1988) has suggested that a part of dominance in humans is taking the initiative. But initiative taking is much more than taking charge in a crises. It is an important social skill and our flow of social interaction depends on it. Depressed people rarely take the initiative (see Chapter 15). Consequently, they are often less rewarding to be with. As we shall see, as we go through this book, there are various reason for this: shame, fear of rejection, or fear of attracting too much attention. Another reason may be high self-focused attention (e.g., see Pyszczynski & Greenberg, 1987). In hedonic groups this is a problem since the relationships depend on mutual interactions.

The inhibition of taking the initiative can be a state effect of low mood but also a trait. Some submissive individuals avoid taking the initiative as a general subordinate style. Of course much may depend on whom one is interacting with and the perception of one's social place. However, lack of initiative taking can cause problems. A woman married to a rather passive man complained that her husband never took the initiative in planning a holiday, nights out, or sex. He would follow along, but not initiate things. At first his passivity and non-competitiveness had been attractive, but not later. Further, she concluded that his lack of initiative meant that he didn't really care about her. When she become depressed he rarely asked how she felt (in part because he thought she would blame him for his passive style).

Individuals who do not take the initiative cannot direct positive social attention to themselves and hence tend to get ignored and are experienced as unrewarding. Moreover, failing to take the initiative can sometimes be read by others as not being interested—which activates resentment. This can set up a vicious circle of needing more cues of reassurance or feeling inferior because one is often ignored. I recently had a powerful experience of this. [3]

Social explorative behaviour shows itself as taking interest in, and showing appreciation of, others. If one is initiating questions, ideas (or even sex) and generally exploring another persons viewpoint, then one is in some sense showing interest (see Heard & Lake, 1986, for the discussion of the importance of this mutual, valuing interactional style). Being the recipient of interest is positively rewarding. It is not uncommon to find that rather passive individuals have histories of authoritarian parenting. Unfortunately, a lack of socially explorative behaviour is unattractive. But if we are correct to link these issues into the ranking system then, as Chapter 6 indicates, low SAHP may block exploration. On the other hand too much initiation (e.g., sexual advances) and following one's own agendas/goals is also unattractive and is seen as dominating. Too much interest in another is intrusive. So it is a tricky balance here.

Culture

It seems to me that the shift from RHP to SAHP has brought with it the major changes in human psychology that underwrite much that humans now regard as our internal theories of mind (Gilbert, 1989), captured so well by Pascal in the passage quoted on page 187. In our art and literature we are concerned with what, how, and why people think, feel, and behave the way they do. To some degree, this is status related for we tend to be more interested in those individuals we regard as being of higher status to ourselves than those of lower status, and the tabloid press relies on this to make its fortune.

The shift to SAHP had major implications for the growth of culture. We cannot here explore the enormous importance of SAHP on the evolution of culture (see Appendix D for further discussion).

It is culture that transmits the rules for gaining SAHP. In a fascinating paper, Rippere (1981) has drawn attention to what she calls socially shared schema. She suggests that human ranking remains linked to more primitive forms, as suggested by Price (1972), but that superimposed on this system is a domain of socially shared information that informs us who we are like and where we stand in our patterns of social interaction. Culture provides our yardstick for self-judgements and also our common sense knowledge about what depression is and how to cope with it. In effect society and culture provide us with our roles and it is culture and social consensus that form the platform from which roles will gain or lose SAHP (e.g., pacifism may lose one SAHP in a war situation but will bring Nobel prizes in a different situation).

THE SELF

At what point in evolution humans developed the capacity for self-reflection, self-awareness, and conscious self-evaluation is unknown. But clearly, the emergence of symbolic reasoning gave rise to new mechanisms for internal self-representation; the self could become an object for its own introspection. The engine of this evolution may have much to do with SAHP (see Appendix D). Once humans could think in symbolic and systemic terms then the individual could conceptualise the role they played in the order of things, their place in the social arena, and the patterns of their relationships. Barkow (1980, pp.323–324) discusses Hallowell's work and puts this point this way:

> Evolving man was selected for the ability to conceptualise the universe and its laws in what may be termed a cognitive map. As he developed the capacity for this internal representation of the universe, he automatically included in it a representation of himself. As the world became "objectified" (Hallowell's term), he became an object to himself. The representation of himself in his own cognitive map may be termed his self.

But by the time humans had this capacity for self-awareness they already had both the motive and the capacity for social comparison, a capacity to be able to judge their relative strengths in relation to others. And so it is logical to suppose that this social comparative ability was shifted (elevated to new forms) into symbolic domains of knowing. We can argue that what we now call self-esteem was a coming into symbolic experience of social comparative information (Barkow, 1975; 1980) on the one hand and the position of oneself in a network on the other. But the data for such social comparisons would now be broad, taking in a perception of how others function in the social arenas (derived from socially shared schema; Rippere, 1981) and matching that with one's own social behaviour. Further, by verbal and nonverbal communication and empathy one would be able to tell how far one deviated from others in this domain or that. Thus, like Barkow (1975; 1980) we can suggest that self-esteem is a mechanism that facilitates judgements about relative standing and in this way the continuity between human self-esteem and non-human ranking behaviour is maintained.

Symbolic representation would also allow us to match our behaviour in an ingroup–outgroup, or them–us, way. Our self-esteem may be raised by feeling part of the dominant group/team and lowered by being a member of an outgroup (see for example, Brown & Lohr, 1987; Abrams et al., 1990). Our symbolic cognitive maps of our social lives not only represent to us how we live in the minds of others of the group we are in but also offer a representation of the rank of our group relative to others. To raise the status of our group is to raise our own self-esteem.

Self–Other Awareness and Social Comparison

The achievement of social goals depends not only on what the individual does but how others react to them. At some point in evolution animals become able to predict the effect their social signals may have on another. Now in chimpanzees it seems that some awareness of self in interaction does exist. Consider the following from Chenery et al. (1986, p.1364):

> In a captive group of chimpanzees two adult males Nicki and Luit were engaged in a prolonged struggle for dominance. During one fight Nicki was driven into a tree. As Luit sat at the bottom of the tree, he nervously "fear grinned". He then turned away from Nicki, put a hand over his mouth and pressed his lips together to hide a sign of submission . Only after the third attempt when Luit succeeded in wiping the grin from his face did he once again turn to face Nicki.

So Luit seems to have some kind of awareness that he should conceal certain kinds of social signal in order to advance his dominance chances. Basically, in humans, this becomes efforts to inhibit negative information about the self—inhibiting/concealing signals or behaviours that might elicit negative responses from others.

When the depressed patient is invited to the party they predict that they will not be able to conceal some perceived deficit on their part; their negative self-attributes will be plain to see. They will either be viewed negatively (i.e., as boring, dull, empty, ignorant, ugly, etc.) or they will (unlike Luit) be unable to conceal their fear, unease, and discomfort. These are recognised to be unattractive signals to be sending. Further, patients identify these as inferior attributes. Submissive behaviour may not be successful for, although it may head off any threat, it is not attractive. To make the point in a different way, Baumeister (1982) notes that, whereas we wish to be seen as conforming and agreeable, it is not desirable to be seen as too conforming, yielding, and weak-willed. It is one thing to be seen as "easy to get on with" but another to be seen as submissive. An individual who exhibits submissive behaviour may be less attractive a target to invest in. Depression-prone subjects can get this equation wrong and inhibit self-assertive needs in order to appear more attractive. Hence, to impress, humans must not only show that they are not frightened but also have more positive attributes to offer.

If we need others to invest in us, without having to coerce them into it, then we need to create in the minds of others a positive affective experience, one that is disposed to investment in us. For this reason we are also motivated to live in the minds of others, to aspire to create a good impression. The internal representation of a place in the social arena opens up many complexities.

DEPRESSION, SELF-ESTEEM, AND SOCIAL COMPARISON

In the last chapter we saw that social comparison of RHP was the basic social algorithm for dominance-aggression. Social comparison, in its many forms in humans, is one of the pillars of self-esteem (Festinger, 1954; Barkow, 1975; 1980; Brewin, 1988; Swallow & Kuiper, 1988; Robson, 1988). However, we now know that the motive to compare self with others and the mechanisms of self-comparison are much more complex than Festinger (1954) originally proposed. Many of these complexities are excellently reviewed by Wood (1989). For example, it appears that social comparison is used to select and pursue personal goals. Individuals select the sources of their comparison, but often this is not a rational decision but one that is self-serving. On the other hand the environment can impose sources of comparison (e.g., television continually shows us people in better houses and with considerably more resources; it can sell us myths about always-happy families and babies who rarely cry). Individuals may chose to compare themselves in non-matching domains—e.g., one may compare one's intelligence with others that are seen to be physically attractive. Upward and downward comparisons function in different ways. Objective standards are effected by social context, i.e., big fish in a small pond, versus small fish in a big pond. (For a comprehensive overview of social comparison research see Suls and Wills, 1991.)

In a major review of social comparison in depression, Swallow and Kuiper (1988) found that depression was associated with strategies and targets for self–other comparison that tended to produce more negative self-evaluation. They also note that depressives are sensitive to social approval—e.g., as measured by the dysfunctional attitude scale ("my value as a person depends on what others think of me")—and while I suspect that many hold this view (as Cooley suggested) the depressive holds it more strongly, at least as measured by this scale. Brewin and Furnham (1986) measured what they called preattributional variables in depression. These were whether a person thought a bad event was more, the same, or less likely to happen to them. Compared to others, depressives thought bad events were more likely to happen to them. In a comparison study of normals (n=50) and diagnosed depressives (n=28) Gilbert and Trent (submitted for publication) explored social comparison on five dimensions. We found that depressives saw themselves as: more inferior, less competent, less likeable, and more reserved and more left out. All differences reached high levels of significance.

In an important study, Davidson et al. (1989, p.357) explored what they call interpersonal sensitivity in depression. They say:

> Interpersonal sensitivity (IPS) is a construct that refers to an individual's hypersensitivity to perceived self-deficiencies in relation to others. It embraces sensitivity to rejection and criticism on the part of others; it also embodies a sense of personal inadequacy, inferiority, and poor morale. Such individuals are quick to take offense, are unduly sensitive to ridicule, feel uncomfortable in the presence of others, and show a negative set of expectations in their dealings with others. A close relationship with social phobia is suggested.

You may recall from our discussion of this study in Chapter 4, that their measure of interpersonal sensitivity revealed that high scorers, compared to low(er) scorers, on interpersonal sensitivity had an earlier age of onset and more chronicity and more severe depression, as measured by the Hamilton rating scale. These patients were also more retarded, had higher guilt and suicidality, and were more paranoid. Greater impairment of work and interests were also noted.

These findings accord well with the ranking and network theory (derived from sexual selection theory) advanced here. These symptoms and concerns may arise from a general over-arousal of the defense system. It should also be recalled that, in primates, rank stress in subordinates occurs because of the low control over resources and events, and subordinates (especially in agonic groups) are susceptible to unpredictable attacks and aggression from dominants (Sapolsky, 1989). Perhaps the sensitivity of these patients might be related to arousal of the agonic defense system (Gilbert, 1989) consequent to the perception of inferiority or what we have called, involuntary, subordinate self-perception (Chapter 6). It is also interesting that in so far as MAOIs are helpful to this group then a question arises as to the degree to which MAO activity is a general marker for ranking stress and is elevated in subordinates as part of the inhibitory pattern. To what extent does having a view of self as inferior influence MAO? And will MAO change with successful psychotherapy that changes self-esteem? What do findings that some of these patients (Davidson et al., 1989) were uneasy with members of the opposite sex tell us about inhibition of seeking mates? Again the role of subordinate self-evaluation and its linkage with sexual behaviour (free or inhibited) is of interest (see Chapters 5 and 6).

Leaving aside our questions, all these findings are in accord with ranking theory: (1) that there is a basic motive to seek out information on one's relative rank on the one hand and security in a network on the other; (2) evaluations of relative rank have important modulating effects in self-evaluation, the pursuit of goals, biological state, and mood. What has yet to become part of social comparison theory is, first, its evolutionary root in ranking behaviour and networking, and its link with social control. Second, social comparison needs to address the issue of the reassuring (psychobiological) aspects of having self-presentation meet with approval/acceptance and the sense of being like others. We wish to highlight this continuity because it provides us with possible insight into the psychobiological mechanisms of affective and behavioural control which are co-assembled with certain kinds of social algorithm. The affective structures of social comparison have remained linked to the cruder and phylogenetic earlier mechanisms of ranking behaviour. Hence, those with low self-esteem may be expected to behave with some similarities to non-human primates with low status—namely inhibition of (social) explorative behaviour, lack of confidence and a low preparedness to initiate in social situations, high arousal and nonverbal submissive signals such as eye gaze avoidance.

As mentioned above, what determines whether a person is free to act (express or exhibit to others) or not, in a social context, depends on the predictions of the responses of others. Hence there is some internal estimate of comparative SAHP. When this internal estimate is low (unfavourable) we judge that we will make an unfavourable impression on others. Under conditions of involuntary, subordinate self-perception there is likely to be increased inhibition in contexts of uncertainty. There are in fact a variety of reasons why SAHP estimates may be low—e.g., selecting inappropriate targets for comparison; having unrealistic expectations about what is acceptable or will impress others (Swallow & Kuiper, 1988), or having negative self-schema as a result of poor early experiences (Beck, 1967; Kohut, 1977; Bowlby, 1980), or the degree of evaluated competition that is actually going on in relationships (Trower & Gilbert, 1989).

Third Party Comparison

Animals can be very attentive to whether their ally (or mate) is cheating on them or about to defect (Trivers, 1985). This concern is in part reflected in the fact that we can gain "a feel" of how one person values another. For example, a new lover may be concerned that they may be seen less positively by the lover than their previous lovers. Or a student may worry that the professor favours other students more than themselves. This motivates social comparison needs for reassurance: "Do you love me more than Fred? Am I better than Joe?". We form in our minds judgements about how the person we are seeking approval from judges others and we may want to be in the top position of their judgements. "I want you to love me more than all others", to quote a recent song. What we call romantic love is often a form of possessive love (some songs again: "I only have eyes for you", "You are my only one", etc.). This kind of rivalry can play havoc in a network and friends can become enemies via envy (see Chapter 8). Communes often break down because of sexual jealousy, and "free love" tends to be an unstable social structure.

This is an extremely complex form of competition for the investments of others. We are competing with others for the positive attentions of a third party; we want preferential investment from them. This is also a basic narcissistic form of competition, as for example in the case of the therapist who feels secret pride when the patient tells him/her how much better they are than other therapists, or the patient who needs to feel he/she is special in some way, more entitled than other patients.

Various forms of sibling rivalry relate to third party competition, where the competition between siblings is for parental attention and investment (Trivers, 1985). For example in the presence of a parent or other adult, children may interact jointly but also individually—that is there may be little interaction between the children except in so far as they may try to limit access to this third party for attention. I am not suggesting that sibling rivalry originates (phylogenetically) at this point in evolution since sibling rivalry is well known throughout the animal kingdom. Rather my point is that symbolic representation of the self means that we can imagine how a person feels about us and how they feel about some other, and compare the two. In our efforts to gain a preferential position in the minds of others we attempt to outshine our competitors. The resource is the attention and investment of another (usually more dominant or higher rank ally or mate), or a central place in a network.

Reciprocal Altruism

Reciprocal altruism evolved under conditions where help-giving to non-kin gave an advantage in reproductive success, for the receiver would reciprocate at some point in the future (Trivers, 1985). It is assumed that various types of motives and social algorithms evolved to increase the orientation to help-giving and to enable people to make the necessary calculations of benefit to self, and to detect and respond to cheaters (Crook, 1980; Gilbert, 1989; Glantz & Pearce, 1989; Nesse, 1990). This social adaptation may lie behind moral forms of reasoning (Gilbert, 1989). Further, as we discussed earlier, reciprocal and kin altruism may lie behind the motive to form networks with like others.

In regard to depression we can note that the kinds of "trades" an individual gives and receives also affects estimates of SAHP. In some depressions, it is common to hear the story "I give so much to others but they rarely return the favours. I always phone others and take interest in them but nobody bothers to phone me." Such individuals complain of a failure of reciprocation (especially of attention) of others and this may release anger at failed reciprocators. However, it is the ranking implications that are related to depression. If failed reciprocation leads to the idea "others do not reciprocate my actions because they see me as inferior, uninteresting, not worth bothering with", then depression is more likely, especially if the person attributes this to some deficit in themselves.

Such perceptions carry information about how one functions in one's network of primary relationships (i.e., a low ranker). Hence, the perception of failed reciprocation, or being taken advantage of, can lower estimates of SAHP. Again it is the signals of appreciation, acceptance, and worth that are crucial (Heard & Lake, 1986). Although reciprocal altruism has become a key idea in some American theories of psychopathology (e.g., Glantz & Pearce, 1989; Nesse, 1990), these are limited if they do not acknowledge that it is the ranking implications that are the dysphoric mediators.

Self-deception and SAHP

Belief in one's own abilities acts like a first gate, as it were, such that a judging audience can assume (before they invest) that the displayer does him/herself see value in their contribution and talent and displays it with confidence. Indeed, a person may have to present self in competition with others. Even in telling jokes around the camp fire one may have to push in a little, to attract attention, rather than waiting for a space to be created. To see oneself as a failure and inhibiting one's contribution is therefore a way of signalling to others "don't invest or put your trust in me, don't follow or select me".

However, in order to "make space", or push in a little and take the initiative, it would appear that humans have evolved the ability to be somewhat over-confident in their estimations of their own ability and the controllability of things (Krebs, Denton, & Higgins, 1988). We may make estimates of relative SAHP that are not entirely accurate. Self-deception has overcome the potential problem of having to be sure of (honest with) oneself. There is now evidence that humans overestimate their abilities in many situations and see themselves more positively than others see them. The depressed person, however, may be more honest and realistic, not necessarily more negative. In a review of a large number of studies Taylor and Brown (1988) found that in general people tend to: rate themselves above average on various traits (of course not everyone can be above average but much depends on the comparison group one has in mind; Wood, 1989); have exaggerated perceptions of their actual ability to control and master situations and can be unrealistically optimistic.

We may be self-deceptive because our parents treated us as special in some way and we have internalised this rather warm glow of ourselves. Positive distortion must have some evolved usefulness (e.g., see Lockard & Paulhus, 1988). Most are familiar with the advantages of hiding (even from self) exploitative motivation. Taylor and Brown (1988) also note that positive self-deception allows us to care for each other, look forward to the future and work creatively. All these may be extremely adaptive from an inclusive fitness point of view. It also has clear advantages to mental health. But self-deception may also lead to increased explorative behaviour and a greater willingness to show off to each other and take risks. It would not matter particularly if the audience agrees with one's displays for the audience is free to choose what they attend to and what they do not. This makes it easier to learn from others. Indeed, we are so used to this that it is easy to forget just how important this audience participation and selection is.

In other words the audience can chose what to attend to and what to ignore. For example, in writing this book, I share with you my thoughts, explore ideas and then it's up to you to make of them what you will: modify or develop the ideas, take some and leave others or ignore all of them. In this way progress comes from exchange and group interactions to problem solutions. The ideas expressed here may not be right but may spark ideas that move us further. I like to think this is the kind of dialectical process that happened around the camp fires millions of years ago. Audience choice is also important in non-human primates (Dunbar, 1988). If I am too inhibited, then first I may not explore or undertake the project of writing, or second, I will keep my thoughts to myself for fear of being put down. Certainly, the history of science has shown the immense importance of being able to learn from others' mistakes and earlier explorations, to adopt new ways of thinking, etc. Over-cautious individuals may hide talents, be less explorative and take few risks, be less inclined to share and therefore inhibit others from learning from their mistakes. Much depends on the situation, however, for at times a cautious and more obsessional approach is essential (e.g., brain surgery!).

It may be that from an inclusive fitness point of view it has been an advantage to have individuals attempting to perform just beyond the limits of their ability, to reach for slightly unobtainable goals. Unless individuals have some kind of optimism (which may well be unrealistic) then this reaching beyond oneself may not take place. To be told that something can't be done may be taken as a competitive challenge by one person, but discouragement by another. Furthermore, who is to say that people are unrealistic? Envy (see next chapter) is a powerful social emotion. And again in science we have seen that various developments have been retarded for years by other people's envy. In so far as depressed people lose the warm glow of a little self-deception that most of us have, then they are clearly not reaching just beyond themselves, though as we shall see later they can still be idealistic. My main point is that there may be a biological aspect to this desire to reach beyond one's actually abilities.

Hartung (1988) has given an interesting twist to the issue of self-deception in depression. He discusses the possibility that deceiving down (seeing oneself as less able than one is) may be adaptive in situations where it is impossible to rise higher in rank without also incurring losses. For example, a woman may deceive herself down in order to maintain a marriage and/or the status (SAHP) of her husband. In therapy I have seen a number of individuals who self-deceive down from fear of other people's envy. Is this voluntary or involuntary subordination? We would suggest that it is mainly involuntary subordination, i.e., from fear or other reasons, and seeing oneself as having no other choice that produces depression (see Chapter 6).

Overview

In general social comparison is complex. In humans there remains a power/coercive dimension, related to the ability to defend or assert oneself. But there is also an SAHP dimension. SAHP is concerned with living positively in the minds of others and eliciting people's investment in us. We calculate our SAHP in various ways: by direct social comparisons, by competing for third party approval, by identification with groups, by the quality of reciprocating relationships and with a little deception thrown in. All this information bears on our estimates of personal worth/value. But while there are immense complications to how our internal estimates of self in our cognitive maps are calculated, rank and issues of subordinate self-perception are closely tied in with them. Because of this the underlying psychobiological programmes of defeat and submission lie just under the surface. This is the fundamental link I wish to make.

THE SYMBOLISING, INNER SENSE OF SELF

Above, we argued that at some point symbolic forms of processing evolved. This does not mean that our every day social interactions are always mediated by highly symbolic styles of thinking. In fact in direct interaction we tend to respond in more automatic ways. The linkage between the crude automatic forms of processing and the slower more reflective forms of self-representation is complex. It is probable that our internal models of self and others, influenced by previous interactions, act as a biological backdrop that sensitises our more automatic and phylogenetically earlier response options. For example, a person who symbolically represents themselves to themselves as inferior is likely to respond (automatically) with certain visceral and other responses to cues of potential or actual put-down and be selectively attentive to them. This kind of sensitivity and attention structure will be different in the person who represents themselves as superior or more positively.

Our concern with symbolic processing then is the internal representation of 'self to self', that is self as an object for internal evaluation and introspection. At this level the self-representations will include: intentions that are future directed; rules that are socially prescribed; symbols of social interaction and meaning (roles); preferences and needs; likes and dislikes; goals and incentives. Into this symbolic map or model of self comes information on previous self–other interactions noted earlier that will shape these various representations.

But to live in the minds of others as "a being of value and worth" requires more than an innate desire to do this. It requires information that it has been achieved, and only the responses of others can provide this information. One cannot be certain that humans are biologically prepared to think good of themselves or to start off with a basic sense of worth and attractiveness to others. Indeed, Kohut (1977; see also Chapter 10) has argued that children are often grandiose and exhibitionist in their early life. However, it is clear that parents, siblings, and peers can have devastating effects on a child's internalisation of their attractiveness to others (or themselves). Parents may control their children such that they only feel good about (attractive to) themselves if they are performing in certain ways, achieving certain successes or playing certain roles.

The Future and Ideal Self

There is one crucial aspect to symbolic processing that other animals almost certainly don't have. That is, we are able to project self into the future (Markus & Nurius, 1986); to work out plans, to aspire to achieve certain goals. Over and above the wish to form alliances, gain power, feel attractive, able, and so on, there are goals which are not innate but are dependent on an internal representation of cultural values; or what the culture conveys SAHP upon (e.g., see Stigler, Shweder, & Herdt, 1990). Hence we symbolically imagine ourselves in certain future roles and actions, in a pop band, as an author, as scoring the winning goal, as dating Sally; and what will impress Sally? I'd like Sally to know this about me but not that.

Our symbolic abilities open up whole new arenas for developing cognitive maps and fantasising ourselves at different places in these maps. We can, for example, symbolically create a self that we would like to be, fashioned from the models set by others (i.e., we want to be like or better than X or stronger than Y, loved by Z), an ideal self. We can internalise the norms of our social group and judge how far we deviate from these. Or we can have a map of comparisons developed from what others have told us we should be and how we should act. Not only can we make comparisons of self with others but also comparisons can be made on how far self deviates from one's ideals or internalised standards. Again none of this is new (see Ewen, 1988; Robson, 1988; Liebert & Speigler, 1989). If ideals are strongly aspired to but not reached we may feel we have failed, which is equivalent maybe to the animal who experiences defeat. Indeed patients talk exactly in these terms—e.g., "I feel I am defeated in life and cannot go on." So our estimates of SAHP are not purely dependent on the impression we create in the eyes of others; they are also dependent on the impression we create of ourselves in our own eyes. In one sense we attempt to create a good impression of ourselves to ourselves. Be it via our altruistic behaviour, moral actions, intellectual or other talents, when we internalise SAHP it is our way of feeling inwardly attractive.

There is increasing evidence that depressed patients have unrealistic ideal selves. This was a key concept for the ego analytic thinkers (e.g. Bibring, 1953; see Chapter 12). More recently, Moretti, Higgins, and Feldman (1990) have reviewed the literature in this area. Those with chronic conditions can have unrealistic ideals about being non-depressed ("I would never be anxious again, I would always be happy"). Or a patient may have unrealistic views of other people ("they are never anxious or depressed but always cope"). Alternatively, a patient may have a life goal that is unrealistic (Arieti & Bemporad, 1980a,b). Although these fantasies cannot be met patients may spend a long time thinking about them and engage in "if only" reasoning. Also, because they continually fall short they continue to feel defeated, falling short of the mark and feeling inferior. Narcissistic patients can feel terrorised by the dread of being ordinary. In therapy it is always worth getting a clear picture of a patient's view of being well.

SOCIAL ROLES

The issue of roles becomes important because it is via roles that we can gain attention from others and have our SAHP confirmed. Thus, our future directed, symbolic self is a "self as": as a clinical psychologist, as having a house and children, as a man or woman, as a mother or father, as being loved, admired. We can choose (to some degree) the roles we are prepared to invest our energy in. For example, I may invest more in being a clinical psychologist than a father, or more in matching the stereotyped values of manhood. Ryle (1982) has explored the issue of personal plans that centre on roles and points out that interpersonal behaviour can have snags, traps, and dilemmas. (e.g., a dilemma might be, "if I love someone then I can't be assertive"). In my view this "self as" is often associated with self as having either RHP aspects and/or SAHP in some form—to be able to feel achievement in a role. We are not socially decontextualised but very much dependent on our validation in the eyes of others.

As mentioned earlier, roles that convey SAHP can be created for us by parents or others. For example, a depressed lady had a domineering but depressed mother. If the patient tried to break free the mother would sulk and convey the impression that her daughter no longer lived in her mind as a positive being but as a selfish individual, an ungrateful daughter. The idea that in her mother's mind she was selfish set up terrible problems for she so dearly wanted to be seen as the lovable daughter, a valued being of worth. Her mother had arranged it that her daughter's SAHP was conditional on compliance to her (the fulfilment of the mother's wishes). In therapy it turned out that this patient knew only how to live for others and not for herself. She could not plan her own goals or have her own aspirations. She could not decide the roles to invest in for these had been chosen for her.

When our SAHP in our chosen roles is not confirmed we may find a regression to more primitive responses of submissive behaviour, coercion or, at the extreme, depression. The roles that we choose to develop are varied and relate both to genetic influences on personality development and the social world we inhabit. For example, a woman may fantasise about having children and being a good mother, with adoring children. If the children do not attend to her in the way that she wants them to, then coercion or depression may emerge. SAHP is the key here, for patients quite openly talk about the lack of attention that others pay them, how "Nobody pays me any attention, nobody takes my feelings into account, I don't seem to matter to anybody, people take advantage of me", and so on. The sense here is of having low status in the eyes of others, not commanding respect. The "self as" in depression is in my view as inferior, incompetent, rejectable, the self as marginalised, unnoticed, weak, etc.

Oatley and Boulton (1985; Oatley, 1988) outlined very similar ideas. In their important model, roles help define self-worth. Roles enable people to make sense of their interconnectedness with others and operate in networks. Roles provide predictable interactional patterns; they provide the rules for interaction. Further, personal plans for the future often involve the role(s) a person would like to play; we aspire to be a person who does something, achieves something, is loved, etc. Oatley and Boulton (1985) point out that certain types of depression may follow the loss of, or invalidation of roles, especially those that have been endowed with self-worth. Also Leary (1957) has decribed patterns of adjustment which are, at one level, particular kinds of role relationship (see Appendix B). While Westen (1988) has explored how these kinds of interpersonal processes affect information processing and the transference relationship.

Blocked Escape and Entrapments

Depressed people often feel helpless to change and may express this feeling as being in a pit or well, struggling to climb out. Why does escape seem so blocked? One answer is that an individual has too much invested in these roles and incentives (e.g., Klinger, 1977); they have become a central part of the self with no clear alternative. The individual sees no other way to gain rank (SAHP), derive a sense of value and there are no other meaningful or obtainable (potentially reinforcing) roles and goals to pursue.

Alternatively, an individual may be blocked due to powerful conflict, in that to exert the power that is required to move against another or assert the self, or even away from another, may be construed as wicked/shameful/selfish (hence a loss of internal SAHP). The self as A (assertive) conflicts with the self as B (loving and inwardly and externally attractive; Ryle, 1982). Yet again the individual may have learnt to place significant others in positions where they are beyond rebuke (Bowlby, 1980). Or there may be unresolved conflicts from the past that inhibit resolving a depression (Gut, 1989). In psychotherapy it often becomes apparent which of these blocks is working and the skilled therapist sets about attempting to unblock the person, either by reconstruing the situation or by aiding deeper affective processing (e.g., Greenberg & Safran, 1987; Safran & Segal, 1990).

Also, entrapment may arise from real problems in the world: being unable to leave children, being short of money, unable to change home, family conflict, lack of support, and so forth. This may be why in working-class families (e.g., in Camberwell) there are such high rates of depression (Bebbington et al., 1989).

Care Eliciting or Submission?

One of the confusions in the literature is whether depression can be understood as a form of care eliciting. My view is simple, depression is not care eliciting. Children do not get depressed as a tactic to elicit care, and generally depressed people are unattractive to others. Care eliciting is effortful and directed and involves a searching out of others. Depression however blocks exploration. On the other hand many depressed people do attempt to elicit care and search out emotional support (see Chapter 15). How can these two observations be reconciled? In my view care eliciting may be used as a tactic to repair a sense of low self-worth; it is a strategy, to cope with or overcome depression.

We have said that SAHP is aimed at eliciting others' investment in us, to elicit a voluntary bestowing of resources, to become friends, etc. But the care eliciting system is also aimed at eliciting investment from others (Trivers, 1985). Hence, to find that some depressives are care elicitors is not at variance with ranking theory. We would argue that the depressive care eliciting is not necessarily a rerun of childhood dependence but rather an attempt to elicit reassurance, and protection from potential allies or a more dominant figure. If in therapy there are unresolved grief issues from childhood then we find, usually, a lack of support and approval and what is really desired is a repair to self, in Kohut's sense (see Chapter 10).

The care eliciting strategy (crying, etc.) may be triggered involuntarily and some patients frequently tell how they try not to cry in therapy because they feel this puts them in a one-down situation or they are ashamed of it. Like Luit (the chimpanzee described earlier) putting his hand over his mouth to cover/hide his fear grin, tearfulness in humans often leads us cover our eyes with a hand. Young children rarely, if ever, do this. So the strategies to signal no threat and to attempt to elicit investment/support can be quite involuntary. The withdrawn person however has given up trying to elicit investment to compensate for low self-esteem and vulnerability and uses instead the strategy of avoidance. Even those who might be able to help are seen as threatening, untrustworthy or too ineffective to help. This is often associated with the more severe depressed states where we see a complete loss of explorative behaviour and reduced social interaction (see Appendix C).

Put simply, *a person does not get depressed as a way to elicit care.* Rather, as a person becomes depressed they may use care eliciting as a tactic of repair; to increase investment from others. If they fail to receive adequate signals of care or reassurance they may become more care eliciting but provoke more rejection (reduce others' investment). This helps explain why patients are often ambivalent about care eliciting. If a person deliberately attempts to use depressive behaviour, a careful analysis usually finds not a true desire for care and comfort but issues of power, control, and resentment.

DEPRESSION AND SAHP

According to this model there are a number of primary sources of depression which have a final common pathway on the ranking algorithms. Here are some of them:

1. *The relationship of control.* In the agonic mode the dominant is concerned with exercising control over others. He/she wants others to obey him/her and requires submission and compliance. In the human situation this is the dictator. The dictator is not just interested in submission but also wants others to live as he/she orders. "You should be, act, and feel as I tell you."

In depressed individuals it is not uncommon to find this relationship acting either currently or in the past. If there is voluntary compliance then depression rarely results, but if this produces significant internal inhibition and perception of inferior self-appraisal and/or sense of entrapment, then depression will follow. Depression is therefore often found in marriages, families or other relationships where control is restricted by a dominant and usually a "down putting" other. In various ways the individual feels unable to retaliate (Price & Sloman, 1987). There is now clear evidence that spouse criticism is a major factor in relapse (Hooley & Teasdale, 1989). Type As tend to treat their spouses like subordinates (Price, 1982). This theme is explored further in Chapter 15.

There are many cases of abuse that one could mention but these are easily understood I think. Here I give a less obvious example.

A forty-year-old depressed patient complained of anxiety and depression. She found it difficult to do many things that previously she had coped with. Her husband was a high level executive and she always felt rather inferior to him, even though they had met at university. At times he had given her explicit messages that he was disappointed in her, compared her unfavourably with other wives and implied that he should have married a stronger person. To advance his career he had insisted that she stay at home with the children (rather than develop her own career) and also that she be the perfect hostess when his "important colleagues" came to dinner, etc. Over the years her life had become increasingly restricted and controlled by her husband and her self-identity had almost atrophied. I did not view her depression as a kind of protest as some might, or as a way of getting her own back or sabotaging him. Rather I saw it as the result of a slow erosion in her sense of self-value. She found relief from antidepressant medication and dropped out of therapy, feeling that things had gone on too long for her to change now.

2. *Being deviant.* The whole concept of tradition is tied up with the issue of social control. On the one hand tradition may provide for a sense of shared values but on the other tradition can be used as a form of control. When individuals try to break free from a rigid set of traditional values, often religious, the consequences can be severe, such as loss of support, ridicule, or being made an outcast. During the British miners' strike of the early eighties whole families became split and alienated and this undoubtedly caused depression but I know of little research in this area.

Sometimes cultural/family values, as Miller (1983) points out, are enforced with the idea that it is for "your own good". Many cases of depression result from this clash of values. Suicide variation across cultures may reflect these aspects (Haynes, 1984). Hence it is not just individuals that can control us but also systems of cultural values.

A woman had serious doubts about her religious life style and bringing up her children in the same way. When she tried to break free, her parents, husband, and friends turned on her with extreme vindictiveness. Clearly, not having lived in any other social group there were few to turn to for support and these people were part of her everyday life.

When people (be these friends or children) in our own network start to behave in ways that appear deviant, the sense of insecurity this produces activates efforts to exert control over the deviant member. Because humans are such value-needing beings this causes serious problems. One can only remain in these groups if one is prepared to be constrained by them. If one follows with voluntary compliance then one may be spared depression.

3. *The relationship of neglect.* The individual may not be subject to abuse or direct put-downs but suffers a loss of SAHP from the partner/or others. This is the neglectful relationship as opposed to the abusive/controlling relationship. The partner may stay away from home for long periods and even when present may spend little time interacting due perhaps to fatigue and/or lack of interest. Whether a relationship is neglectful or whether the partner needs more attention to boost their sense of being valued is unimportant in theoretical terms (though vital in therapy terms). As a result of the (perceived) lack of attention, resentments build up and in this situation anger is more common but it is a kind of protest anger: "pay attention to me". If this attention is not forthcoming and the individual may attribute this to their own lack of attractiveness. Hence the ranking system is involved and the person feels inferior or unworthy.

A patient married a man who was highly attentive during courting. But within a year of marriage it seemed he "hardly noticed her". She would cook good meals and buy fancy clothes but still to no avail. Gradually, she began to think that either he had found someone else or that she was boring (an idea she had before marriage and one of the reasons that his previous behaviour had been so attractive to her). Her protests of his lack of interest were met by further withdrawal on his part. She had few outside relationships to support her SAHP, having moved far from home. Her inner resentments became further evidence (to her) that she was unattractive to herself and her husband. In these depressions the theme is often: "Whatever I do makes no difference to anyone. I may as well not be here." It is not uncommon to find that some depressives use mixtures of submissive and cooperative strategies in neglectful relationships. There is a basic belief that, "if I invest in this person and show them I care, then sooner or later they will reciprocate." Unfortunately this rarely happens. However, so much of the patients' own investments are focused on the other person that they find it difficult to break away. An evolved adaptive strategy such as "elicit others' investment by altruism" is not adaptive in all situations (see Chapter 5, page 139).

4. *Loss of a significant other.* A person may lack a confidant or discover things about a trusted other that seriously undermines their sense of access to a reassuring other or individuals from whom SAHP was being provided (Brown & Harris, 1978a). However, grief will not turn to depression unless the person comes to think negatively of themselves and/or cannot escape and seek alternative sources of reassurance and signals to boost SAHP. Horowitz et al. (1980a) have also drawn attention to the fact that in some cases loss reawakens negative self-beliefs. This is the person who had low self-esteem before marriage but was given some protection from the spouse (see also dominant other types, Chapter 12). With the loss the spouse these negative self-images re-emerge.

5. *Loss of roles.* An individual may lose access to roles that convey SAHP (e.g., at retirement or when children leave home) and become depressed when there is nowhere to gain a sense of SAHP or appreciation. We can become socially decontextualised. In this situation it is often a loss of a place in a network. I have called this the outsider theme (see Chapter 11). The point is, it is difficult to have status outside of meaningful relationships.

An eighty-year-old came to see me for depression. She had had an illness that had kept her in bed for a month. When she felt well she found that her husband had (in an effort to be more caring) taken over many of the household duties. Her place in the church (as flower arranger) had been taken over by someone else (again because it was thought that the duty was getting too much for her). Her GP warned her that at her age she could not expect to do what she did at sixty and to slow down. There were various other examples. She was depressed and felt that she had no place any more and maybe she was indeed now too old. The question for me was, should one help to accommodate her to this new situation and the death issues that were clearly around or fight it. Rightly or wrongly we chose the latter. I sensed that she needed validation from me that she wasn't finished and that it would be better to go on "shining brightly". Two months after therapy I received a call to tell me that her church had asked her to help with the summer fête, that she was back flower-arranging and felt very well.

6. *Loss of self-identity.* We often have images of ourselves as being a certain kind of person (Gilbert, 1989). We may become depressed when our own behaviour invalidates this. Discovery of our own vengefulness or sadistic behaviour is one common event. But there are other examples. A depressed therapist had always prided himself on being caring of others. One patient was difficult and frequently making demands but he liked her and thought she was doing reasonably well.

Over many years she had threatened suicide and in consultation with others involved in the case, he felt he shouldn't overreact to these threats. Six weeks into therapy she killed herself. Her death devastated him. He felt he had not helped her enough, was incompetent and that he not longer deserved the title of caring psychotherapist. He even thought about giving up the profession altogether. Later he said: "I guess at that moment I lost my naivety and realised that my previous self-confidence was based on a certain artificiality. When she died something in me died also, a certain confidence maybe or innocence."

The loss of self-identity via one's own actions can at times be painful and causes a massive loss of internal SAHP. Various defenses can be used to protect self but the sense of inadequacy can remain. This kind of loss can recruit many of the global self-downing (or what we might call internal, subordinating) systems that cognitive therapists have explored (see Chapter 13). Another typical example arises from war trauma when one believes one has let others down, friends have died or been injured or one has done things that seem so in conflict with one's previous self-identity. In a sense we lose that warm glow we may have had of ourselves and it may take some time to put it back again. The loss of our inner warm glow is nearly always dysphoric. If a defense like "I will never allow myself to become that close to anyone so I will never hurt them or be hurt myself," arises, then depression can remain. Some chronic mild depressives often have this defensive style.

7. Feeling different. An individual may compare their inner experience with those of others and conclude that what they are experiencing or the way they are coping is a mark of inferiority (Brewin & Furnham, 1986).

A twenty-two-year old patient became depressed when her emotional conflicts with her parents were not shared by her siblings. When she went to her siblings in a tearful state about her mother's lack of love, her siblings responded, "I don't see why you get so upset. You know how mother is. Why don't you do what we do and just not visit anymore. Just ignore her." The fact that her siblings were married and had moved away from home was not mentioned by her siblings. Also discussion of "mother" stirred up their anger and they didn't want to hear about her. My patient however concluded there must be something wrong with her, because unlike her siblings she could not cope (i.e., not be emotionally unaffected). Therefore, she concluded, she was emotionally weak and dependent and became fearful of sharing her experiences with others in case they came to the same view of her. She was able to come to terms with her mother's lack of love once she no longer put herself down over her emotional responses.

After quite a long time in cognitive type therapy I asked this patient what had helped (expecting to hear that it was the skills of testing the evidence, learning not to self-label, and so on). In fact she said that it had been her gradually learning to trust me and my validation and acceptance of her experience: that there was nothing weak about her to feel so affected by her mother. Such experiences have such resonance with self psychology (Kohut, 1977) and the key elements of other therapies (Frank, 1982) that it is difficult to believe in the purely cognitive (re-)educational models of change.

Overview

All the cases just described are of course a little more complex than I have suggested. As we go through the rest of this book we will put some flesh on these bare bones. However, they convey how ranking theory might be applied in helping our understanding of depression. Ranking theory suggests that depression is not one thing or entity but that there are some commonalities. In ways that are still obscure to us, self-worth is a phylogenetic adaptation to more primitive ranking and group identification issues. It engages the notion of freedom to act versus a sense of inhibition. In understanding how ranking tactics have changed over millions of years it becomes possible to focus on aspects of social comparison, the roles of alliances and networks that support self-values, and internalised maps of self in a social arena. Ranking and network theory suggests that "relatedness" is a key variable in depression. However, while depressed patients may want investment and reassurance from others, it may be a mistake to equate this with child-like needs for nurturance (Gilbert & Trent, submitted for publication). Rather it is more a matter of a sense of self-worth and attractiveness to others (and oneself), not as someone who needs looking after, but as someone who has a positive contribution to make, someone of value and worth.

SUMMARY

In this and the proceeding chapter we have outlined the following ideas:

1. Ranking behaviour evolved from breeding strategies.
2. The most primitive form of ranking (territorial) involves the capability to judge relative strength (derive estimates of relative RHP).
3. These estimates act as internal modulators of social behaviour and biological state: submit to stronger individuals, challenge the weaker. They are linked into internal inhibitory systems.

4. A vast number of evolved changes in social behaviour on route to becoming human have resulted in a shift from asymmetries of aggression and estimates of one's own power/strength to asymmetries derived from the demonstration of attractiveness (e.g., via talent, ability, physical attributes, and so forth) and allowed for estimates of our own attractiveness/competency, SAHP; this is an important evaluative component. Furthermore, networks and alliances became important in chimpanzee and human social life and self-esteem is also effected by group membership.
5. A consequence of this shift is that we seek to live in the minds of others, to elicit their investment in us and to have them confer on us a sense of our own value/worth. This sense of value reduces internal inhibition, promotes exploration and positive affect.
6. Both estimates (power and attractiveness) can be internalised such that we can appear strong and attractive to ourselves and others, or on the other hand weak and unable, in which case we can describe the internal estimate as involuntary, subordinate self-perception.
7. These internal estimates are co-assembled with ranking psychobiological functioning and as such act as modulators of biological state. Depressive brain state patterns may reflect either a primitive defeat-like state which involves loss of feeling and social withdrawal; or a more submissive pattern with various efforts to elicit investment from others; or some combination of the two. In actual cases one can see blends of these two strategies for dealing with depression.

Ranking and networking theory help us to set up a theory for understanding why depression is often associated with a number of psychological aspects: an appraisal of powerlessness and lack of attractiveness (to ourselves and others); reduction in explorative behaviour and changes in cognitive processes such as the ability to remember positive information about the self, or problem-solve. In effect the changes of biological state reduce competency and hope (the yielding subroutine was evolved to keep an animal out of action, to behave like a loser). In the next chapter we shall look more closely at patterns of experience. These are co-assembled with affects and behaviours that are part of the ranking and networking systems.

CONCLUDING COMMENTS

Our human needs are social. We want to find a place in the world where we can engage our inner talents and attributes and be reinforced for so doing. In this chapter we have argued (as many others before Ewen, 1988) that self-worth is the most basic of needs for humans. We have explored the evolutionary root of self-worth from the primitive ranking system through to the need to present self as attractive to others and seek reassurance, approval, and acceptance. That these latter evaluations are still linked to the more primitive ranking systems can be seen by the fact that the nonverbal behaviour of those with high status and value demonstrate confident display (upright posture, met eye gaze, taking the initiative, etc.), whereas those who feel they have little worth or rank are inhibited, tense in the presence of others, and submissive. Others may become aggressive to inhibit others if they think they can win. Whether it be the subordinate feelings of women, children or ethnic minorities; whether it be in relationships with our intimates or in our place of work; whether it be our aspirations, goals and plans, the one thing that causes so much distress is when we seem to fail to obtain for ourselves a sense of value.

Depressives are concerned with their self-value/worth because we are internally constructed to be worth-seeking animals, to live in the minds of others. The reader may now say, "Yes, but some seem much more preoccupied with their self-worth than others," which is of course true. So we need to understand how some people manage to store self-worth somehow and appear more robust to the ups and downs of life. This will be explored as we go through other theories of depression, especially those of Bowlby and Kohut (Chapter 10). In good measure our early life seems to provide the sense of self-worth that we will carry throughout our lives. Indeed our early attachments may be the most salient influence determining whether we will engage the social world as a highly ranked system or in a more affiliative, cooperative manner. In the former case the person is often defensive and controlling or easily controlled. In a small minority, however, ranking systems may be unstable for genetic reasons.

Finally a note about independence must be made. To live in the minds of others can cast a shadow; we can become too dependent on it and inhibited. But to be totally unconcerned with the feelings and opinions of others is to be psychopathic. This balance is no mean achievement in human development. In some ways the RHP and SAHP systems must be integrated. The myths through the centuries tell the story of the warrior or hero who at some point must strike out on their own, find their own way and (something that science cannot define) their own centre. This sense of security and confidence in self (aided perhaps by a little self-deception) is neither an arrogant over-compensation for inferiority nor fear of attack, but a quiet, inner sense of self. Perhaps as Kohut (1977; see Chapter 10) suggests it relates to the cohesive self-structure. Furthermore, while we have emphasised the importance of connectedness, humans also have desires for solitude, to be alone, and it is often at these times we are at our most creative (Storr, 1989).

I do not want to leave the reader with the impression that we are all nothing but reflecting mirrors (see Chapter 11 and Jung's ideas). However, here, we are concerned with depression and I hope I can be forgiven for passing over the equally complex subject of what Maslow called self-realisation, what the Taoist's call the centre and others may refer to as the independent, integrated personality.

NOTES

1. A similar situation may pertain in humans in that some conflict actually strengthens a relationship. Although conformity and sharing of goals and plans is attractive, too much fear and compliance is not. This is often a mistake that some depressive-prone individuals make. In an effort to be attractive to others they inhibit their dissatisfactions (follow a subordinate strategy), store up resentments which may become a source of inner rumination and then explode inappropriately over minor things. Because this exaggerated response can be demonstrated to be inappropriate, the person feels guilty and even more subordinate. As pointed out elsewhere (Gilbert, 1989), cooperative behaviour is not conflict-free but obeys different rules. There may be a wish to be noticed, respected, understood but not a wish to force the other into an inferior/subordinate position. If one wishes to be respected then it is recognised that this goes with respecting the rights and values of others.

   The manner in which conflict is conducted is crucial, and especially how conflict is reconciled. Does a person support an individual that they have just gained an advantage over or are they intent on pushing home their advantage and at the extreme attempting to humiliate the other? None of this is unknown to us and in our international politics it has become clear that one should not seek to humiliate a defeated foe but reconcile and offer help. Had this been followed after the first world war, the second may never have happened. Reconciliation is a crucial issue. It has become clear to me over the years that some families have poor reconciling behaviour and after punishment a child is left clearly in the position that the only way to stay safe is to submit and comply. But without some reconciliation then the social affiliative behaviour may not develop.
2. Reassurance is not the only way animals and especially humans can feel safe in the world of course and the internalisation of self-efficacy is another very important dimension (Bandura, 1977). Hence via evaluating our own efficacy and ability to control outcomes we can, as it were, reassure ourselves. Nevertheless in my view, despite the current trend in psychology

to stress the individual as a bestower of his/her own value and competency, humans cannot socially decontextualise themselves (Wenegrat, 1984; Hinde, 1987) and a good deal of our ability to feel safe in the world (and hence explore it and display to others) comes from the comfort we feel and the value that is bestowed on us by other human beings. In so far as others reassure us when we are young then we will develop internal models of ourselves and others as sharing reassuring interactions—or what the self psychologists would call an internal reassuring self-object which has a soothing quality when under stress (see the section on Kohut, Chapter 11). Throughout this book we will have reason to return time and again to the importance of reassurance that is both internally and externally given as a way of calming and reducing defensive arousal.

3. I was doing a day's course on depression and the clinical students were as dead as dodos. Their nonverbal behaviour expressed disinterest. Getting these kinds of signals I could feel my own energy draining away. Eventually, I decided to stop the seminar and look at what was happening. Far from disinterest they gradually revealed intense social anxiety with each other, had not jelled as a group and, early in the group formation, there had been various unresolved competitive conflicts. There were all kinds of negative cognitions like: "If I say something the others will jump on me, or make me look stupid". Many of them felt rather depressed by their training, and the loss of energy and sense of not being part of what was going on (e.g., the seminar) was all tied up with this. Over the years I have seen students who in class appear timid and uninterested and rarely ask questions. However, in individual supervision (with a little mirroring or positive reinforcement) they come alive, are keen, explorative, and open. Their explorative side is switched on.

CHAPTER 8

Patterns of Depressive Self-organisation: Shame, Guilt, Anxiety, Assertiveness, Anger, and Envy

> If I were to reduce all my feelings and their painful conflicts to a single name, I can think of no other word but: dread. It was dread and uncertainty that I felt in all those hours of shattered childhood felicity: dread of punishment, dread of my own conscience, dread of the stirrings in my soul which I considered forbidden and criminal.—Hermann Hesse (1971, p.13)

Any psychological theorist of depression must not lose touch with experience. How simple it is to talk of genes and innate algorithms and to feel detached from the experience of our subject matter. Yet, for me, Hesse sums up eloquently the core of the depressive experience, that of dread. Today we may begin to see exactly how this dread is constituted and to recognise the burden humans carry by virtue of their social evolution.

In various states of mind we experience patterns of thoughts and feelings. As we pointed out in Chapter 5 the mind is a system of mixed modules that becomes organised in certain ways. In our psychiatric phenomenology and classification of depression not enough consideration has been given to the various patterns of experience of depressive self-organisation. Depression is often associated with various patterns of affects and behaviours and very few assessment instruments tap this complexity. This complexity can be seen to relate to various sub-components of ranking behaviour and sense of belonging.

SHAME

During the last decade shame has finally become a central concern to some psychopathologists (see for example Lewis, 1987 [Ed.]; Nathanson, 1987; Schore, 1991). Unfortunately, much of the cognitive work on self-schema and self-worth (e.g., Kuiper, Olinger, & Martin, 1990) continue to ignore this area. Scheff (1988) suggests that shame is part of a bipolar affect system (called the social deference system), with shame at one end and pride at the other. In shame we evaluate that we have courted others' negative evaluation of ourselves. In pride we have courted their positive evaluation. He links both Lewis's (e.g., 1986) psychological theory of shame with Goffman's (1968) sociological view of stigma. If you accept the idea that a deference system probably evolved for ranking behaviour (Barkow, 1980) then shame arises as an affect of the submissive pole of interaction and is associated with a sense of inferiority and involuntary, subordinate self-perception. Mollon (1984, p.212), in a fascinating paper on shame, captures the essence of how shame involves an awareness of living negatively in the minds of others with a quote from Sartre:

> To see oneself blushing and to feel oneself sweating, etc., are inaccurate expressions which the shy person uses to describe his state; what he really means is that he is physically and constantly conscious of his body, not as it is for him but as it is for the Other. This constant uneasiness which the apprehension of my body's alienation as irredeemable can determine ... a pathological fear of blushing; these are nothing but a horrified metaphysical apprehension of the existence of my body for the Other. We often say that the shy man is embarrassed by his own body. Actually, this is incorrect; I cannot be embarrassed by my own body as I exist in it. It is my body as it is for the Other which embarrasses me.

Shame and Guilt

Perhaps one of the common confusions is between shame and guilt in depression. Although much depends on the definition one chooses, it is useful to clarify their distinction since much that we call guilt can in fact be more usefully investigated as shame. Lewis (1987a) called shame the "sleeper" in psychopathology and clearly distinguished it from guilt. Lewis (1986, p.329) says "I use 'shame' to refer to a family of affective-cognitive states in which embarrassment, mortification, humiliation, feeling ridiculed, chagrin, disgrace and shyness are among the variants. 'Guilt' is a family of affective-cognitive states that share the themes of responsibility, fault, obligation and blame for specific events." Lewis points out that not only personal transgressions (deviating from an evaluation of how one should or ought to have thought, felt or behaved) but also defeats and disappointments can activate shame. Guilt, however, is entirely related to personal transgression. In Lewis's view, guilt is always about moral issues whereas shame is not. The distinctions she offers may be summarised as follows:

1. In shame the physiological arousal evokes blushing, sweating, and tears whereas this is less so for guilt. (In my view the physiological arousal is related to both anxiety to do with being overpowered and/or rejected/expelled and also the physiological shifts that take place in the activation of submissiveness.)
2. Shame evokes a sense of helplessness, as if paralysed and impeded in movement. Shame is about the self, about the "I", whereas guilt does not involve the same sense of helplessness and is about "things" done or undone in the world or to others.
3. Shame evokes, and is related to, rage, fury, and resentment (I see these as related to hostile submission as in Leary's model of 1957). These affects may be perceived as inappropriate. They are experienced as threatening in so far as if they became known it would result in estrangement and loss of the significant other. Because of this, these experiences can be held in a state of inhibition (concealment/denial), which makes them difficult to communicate. This can cause some difficulties in psychotherapy. Guilt, on the other hand, relates far less to aggressive emotions and desires for revenge but rather to regret and remorse with desires for reparation. In therapy patients will often talk a great deal about the things they feel guilty about in an effort to seek forgiveness and redemption. This is not the case for things that shame them.
4. In shame, the other is perceived as a source of scorn, contempt or attack and at the same time is viewed as being fully intact but threatening a separating, abandoning or overpowering response. In guilt, the other is perceived as injured, needful, suffering, and hurt. In other words, shame and guilt relate to different ways of viewing the self–other power relationship.

These distinctions are outlined in Table 8.1.

Mollon and Parry (1984) and Lewis (1987a) suggest that shame rather than guilt is the more important in depression and this seems borne out by current evidence (Hoblitzelle, 1987; Gilbert & Trent,

TABLE 8.1
Shame and Guilt

	SHAME EXPERIENCES	
	Self (Unable)	*Other (Able)*
1.	Object of scorn, disgust, ridicule, humiliation	The source of scorn, contempt ridicule, humiliation
2.	Paralysed, helpless passive inhibited	Laughing, rejecting, active uninhibited-free
3.	Inferior, smaller weaker	Superior, bigger, stronger
4.	Involuntary body, response, rage, blush, tears gaze avoidance.	Adult and in control
5.	Functioning poorly, mind going blank, desire to hide, conceal	Functioning well but experiencing contempt
6.	Self in focal awareness	Other in focal awareness
	GUILT EXPERIENCES	
	Self (Able)	*Other (Unable)*
1.	The source of hurt, let down or failure	Injured, needful, hurt
2.	Intact and capable	Incapable, needing
3.	Focus on self actions and behaviours/feelings	Focus on let-down/injury from other and own needs/losses
4.	Efforts to repair	Efforts to elicit reparation or rejection/contempt leading to shame.

(Adapted from Lewis, 1986). Self-blame does not distinguish shame from guilt but the power relationship does.

submitted for publication). Shame involves, as we have seen, a sense of helplessness, inferiority, and being overpowered by others. In two studies, Wicker, Payne, and Morgan (1983) asked 152 students to recall personal experiences of shame and guilt, and rate them according to a number of characteristics and attributes. Many similarities, especially in relation to pain, tension, and arousal were found between guilt and shame. However, there were also some significant differences:

1. There was strong agreement that shame was the more incapacitating and overpowering emotion.
2. Shame related more to feelings of inferiority, submissiveness, and being smaller.
3. Shame was associated with a sense of weakness, encouraging hiding rather than (as for guilt) reparation.

4. Shame produced more confusion over how to act appropriately.
5. Shame involved greater self-focus (e.g., physical sensations) and self-consciousness.
6. Shame produced a greater sense of being under scrutiny.
7. Shame invoked more anger with a greater desire to punish others, compete and/or hide with desires for revenge.
8. Guilt was more likely to be linked with moral and ethical evaluations.

However, shame did not last longer than guilt. Furthermore, there was a tendency for both to fuse and co-exist. In a recent study of students Pehl (1990) explored some of the ideas of Lewis's theory and Gilbert's (1989) evolution theory (e.g., that shame is associated with feelings of helplessness and inferiority and evolved from submissive action patterns). Pehl took items (ten of shame and ten of guilt) from the Johnson et al. (1987) shame–guilt scale and constructed a self-report questionnaire that asked students (N=126) to rate the degree of helplessness, anger at others, anger at self, sense of inferiority, and self-consciousness that they might experience to each item. She then correlated each item with the total shame score and the total guilt score. As predicted, shame was highly (significantly) correlated with each of these items. The findings were: shame—with helplessness $P<0.56$, with anger at others $P>0.3$; with anger at self $P<0.57$; with self-consciousness, $P<0.70$; with inferiority, $P<0.57$. Guilt on the other hand did not seem so clearly related to these variables and correlations were of a much lower order. Here the findings were: guilt—with helplessness $P<0.14$; with anger at others, $P<0.17$ with anger at self, $P<0.36$; with self-consciousness $P<0.36$ and with inferiority $P<0.18$. These variables (e.g., helplessness, inferiority, etc., to shaming events) were also significantly correlated with submissive behaviour and depression although the latter finding is dubious because of low depression scores. The high correlation of self-consciousness with shame, in this group, might suggest that it is shame rather than depression that accounts for the high self-consciousness in depression (Pyszczynski & Greenberg, 1987).

Essentially, from an evolutionary point of view, shame is about power and dominance conflicts in a way that guilt is not. Guilt focuses on harm done to others and breaking internal moral codes (Crook, 1980; Gilbert, 1989). The evolutionary root of guilt is probably from cooperation, reciprocal altruism, and care-giving. Shame however, centres on issues of defeat, intrusion, encroachment, injury, and ultimately destruction of the self. The guilty need not feel defeated or encroached upon. In shame one lives in the minds of others as something smaller, inferior or undesirable. Again it is inferiority and its link with social comparison that is crucial to ranking theory.

Shame and Disgust

However, there is an important addition to the evolutionary view. It seems to me that shame as a human experience is only possible with the SAHP system since it involves some kind of awareness of how the self exists in the minds of others. Non-human forms are probably related to social anxiety. Furthermore, shame is often associated, not with the expectation of aggression from others, but of being treated "with contempt". I doubt that non-human primates would have an equivalent concern. This "being treated with contempt" is associated with the experiences of being pushed away and, in the extreme, an object of disgust, i.e., causing the affect of disgust to oneself in the minds of others. It may be true that this links with inferiority feelings but it also links with the concept of being separated from others, cast out, rendered an outsider (outgroup person), expelled in some way. Certainly in cases of sexual abuse the experience is often one of disgust, of becoming inferior by having been contaminated. Therapists need to be extremely sensitive to this "feeling of disgust", this "fear of expulsion". In some cases the fear of invoking disgust is more powerful in depression that the fear of invoking aggression from others.

It may be therefore that there are different types of shame. For example, one that is related to inferiority and being seen as inadequate. In this situation one is simply ignored, or perhaps laughed at. But another form seems more related to experiences of the physical self and is associated with the fear of engendering disgust and expulsion, a pushing away from/by others. Here one is not just inadequate but something (or someone) positively "distasteful". In both cases we may fear the loss of investment from others, as is the sense of creating a negative image in the minds of others, but the experiences may be different.

As far as I am aware this distinction has not been explored by researchers. My clinical experience would suggest that women are particularly vulnerable to shame/disgust. Depressed men sometimes talk about themselves in terms of disgust but in general are less cognitively and emotionally focused on their bodies as objects of attraction. I am not sure if this is a biological difference (e.g., arising from sexual selection strategies) or whether it arises because women are made more aware of their bodies, by families, culture, and the attentions of men. Male therapists should be aware of this possible distinction and one must be sensitive to the feminist claims that perhaps men do have difficulty in understanding this aspect of female psychology. When exploring this aspect of shame one can sometimes have the sense of encroaching "into" a person. When the shame is inadequacy one does not have quite this sense of "intrusion into".

Another aspect is whether this distinction has anything useful to say about the prominence of eating disorders and problems of weight in females (Silberstein, Striegel-Moore, & Rodin, 1987). Certainly bingeing and purging are often associated with disgust/shame. The (evolutionary) links between the affects of disgust, expulsion, and notions of "getting rid of", with what is going on in one's body can only be speculated on at the present time. Also it may be that males have ignored these issues (Silberstein et al., 1987) because they do not have the same experience of shame/disgust or the same orientation to the physical self. Rather, they are more into issue of power, strength, and competency (or its opposite inadequacy and weakness). Greenberg et al. (1990) bracket the experience of the weak/bad self together (see below) but I think the experience of badness is different to the experience of weakness. Badness is associated with fears of being expelled whereas weakness is associated with not eliciting any interest, with a feeling that one is not worth bothering with.

It is women who flock to plastic surgeons, diet excessively and focus so much attention on their physical appearance for others, not men, and this must say something about their tactics for attempting to "live positively in the minds of others." At the present time more research is needed in this area of gender differences in the shame experience.

Shame and Concealment

Individuals may fear revealing those parts of themselves they feel ashamed about if, in so doing, they make themselves vulnerable to attack/ridicule (Gilbert, 1989). This is, in a sense, to do with the issues of how and what we display of ourselves to others (see Mollon [1984] for a discussion of sexual shame) and also with how we are internally represented to ourselves. A patient felt unable to cry in therapy because this made her feel weak and inferior. In her early life she had been criticised for crying. With her friends she maintained a coping persona, but became angry when her friends gave her messages like "things can't be too bad for you because you always cope and look fine". Before she could face the world she paid particular attention to make-up and social presentation. Although she was lonely, she hated people dropping in on her in case they found her with her "guard down".

The anticipation of shame and producing a negative image of self in the eyes of others motivates concealment (Gilbert, 1989). Pennebaker and O'Heeron (1984) and Pennebaker and Becall (1986) have argued that failure to reveal past traumatic events (e.g., abuse) has biological consequences and involves internal inhibition. Pennebaker and Becall (1986) found that college students who had been unable to reveal and discuss childhood traumas (e.g., abuse or loss of a parent) had more health problems than those with similar experiences that had been able to disclose them. This inhibition acts to keep the person on the defensive in certain areas of social life and can in some cases lead to secret fears of being found out and rendering the person subject to intense experiences of shame.

Brewin and Furnham (1986) explored what they called pre-attributional variables in depression. They found that depressives often fail to reveal experiences and fail to gain consensus validation for experiences leading to a sense of isolation and difference from others. This failure may be related to fear of scorn (shame) and the idea that their experiences or ways of coping were different from others and probably inferior in some way.

As Mollon and Parry (1984) suggest, shame associated with depression can be seen as a form of self-protection. However, it is not the depression that is protective but rather the tactics used to conceal and protect the self from ridicule that are the protective elements. Unfortunately, these tactics may actually produce the depression. This is because, in the main, it is mechanisms of inhibition (Pennebaker & Becall, 1986) that block exploration, and carry with them the idea of inferiority and a sense of negative difference/separation from others.

Shame and concealment are very under-recognised throughout the psychiatric spectrum of disorders. The consequences of shame vary from difficulty in expressing negative affects to feeling vulnerable/ inferior to the confiding relationships. Shame maintains defensive self-processing.

Shame and Self-Blame

Janoff-Bulman (1979), in exploring the relationships of depression to rape, found that there was an important distinction between the types of blame people ascribed to themselves. Behavioural self-blame was focused on actions and related as "I should have done; I should not have done X, Y, Z." Characterological self-blame, however, was related to personal qualities, "I am or am not". When victims blame something about themselves rather than specific actions they are more likely to become depressed. Janoff-Bulman and Hecker (1988) have reviewed their work and accommodated it within the attributional model of learned helplessness. They argue that blaming one's character tends to reduce the chances for change whereas actions can be changed in the future. Hence the former leads to greater hopelessness. However, one needs to remain aware that there may be gender differences here. Furthermore, the self-blame literature is poorly integrated with the shame literature and hence does not make a distinction between blaming one's lack of skill or intelligence, which is focused on personal inferiority, and the more disgust type affects of shame.

Second, Brewin (1988) and Hammen (1988) have pointed out that not all studies have shown that depression is associated with the perception that events are uncontrollable. Rather, failing to control what others may be able to control is also an important depressogenic aspect. This fits well with ranking theory that places social comparison at the heart of self-evaluation. After all we learn what is controllable or not by observing others. If everyone is doing badly (failing) then we are less likely to be depressed because this carries no sense of inferiority. Time after time in therapy one hears this aspect: "But my mother coped well; my friends don't seem to be like this, it's only me." It is not just the controllability of things in themselves that is a problem but how others are (perceived to be) doing. It is often this perception of an (inferior) difference that leads to a secondary evaluation of "well they are okay so it must be something about me" (Brewin & Furnham, 1986). And in ranking theory it is this (social comparative) evaluation that takes us into inferiority preoccupations, self-blame, and all the inhibitory processes we have spoken about in the last two chapters (e.g., on exploration, initiative taking, and so on). Although Teasdale (1988) has suggested that people can be depressed about being depressed it is also common to find shame about depression.

Shame, Humiliation and Revenge

The third aspect where self-blame may be important in shame research in depression is in the difference between humilation and shame. I may well be humiliated by others but not get depressed, but strive for vengeance. This is because my own judgement of myself does not concur with those of the humiliator. Hence shame also requires that in some sense we accept the judgements of others (or they become our own judgements). Thus shame which has any depressogenic quality is probably associated with some negative lowering of SAHP and self-esteem. Those who remain robust in the face of torture are noted to say "they could break my body but not my spirit." Hence self-blame and self-evaluations are probably associated with the depressogenic aspects of shame and we should, on psychological grounds, distinguish more clearly between shame and humiliation. In those that have been treated as subordinate but smell the possibility of revenge, the fight can become savage and we say "the knives are out" or, "the back stabbing has begun". Of course the desire for vengeance is not without its own problems, even though it may protect a person from depression by giving them a certain degree of power.

Humiliation can lead to shame, however, as a patient who had been abused explained to me. Although her experience of her abuse was one of humiliation and she blamed her father, the consequence was that she was left feeling contaminated and feeling inferior and tainted—the soiled and spoiled syndrome. This is sometimes experienced as having some of "the good self" stolen from one. "I can now never be like others," she said. "I have lost my self-respect. He took all that away."

Reputation and Shame

Also, shame can be experienced as a result of other peoples' actions. A patient whose family had a bad reputation in the local community said, "I feel so ashamed of being one of them. All my life I have struggled to prove I was different but people tar you with the same brush." People may feel ashamed of how members of their group behave (e.g., football hooligans). A politician on television revealing what his country had done during the war said, "You know I still feel a deep sense of shame about all that. It is something I can't get rid of I suppose. It's just there, a reminder." (He was two years old when the war broke out.) Children of parents found guilty of war crimes have also suffered much shame (e.g., Serney, 1990). Hence, shame can be felt for other reasons apart from personal actions. We can also feel embarrassed for someone else—e.g., when we see someone making a fool of another and this can even be from watching it on television. In real life, we may feel anxious observing these events because we know we should step in and stop it, but we do not want to become the centre of attention and possibly be put down. We don't want to signal possible outgroup membership.

Internalised Shaming

Can one be ashamed of oneself even though others are not being critical? Can one have an internal relationship of persecutor–victim? Well, certainly this kind of internal, split relationship has been written about in object relationships for some time (Greenberg & Mitchell, 1983). We may have a relationship with ourselves that is a mirror of our relationships with others. For example, a depressed patient recently told me that in her head she attacks herself. "It's like there is a part of me that whips me with a stick and says, 'Get down. You are a lazy good for nothing. You are an inferior weakling, fit for nothing.' When I can't fight back these feelings I just want to crawl away and hide in bed, which I often do." This hiding away of course convinced her further that she was lazy. (Firestone, 1985, noted a similar internal relationship; see Chapter 6). Moreover, interestingly her response to this internal attack was (before therapy) to try to prove this attacking part of her wrong, and, when she felt able, she would throw herself into things more and become very competitive and perfectionistic. Using the two-chair technique (Greenberg, 1979; Greenberg et al., 1990) it turned out that the shaming part of her believed that she would be unwilling to do anything without a constant attack and pushing. Freudian therapists would call this a harsh super-ego (see Schore, 1991). Indeed the two chairs approach revealed the voice to be that of her mother. This activated much affect and an opportunity to learn that she had nothing to prove.

Hence, as discussed elsewhere (Gilbert, 1989) it seems that we can play out the agonic (hostile dominance–submission) relationship in our own heads. Just as we can be hammered into submission by others we can hammer ourselves into submission and states of defeat. The two chair technique is possibly one of the best techniques for getting at this kind of internalised shaming system. As an aside, it may be that in some forms of schizophrenia this internal shaming system is externalised somehow (see also Morrison, 1987). What the depressive fears (others running them down behind their back), or what they think about themselves, is experienced as coming from outside, as external voices of condemnation. The whole issue of how these sub-components of the mind work is still under research, but the syndrome of schizophrenia seems similar to the behaviour of defeated animals (e.g., low exploration, psychobiological retardation and so forth). Hence, again, thinking about how the evolution of social dominance has shaped psychic structures may pay dividends.

Shame and Fear of Failure

The fear of failure (Birney, Burdick, & Teevan., 1969; Sadd, Lenauer, Shaver, & Dunivant, 1978) or of being different is rife in our society and this is about social power. The point is that effort and the preparedness to make mistakes are vital for growth. Without a preparedness to risk being wrong learning becomes more concerned with self-protection. Shame however can arise unintentionally. Holt (1969, p.55) points this out clearly:

> Note the danger of using a child's concept of himself to get him to do good work. We say, "You are the kind of sensible, smart, good, etc., etc., boy or

> girl who can easily do this problem, if you try." But if the work fails, so does the concept. If he can't do the problem no matter how hard he tries, then, clearly he is not sensible, smart, or good.
> If children worry so much about failure, might it not be because they rate success too highly and depend on it too much.

Holt goes on to suggest that most strategies that children use in school are self-protective, to avoid embarrassment, disapproval, and loss of status. Children try to create a good image in the eyes of others and are fearful of not doing so. Sadd et al. (1978) factor-analysed various measures of fear of failure. These were related to measures such as self-depreciation and insecurity, failing to live up to internal standards, unassertiveness, and self-consciousness. These were significantly associated with a number of symptoms including feeling low in energy, guilt, worthlessness, difficulty in making decisions and concentrating, and various others. Gilbert (1980) found that fear of failure was associated with higher depression and anxiety and a more negative thinking style.

The Shamer

It is common in psychopathology research to focus on the one that suffers. However, if we are to be effective in prevention then we cannot escape the fact that others can cause distress and pathology. In therapy we hear time and again the stories of the experience of shame. One patient spent a year with a teacher who would constantly punish him by calling him to the front of the class and ridiculing his work in front of others. There is little doubt that shame induction has been used as a way to control children for centuries (see Miller, 1983). Many junior doctors over the years have told me that some of their educators used shame and ridicule as a way to advance learning. My daughter came home from school in tears at the start of a new school year. She had been told off. When my wife went to ask what this was about the teacher said " Well she had not been working as I wanted. But I am often harsh to begin with. Sometimes you have to knock children down before you can build them up again." Amazing isn't it? If we wish to study shame then we should also look at those that cause it.

Cultures throughout the world understand, at least intuitively, the need to be valued and have a sense of belonging and play cruelly on the shame-fears to effect social control. In small measure shame may well be helpful in some situations but it would be so much more desirable if people learnt how to value themselves and others rather than comply from a sense of fear. In the behavioural theories of Skinner this is via positive reward rather than punishment, a position he always advocated.

Guilt, Shame, and Entrapment

Many authors believe that a sense of personal responsibility defines guilt in contrast to shame but from the analysis given above this would seem unlikely. Elsewhere (Gilbert, 1989) I have suggested how guilt may reduce a person's sense of entitlement and is linked to moral and existential issues. Here I would simply add to this discussion by pointing out that guilt unlike shame is often associated with an internal sense of entrapment (Trent, personal communication). Shame on the other hand tends to motivate withdrawal and avoidance. It may be guilt and the fear of hurting another that stops us from breaking off relationships that are in fact detrimental to us. It may be guilt that stops us from allowing ourselves certain pleasures. In these situations a person says "I would like to leave or do this, but I would just feel too badly about myself if I did." Marriages and parental relationships seem particular areas for this type of personal conflict.

Hence guilt is often linked with what a person feels they are entitled to do or what they (think they) have a right to do and this is an internal judgement. This can sometimes link with the martyr theme or caring guilt theme (see Chapter 11). Not letting others down can be a major source of self-esteem. Guilt-prone people often think in terms of selfishness and make judgements of themselves and others with this construct. Behaving towards others out of guilt turns relationships into burdens, fuels (secret) resentment, and increases the sense of being trapped and unable to escape from the burden. If resentment shows, this can be taken as further evidence of personal selfishness, fuelling the "bad self" image. However, we should not make the distinction between shame and guilt too acute at this point since both may be involved in our internal sense of entrapment and these are not the only sources of social entrapments (e.g., blocks to breaking away from others). Fear is also common.

SOCIAL ANXIETY

What is the link between social anxiety, depression, and shame? Social anxiety is highly represented in many depressed patients and often high enough to reach diagnostic levels (Sanderson, Beck, & Beck, 1990). Pilkonis and Frank (1988) found that avoidant personality disorder was the most common personality disorder in hospitalised depressives. To explore the relationship of shame and social anxiety Pehl (1990) noted that a lot of the social anxiety literature used a concept called fear of negative evaluation, FNE. Using a FNE evaluation scale (Leary, 1983) and the Johnson et al. (1987) shame–guilt scale in a group of students

(N=93) Pehl found that FNE and shame correlated $P<0.55$, but FNE and guilt were not significantly associated. A median split of FNE into high and low scorers showed that the high FNE subjects scored significantly higher on shame variables: helplessness; anger at others; anger at self; self-consciousness and inferiority feelings and also depression and submissiveness. This research like others, indicates that social anxiety, shame, and depression are related. Further work with a patient group is now required.

Like the subordinates of most species, humans who feel subordinate in groups are generally more tense and anxious, especially if called on to "display" to the more high ranking individuals. For example public speaking seems to be far more anxiety provoking in the context of others who have higher status than the speaker, compared to contexts where the speaker is of equal or higher status. Giving a talk to a group of new students may be far less anxiety provoking than giving the same talk at a world conference. Indeed social anxiety relates to the degree to which individuals see situations as a ranking encounter where others (evaluators) can add or subtract from status, i.e., they have potential to "spoil" the display of the speaker and hence reduce SAHP. In fact ranking evaluations seem to lie at the heart of social anxiety (Beck, Emery, & Greenberg, 1985; Trower & Gilbert, 1989; Gilbert & Trower 1990).

The role of loss of SAHP rather than fear of aggression in social anxiety can be seen most easily in the sexually anxious. The man who fears that his sexual body will fail him is not worried about the aggressions of his potential partner but about the loss of her attentions. Hence social anxiety is much concerned with self-presentation. In Chapter 2 we explored the relationship between depression and anxiety and noted a high association (e.g., Kendall & Watson, 1989). What has yet to be done is to explore in more detail specific forms of anxiety. Gilbert and Trent (submitted for publication) found that social anxiety correlated with depression at 0.56.

Beck et al. (1985) point out one crucial difference between shame and social anxiety. While social anxiety may fall after an encounter, i.e., when we have left the social situation, a sense of shame may increase. In other words there is a post-event ruminative aspect to shame which is not evident in social anxiety. This ruminative quality of shame may stay with us years after an event. Hence although shame and social anxiety are linked they function in different ways. This may be because, whereas in social anxiety we are concerned with the approval of others, in shame our approval of ourselves is also at stake. In other words I may fear that others may find me unattractive which, if I desire their approval, may lead to social anxiety, but feel that I am basically an okay person. In shame we, ourselves, have become inwardly unattractive and in shame we attack ourselves in some way.

Social Anxiety or Depression

Ranking theory and network theory would suggest that social anxiety and depression follow similar paths. In both there may be negative social comparison, a sense of inferiority and fear of shame in social situations (Trower & Gilbert, 1989; Gilbert & Trower, 1990). However, in social phobia feared situations are normally fairly specific and when out of the situation the person does not feel badly about themselves. Hence the socially phobic lacks the global sense of weakness and inability or inferiority of the depressed person. Second, the socially phobic does not feel incapacitated to reach goals and rarely has a global view of themselves as being trapped in an unfavourable life style from which they cannot escape. Third, although the socially phobic is easily tipped into submissive responses in social situations they do not feel defeated or burdened down and do not experience the pervasive loss of energy or pleasure as does the depressive. Fourth, they do not show the general losses of energy and information processing dysfunctions of the depressed person (see Chapter 6).

If these conditions change, such that the socially phobic does start to feel a greater sense of personal failure and inadequacy, then depression is more likely. And as we have mentioned, when social phobia is highly generalised, as it may be in avoidant personality disorder, depression is more likely (Pilkonis & Frank, 1988). Hence many depressed patients are socially anxious (Davidson et al., 1989; Kendall and Watson, 1989), depressed children and adolescents are particularly fearful of social evaluation (Ollendick & Yule, 1990) and, as mentioned above, in our study, social anxiety correlated with depression 0.56. One difference between endogenous and neurotic patients may be in the degree of their pre-depressive social anxiety. We are currently investigating this idea.

ASSERTIVENESS

Ranking theory would predict that depressives are likely to be relatively unassertive (more inhibited) and certainly not likely to behave as dominant or confident. However, much will depend on how relationships are construed. Depressives may be aggressively irritable with those they regard as more subordinate than themselves, but more of this later. Certainly one of the predictions of ranking theory would be that depressives would be inhibited in situations of (potential) agonism that they felt they could not win and would tend to select submissive responses in those situations. There is evidence that this is indeed the case. Forrest and Hokanson (1975) investigated the propensity for depressives and non-depressives to use self-punishing behaviours in response to interpersonal conflict (confederate aggression). They examined the rates of self-administered electric shock in response to aggressive behaviours. It was found that baseline rates of self-punishing responses were much higher for the depressed group. They suggest that this indicates a previously established repertoire for dealing with aggression from others (although it cannot be ruled out that such behaviours become manifest as a consequence of the biological change associated with depressed mood). They also found evidence to suggest that self-punishment or the emission of a friendly response, in the face of aggression from another, had significant arousal-reducing properties. In other words, "avoiding attack responses" reduced the arousal associated with confrontation in the depressed, but not the non-depressed group. Forrest and Hokanson (1975, p.355) state:

> ... The experimental findings indicate that the greatest plethysmographic arousal reduction takes place in the depressed group when a self-punitive (or friendly) counterresponse is made to the aggressive confederate. The nondepressed group exhibited comparably rapid reductions only following an aggressive counterresponse.

More recent work now confirms that depressives are unassertive (e.g., see Kuiper, Olinger & MacDonald [1988], and also Chapter 4 this volume on personality). A number of theorists have speculated that this arises from the depressive need for approval. Ranking theory suggests it relates to fear of rejection, or of invoking an overwhelming counter-attack. It may also be that there is something about assertive behaviour that depressives experience as undermining of their positive self-beliefs: i.e., it is not nice to be assertive. For example, Schwartz and Gottman (1976) demonstrated that, compared to high and moderately assertive subjects, low-assertive subjects seemed to be inhibited in the delivery of an assertive response to an unreasonable request. The cause of this difficulty was not a lack of knowledge of what to say or do. Rather, it lay in their significantly higher degree of intrusive negative thoughts about responding assertively. Low-assertive subjects scored significantly higher for responses such as "I was worried about what the other person would think of me, if I refused; I was thinking that it is better to help others than to be self-centred; I was thinking that the other person might be hurt or insulted if I refused" (Schwartz & Gottman's test example, p.913). Such data suggest that it is not only aggression that is feared but the loss of SAHP. However, this view would only be supported if depressives were equally unassertive with everyone. My hunch is that it is with those they feel lower in rank to that they behave non-assertively.

My colleagues (Gilbert & Trent, submitted for publication) and I wished to explore submissiveness in depression (rather than lack of assertiveness) and have developed a scale from the work of Buss and Craik (1986) called the submissive scale. We found that self-rated submissiveness correlated with BDI 0.47 in students and 0.52 in a depressed population (ICD 9 neurotic depression). Pehl (1990) found that in a large group of psychology students submissiveness correlated 0.33 with BDI. A median split of students into high and low BDI responders found that the high scorers had significantly higher submissive ratings. Using the component measures of shame mentioned above it was also found that submissiveness correlated $P<0.44$ with helplessness, $P<0.29$ with anger at others, $P<0.39$ with anger at self, $P<0.43$ with self-consciousness, and $P<0.49$ with inferiority. Hence inferiority comes through again as an important variable in submissive behaviour.

Does one need a ranking theory to explain these findings? Well actually, no. Animal conditioning work has shown that noxious events can become reinforcing, if they are associated with the avoidance of even more aversive events. Animals can learn to direct their behaviour to the lesser of two evils. Forrest and Hokanson (1975, p.356) suggest that such learning has been developmentally important in depressives. They suggest that:

> ... depressed patients have learned to cope with environmental and interpersonal stresses with self-punitive and/or nonassertive behaviours and these behaviours have been successful in dealing with their normal day-to-day existence. At times when situational stresses become great, this limited behavioral repertoire may be invoked to a degree that may seriously impair adequate functioning and these people may manifest a clinical depressive or masochistic episode.

Similarly, the behaviour theorist Ferster (1974) argued that depressives demonstrate significant passivity in response to aversive events and that this arose from early conditioning experiences. Ranking theory would not deny the enormous importance of early learning to depressive proneness but it would also argue that since yielding and submissive behaviour is an innate potential, early learning is not necessary. Individuals with relatively favourable estimates of RHP and SAHP can still get depressed by life events, head injury, hormonal disturbance, and so on. It would be interesting to know whether Forrest and Hokanson's work had particular relevance to the concept of dysthymic personalities/disorder outlined by Akiskal (1988, Chapters 3 and 4, this volume).

Is submissiveness the same as lack of assertiveness? Here one must be cautious. In a factor analysis Arrindell et al. (1988) found that assertiveness had at least four components: (1) display of negative feelings, involving standing up for oneself and engaging in conflict; (2) expression of and dealing with personal limitations, involving a readiness to admit mistakes and deficits; (3) initiating assertiveness, involving making one's opinion known; (4) praising others and accepting praise. We do not know how submissive behaviour would relate to these factors. Equally, new scales have been developed to measure how people try to influence others, which Buss, Gomes, Higgins, and Lauterbach (1987) call tactics of manipulation. They devised a scale to measure these six basic types: (1) charm; (2) silent treatment; (3) coercion; (4) reason; (5) regression; (6) debasement. These researchers found that charm was often used when trying to get others to do something, but coercion and silent treatment were used when trying to stop/terminate people from doing something. Hence, our tactics interact with what outcome we want. Also, extraversion and neuroticism were correlated with different patterns of manipulation. The highest correlation at 0.33 was with neuroticism and the use of silent treatment.

We do not know if it is a mood effect or ranking effect that accounts for Buss et al.'s findings. In much of these research areas there has been little control for the rank issue, i.e., to whom assertiveness may be inhibited or expressed and when, or how people try to manipulate those seen as higher in rank compared to those seen as lower in rank. Hence the issue of how assertiveness relates to submissive behaviour is complex. Is submissive behaviour associated with tactics of manipulation (e.g., silent treatment) that are likely to lead to more negative feelings between people? If so then the submissive strategy to avoid trouble may be counterproductive.

The implications of ranking theory however must be seen against the backdrop of evolutionary processes, for it is not simply that submissiveness may succeed as a coping response. Rather, it is the fact that such responses carry significant information about one's standing in the social hierarchy. The relationship between depressed or angry moods when one is forced to "eat humble pie" bears close examination! The experience of "having let oneself down" or "sold oneself short," or "let someone get away with something, take advantage" etc., can produce powerful, unpleasant emotions including shame. How we see ourselves as a result of such inhibitions, be they internally or externally imposed, can have a powerful impact on mood state, depending upon the importance we place on the encounter. We may brood on resentment and/or become angry with ourselves over our fear of lack of assertion. We may attempt to manipulate in a negative way (e.g., silent treatment). Thus, although the depressed individual may feel relieved by their self-punitive responses (Forrest & Hokanson, 1975), self-esteem and perceived place in the hierarchy are likely to suffer. This will be counterproductive since it may increase dependency needs.

Dependency Needs and Assertiveness

It is currently believed that dependency needs and needs for approval are related to the needs for nurturance and fears of abandonment (Nietzel & Harris, 1990) and are part of an attachment system. However, we have reason to doubt this view at least in part (Gilbert & Trent, submitted for publication). Needs for allies, as part of sexual reproduction strategies, are now well recognised in animals (Trivers, 1985). Also, according to the investment theory of self-presentation outlined in Chapter 7 we are all, to some extent, dependent on each other to maintain a positive sense of self. We suggest therefore that distinctions should be drawn between different needs for social relationships as outlined by Weiss and others (see Chapter 15). A theatrical actor may need the admiration of his audience but not wish to form an attachment relationship with them. As discussed earlier (Gilbert, 1984), humans want to feel valued by others, they want to be acknowledged, to believe that what they are or can do is useful, and in this way can elicit others' investment in them.

In behavioural terms we not only want to receive positive reinforcement from others but it is positively reinforcing to know that we are reinforcing to others, that we have value in their eyes. When the lover gives you up it is not just the loss that is important but also the implications that you may no longer be reinforcing to her/him. One loses one's sense of reinforcement to others, one's sense of being attractive.

How do assertive problems relate to these concerns? As noted in the last chapter this is a tricky dilemma since to be assertive we must at times risk not being valued by others and losing (at least temporarily) their support. At this point the depressive must choose the lesser of two (potentially) negative outcomes: either (a) be assertive, go with conflict but risk a loss of approval, support and/or an increase in hostility, or (b) submit to others but then lose the incentive that they wish to pursue. The depressive tends to choose the latter strategy. (Aggressive and more dominant individuals on the other hand tend to choose the former and devalue the need for support.) This dilemma and the biological ramifications are outlined in Fig. 8.1.

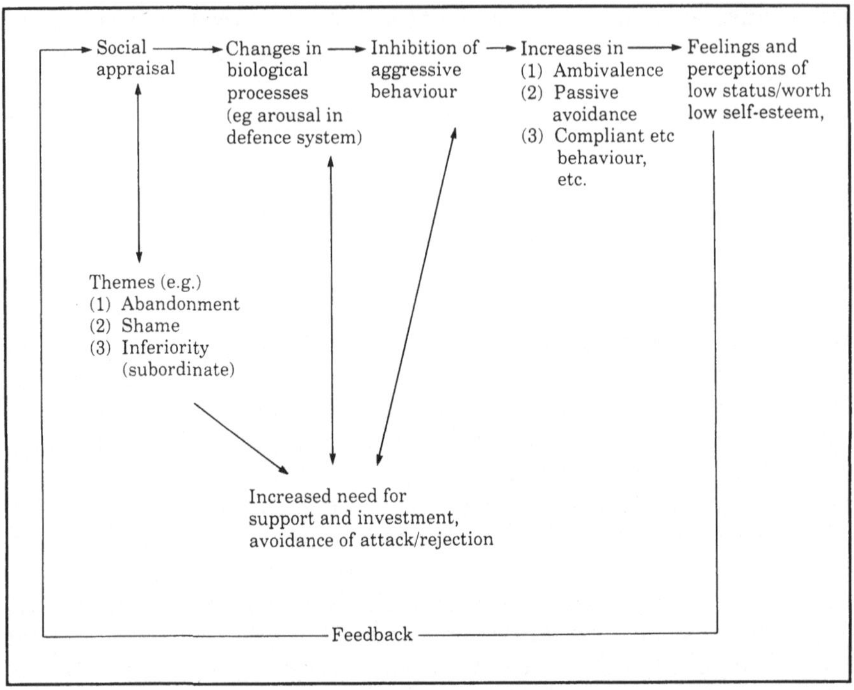

FIG. 8.1. Model of the interaction between social evaluation, biological change, and cognitive-behavioural change.

Some patients hate the feelings of neediness of depression whereas others are all too ready to elicit care at every turn. The therapist who has unresolved problems in needing to be seen as a "caring person" to support their self-esteem may find the latter patient idealising him/her. The problem here is that this keeps them in an inferior position to the therapist. Rather, they should come to value themselves and, as Arieti and Bemporad (1980a) point out, avoid continually entering into "bargain relationships". Hence the role of therapist mirroring and helping a person to internalise a sense of their own value is important, but an eye should be kept on dependency.

Reputation

As we argued in the last chapter networks are very important to chimpanzees and humans. Depressed patients sometimes discuss the possible impact of assertiveness on networks; a useful term is reputation. A patient felt that an old friend was taking advantage of her. They shared the same network of friends however. At one point the friend asked to borrow some money. The patient refused and was confronted by an attack on the lines of "I've known you for so long. How can you not help me now? I'm very disappointed in you", etc. However, despite high arousal and some shock at the friend's outrage she continued to refuse. Later that night she felt very tearful and had images of the friend going around their shared network telling all her friends how bad and horrible she was. She was sure her friends would side with the accuser and became more depressed. Whenever she met members of her network she thought, "I wonder if X has told them? I bet they think I'm horrible". Hence human assertiveness can involve fears of how a reputation may be changed and how this may result in a feeling of alienation (see also Baumeister, 1982). Needless to say the patient saw the friend who had asked for money to be one of the more dominant members of the group of friends and certainly more dominant than herself.

ANGER

Although during the first part of this century anger and rage were centre stage in theories of depression (see Chapter 9), some of the newer approaches (e.g., cognitive and behaviour theories) are unfortunately negligent on the issue of anger in depression. This is a problem, for new therapists may be quite unprepared for the hostility that can lurk in some depressions. Indeed, in some cases, anger and resentment are the key affects that require help. It can sometimes be a person's inner resentment and the ease by which it is aroused that stops them from developing stable hedonic/affectionate personal relationhips. On a number of occasions I have had cause to reconsider a diagnosis of depression in terms of anger and resentment being the more primary problem. Many patients talk of "having to sit on my anger" and the fear of 'exploding'.

Assertiveness and anger are not the same thing as assertiveness trainers frequently tell us. Hence we should clearly distinguish the problem of assertiveness in depression from that of anger. Explosions of anger or instability in mood states (e.g., irritability) can occur because of lack of assertiveness and a build-up of resentments. The relationship of anger to depression is complex and not all depressives have the same types of anger. Second, there are two kinds of question: (1) the degree to which depressives actually experience anger or aggressive feelings and (2) if experienced, how and to whom are they expressed.

The way depressed individuals actually handle anger is complex. Blackburn (1974), using questionnaire measures of hostility, found high intrapunitiveness in both unipolar and bipolar depressives. Unipolars, however, also had higher extrapunitive scores. Lyketsos, Blackburn, and Tsiantis (1978) observed cultural differences in hostility patterns during recovery from depression. A reduction in intrapunitiveness was associated with recovery.

Cochrane and Neilson (1977) found that inhibited aggression was especially marked in endogenous depression. Pilowsky and Spence (1975) found that hostility was rarely expressed in the presence of vegetative symptoms (if vegetative symptoms are indicative of a primitive defeat algorithm then this is an important finding). Riley et al. (1989) have reviewed the theories and evidence concerning the role of anger in depression and found depressed patients suppressed anger more than normals or a post-traumatic stress group. As they point out however, individuals must be aware of their anger to be able to acknowledge suppressing it. Fava et al. (1987) found there were differences in hostility in patients who had experienced losses compared to those who had not. Loss patients rated themselves as more friendly than non-loss patients. Thus the relationship between friendliness and hostility is complex. It may be that, as depression improves, some patients switch from a previous (depressed) agonic state to a more hedonic one. Other patients may not have (as their basic interpersonal style) a particularly friendly orientation. Another interesting finding is that in depressed children expression of anger is more common and this has been put forward as an important distinction between child and adult depression (Izard & Blumberg, 1985; see also DSM-111-R). The probability is then that we are dealing with different types of anger in depression.

Ranking theory suggests that aggression is rarely directed up the hierarchy. So as Price (1988) suggests depressives may be responding to the internal dictates of an unfavourable perception of rank and negative social comparison, i.e., the biological response rule "don't express aggression to those that are more powerful than you". It would not be surprising however if depressives were more expressive of anger to those that are seen as subordinate in some way or unlikely to fight back (e.g., children).

Weissman, Klerman, and Paykel (1971) found depressed women had greater hostility towards those with whom they shared a close relationship. But according to Price (1988) this would only be expressed if the patient saw the other as subordinate. Against this view is the observation that in chimpanzees angry tantrums can be aimed at a dominant who does not offer reassurance (Goodall, 1975). Also in some primates, infant temper tantrums are met with stroking by others and calming. Hence another possibility is that "tantrum anger" may be elicited when a person needs reassurance/support and is not getting it.

This might be the anger directed at a neglectful or unreassuring partner. Price (personal communication) has been exploring tantrum anger in children and feels that the evidence supports the view that tantrum anger is usually expressed by the subordinate in the relationship.

Anger may be a consequence of a change in state; the depressed state may actually reduce frustration tolerance in some individuals. Fava, Anderson, and Rosenbaum (1990) have drawn attention to a fascinating element of anger control in depression. They document a number of individual cases in which people literally had "attacks of anger". For some these seemed out of line with previous personality. One patient described himself as "being on a short fuse" and losing his temper quickly and becoming enraged, or going well over the top. The researchers think these anger attacks may be like panic without the fear. Is it possible that this is triggered by some ranking threat? It has been noted that, in non-human primates, unpredictable attacks from dominants may do much to keep subordinates fearful and compliant (Trivers, 1985; Sapolsky, 1989; Chance, personal communication).[1] As far as one can tell these patients' anger attacks were always elicited in the presence of others or when thinking about others. Ranking theory would be interested in looking at the subordinate–dominant relationships and making a distinction between subordinate temper tantrums and those of more dominant individuals who may feel their rank is under threat and switch to primitive attack options to exert control. In the former it is a seeking for reassurance, in the latter it is related more to a desire to "push way" (out of the territory?) and to subdue others or force them into compliance. Maybe these will be difficult to separate.

Depression may, then, produce instability in the primitive fight/flight mechanism. The anger outbursts of Fava et al.'s (1990) patients (which were helped by antidepressants) were also most distressing to them. (Aggressive dominants on the other hand are rarely distressed by their displays of anger and often have all kinds of self-justifications for them.) So to say it again, we are confronted with two issues: (1) what type of anger is felt and (2) when, how or to whom is it expressed? Certainly anger control should be clearly separated from problems of assertiveness.

Finally, we should note that some patients do carry a lot of anger with them about past events and various grievances. Sometimes these can relate to poor parenting. The problem is that carrying this anger may reduce the chances of developing smooth interpersonal relationships and leads one to feel misunderstood and separate from others, and often feels unpleasant. It is sometimes associated with feeling a victim and a need for revenge (see Chapter 11). However, in these cases it is not sufficient to use anger control methods, but one must help the patient to forgive, though not condone (Fitzgibbons, 1986), and come to terms with the past and let it go rather than stay preoccupied with it. Fitzgibbons (1986) notes how this can be very difficult but often helps to put patients in touch with a deep underlying sense of disappointment, hurt, and vulnerability that has been defended against via the anger. Kohut (1977) regards anger as a secondary event to fragmentation (see Chapter 10 for a further discussion of narcissistic rage).

ENVY

Envy is another of our primitive responses to the problems of ranking, competition, and social control. Its role in depression is complex and often (like shame) unrecognised. I am indebted to my colleague Dr Ghadalai for many discussions on this topic and for indicating how envy is often involved in depression. Klein (1957/1975b) made envy an important aspect of object relations theory but confused frustrative aggression with envy (for a review of the psychoanalytic concept of envy see Joffe, 1969; Horner, 1989). Although her distinction between envy and gratitude is an important one, I do not believe young children are capable of envy but do suffer frustrative aggression (Mandler, 1975). Whether or not frustrative aggression is a forerunner of envy is unknown. However, Kohut makes a clear distinction between frustrative anger and narcissistic anger (see Chapter 10). It is the latter that is associated with envy.

Nevertheless, Klein introduced many important concepts on the relation between envy and gratitude. She argues, "I believe that envy is an oral-sadistic and anal-sadistic expression of destructive impulses, and that it has a constitutional basis." Hence, envy could be heightened in situations of need, but where the person lacks the capacity for gratitude. Envy is sometimes confused with greed, jealousy, and shame. Berke (1987) made a distinction between the greedy thief and the envious thief. The greedy thief breaks into a house carefully and takes only the most precious and valuable items. The envious thief, however usually smashes his way in, leaves the most valuable items but is intent on messing/spoiling, even defecating and urinating about the place. In academic contests things rarely go this far, but individuals often talk of "rubbishing" the ideas of others, etc., and undermining the efforts/ideas of a competitor. Greed, however, is life-affirming, a reaching out with desire. Destructive envy is the opposite.

Although jealousy and envy often overlap, jealousy is aroused in a triangular relationship where hostility is expressed at the competitor, e.g., a man may be jealous of other men who show his wife attentions. If he wanted those attentions for himself then this would be envy of his wife. Envy, unlike jealousy, involves hostility at the desired object itself.

There is no clear ethological or evolutionary account of envy. Yet it is perhaps one of the most unresearched areas of human life. I have tried to find examples of animals destroying/spoiling resources of others if in the process this reduces their own access to the resources. The idea that "if I can't have it then I will destroy it so that others can't" is not seen in animals as far as I know.

A ranking and evolution theory might suggest that envy relates to rank and the recognition that someone has resources or qualities (e.g., SAHP via beauty, competence) that one wants for oneself. We do not envy the painting but the person who owns it. It can also relate to what I have called third party competition (see Chapter 7). Envy can have positive and negative consequences. Envy may lead us to aspire to be like someone else that we admire or idealise (our heroes). Indeed it may be our admiration that turns envy into something positive. Positive envy may better be called idealising. These distinctions are outlined in Table 8.2.

The aggressive (fight) for a dominant position to that of the envied may not be expressed directly, but can be expressed indirectly. It may be envy that motivates us to go behind someone's back and attempt to spoil their display and achievements in the eyes of others (i.e., reduce their SAHP): "Fancy him getting the prize; of course he's only an upstart, more mouth than brains. Personally I wouldn't trust him to mow the lawn, let alone be in charge of the team, etc.". This kind of envious

TABLE 8.2
Positive and Negative-Destructive Aspects of Envy

THE OTHER HAS THINGS, ATTRIBUTES, TALENTS, POWER OR RESOURCES THAT ONE WOULD LIKE FOR ONESELF.	
NEGATIVE	*POSITIVE*
Spoiling	Treasuring
Devaluing	Valuing
Destructive	Protecting, Defending
Rage, Resentment	Love, Adulation, Admire
Stealing	Modelling, to become like
Pull down	Build up
Distance	Closeness
Self feels vulnerable— Inferior in presence of	Self feels accepted — superior in the presence of

spoiling is directed at reducing the positive image of a person (or group) in the eyes of others. We are using catathetic signals (see Chapter 6) to bring down another but in an indirect way and when we meet the object of our envious attacks we may behave with politeness and present ourselves as a friendly ally. We may use humour to put others down. This tactic is difficult to deal with because one's natural inclination is to be aggressive or feel embarrassed if one is the butt of downing and shaming jokes, but both responses can reduce one's SAHP if others are present. Some individuals who believe themselves to be caring can nevertheless have a downing "sense of humour" if one could call it that.

The envious person begrudges the attributes, success, rank or status and attention accorded to the other. He or she may fail to offer assistance to those that succeed and be undermining of their efforts. Such behaviour has been noted in Type A personalities (Price, 1982) but often the role of envy is only mentioned in passing. According to DSM-111-R the narcissistic personalities are also prone to significant envy. And in narcissistic depressions envy is rife.

Envy and attempts to maintain the rank order in marriage can also be the source of a spouse (usually the husband) belittling and undermining achievements of the partner (usually the wife) especially if these appear to raise her status position or facilitate more control (see Chapter 15). Sometimes these battles over rank/dominance and the subtle signals aimed at maintaining the wife in a subordinate and compliant position can lead to significant hostility and depression in the wife (Price, 1988).

Another side to envy relates to stealing. There is no research evidence to support this view but it seems likely that envious people are more prone to stealing (e.g., other people's ideas) in an effort to increase their relative rank. It is likely that envy increases as a function of the size of rank differentials and shortage of resources, but such a view awaits research. Nevertheless, at both the individual and group level, anecdotal evidence suggests that the greater the potential rewards (e.g., Nobel prizes, research funds) and the more these rewards are idealised, the greater the potential for envy between competitors. The biblical name for envy is covetousness, which is regarded as one of the basic sins.

Envy and Depression

The expression of envy differs according to whether it is up rank or down rank directed. The attacks of spouses, bosses, or others who are envious of those they see below them are often direct, aggressive, and open. Their reliance on the subordinates for support is often denied. Those whose envy is directed up the hierarchy tend to be passive and express their envious attacks behind backs, and in various ways to avoid outright agonism or risk separation/rejection.

Envy relates to depression in at least three complex ways:

1. *Fear of exciting other people's envy.* A patient had recently saved money over a number of years to buy a very fine car. To his surprise he never felt comfortable driving it and within three months sold it and became more depressed. A cognitive exploration of "what was going through your mind when you drove around" revealed, "I just had this sense of people looking at me and thinking 'look at him in that fancy car. Where did he get the money? Who does he think he is?' I felt people wanted to bring me down somehow, that they didn't like me for having it." The patient articulated very clearly a feeling of being persecuted for having (in this case) a fine car and was so disturbed by it that he sold it.

In another case a patient had won a scholarship to a grammar school. However, her friends all went to a secondary modern school. She found that her new school friends did not fully accept her (because she was from the poor area of town) and her old friends thought that she was "snooty" and above them. Throughout life she had engaged in a self-handicapping strategy to avoid eliciting other people's envy. For example, she told me that when playing tennis (she was a rather good tennis player) she had difficulty in playing to win for fear of the others disliking her for winning. When playing doubles it was different because then she felt she shouldn't let her partner down. Many times in life when success was in her grasp somehow she would sabotage it. Nevertheless, she was very rank conscious and only felt attached to people who were of "higher status" than herself. The (often female) fear of success is often linked to the fear of eliciting other people's envy. Women in professions often complain of having to put up with male envy and attempts to run them down (see also Welner, Marten, Wochnick, Davis & Fishman, 1979). Because men see themselves as (at least physically) superior to women, men are more likely to express their envy openly.

False modesty can also be a tactic to avoid eliciting envy in others. In these cases much work may be necessary to help the person cope with others' (possible) envy and the issue of separation it can sometimes entail. It is true, unfortunately, that via envy we can lose friends and disrupt relationships (Gilbert, 1989). Also, as Horner (1989) points out, sometimes people are themselves envious and follow the rule, "if I envy and hate others then they will envy and hate me if I move above them in some way". However, some people can feel so ashamed of their own envy that it is very difficult to research.

Sometimes the fear takes a more sadistic turn. Remember the person who refused to give money to a friend (see p.243). This patient has spontaneous images of her friend breaking into her house and destroying things or putting glass in her food. At one level she knew this was illogical but found the images upsetting and frightening none the less. When working cognitively with these images it is important not to step too quickly into disputing. Rather, the therapist can help the patient understand the nature of the fears and the underlying sense of helplessness and persecution they involve.

2. *Fear of one's own envy.* A patient told me: "You know I hate other people coming to the house and seeing me like this. I really feel vindictive towards them. I feel my depression gives them a power over me. I want them to go through what I am going through. I want to wipe the smiles off their smug consoling faces. I am sure they talk about me behind my back. It's awful. I never used to feel so vindictive and I hate myself for it. I have come to the conclusion that underneath I must be a pretty rotten person."

In another case a person had been passed over for promotion. "I sit at home and think why them? I compare myself with them and I begin to think of how they are no good. I think they got there because of their hob-nobbing with powerful friends and that they have never liked me because I didn't fit in. I make plans in my mind to bring them down, to squash them in some way. I don't want to see them anymore because I feel this bubbling sense of resentment. I begin to hate the world. This is a terrible way to live. I feel so bitter and there is no way out. I used to be so outgoing. I used to like people. Now I hate them and I detest myself for feeling this way."

Both cases reveal the resentment that is part of envy, the terrible inner experience of it, and the self-dislike. Also the experience of one's own envy can be a very separating and lonely experience. If one's hate destroys the world then one is alone. If one's resentment becomes known then one may be rejected. Envy cuts one off from valuing others. This kind of envious difficulty can leave one feeling very lonely and an outsider, compounding a depression.

Envy, then, can be linked to shame/guilt (recall that the early analysts did not separate them as we have done here). Klein (1957) noted: "It appears that one of the consequences of excessive envy is an onset of early guilt. If premature guilt is experienced by the ego not yet capable of bearing it, guilt is felt as persecution and the object that arouses guilt is turned into a persecutor." In the above two cases—fear of others and fear of one's own envy—we have taken an essentially cognitive-ranking theory view. However, it obviously resonates with Klein's ideas except that it is stripped of libido theory of course. But the "felt experience" aspect of persecution is of interest, although how one would test this idea is unclear.

3. *Envy and separation.* Dr Ghadiali has suggested that envy begins with separation. If a child is in a relationship with an idealised other then the qualities of the idealised other are available for the child (as Kohut [1977] suggests). However, with separation the other takes those qualities and keeps them for themselves or gives them to others. In his view envy is often elicited via separation or the unavailability of the qualities of the other. The essence here is "if I could be like you I would not need you. If I didn't need you I wouldn't feel so vulnerable with you leaving me." The destructive aspect relates to a desire to stop the person having/keeping those qualities for themselves or giving them to others. This, as a primitive tactic of self-interest, is fairly clear to see. As Klein (1957;1974;1975b) suggests this kind of envy relates to a form of dependency and the desire to have (oneself) what one is dependent on the other for, or at least have complete control over it/them.

This kind of envy is also noted in sexual problems. A man who visited prostitutes told me that at first he feels great desire but after he has finished he begins to feel contempt for the women. This is also a kind of envy because he cannot control the object of his desires and therefore belittles what he has just received. He also feels contempt for himself for needing and desiring a sexual partner. As Horner (1989) suggests, devaluation of that which is desired is a defense against recognition of envy and need.

A patient had just gone through a painful divorce. Her ex-husband had quickly found someone else and had set up home. Sometimes she saw him in the street. "When I see him I think, you shit, you have got away scot-free whereas here I am alone and depressed. I would like to go round and smash him, I would like to tell his new woman all about him. I want him to suffer like me. I just can't stop thinking about it." She was clear that if he suffered too she would feel better, although she acknowledged it would not do any practical good. Sometimes she felt that suicide was the only way to get back at him, to make him pay.

A patient who had done quite well with cognitive therapy was approaching the end of therapy. To the puzzlement of the therapist she came to one of her last sessions in a very aggressive mood. "I now understand everything that you have been saying but I am so angry with myself for not working this all out myself. I just can't understand why I have been so stupid all these years." This "I should have seen this for myself" is a way of denying the skills and talents of the therapist, and of course the years of research on methods of treatment. It dawned on the therapist (me, unfortunately) that we had not addressed at all her problems with envy, and how this belittling of other people who had been helpful to her, was a part of her problem.

So it is understandable why the analytic therapists link envy with its opposite, gratitude. In gratitude we are able to feel a positive feeling of having received something that we could not have done for ourselves. We recognise the talents and attributes of the other.

Overview

The main concepts in (negative) envy are the spoiling, bringing down, destroying and/or stealing, and lack of gratitude. We may denigrate that which is envied or engage in "third party competition" (see Chapter 7) to destroy a positive image of a person in the eyes of others.

Horner (1989, pp.56–57), who has written on the issues of power and envy, gives this example:

> A woman who characteristically clung to a powerless position in order to force her mother to take care of her, as well as to protect the mother against the hate of her own envy of the older woman's power, said of an associate, 'I hate her, and there's nothing that can be done about it. I spoil her by thinking her seams are crooked or that she only seems nice because she is so shallow. I am powerless with her. I do want to smash her, to get rid of her, to tell her what I think of her. And I hate you (the therapist) for being so strong. I feel impotent. I can't change you. I kiss ass and walk away hating you. It's a passive ragefulness.'
>
> Although she used to think of herself as competitive, she came to understand the critical difference between competitiveness and envy. This difference resides in the degree of hostility and the wish to spoil or destroy that go with envy. One can value the competitive rival and have no wish to harm that person. In competitiveness, unlike envy, the only wish is to win.

It should also be noted that it is not necessarily the case that the negative (anger and efforts to spoil the SAHP of the envied) and positive (idealising) aspects of envy are mutually exclusive. Indeed, in therapy both the positive and negative components of envy can be directed at the therapist. Unfortunately, a depressed patient who is very envious of the therapist will have difficulty in accepting help from them since part of their orientation is aimed at undermining the therapist efforts, "to bring them down, to rubbish their efforts". This can also be a power ploy "I'm too difficult a case to be treated. This therapy is okay for them other dudes but I'm more complex." Envy is about power, rank, and social control and though the activity of negative envy may be over-all counter-productive it arises from the desire to be top dog and destroy competitors.

THE SELF

The above aspects can all be regarded as part of the depressive experience of dread. Further, they are all aspects of ranking and the need to accommodate oneself to group and ranked social living. They form different patterns, however, for each individual case. A central question is how these various aspects (shame, anger, assertiveness inhibition, envy, and so forth) are organised. Various theorists following the work of Beck (1967; 1976) have developed the notion of negative self-schema as part of the constellation of depression. Among the most important theorists are Kuiper and his colleagues, (e.g., Kuiper & Olinger, 1986; Kuiper et al., 1988). In their view the above aspects (shame, envy, etc.) would constitute aspects of a generalised negative self-structure (schema).

This is like the legc model of personality (see Chapter 4): different schema are built up over time and shift about in the psyche, some are latent others are active. Unfortunately, it is difficult to find convincing evidence for there being consistent and coherent negative depressive self-schema (e.g., see Spielman & Bargh, 1990, for a review). Depressive self-schema are difficult to find in individuals who have not been depressed but will become so (Lewinsohn, Steinmetz, Larson, & Franklin, 1981).

An alternative view is like the recipe model of personality: that there are various potentials, algorithms, and archetypal themes (see Chapter 11) that at different times can become mixed together to form a particular self-organisation. Individual aspects (or ingredients of the recipe) may emerge but not produce depression. Depression arises from a particular organisation of these elements. Hence like a cake mix it is the way various elements in the system interact; what emergent patterns arise from the interaction of these elements (Gilbert, 1989). It is from the interaction that various feedback and amplifying mood destabilising processes may form (see Chapter 13). This view is articulated by Greenberg and his colleagues (e.g., Greenberg et al., 1990).

Perhaps this problem can be resolved by suggesting that the self is a fluid system that becomes organised in different ways at different times. In other words there are no permanent schema stored in the brain some place but rather there is the potential for certain kinds of self-construing patterns. Hence we may speak of patterns of experience that represent the activation of various archetypal potentials (which are shaped by learning and memory). In depression what emerges is a pattern of interaction of different memories and self-constructs. Such a view is implicit in archetype theory and mentality theory (Gilbert, 1989).

A key question is, does the brain have within it a preparedness to bring together certain of its internal algorithms and response options, to access various affective memories, to form the depressed state? The ranking theory answer is yes. Under conditions of low self-efficacy and negative social comparison the brain evolved to switch to particular patterns, that of the inhibited, which gives rise to subordinate or yielding routines. Greenberg does not follow an evolutionary view but his approach is consistent with this idea. Greenberg et al. (1990, p.170) suggest:

> Based on our clinical observation, it appears that depression is much more likely if a person's weak/bad, hopeless, self-organisation is triggered, than if the critical self and negative cognitions alone are activated. It is much more the person's response to the negative cognitions and their inability to cope with the self-criticisms, than the cognitions and criticisms alone, that lead to depression. People are unable to counter or combat the negative cognitions when the weak/bad helpless state has been evoked. This is when depressed affect emerges.
>
> It is thus the combination of the hostility of the critic and the activation of the weak/bad self which constitutes the experiential vulnerability to depression, and it may well be that the hostility is the crucial variable in invoking the weak/bad organisation. The weak/bad organisation, although it is a recurrent, possible self-organisation and therefore possesses some degree of structuralization, does not predominate in the person's every day functioning and is not necessarily accessible under normal circumstances. Other forms of self-organisation develop and help the person function in the world.

Above we noted that the weak self should be separated from the bad self and not bracketed together. There are some depressives who do not see themsleves as bad but as trapped in unfavourable situations and unable to change the situation (i.e. the helpless self). Prison camp victims would be an obvious example. These are forms of involuntary self-perception but not necessarily with low self-esteem. Nevertheless, the internal referee is activated in depression (see Chapter 6) as a consequence of feeling overpowered or without control.

In the majority of depressions, however, the internal referee is also experienced as an attack on the self (you're no good, useless, etc.) and self-esteem is low. Another key issue is whether these kinds of self-attacking processes are already formed in some way and are structuralised (e.g., negative self-schema exist but are latent when not depressed) or, alternatively, whether the brain is a pattern-generating system such that various (and new) self-organisations can "materialise". Brain state theory (Reus, Weingartner, & Post, 1979a; Gilbert, 1984, 1989) has tended to support the latter view.

This view is in keeping with the evidence that: (a) various forms of damage to the CNS, (b) genes, (c) various kinds of hormonal and other biologic difficulties, (d) viruses, and so on, can produce depression. None of these factors require that there is some latent depressive self-schema. Rather, the potential for shame (evolving from social dominance) and all the other aspects spoken of earlier are part of our innate set of possibilities. Under certain kinds of biological influence these may be organised (brought together), including styles of information processing, to inhibit the person from taking part in the challenges of social life and switch them into subordinate and/or defeat routines.

We may speculate that certain kinds of biological change (e.g., hormonal, viral) signal to the brain that we are unlikely to succeed and that a better option is to become more attentive to threat and stay out of action or switch to alternative strategies for eliciting other peoples' investment (e.g., care eliciting). For my part at least, these remain extremely crude approximations to what is actually happening at a psychobiological level when an individual is depressed. Furthermore, it is often the case that in therapy we find the person has had repeated experiences from parents or others of being "put down" or in a weak/bad position. However, we also find people who have had reasonable childhoods and, until they became depressed, functioned perfectly adequately.

To summarise: all the aspects referred to here (shame, envy, etc.) exist as potentials of "self-experience", they are archetypal themes (see Chapter 11). However they can be over-developed by life experiences and/or recruited via brain dysfunction, life events, and so forth. Ranking and network theory suggests that the depressed patterns arise from various forms of an involuntary, subordinate routine.

SUMMARY

1. The depressive experience is often one of dread, emptiness, and anxiety. Many aspects make up this experience of dread and for the most part these can be understood in terms of ranking and network theory.
2. Ranking theory, attachment theory, and needs to belong (ingroup identification) help to explain the experiences of shame, lack of assertiveness, poor anger control, and envy. These relate to underlying components of mind that we all share by virtue of our evolution.

3. Shame relates to many factors such as perceived inferiority, fear of rejection and of being held in contempt, concealment, and self-blame.
4. Evidence suggests that depressives are not adaptively assertive and are mostly submissive. Also, they are not reinforcing to others, and certainly to do not elicit others' investment by a free, confident, and open display of talent.
5. The role of anger in depression has fascinated researchers for many years and there is now little doubt that depression is associated with a disturbance in anger control. However, there may be different types of anger. Some may have anger attacks, others may have temper tantrums, and others may suffer from an elevated threshold for frustrative aggression. The role of rank (when and to whom anger is expressed) is still to be fully researched.
6. Envy is a serious but often unrecognised problem in depression. Like so many other experiences, it seems related to evaluations of relative rank. Those that feel inferior may express their envy "behind backs" and try to destroy the SAHP in a third party competition (see Chapter 7). Fear of eliciting others' envious attacks can inhibit us. We can also be depressed by the strength of our own envy. Strong experiences of envy/resentment leave us feeling separate from others and alone and can make it difficult to develop affiliative relationships.
7. Self-organisation derived from innate and experiential modified components seem to come together in depression although there are wide individual differences in their actual pattern.

CONCLUDING COMMENTS

The processes, affects, and behaviours that have been discussed here are so important in depression that it is worrying that researchers have not addressed them more fully, except in a piecemeal fashion. Perhaps part of the problem is that we are so dominated by psychiatric phenomenology for medical diagnostic purposes. At the present time we have no good measuring instruments that are able to look at complex state change patterns.

All the above aspects are related to the evolution of rank and the need to form ingroups and the subsequent modification of strategies for controlling others by eliciting their investment via creating a good impression. The problem is that the aggressive options for social control live with us still. Interpersonal schema theory (e.g., Safran & Segal, 1990) is negligent on the schema of power and control, perhaps because it has been so dominated by attachment theory. This is not so much a rebuke as a plea to take on the issue of social power as it exerts itself in all facets of our lives. It is likely that early attachments significantly determine whether we are orientated to the social world in an agonic or hedonic manner. In the former case we enter the world in a controlling way and our symbolism is in terms of power (or the lack of it). Problems are solved by the demonstration of strength.

In current political arenas the agonic style is prominent, with its focus on strength, power, need to punish those who are too deviant, and stress on individualism, winners and losers. Other political systems are organised around envy and limiting others (e.g., the rich). At the present time we have no clear hedonic political system and it is difficult to know what it would look like if we did. But, as we shall argue in Chapter 15, cultural values are the yardstick by which people come to judge themselves. Since psychopathology is concerned primarily with brain function and since the brain evolved as the organ for tracking social success (Vining, 1986; Nesse, 1990) then it follows that at some level the social milieu in which we grow and live must enter our research endeavours and theory building.

NOTE

1. In many animals ritualistic aggression is not designed to injure but intimidate. Thus what evolved in a dominance action repertoire was "ferocious display". In primates there is much psychomotor discharge (e.g., running, screaming, charging, banging the ground, throwing things, stamping, etc.). The experience of rage may have evolved from this action pattern—to intimidate. Thus in depression, rage attacks may suggest the activation of a primitive intimidation display. In today's environment these may not be adaptive, but intimidation displays may have been adaptive earlier in our evolution. I am grateful to Dr Leslie Greenberg for asking the question "How is rage adaptive?"

PART III

PAST AND CURRENT THEORIES

INTRODUCTION TO PART III

In the first section of this book we explored types and classifications of depression. In Part II we explored an evolutionary approach and put forward the basic axioms of a ranking theory and our need to belong. In the next seven chapters we explore current psychological and social theories of depression. At appropriate places we will note how each theory compliments or is in conflict with our evolution derived theory. I have tried to follow a logical sequence, which hopefully will become clear as we move through the different approaches. Basically this is a journey from the inside (the role of innate aspects of mind) through to the more cognitive and behavioural theories and finally to theories that focus on the outside or the (social) environment. In the last chapter we shall try to pull various themes together. As with all journeys there are places where lack of time and the lack of expertise of the guide prohibit exploration.

CHAPTER 9

Psychoanalytic Theories of Depression: The Early Schools

HISTORICAL BACKGROUND

Before we proceed with our exploration of early psychoanalytic theory it should be remembered we will be considering theories that had their origins in the immediate post-Darwinian period. This period provided the historical-cultural background for analytic thinking. Without this awareness various concepts may seem bizarre.

The interaction between psychological and biological processes became especially problematic with the emergence of psychoanalysis, but the origins of these difficulties predated Freud. For example it had been known for centuries, and in many cultures, that trance-like states altered pain perceptions. Charcot (1825-1893) and Janet (1859-1947) moved these observations forward with the concepts of disassociation (Ellenberger, 1970). Freud, heavily influenced by Charcot's demonstrations of hysterical paralysis, became fascinated by such phenomena and sought explanations of how the psyche could be influenced by processes that were outside a person's conscious awareness. But neither the idea of the unconscious nor the idea that unconscious processes were involved in neurosis were original to Freud (Ellenberger, 1970). Although many of the concepts utilised by Freud had existed as isolated ideas for some time, Freud secured himself a place in history with his ability to bring such ideas together and develop them into a comprehensive theory of mind. He attempted to establish a systematic theory, able to explain mental pathology as the interplay of psychological processes on physiological ones, and, Freud hoped, one day vice versa.

Psychoanalysis was very much a consequence of Darwin's evolution theory. With Darwin came the greater certainty that humans are evolved animals whose superiority (if it be such) lies in their history and not in the hands of God. This allowed Freud to suggest that the study of the disordered mind (via psychoanalytic theory) was biological psychiatry; for in neurosis, Freud believed, the interplay between the preservation of the individual and the preservation of the species were central. As evolution theory is important to all early analytic theories, further attention is given to it here.

Darwin's influence on psychology and psychopathology was immense but indirect. In suggesting and substantiating the view that humans and animals share a common history, shaped by the forces of evolution, the classical discontinuity view of humans and animals, proposed by Descartes, could no longer exist. Humans had finally lost their souls. For psychology, three major implications of Darwinian theory became evident. Atkinson (1964) and Weiner (1972) outlined these as follows:

1. Darwin and later researchers demonstrated the existence of intra-individual differences in the ability of organisms to adapt to their environment. Thus the study of individual differences in terms of psychological ability (e.g., IQ and personality) and physical ability became of major importance. Indeed, the study of the causes of individual differences (the nature–nurture debates) has been a cornerstone of much work in clinical psychology and psychiatry. The genetic versus the environmentalist controversies in the classification debates owe much to this concept of intra-individual differences in the adaptive ability of conspecifics.
2. Darwinian principles reaffirmed the idea that laws of adaptation and learning exist in other species apart from humans. Such a view provided the theoretical rationale to study the laws of learning in animals, both for their own intrinsic interest and as a means for offering insights into learning mechanisms in humans. Weiner (1972) suggests that this led directly to Thorndike's experiments and the operant principles of the laws of effect. Also, of course, the study of physiological and anatomical mechanisms of learning in animals rests squarely on this principle. Should it have been shown that the non-human primate brain (say) operates radically differently from the human brain, this line of research would have been much less interesting and useful

and, of course, would have challenged Darwinian principles. As it is, many of the neuroanatomical and biochemical insights (including the mapping of neurotransmitter pathways in the brain and the development of many drugs) have been possible as a result of the study of non-human brains.

3. Darwin's view of a continuity between humans and animals lent itself very directly to the idea that humans, like animals, are (to some extent) driven by instincts which are primarily concerned with survival rather than rationality. Rationality will develop if it bestows advantage in the struggle for survival. Further, there is no particular reason why humans should be conscious of all that goes on in their minds.

This third implication leads directly to Freud's id psychology and indirectly to various drive reduction theories of learning. Even today, this area of psychology remains one of the most conceptually complex and controversial. Some modern theories of psychopathology ignore the difficulty of inherited psychobiological response patterns completely and suggest that it is only the laws governing the development of beliefs and attitudes that are necessary for understanding psychopathology.

At the turn of the century, however, this would have been considered naive indeed. For this was a time when questions of how humans could deal with their (then accepted) primitive and savage past abounded. It was a time of Frankenstein and Dr Jekyll and Mr Hyde and also when Nietzsche was at his most popular. It was a time when we began to replace our fear of external demons and Gods and become preoccupied with the beast within. What evil existed in the world arose from the actions, desires, and motives of people, not supernatural forces. Although Freud apparently put off reading Nietzsche directly for some time, as Ellenberger (1970) points out, Nietzsche was so well discussed at the time of Freud's early maturity that it was not necessary to have read him directly to be permeated with his ideas and the cultural preoccupations. To be able to appreciate some of the parallels of Freudian thought with Nietzsche's ideas, it is worth quoting Ellenberger (1970, p.277) at length:

> Psychoanalysis evidently belongs to that "unmasking" trend, that search for hidden unconscious motivations characteristic of the 1880s and 1890s. In Freud as in Nietzsche, words and deeds are viewed as manifestations of unconscious motivations, mainly of instincts and conflicts of instincts. For both men the unconscious is the realm of the wild, brutish instincts that cannot find permissible outlets, derived from earlier stages of the individual and of mankind, and find expression in

> passion, dreams, and mental illness. Even the term "id" (das Es) originates from Nietzsche. The dynamic concept of mind, with the notions of mental energy, quanta of latent or inhibited energy, or release of energy or transfer from one drive to another, is also to be found in Nietzsche. Before Freud, Nietzsche conceived the mind as a system of drives that can collide or be fused into each other. In contrast to Freud, however, Nietzsche did not give prevalence to the sexual drive (whose importance he duly acknowledged), but to aggressive and self-destructive drives. Nietzsche well understood those processes that have been called defence mechanisms by Freud, particularly sublimation (a term that appears at least a dozen times in Nietzsche's works), repression (under the name inhibition), and the turning of instincts toward oneself. The concepts of the imago of father and mother is also implicit in Nietzsche. The description of resentment, false conscience, and false morality anticipated Freud's descriptions of neurotic guilt and of the superego. Freud's "Civilization and Its Discontent" also shows a noteworthy parallelism with Nietzsche's "Genealogy of Morals". Both give a new expression to Diderot's old assumption that modern man is afflicted with a peculiar illness bound up with civilisation, because civilisation demands of man that he renounce the gratification of his instincts. Scattered throughout Nietzsche's works are countless ideas or phrases whose parallels are to be found in Freud. Nietzsche taught that no one will complain or accuse himself without a secret desire for vengeance, thus, "Every complaint (Klagen) is accusation (Anklagen)." The same idea with the same play on words is to be found in Freud's celebrated paper "Mourning and Melancholia": Their 'complaints' are actually 'plaints' in the older sense of the word.

Outlining the parallels between Nietzsche and Freud helps to put Freud in some philosophical and historical perspective. It is clear that social Darwinism and Nietzsche's philosophy had an enormous impact on Western thought at this time, and Freud could not have avoided being influenced by it. Jung (1963), for example, unlike Freud, clearly outlined the influence Nietzsche had on his thinking.

Today these influences on our thinking are less acute, and we leave consideration of the beast within to the writers of horror fictions. Perhaps our models of human behaviour are more influenced by current developments in the technical fields and metaphors of the computer, and the fact that we desperately wish to see ourselves as rational. Thus computerisation has brought with it psychological ideas of information processing and feedback systems, circuit loops, and we map out mental processes like a circuit board. These reflect the rather cold and lifeless aspects of the computer. It would seem unfair, however, to introduce analytic ideas without some recognition of the cultural background from which they emerged and the kind of issues that were of central concern. It is with these thoughts in mind that Freud's ideas on depression are introduced.

THE INFLUENCE OF FREUD

Energy

A key idea in Freud's thinking was that of psychic energy, that which moves from within. As a neurologist, for the first forty years of his life, Freud was keenly aware of the need to offer up a psychobiological theory of mind. The *Project for Scientific Psychology*, written in haste in 1895 but never published, formed the neurobiological framework from which Freud was to postulate various energy-based mechanisms in the formation of psychological symptoms (Wollheim, 1971). He believed that neuronal energy was excitatory, could be diverted or repressed, but not destroyed (all in agreement with Nietzsche). Such a view may also have been stimulated by his experiments with cocaine. For Freud, the mind was a system of flows of energy. In consequence the idea that quantities of energy could be shunted around the central nervous system according to the vicissitudes of mental mechanisms appeared tenable. Indeed, it leads directly to the concept of symptom substitution and the importance of catharsis (the release of repressed energy) for recovery (McCarley & Hobson, 1977). Much of Freudian theory is therefore a theory of how energy is working within the psyche. To misunderstand this is to misunderstand the very basis of Freudian theory.

Instinct

In the first instance energy is needed to carry out the internal dictates of the instincts, the inborn patterns of object seeking. Freud argued that each instinct has a source, an aim, an object, and an impetus (Hall, 1979). In Freudian theory energy is bound up with instincts, for without energy instinctive behaviour (e.g., seeking food to reduce hunger-tension) would not be activated. The basic drives of the id were seen as primarily sexual (for reproduction of the species à la Darwinian theory) and self-preservative. In 1920 in *Beyond the Pleasure Principal*, Freud reviewed these ideas and suggested eros and thanatos drives, the life and death instincts. (See Erdelyi [1985] for a fascinating discussion of how these drives are believed to operate in the formation of symbols and dreams, and the controversies of the theory.)

The Id and Primary Process Thinking

Freud, then, was writing at the turn of the century, a time of the unmasking of human nature as Ellenberger (1970) calls it. Consequently it is no surprise to find a concept like "id", possibly borrowed from Nietzsche. The id represented the innate/instinctive aspect of the personality. It is the realm of the impulses; it is irrational, demanding, selfish, and pleasure-seeking and tension-reducing. It seeks immediate gratification. From the id comes primary process thinking. With experience the baby is believed to form an image of objects that provide gratification (e.g., food for hunger) and this memory of the objects that are gratifying are stored in the id as memories. "The process which produces a memory image of an object that is needed to produce gratification is called the primary process" (Hall, 1979, p.25). In behavioural language the primary process might be simple conditioned associations. It is a direct linkage of need with desired object. For example, the baby who is not fed may generate images of food. "The investment of energy in the image of an object, or the expenditure of energy in discharged action upon an object that will satisfy an instinct, is called object-choice or object cathexis. All energy of the id is expended in object cathexes" (Hall, 1979, p.39).

When energy is moved from one object of potential gratification to another, this is called displacement. The notion of catharsis is another concept central to psychoanalysis for it relates to the flow of energy towards its object. This concept was used in various ways . For example, catharsis as cure can take place when a memory has been repressed and is made available again, leading to an outpouring of anger or grief for example. Displacement can occur as in the sexualisation of oral dependent needs to be loved and cared for. Sometimes analysts talk of decatheted memories. By this they mean the kind of person who can reel off a horrific story of (say) childhood abuse but in a totally unemotional way.

The treatment for neurosis, then, rests squarely on the idea that energy in the system is literally flowing (or residing) in the wrong place and the object of therapy is to enable the person to work through various defenses so that psychic energy is not diverted into symptoms. This view is in complete distinction to the cognitive view which has little concern for energy but argues it is the constructions we make of events that leads to neurosis and other psychopathologies. In such a view symptoms are not the result of wayward energy or thwarted drives but a natural consequence of personal meaning and beliefs. However, Erdelyi (1985) has argued that Freud's theory is also a cognitive theory in that it is concerned with internal/mental representations of objects, fantasy, and the production of meaning-creating contents. The other basic mental mechanisms, ego and superego, represent similar ideas which can be found in cognitive thinking. Indeed, in the immediate post-Freudian area a new school of psychoanalysis (which was to be a powerful influence on cognitive theorists), ego analysis, dropped the whole concept of drives and energy, but retained the ego and superego as fundamental concepts (see Chapter 12).

The Ego and Secondary Process Thinking

The id discharges tension via direct motor action and/or image formation (e.g., wish fulfilment, seen commonly in dreams). However, these by themselves are not likely to be successful in survival and Freud argued that the person had to take account of the reality of the world in which they lived. For example, one might feel sexually aroused by a stranger but it would be inappropriate to immediately seek to copulate (though one might have various primary process images of so doing). Hence, the pleasure principle is given over to the reality principal (awareness of obstacles to a goal); and primary process thinking is modified by secondary process thinking. Secondary process thinking acts to monitor the outside world, postpone or abandon actions or work out strategies for securing goals (e.g., planning a strategy to chat up the sexually arousing stranger). Hence it takes account of reality and of course this "taking account" of reality may mean that the goal is deemed by the ego to be unreachable. The id and primary process thinking is purely internal with no account given to the realities of object seeking. Secondary process thinking is what cognitive theorists might call coping strategies.

Both the reality principal and secondary process thinking are part of the functions of the ego. Because the ego is aware of all the dangers of pursuing impulsively desired goals it can block the id. It is this process that gives rise to the various defensive mechanisms, such as repression, denial, reaction formation, regression, projection, and sublimation. The ego can in effect become overwhelmed by the energy of the id seeking for gratification and seeks to repress or divert that energy. For example, via sublimation, aggressive, impulsive energy can be harnessed into carpentry or surgery. We cannot here go into all the ways these defensive operations are performed but the interested reader can find easily understood formulations in Hall (1979) and more recently Liebert and Spiegler (1990) and a more complex treatise in Greenberg and Mitchell (1983).

The Superego

The superego is the third major component of Freud's tripartite system. "It develops out of the ego as a consequence of the child's assimilation of his parents' standards regarding what is good and virtuous and what is bad and sinful" (Hall, 1979, p.31). In essence the reality principal modifies the id and the superego helps direct behaviour in order to obtain parental approval. Later this modification is related to any who are in a position to offer social rewards. In other words, to obtain social rewards the child learns that one has to take account of parental wishes. Over time the punishments and rewards that are contingently given to the child become internalised such that the child can feel good or bad about his/herself for behaving in approved or disapproved ways. Again there is some resemblance to learning theory here.

There are two sub-systems of the superego: the moral conscious which is the source of guilt, and ego ideals. Hence the superego also contains within it a striving for perfection. When a person is said to have a harsh superego it means that they set high stands for themselves and are driven to achieve and may attack themselves for failure—called a superego attack. Later Bibring (1953; see Chapter 12) argued that ego states and ideals caused depression, and Karen Horney coined the term "the tyranny of the shoulds". The cognitive elements of the musts, shoulds, and oughts are, in Freudian theory, the result of a harsh superego.

Anxiety

In many ways Freud's theory is an anxiety or fear-based theory for it is fear that resists and gives rise to conflict. Freud recognised that humans can be fearful of things both external and internal. Hence he distinguished three kinds of anxiety (1) Reality or objective anxiety, arising from things in the world such as snakes, heights or terrorists. (2) Neurotic anxiety, fears arising from doing, thinking or feeling something that was threatening to the self (e.g., being aggressive to needed others and being abandoned or attacked back). In other words id-based impulses and primary process thinking give rise to neurotic anxiety since primary process thinking and secondary process thinking are in direct conflict. At times the conflict can be such that the impulse is kept unconscious. (3) Moral anxiety, fear of doing something that contravenes the superego, or failing to live up to ego ideals with the risk of internal punishment (e.g., guilt, self-dislike; see Hall, 1979, for further discussion).

PSYCHOSEXUAL DEVELOPMENT

In many ways the above outline is not very remarkable or controversial perhaps. We can find some kind of intuitive sympathy with it. People can be impulsive, can scheme and be deceitful to secure their goals, to which they may or may not admit or be conscious of, and people can be fearful of their own thoughts and feelings and block out further processing (Greenberg & Safran, 1987). The degree to which id impulses can be diverted into defense mechanisms might be more troublesome but most trouble begins with Freud's theory of psychosexual development and even more with his ideas of how to heal a psyche in conflict with itself.

The Oral Stage

In his three essays on sexuality Freud argued that what is experienced as pleasurable is determined by the location of libidinal energy. Libidinal energy is distributed in body parts and functions and it changes during development. In the oral phase it is the taking in which is both pleasurable and tension-reducing. In this stage it is external supplies that are the sources of wishes from the id, and the mouth particularly is an outlet for oral-libidinal energy. Under stress people can regress to oral means of reducing tension, e.g., smoking, drinking, eating or oral aggression, e.g., nail biting. As Liebert and Spiegler (1990) point out, while Freud focused on the biological aspects of the oral phase, later analysts focused on the psychological aspects—namely the need to be mothered, cared for, held, dependent, being given to, receiving.

The fixation of libidinal energy at this stage gives rise to the oral personality. The oral personality is one who is preoccupied with these themes, and the id and ego work together such that the person is constantly striving to maintain contact with those who can fulfil their (receiving from the outside) needs.

An oral personality may however deny or repress their needs and become superficially autonomous, or may become more orally aggressive with intense anger directed at those who do not supply their dependent needs. If id-based aggressive energies are experienced as too great and threatening to plans to obtain gratification from others, they may be repressed or displaced or diverted to the ego itself. This, as we shall see shortly, is the basic Freudian view of depression.

The Anal Stage

The second stage of libidinal development is the anal stage. This is the stage where pleasure is obtained from retaining or eliminating faeces (and later the need to have things for oneself and keep them for oneself). Power comes from having/owning and controlling (e.g., secrets, worldly goods, lovers). More generally the child is learning about his/her own mechanisms of control over his/her own body and social control over others. At this stage the child is becoming less dependent and more power-seeking and autonomous; this is the stage of power struggles for the child. If the libidinal developmental process becomes fixated at this stage the personality may become focused on needs to hoard and retain things, becomes secretive, stubborn, and a "you can't make me do that" attitude develops. The person has difficulty with cooperation and sharing. Two types of character formation are possible: anal retentive—stubborn, ordered, obsessional careful, withholding; and anal expulsive—messy, chaotic, reckless, wasteful. To date no study has found that these personality traits have anything to do with toilet training however.

The Phallic Stage

The third stage is the phallic stage where libidinal energy becomes invested in the genital region as a source of pleasure. It is a time of awareness of different sexual characteristics of the self and parents and also the potential of the oedipal complex. Basically this is the desire to be rid of the father so that the child can have the mother to himself. But this desire ignites the fear that the father may castrate the child. Now most parents are well aware of the child's competition for attention, and in bed how a child may push in between two parents. It is also clear that infant sexuality exists (Hofer, 1981; Efron, 1985). While it may be true that some fathers can react angrily in the competition for the mother's/wife's attention the idea that the child has a castration anxiety seems extremely unlikely. Speaking as an evolutionist there is one very good reason for this. This is, in no species has it been found to occur. Yet there is mounting evidence that most of our primitive fears arose from actual possibilities in phylogenetically earlier times (Nesse, 1990). Certainly in many species infants can be injured or even killed by older males but this is an issue of awareness of power. If castration anxiety exists it is a highly symbolic fear; a metaphor of the loss (or lack) of power. It is also true that sexual signalling is prominent in threat behaviours and phallic symbols as symbols of potency and power exist in many cultures. (Eibl-Eibesfeldt, 1989). In our everyday language we talk of feeling impotent to act, and so on, but none of this points to actual castration fears.

Overview

I hope enough has been said to help with understanding the analytic view on depression. Also, as we move through the book we will see how often the themes of dependency and autonomy crop up in theorising on depression. The basic concepts to recognise are related to those of energy and how these are moved about within the psyche.

FREUD AND DEPRESSION

As we saw in Chapter 1, Kraepelin was the first to systematise the distinction between dementia praecox (schizophrenia) and manic-depressive psychosis. But the phenomenology of the manic-depressive complex changed throughout the course of Kraepelin's publications. Indeed, it was this tendency to broaden the concept which enabled Hoche and others to accuse Kraepelin of making woolly and ill-defined distinctions. Although these disputes raged in the background, it seems that Freud generally accepted Kraepelin's classification system, despite the fact that it managed psychogenic factors poorly or not at all. Of major importance was Freud's apparent belief (in which he was not always consistent) that psychoanalytic theory should address itself to mild and severe forms of the disorder, including manic-depressive illness. That this is so can be seen from the following extract taken from *Mourning and Melancholia*, first published in 1917. Here (at p.253) Freud makes clear his concern with the manic episode:

> The most remarkable characteristic of melancholia, and the one most in need of explanation, is its tendency to change round into mania—a state which is the opposite of it in its symptoms. As we know, this does not happen to every melancholia. Some cases run their course in periodic relapses, during the intervals between which signs of mania may be entirely absent or only very slight. Others show the regular alteration of melancholic and manic phases which has led to the hypothesis of a circular insanity. One would be tempted to regard these cases as non-psychogenic, if it were not for the fact that the psycho-analytic method has succeeded in arriving at a solution and effecting a therapeutic improvement in several cases precisely of this kind. It is not merely permissible, therefore, but incumbent upon us to extend an analytic explanation of melancholia to mania as well.

There are a number of elements in this passage which should be considered. If Freud is talking about true manic-depressive illness, then he may have had psychoses in mind. However, it is unclear how familiar

Freud was with the true psychoses. For example, his analysis of paranoia did not arise from directly observed data, but from Schreber's book on the subject. On the other hand, Abraham (1911) clearly stated his concern with depressive psychoses and offered an account of a case which today would most probably be considered a bipolar affective illness. Abraham postulated a connection between obsessional neurosis and depression, and in regard to the manic-depressive cycle he argued that: "Psychoanalysis shows, however, that both phases are dominated by the same complexes, and that it is only the patients' attitudes towards these complexes which is different" (p.149).

It seems fair to conclude, then, that early psychoanalytic views had a rather inclusive notion of depression and were not simply concerned with mild neurotic states. It is interesting to note Freud's rejection of the "cyclical insanity" view of manic-depressive illness on the basis of the reported efficacy of psychoanalytic treatment for some cases. The possibility that spontaneous remission may have played a role is not considered. Moreover, a certain element of doubt about the generality of an analytic explanation is also evident in *Mourning and Melancholia* where (p.243) Freud wrote: "Our material, ... is limited to a small number of cases whose psychogenic nature was indisputable. We shall, therefore, from the outset drop all claim to general validity for our conclusions ... ."

This was to create a problem for subsequent psychoanalytic theory, for having acknowledged a probable lack of generality, the phenomenology to which Freud addressed his theory was very wide indeed. In general, the limiting factor was a kind of diagnosis by prognosis. If manic-depression responded to psychoanalytic therapy, then it was psychogenic. If a case did not respond to such treatment, few conclusions were drawn regarding etiology. More recently, some psychoanalysts have agreed that even in severe depression psychogenic elements are of the utmost importance (Arieti, 1977; 1978) and most now agree that, regardless of cause or type, psychological and social difficulties accompany depression.

There is much that can be written on the various aspects of the generality of psychoanalytic theory and the patients from whom the ideas developed. Such considerations should be borne in mind when considering Freud's view of melancholia.

Mourning and Melancholia

Mourning and Melancholia was undoubtedly a landmark in psychological theorising on depression. By the time of its publication in 1917 many events in the history of the psychoanalytic movement had already occurred. Jung and Adler had disaffected themselves from Freud, the First World War was well under way in all its tragedy, and Freud himself, now into his sixties, had experienced his own personal depression. Moreover, psychoanalytic theory had erected a complex and powerful set of axioms for explaining the development and cure of neuroses. Although Abraham had offered a psychoanalytic theory of the manic-depressive complex some six years earlier (from which Freud borrowed and which he acknowledged), it was *Mourning and Melancholia* which was to shape many of the subsequent views on the subject.

Freud had touched on the problem of periodic depression some years earlier, believing it to be a third form of anxiety (Goldberg, 1975). But it was in the comparison of mourning with melancholia that Freud directed his attentions to a systematic explanation of depression. As psychoanalytic theory was already well developed, Freud's analysis was much more than a simple comparison of these two states. Hence *Mourning and Melancholia* is a complex work incorporating many aspects of general psychoanalytic theory, including libido theory, narcissism, ambivalence, the oral personality, regression, the process of identification, and so on. It needs to be emphasised, therefore, that a complete understanding of Freud's theory of depression requires a good, general grasp of psychoanalytic theory. As such an exposition cannot be undertaken here, the reader interested in this approach should consult psychoanalytic literature directly (e.g., Anthony & Benedek, 1975; Hall, 1979; Wollheim, 1971; in regard to depression specifically, see Volkan, 1985). Only the central elements of Freud's position will be discussed.

In *Mourning and Melancholia*, Freud proposed that loss was central to both these states. Both are painful states of mind which focus on a lost object. However, loss may be of a more ideal kind or the patient may be unsure about what is actually lost. Thus, there is the suggestion that for some depressed individuals the object lost is unconscious. In mourning, however, the loss is very much within consciousness. Freud highlighted a further important distinction between mourning and melancholia by suggesting that in melancholia there is "an extraordinary diminution" in self-regard, which is not present in mourning. *In mourning, it is the external world which has become impoverished and empty. In melancholia it is the internal world, the ego itself, which has become poor and empty.* This is because rage and anger at the (now) unavailable object cannot be expressed and is diverted from the object to the ego: i.e. the individual represses his rage to a loss. It is in the explanation of the relegation of loss to the unconscious and the lowering of self-esteem that Freud turned to psychoanalytic theory. Here we should note the distinction between "observations" of phenomena (in this case psychological events) and the "explanation" of how these events came about. Many writers agree with Freud's observations on the importance of loss and a lowering of self-esteem in depression, but disagree as to the mechanisms.

Comment

In the years that followed, many theorists focused on the issue of anger against the self. As Deitz (1989) points out, rage was centre stage (as for example in Rado's work of the 1920s) and the idea of depression as diverted rage, a drive that should have been directed outward but due to various fears (e.g., dependency) was not, became the starting place of many theories. In Freud we hear an echo of Nietzsche's claim that "no one accuses themselves without a secret wish for vengeance".

As we saw in Chapter 8, anger is certainly an element of depressive experience but it may be expressed (e.g., increased extrapunitiveness) or inhibited. However, many other affects are similarly affected. Furthermore different types of anger may be involved in different people and assertiveness and anger should be clearly separated, which in depression theory they often are not. Still the issues of anger inhibition and dependency remains a prominent aspect of many theories—e.g., Arieti and Bemporad (1980a,b), Blatt et al. (1982). Further, we know that depression is often associated with hostile, self-blaming or negative attitudes to the self, that is few if any depressives feel good about themselves.

The concept of "energy flow" is now rarely accepted as valid even though the concept of energy is useful at a descriptive level (see Chapter 6). For example, patients talk about getting their energy back as they recover. However, such descriptions should not be confused with actual internal processes. At this level it is more accurate to think in terms of inhibition and excitation and ponder actions at the level of neurochemical action (e.g., Weiss & Simson, 1985). If energy does not "flow in the system" (and thus cannot be dammed, or diverted or repressed, etc.) then many of the basic psychoanalytic concepts for change break down and catharsis is unlikely to cure. In regard to unconscious processes scientific exploration reveals that much of our processing and decision making may indeed not enter consciousness (Brewin, 1989; Power & Brewin, in press; and see Chapter 13). However, in my view, interpretation is a poor treatment mode; too dependent on the whims of the therapist, it is too passive and many patients find it unhelpful when depressed. Rather the therapist should come to the rescue of the self and do what they can to break up the various forms of inhibition associated with subordinate self-perception, shame or loss of ability, be these arising from the past or currently. More often than not this requires a caring, non-passive therapeutic relationship and action-focused interventions.

OBJECT RELATIONS THEORY

The work of Melanie Klein (1957/1975a) came eventually to represent a major departure from Freud. In the early days, however, during the 1920s, Klein regarded her work with children as an expansion and development of drive-libido theory. Subsequently, it became clear that her later formulations constituted radical changes in psychoanalytic thinking and led to a further fragmentation of adherents, especially in Britain. Like other developments in psychiatric thinking, Kleinian ideas have influenced therapy concepts in ways which are obscured by history. The most notable departure of object relations theory from Freudian theory is the shift away from drives to the concept of internalised representations of others, called self-objects. As Greenberg and Mitchell (1983) make clear, object relations theory is primarily a "relational/ structure" theory rather than a "drive/structure" theory as in Freud.

Object relations theory is now not one school, and there are many debates, disputes, and alternative formulations within it (Greenberg & Mitchell, 1983; see Hamilton, 1989, for a critical overview). The basic core of object relations theory is that of internal, mental representations of self and significant others. Much of how we feel about and behave towards others reflects our internal relationships derived from experience. Horner (1989, pp.28–29) gives a comprehensive summary. She says:

> The patterning of the mental schema we call "self," and the patterning of the mental schema we referred to as the "object" take place in predictable, hierarchical stages. We used the term "object," rather than "mother" because this particular mental image is in part *created by* the child in accord with his or her limited mental capabilities, and with his or her own unique experience of the early caretaking environment. In a way, the child creates a kind of metaphor or template for the significant other from his or her interpersonal experiences. In turn this metaphor, or template, reciprocally shapes the child's perception of and expectations of the interpersonal environment, along with his or her behaviour towards it. Through its genetically endowed intrinsic creative capacities, its inborn intrinsic power, the infant creates an inner image of itself as well. "Object relations" refers to the dynamic interplay between the inner images of both self and other. This interplay entails

the perception and experience of power along with feelings, wishes, thoughts and impulses. [1]

Basic Theory

Of all the individual divergences from classical psychoanalytic thinking (e.g., Jung, Adler, Reich, Rank, and so on), Kleinians have been among the foremost in advancing a therapeutic technique based on the transference relationship (the feelings and attitudes stirred up in a patient towards the therapist). Unlike the Freudian approach, which suggests the transference develops slowly, Kleinians believe that it occurs immediately, brought by the patient at the start of therapy, the product of previous stored object relationships. In other words an individual cannot come to a new relationship as if neutral, that is without hopes, expectations, fears, and so forth. This allows for early interpretations and opens the possibility for short-term, focal psychotherapy. This appears odd to non-Kleinians because of the potential number of possible interpretations. However, Klein's system acknowledges only a few fundamental forms of maladaptive mechanisms relevant to pathology. Both are related to processes which are inevitably confronted during the first months and years of life. Given this, the style of interpretation is guided by which of the two types of mechanism seems responsible for the patient's difficulty.

The mechanisms of pathology relate to two developmental stages or positions; the paranoid–schizoid position and the depressive position. The relationship between positions and mechanisms is complex. Generally, "positions" refer to developmental stages whereas "mechanisms" refer to the psychological processes (defense mechanisms) used at these stages. Thus it is possible that individuals use paranoid-schizoid mechanisms for coping with conflict even though they may be well into maturity with the cultural standards of success behind them. In regard to depression, there is sometimes the confusion that depressive illness relates to mechanisms associated with the depressive position. This is inaccurate, since severe and psychotic depression can relate to paranoid–schizoid mechanisms (or defenses). In such cases the severity of the depression relates to the engagement of primitive, intense, paranoid–schizoid splitting mechanisms associated with the very first phase of life. Mechanisms associated with the depressive position are likely to relate to milder forms of pathology. One aim of psychotherapy is to interpret and hence help the patient avoid the use of paranoid–schizoid mechanisms, which can bring about detachment from reality. This system of thinking can be made clear by considering the two developmental stages and positions in more detail.

The Paranoid—Schizoid Position

Kleinians start with the hypothesis that at birth there is a complete projection of all bad feelings associated with inevitable frustration. To put it another way the baby is unable to conceive that bad feelings actually originate from or are caused by the self. If the baby bangs its foot against the cot it was the world that did that not the baby's erratic movements. The origins of bad feelings must therefore have a source outside of self. Thus, aggressive impulses experienced at points of frustration are not seen as arising from self but from outside self. It is assumed that the newborn baby is totally incapable of integrating self-generated, aggressive impulses within its own ego structure. Clearly, there can be no guilt at this point since there is nothing to be guilty about; all badness and aggressiveness are outside. Thus, there is an inner–outer splitting of good and bad. In the beginning the bad is always outside. Use of this paranoid–schizoid mechanism has the patient making absolute judgements and projecting all the cause of badness outside of self: "It's your fault I failed my exams". This is related to the person who never takes responsibility and bad things are seen as other people's fault. It is also the position of paranoia since the world is the source of harm. The first splits then are inner and outer—good and bad.

Part Object Splitting. There is another innate mechanism for dividing up experience, called part object splitting. It is assumed that the baby can only relate to part objects—e.g., to the breast or face—which are not integrated into any complete whole object, e.g., the mother. Again, through inevitable frustration, the baby experiences good part objects (e.g., the good breast, giving fulfilment and comfort) and bad part objects (e.g., the bad breast, empty, absent, non-fulfilling, frustrating, not capable of satisfying). This constitutes an external splitting of good and bad. This kind of splitting is quite common especially under stress. It is represented in the person who cannot relate to people as whole persons but only as parts. And indeed they may say, "There are bits of you I like and bits of you I hate." Instead of trying to understand that part of the person they dislike and seek the reasons for the dislike or realise that people are multi-faceted, they try to relate only to the good bits. For such individuals, where such splitting is pronounced, they may only relate to others who can furnish their needs and see as bad that which is not satisfying. The idea that in pornography and prostitution women are portrayed as only "a body or flesh" is to accuse men of part object relating. This style is also highly egocentric.

The mechanisms of the paranoid–schizoid position are of a splitting of good and bad, all or nothing, absolute dichotomies. Use of this paranoid–schizoid mechanism has the patient making absolute judgements, and projecting all the causes of badness outside of self. Where badness is identified it is outside self, threatening to destroy what is inside, and thus forming the basis of paranoia.

The Depressive Position

As the child develops (possibly at about six months and onward) there is an awareness that both the internal split, of good inside and bad outside, and the external split, of good and bad part objects, is not a reflection of reality. The child comes to realize that the good and bad part objects are actually part and parcel of the same whole object, e.g., the mother. Thus, the whole object is both loved (for being at times good) and hated (for being at times bad). In addition there is a growing realisation that some of the aggressive (bad) impulses do arise from within. These two realisations, which occur at an unconscious level, set up a terrible problem. It is suggested that the baby now comes to fear the strength of its own aggressive impulses toward the bad parts of the whole object, lest in the process the good parts of the object are also destroyed. Entry into this stage of development constitutes the depressive position. Problems at this level manifest as needs for reassurance that the good has not been destroyed. Separation anxiety originates here. In therapy patients who have not successfully negotiated this stage of development will experience intense anxiety about their own aggressiveness toward loved objects, including the therapist. It is hypothesised that patients using mechanisms relating to this position will have unconscious fantasies that they may, or have, destroyed the therapist with their own badness. To put it another way there is a fear that the bad feelings/ impulses arising inside of one (e.g., anger, rage) may destroy or push away those that are also needed (similar to Freud's view). This is also a source of shame (see Chapter 8).

Entry into the depressive position also marks the first experiences of guilt. There is an unconscious awareness that what the self does in the world has an effect on the whole object. Thus, there are instinctive aggressive impulses both to destroy the object of badness, but also to keep it intact and put it back together. Segal (1975, p.75) states that:

> . . . his (the baby's) concern for his object modifies his instinctual aims and brings about an inhibition of instinctual drives. And as the ego becomes better organised and projections are weakened, repression takes over from splitting. Psychotic mechanisms gradually give way to neurotic mechanisms, inhibition, repression and displacement.

Although successful negotiation of the paranoid–schizoid position is possible, there is doubt whether the depressive position is ever fully overcome. As with Jung's concept of individuation, there is a movement towards it perhaps, but without complete success ever being assured.

Another form of part object splitting that is a development of Klein's basic theory is internal or self-splitting. Once a person recognises that they are the source of bad feelings and sadistic impulses and can experience guilt, a person may come to sees themselves as split up and fragmented. They may talk of themselves as having good and bad bits or good and bad sides (Greenberg, 1979). There is a difficulty in forming a sense of self-coherence. In cognitive therapy this splitting is well recognised but not spoken of in this way. Rather, it is the attitudes to aspects of self that are seen as responsible for the splitting—e.g., a person may label themselves as evil for having hateful feelings or sexual homo-erotic desires. In object relations theory however the experience can be one of trying to bring these various (split) aspects of the self under control, inhibiting them or keeping them hidden. Further, unlike cognitive therapy much of this conflict is seen as unconscious. Under strong arousal the person may fear fragmenting, literally falling to pieces, out of control or being taken over by the undesirable attributes within.

It follows from this model that mild (neurotic) depressions revolve around mechanisms of the depressive position. The patient experiences intense anxiety about his own destructiveness and his capacity to be loved and wanted. The experience of internal, destructive impulses produces significant guilt and constitutes a threat to the loved object, by possibly (in unconscious fantasy) destroying what is also loved and needed. Here we see a reworking of Freud's concept of dependency needs and anger turned inward. More severe depressions, however, relate to earlier paranoid–schizoid mechanisms where internal and external, and good and bad, part objects are profoundly split up and separated. Severe depressions are different from mild depressions in their propensity to use these primitive (early) coping mechanisms.

Comment

Anyone who has tried to study Kleinian theory and ideas relating to object relations theory (of which there are many forms; see Greenberg & Mitchell, 1988) will know that this summary is a gross over-simplification. Also the language is extremely obscure and bogged down in symbolic over-sexualized terms. However, although it is easy to find fault with the theory and the way it is expressed, it has none the less been a rich source of ideas and it is dishonest not to recognise how often these ideas have been taken up with a change of language and description and fed back under a different disguise. The cognitive idea of black–white or absolutistic thinking is in Klein's theory splitting.

Also, a number of therapists working with very disturbed people have suggested that the greater the disturbance the easier it is to recognise part object styles of relating, and I tend to agree. However, I would like a rather different theory, possibly derived from modular processing theory (see Chapter 5 and Power & Brewin, in press). In my view, as patients become more psychotic we see phylogenetically earlier (more segregated, less integrated) processing modules coming to dominate thinking and experiencing.

To be able to cope with primitive innate (archetypal) fears we need various forms of symbolic knowledge. In some cultures rituals are used to provide this knowledge. For example, Jung noted how one Mexican Indian tribe thought they should perform rituals to ensure that the sun came up each day. Not so long ago humans would not sail beyond a certain point for fear of falling off the edge of the world. Ideas that gods and demons exist in the forest is not unusual in some (now fading) hunter gatherer groups.[2] In fact rituals played a large role in alleviating various innate types of fears in hunter gatherer bands and some of these fears may, in our cultural context, be regarded as psychotic. If patients have such fears maybe this is because our shared cultural knowledge that tells us that these things cannot happen is not operating in the psychotic mind. Thus, there may be a deficit in the ability to integrate symbolic operations into experience and this leads to various forms of more primitive construing. However, this is a complex story that we cannot discuss further here.[3]

Klein's views are far more instinct related than those of Freud. Moreover, they reflect her work with children, in that they are concerned with mechanisms which are an inevitable consequence of limited cognitive development. Klein attempted to consider the ways a young child may work through a love–hate (aggressive) conflict. One may agree that this type of conflict, as Freud and others suggest, is often evident in psychopathology. It is also true that some theorists do not pay nearly enough attention to it. Hence in Chapter 6 it is considered from an evolutionary and ethological perspective. More recently Horner (1989) has discussed the nature of power from an object relations theory point of view. Apart from her inclusion of penis envy there is much that might resonate with the ethological ideas of Chapters 6 and 7.

However, it can be suggested that behavioural theory, as advanced by Ferster (1973; 1974; see Chapter 14), and possibly Solomon (1980), offers a more rational basis for discussion of love–hate conflicts. It should also be considered that much of the difficulty the child faces has to do with attributions, that is, who or what causes this or that to happen. Thus perhaps an attributional analysis of some of Klein's concepts would provide a more comprehensive framework for considering these issues. Indeed, the relationship between attributing a quality to someone and projecting a quality onto that person needs to be explored (see Holmes, 1978; 1981; Sherwood, 1982). As yet cognitive theory has not given the necessary attention to mechanisms such as projection.

Klein, like Freud, had a developmental view of psychopathology. That is to say, vulnerability was laid down during the child's navigation of various developmental periods or stages. Although Klein worked especially with children, while Freud did not, both argued that vulnerability arose from childhood experiences or fantasies. Jung, however, is one of the few analytic theorists who does not specifically relate vulnerability to childhood.

Object relations theory is now a vast area of different schools and approaches (Greenberg & Mitchell, 1983). What all have in common is the idea that interactions with others become part of an internal system of representations of self and others and that much of our emotional life is organised around our internal object relations.

THE ROLE OF FANTASY

In Freudian and object relations theory, fantasy takes on special importance. Both suggest that our fantasy lives are of paramount importance to our everyday living. Object relations theorists spell fantasy as "phantasy" to emphasise this issue (J. Segal, 1985). Now there have been many attacks on psychanalytic theory for just this reason. Indeed, Freud at one time adhered to a seduction theory of neurosis but heard so many stories of sexual abuse that (some say) he just could not believe it. So he changed a real event theory into a fantasy theory with, as we now know, serious consequences. Furthermore, some of the "phantasies" the Kleinians suggest are, frankly, bizarre (e.g., of internal persecutory part objects, breasts and penis, and savage sadistic impulses directed at part objects, e.g., to rip up the breast). It may be true that some of our fantasies are linked to affects and their evolved action tendencies. For example, the affect of disgust may be linked with the wish to be rid of something within oneself, as in shame (see Chapter 8), or the experience of frustration may activate aggressive action tendencies (hence it is often called frustrative aggression). But in my view this is as far I would go. Many of the Kleinian phantasies simply do not make sense from an evolutionary point of view.[4]

On the other hand, much of our life is spent in fantasy and imagination. When we think of future goals, plans, and intentions we fantasise our success, we anticipate. When we are anxious we fantasise the world as populated by shaming others. When we are depressed we fantasise that nothing can change and all is hopeless.

It is surprising, but true, that very few theories of depression pay much regard to our inner fantasy life or the underlying systems that make fantasy possible, or if they do it is rather indirect (e.g., Klinger, 1977, talks of current concerns; see Chapter 12, and cognitive therapists recognise the importance of internal imagery and ideals). Yet affective consequences often follow from the pursuit or loss of fantasy. For example, a twenty-year-old student developed a fantasy about her lecturer. She thought about him constantly and all kinds of possibilities were played out in her mind. At one level she knew these would never happen in reality and she knew that when she left college she would say goodbye. One day she mentioned her crush to a friend. Her friend responded, "Oh, didn't you know he doesn't fancy women. He is homosexual." At the following therapy session she cried for her lost fantasy and became more depressed for a while. There had never been any real relationship and he knew nothing of it, it had all been in her head, as hopes maybe. Of course this begs other questions of why she found him a target for fantasy, etc., but the point is that grief can arise from a lost fantasy. We have to consider therefore how far is a hope a form of fantasy?

Fantasies can be a way of relating at a distance and/or maintaining control; they can be the source of inspiration and pleasure/excitement or traps from which we will always be disappointed by reality. Also when we fantasise about an ideal person (our ideal lover) we fantasise about them as part objects rather than real whole persons. For example, we imagine how they will look or how they will be in bed. We exclude their other human characteristics such as their bad moods or their tendency to fart after eating beans. Often, our fantasies are like mini-scenes from a film that are played out in our heads.

As pointed out elsewhere (Gilbert, 1989) Type A and narcissistic personalities can have various fantasies that if only they could work hard enough, then they will be accepted or somehow win (see also Arieti & Bemporad's [1980a,b] description of dominant goal types; Chapter 12). Even though they could avoid a sense of low self-worth by not putting themselves down they often have difficulty in giving this up. Part of the reason is that self-punishment has been used as a tactic to force themselves to pursue various standards and goals, maintain a fantasy of potential superiority over others and avoid weakness. If the therapist is not aware that to give up self-downing often (in their minds) involves giving up also the idea that one day they will make it and fall over the winning line, then the therapy can get very difficult. Hence fantasies often have a major impact on ideals. The problem is that when ideals are not met then self-downing may begin. Few patients will change unless the therapist also addresses this issue of the fantasised ideal and allows the patient to mourn the loss.

Fantasies are richer than automatic thoughts (see Chapter 13), can operate in the absence of any specific event, can be elaborated over months or even years, and are active in our dreams and may not be easily available to consciousness. For example a patient had a fantasy that he could overcome his anxiety, become successful, and out compete his brother for parental attention. It was some time before this fantasy became clear in the therapy. In therapy when we elicit (e.g., by working with images) a person's fantasy and imaginary lives we become aware of how much of our lives are spent in fantasy; how important they are to us and the underlying structures, processes, and memories that bring them to life (Segal, 1985). For me, fantasies in depression are often linked to issues of control, power, escape, success, and love—i.e., gaining, or the fear of losing, social success.

One has to ask therefore, why, in so many of our theories, has the inner realm become cold and barren of its essential internal creative life. One reason maybe that our imagination has been taken over by the wonders of the computer. But computers do not dream of falling in love, making friends, scoring winning goals or being awarded prizes. Our cultures shape our theories and these in turn shape our metaphors and conceptual systems.

SUMMARY

1. Early psychanalytic theory struggled to make sense of human behaviour and mental disorder in the immediate post-Darwinian era. This was a time of fear of the beast within. While Nietzsche stressed aggressive drives and the will to power, Freud focused on sexuality as libidinal energy.
2. Freud used his observation of hidden anger in depression to fit his own theory. Hence depression was seen as an internal, aggressive drive that was diverted back against the self. It was not fear in a ranking sense that inhibits (as implied by Nietzsche) but oral dependent needs.
3. Freud's basic dictum of "empty world, empty self" as the primary distinction between mourning and melancholia has stayed with us ever since, although we now know that this is not as simple a categorical distinction as he suggested.
4. The object relations theorists changed the basic Freudian model from a drive/structure model to a relational/structure

model. Their concern was in understanding internal representations of self and others and they used term self-objects.

5. The object relations theorists were also concerned with the psychological mechanisms that infants and adults bring to their construction of social life. The basic mechanisms were in terms of splitting, e.g., good inside, bad outside; and also part object splitting, e.g., relating to self and others having different 'bits'; some good, some bad.
6. The type of depression relates the type of the defenses that are brought to bear on the construction of events. Schizoid–paranoid mechanisms give rise to psychotic depression. Defense mechanisms of the depressive position give rise to feelings of guilt, fear of one's own destructiveness and excessive responsibility for bad events.
7. More than any other theory psychoanalytic theory has focused on internal fantasy as a source of mental life. Although many other types of theorist rarely use these terms, ideas regarding ideals and images (e.g., self-image, future self-image, etc.) remain. The internal life is a highly creative life.

CONCLUDING COMMENTS

It is sad that today many working in psychopathology are unfamiliar with the history of ideas and their cultural context. The problem is that new schools spring up at a constant rate with little recognition given to their students of how ideas have been taken from somewhere else. For me, scatterings of object relations theory turn up in different disguises constantly. Nevertheless it is important to recognise where theories differ. There are a number of issues that separate psychoanalytic and other types of theory. The first is the degree and form of innateness of psychic structures and the implications these may have for both theory and therapy.

It is this aspect that leads to interpretation since the analysts believe that they can recognise the basic structures and contents of unconscious material. They also believe that insight is a powerful vehicle for change. Cognitive therapists however are deeply suspicious of this view and prefer guided discovery (Chapter 13), preferably in the context of an empathic relationship; whereas behaviourists are very action and skills focused. So in regard to innateness and interpretation there are major differences. On the other hand, it has been the analysts that have drawn attention to the issues of: guilt, shame, rage, grief, envy, and power in depression and these are yet to be fully explored through other theories.

Second, as we shall see in subsequent chapters, there are major differences in the role and type of the therapeutic relationship as the vehicle for change. I think that nowadays most agree that therapist passivity is not a good treatment stance for depression. Indeed, it is doubtful whether Freud himself was as passive as his writings suggest (see Yalom, 1980). Hence some form of an action or performance based component and a re-educative aspect seem important for change in depression and insight is rarely enough. Family members may need to be involved. Nevertheless we cannot avoid the fact that humans have rich internal lives and here lies one source of suffering.

NOTES

1. To put this in a more concrete way; suppose I experience a very hostile father as I grow up, then in so far as he also represents authority I may be inclined to approach others in authority with timidity or counter hostility. Also, according to how I have experienced self-objects I will come to experience myself (e.g., as timid or hostile in the face of authority). It is not the others' behaviour that dictates my behaviour but the internal memories of myself in interaction with others (e.g., father). Thus there are three components here, representation of self, representation of other, and representation of interaction (i.e., whether my experience of the interaction was loving, giving, fun, soothing or hostile and withholding). Hence it is the experienced interaction that is internally stored and important. This may or may not be an accurate reflection of actual characteristics of the other. As we shall see in Chapter 10 this is the essential approach adopted by the self psychologists.
2. A Kleinian with whom I once debated these things asked if I had seen the film *Alien*. In one scene a creature looking like a small penis burst from the chest of an actor. My conclusion: "Ah so aliens are the source of the persecuting penis", I think I missed the point. The repetitive themes of fantasy are indeed food for thought. Horror writers know well these themes. Brant Wenegrat at the APA Conference in New York (1990) analysed the themes of 100 horror movies. Themes of having one's mind taken over by external forces, or loved ones being replaced by copies (capgras), zombeism, fear of the outgroup, "them" and the aliens are all prominent. His point was that some of our fantasies appear to track evolutionary relevant fears (fear of the outsider, of difference, of being controlled) and it is in this way that the writer is able to pull us into his/her fantasy world. Also it is these themes of fantasy that are often activated in psychotic experience.
3. A few years ago at a conference a person, whom, sadly, I can't recall and credit, told an interesting story over a couple of beers. He had been asked to go to see a family with a rather disturbed girl. The mother showed him in and then with pride showed him a video set up in the kitchen. On the screen was the daughter playing in her bedroom. At one point the daughter did something the mother did not agree with, and the mother spoke into an intercom, "Emily don't do that now." The daughter looked shaken at this

voice appearing out of nowhere. He then mused about this as an obviously abnormal situation but also wondered how much children actually (over)hear the voices of their parents speaking about them in the third person, and whether such early experiences in sensitive individuals may increase vulnerability to auditory hallucinosis under stress. Can we be sure that when parents speak about their children in the third person and may be out of the visual field that the child (below a certain age) can identity the source of these voices? I really don't know. What if there are biological differences in the ability to identify the source and origins of sounds at a certain age? It is an intriguing idea that I think requires research.

4. The object relations theorists suggest that phantasies can be unconscious, but some of them seem very bizarre and not open to scientific testing. I am not against the idea in principle since a scientific approach requires an open mind in the absence of evidence, but a decent methodology and evidence are necessary before we can proceed further. Also and I am not sure how much this would add to the therapy over and above what can be achieved with guided discovery (see Chapter 13).

CHAPTER 10

Depression as Thwarted Needs

The idea that animals and humans have certain needs, and that a failure to secure these needs results in difficulties, has a long history in psychology. It is evident in Murray's work of the thirties, Maslow's concept of a hierarchy of needs and many psychoanalytic therapies (see Liebert & Spiegler, 1990, for a comprehensive overview). Cognitive, behavioural, existential, gestalt, psychoanalytic drive reduction, and various other theories do not articulate a theory of basic needs. Yet over the past thirty years the role of interpersonal needs, to facilitate the process of human development has been well researched.

Needs are different from goals. Goals and plans are internal orientating mechanisms, whereas needs focus more on an environmental requirement to grow and function. Of course they interact in that to secure a goal the environment must respond in a certain kind of way. However, from an evolutionary point of view individuals have basic requirements that the environment must serve. It must, for example, provide access to social others to allow social learning. Certain types of interaction are essential if the maturing nervous system is to come to function in a species-typic way. For example, the disruptive biological consequences to separation are now well established (e.g., Reite & Field, 1985). Thus, human gene-neural structures have evolved which anticipate and require certain kinds of social, holding, supporting, and mediating environments/relationships (Gilbert, 1989). Failure in provision, at the extreme, means death, and, less extreme may lead to psychopathology and defensive self-organisation. This view leads to an evolutionary ecology of human development (Chisholm, 1988) where innate possibilities are actualised via life history (see also MacDonald, 1988; 1988, ed.).

In this chapter we will explore two recent developments of psychoanalytic theory, attachment theory and self psychology. These vary from other theories (at least to the degree to which they focus) on vulnerability to depression as arising from the thwarting of early developmental needs. This orientation has very important consequences to our theories, treatment methods, and ultimately preventive programmes.

ATTACHMENT THEORY[1]

Bowlby's (1969; 1973; 1977a,b; 1980; 1988) development of attachment theory constituted a major advance to the understanding of psychopathology. Like Freud, Klein, and Jung, Bowlby's concern is with the activity of inherited psychobiological response patterns. But for Bowlby, the most important response patterns are those guiding the formation and development of attachment bonds, not those governing aggressive and sexual impulses or drives. Indeed, Bowlby (1969) offers a major critique of Freud's energy concept of mind and presents an alternative explanation of how evolved, instinctive behaviour operates. Also of significance, Bowlby points to real, not fantasy events as the basis for vulnerability.

Unlike some theories of depression, the central factors of Bowlby's theory—disturbances in the development, maintenance, and/or termination of attachment bonds—are seen to underlie a variety of psychopathological disturbances. The basic biosocial goal (Gilbert, 1989) that is frustrated in the maturation process is care eliciting and the basic needs are nurturance and safety. The general assumptions of attachment theory can be summarized as follows:

1. Attachment behaviour is instinctive and goal directed. There is an inherited predisposition to behave in a way which maintains proximity and communication with attachment figures. This inherited predisposition has survival value (is probably a K-selected strategy, see Chapter 5) and as a consequence it has evolved in a variety of species. Thus infants need relationships with attachment objects to survive and prosper (i.e., they need investment from others).
2. The internal psychic mechanisms (e.g., affects, cognitive orientation, and behavioural patterns) which mediate

attachment behaviour may only be activated under conditions where the functions of attachment behaviour (e.g., to be nurtured and protected) are threatened—in other words, situations which are potentially threatening to survival (e.g., aloneness, separateness, strangeness, noise, strangers) will activate a sequence of behaviours (e.g., distress calling, searching, clinging), which are designed to maintain proximity to, and protection from, care-givers.

3. Many affective consequences are related to the making and breaking of attachment bonds. For example, uninterrupted, stable attachment may be experienced as security; threat to attachment bonds, as anger and/or anxiety; complete loss of attachment bonds as depression; regeneration of attachment bonds as joy. The actual affective consequences will be a function of many variables, antecedent and subsequent to the actual changes in attachment.
4. Attachment behaviour is a source of varied emotional experience. It is present through all stages of life and is not a sign of pathology or regression.
5. In addition to offering survival advantage, by protecting the young infant from predators (and diseases—the mother's milk contains antibodies, and her body is a source of warmth, Hofer, 1984), attachment objects also provide a secure base from which to explore the environment, a source of reassurance and calming, and also stimulation. The ability to explore safely conveys considerable advantage in that it facilitates discrimination learning and the development of necessary skills for adaptation. In depression exploration is significantly reduced.

Gilbert (1989) reviewed the evidence that secure attachment relations exert psychobiological effects in that the presence of (and reassurance given by) attachment objects maintains low defensive arousal and increases safety-explorative behaviour. Security, as may be provided by attachment objects, therefore affects the internal biological environment of the developing child's CNS (Hofer, 1984). Development proceeds under the psychobiological conditions of safety (e.g., low cortisol and other stress hormones, etc.). Kraemer (1985, p.141) notes that isolated primates (those deprived of necessary social input) show disturbances in "(1) abnormal posturing and movements; (2) motivational disturbances (excessive fearfulness or arousal); (3) poor integration of motor patterns; and (4) deficiencies in social communication, such as failure to withdraw after being threatened by a dominant animal." Hence, as argued in Chapter 5, safety is necessary to help the various modular processes become integrated and coordinated. Further, Gilbert (1989) speculated that this may relate to opiate tone in the brain which may be raised by access to and comfort (holding, stroking) from care-givers.

It is also now known that poor social conditions in early life may sensitise neural systems such that even if an animal appears to make a satisfactory adjustment this is only maintained in states of relative calm. The animal's behaviour may become dysfunctional under stress (possibly due to some synaptic receptor sensitivity). Hence previous social experience will exert an influence on self-organisation in different states. (See Kraemer, 1985, for a review of the biological consequences of poor early social environments and Coe, Weiner, Rosenberg, & Levine, 1985, for the interaction between hormonal changes and separation. Mineka & Suomi, 1978, provide a review of the primate research on separation.) Rasmussen and Reite (1982) suggest that subordinate animals are more at risk to depression following loss of attachments and relationships.

Development

Right from the start infants are born to target responses to adult others. They are innately prepared to learn and take interest in the social environment (for example, interest in faces, smiling, seeking to be and being reassured by physical contact, suckling, and so on). The role of touch and tactile input is of major importance (Montague, 1986). In fact we now know that the neonate is extraordinarily talented at birth and is already a social being. Chamberlain (1987, p.51) says:

> Newborns have impressive resources for communicating actively with people around them. They express strong personal feelings facially and vocally, listen with unbelievable precision, and show perceptive awareness of important changes as they scan the environment. Not only are they equipped to sense people but they respond strongly to social stimulation, prolong such stimulation, and what is more, initiate social interaction. Relationships are not static or one sided but dynamically changing, influential and reciprocal in nature.

Styles of Interaction

Considerable work has explored the quality of infant/mother relationships and subsequent relational styles of the child. One of the most researched paradigms has been the infant's response to separation (Ainsworth, Biehar, Waters & Wall, 1978). Sroufe and Fleeson (1986) suggest that the behaviour of infants in these situations represents a test of the relationship between child and care giver (although not all researchers agree on this). The general procedure is to stress the infant in various ways, usually by brief separations, and then observe the behaviour of the child during the separation and on the mother's return. In brief, the behaviour of the infant can be classified

TABLE 10.1
Patterns of Attachment

Pattern A: Anxious/Avoidant Attachment

A.
Exploration independent of caregiver
1. readily separate to explore during preseparation
2. little affective sharing
3. affiliative to stranger, even when care giver absent (little preference)

B.
Active avoidance upon reunion
1. turning away, looking away, moving away, ignoring
2. may mix avoidance with proximity
3. avoidance more extreme on second reunion
4. no avoidance of stranger

Pattern B: Infants Secure in Their Attachment

A.
Care giver as secure base for exploration
1. readily separate to explore toys
2. affective sharing of play
3. affiliative to stranger in mother's presence
4. readily comforted when distressed (promoting a return to play)

B.
Active in seeking contact or interaction upon reunion
1. If distressed
   (a) immediately seek and maintain contact
   (b) contact is effective in terminating distress
2. If not distressed
   (a) active greeting behaviour (happy to see care giver)
   (b) strong initiation of interaction

Pattern C: Anxious/Resistant Attachment

A.
Poverty of exploration
1. difficulty separating to explore; may need contact even prior to separation
2. wary of novel situations and people

B.
Difficulty settling upon reunion
1. may mix contact seeking with contact resistance (hitting, kicking, squirming, rejecting toys)
2. may simply continue to cry and fuss
3. may show striking passivity

Source: Sroufe and Fleeson (1986). With kind permisson of Lawrence Erlbaum Associates Inc.

into three basic groups. Sroufe and Fleeson (1986) have summarised this in Table 10.1.

What we may be observing here are differences in the psychobiological activation of defense–safety systems (see Chapter 5). Secure infants seem to be able to use care-givers to instate safety and reduce arousal, often via physical contact, if threatened or anxious (Gilbert, 1989). Based on a review of a number of studies, Campos et al. (1983) suggest that 62% of children tested in this way met the criteria for secure, 23% avoidant, and 15% anxious. These patterns may vary with parents, i.e., a secure attachment to a mother maybe not be mirrored to a father. However, there have been some critical reviews of some of the conclusions derived from the strange situation methodology (Kagan, 1984; Lamb et al., 1984). Nevertheless, it is now generally accepted that children do vary in their attachment relationships and these have consequences for subsequent development. We remain unsure how these patterns and styles of attachment lead on to subsequent relational styles (but see Collins & Read, 1990). One possibility is that poor attachments relations lead to overdeveloped defensiveness showing itself in needs to control others in a more agonic style (i.e., dominant or submissive), thus such children may become either hostile dominant or victims and subordinate.

The Nature of Early Relationships

While it would be very good if we could separate clearly the issues of rank from issues of attachment and needs for nurturance, in reality this is not possible. The problem is that early attachment relationships are also rank relationships. Hartup (1989, p.120) puts this issue very clearly:

> Experience in two major kinds of relationships seems to be necessary to the child's development. First, children must form vertical attachments, that is, attachments to individuals who have greater knowledge and social power than they do. These relationships, most commonly involving children and adults, encompass a wide variety of interactions among which complementary exchanges are especially salient. For example, adult actions towards children consist mainly of nurturance or controlling behaviours, whereas childrens actions toward adults consist mainly of submission and appeals for succorance.... Second, children must also form close relationships that are horizonal, that is, relationships with individuals who have the same amount of social power as themselves. Ordinarily, these relationships involved other children and are marked by reciprocity and egalitarian expectations. The social exchanges occurring within child-child relationships,

however, vary greatly in the extent to which they manifest these characteristics.

So it is likely that experience with care-givers may set the basic style of the child and later adult (i.e., highly rank and control orientated versus more cooperative and affiliative). Since the agonic styles of relating have not been removed by recent evolution it would seem that parenting style may do much to activate them or, alternatively, bring out the more hedonic possibilities of the child. For Bowlby, it is child–parent relationships which determine subsequent vulnerability and it is the capacity to secure and maintain attachment bonds that are crucial to mental health. Bowlby (1977a, p.206) puts it:

> The key point of my thesis is that there is a strong causal relationship between an individual's experiences with his parents and his later capacity to make affectional bonds, and that certain common variations in that capacity, manifesting themselves in marital problems and trouble with children as well as in neurotic symptoms and personality disorders, can be attributed to certain common variations in the ways that parents perform their roles.

Unlike the self psychologists (see further on) who outline the needs to be approved of and to find idealising others, these aspects are not given special emphasis or separated out in attachment theory. Although Bowlby often emphasises the view that early attachments are to those who are seen as older, wiser, and stronger, this rank aspect of the theory has not yet been fully integrated into therapy considerations in the same way as it has for the self psychologists. Therefore, Bowlby's (1977a) focus is on different aspects of maladaptive early attachment behavioural interactions. He suggests (see pp.206–207) that many psychiatric patients (especially those with neurotic and personality disorders) have histories which include:

> ... one or both parents being persistently unresponsive to the child's care eliciting behaviour and/or actively disparaging and rejecting; discontinuities of parenting, occurring more or less frequently, including periods in hospital or institution; persistent threats by parents not to love a child, used as a means of controlling him; threats by parents to abandon the family, used either as a method of disciplining the child or as a way of coercing a spouse; threats by one parent either to desert or even to kill the other or else to commit suicide (each of them commoner than might be supposed); inducing a child to feel guilty by claiming his behaviour is or will be responsible for the parent's illness or death.

All these distorted attachment relations plant the seeds for significant emotional conflict between what is felt to be needed and what is available. In evolutionary terms these are abnormal deviations from the environment of adaptedness. Also, a child may experience powerful demands from a parent for love and affection which are unrealistic and impossible. The mother may express the idea that her child(ren) is all that is important to her, thus generating considerable conflict for the child, predisposing her/him to guilt when the child tries to fulfil his/her own needs and separate from the parent. This is often the case for children of depressed parents or where low self-esteem and marital difficulties dominate. Or children may be brought into marital conflicts and used as allies against the other parent. The result is the generation of significant conflicts in later life over developing and maintaining attachment bonds on the one hand, and becoming independent on the other. As a result of the attachment relations children experience, they come to develop certain kinds of *internal working models of self and others.*

Abuse

We also now know that various forms of abuse should also be considered. In a group of abused women treated for depression Jehu (1989) found that, "92% reported low self-esteem, 88% feelings of guilt, 70% depressive episodes, and 92% had at least one of these mood disturbances". Further in regard to family background Jehu (1989, p.167) notes that:

> Male supremacy was featured in the families of origin of 58% of victims, and around half the father figures exhibited the problems of anger/hostility/violence, physical abuse of spouse, and physical abuse of children. These fathers were variously described as tyrannical, imperious, autocratic, patriarchal, or dictatorial. Many of the problems exhibited by the victims' mother figures are the obverse of those displayed by supremacist father figures. The mothers tended to be overdependent (68%), oppressed (64%) and depressed (53%), with limited social skills, including unassertiveness (76%), low self-esteem (35%) and poor physical health (35%).

There is growing evidence that abuse can result in a borderline pattern of symptoms (see Chapter 4) and that it is not only abuse from fathers that is important but also from siblings, uncles, and cousins, and there may be abuse from more than one individual (Ogata et al., 1990). Systematic abuse (e.g., in boarding schools) goes on but has been less well researched. Abuse gives rise not only to mood disturbance but a variety of other difficulties (e.g., sexual difficulties, alcoholism, social anxiety, self-mutilation, and others). There are major disturbances in: self-identity (e.g., a bad self) and self evaluative cognitions (Jehu, 1988; 1989); the capacity to deal with emotional arousal (Ogata et al., 1990); and major disturbance in the capacity for interpersonal relating (see Alter-Reid, Gibbs, Lachenmeyer, Sigal, & Massoth, 1986, for a review of sexual abuse, and Ammerman, Cassi, Hersen, & Van Hassett, 1986, and Rohner, 1986, for a review of physical abuse and neglect).

As Ogata et al. (1990) point out, this evidence suggests that abused victims come from very disturbed families who, "do not protect their members and fail to attend to the needs of their children" (p.1011). In general these families can be seen as suffering from severe distortions in power behaviour (Gilbert, 1989), do not provide safety and soothing self-objects and distort the formation of self-systems towards a fragmenting, self-defensive style of processing. Not surprisingly therefore, these people feel vulnerable to both internal and external persecution.

Overview of Basic Concepts

The basic concepts of attachment theory are:

1. The innate need to form attachments who provide special types of input (i.e. availability of attachment objects and their sensitive attunement to the child).
2. The way parents perform their roles to meet these innate needs facilitates positive or negative experiences which influence subsequent development.
3. The threats, or actual experience, of abandonment, separations or discontinuities, reversals of care provision, and/or various forms of abuse are the crucial events in the development of psychic structures that will lead to later, maladaptive styles of social relating and vulnerability to psychopathology.
4. Experience of attachment objects leads to the development of internal, self–other schema. These cognitive representations (beliefs), often referred to as internal working models, significantly influence how information about relationships is interpreted and, therefore, shape consequent emotional reactions to disturbed attachment bonds.[2]

One way of thinking about these issues is that parents orientate the child to either an agonic or hedonic social structure. In a sense the parent is educating the child according to how they (the parents) experience relationships. This basic orientation is carried over into peer group relationships. The parents can over sensitise the child to (agonic) ranking. Hence even in someone who is outwardly polite, this may not be a genuine hedonic behaviour but a form of defense, and the underlying orientation is concerned with rank (and the avoidance of threat/shame/put-down). Second, parental authoritarian behaviour or over-protection may reduce the exploration of the child. At an internal level this reduces the likelihood of integration, of hedonic social behaviour. In more general terms the parental relationships may provide the "affective climate" of development (see Tronick, 1989, for a fascinating discussion). Those who grow with high levels of emotional support and pleasure develop a more integrated, explorative and optimistic orientation compared with those who grow in an environment with greater negative affect. This will affect the self-organisation and "pattern generating" processes of self-construction (see Chapters 8 and 16).

Belief and Construct Systems

The experience of care receiving has powerful effects on the development of beliefs and attitudes about the self. Via interaction with others the child develops *internal working models* or schema about his/her acceptability, lovability, self-esteem, and personal competency and power on the one hand and the availability and supportiveness of others on the other. Under threat these internal models are activated. For example, hearing that one's lover no longer loves one, an individual may conclude that this is because they are in fact unlovable (as perhaps a parent had previously indicated to them) and/or they may conclude that others are fickle and cannot be trusted, mobilising action tendencies of anger and avoidance. But even before such a threat arises they may carry this orientation into their key relationships. Thus, even if someone acts in a loving way towards them they may seek continual reassurance of their lovability (to the eventual irritation of the other). Alternatively, loving acts from others may activate the belief "they are only doing this to get around me and will eventually turn on me when I no longer satisfy them." Hence as Leary's (1957) model suggests (see Chapter 4) we can actually elicit those behaviours in others that (we say) we dislike. A patient fears rejection but behaves in a way that makes it more likely.

Guidano and Liotti (1983), Liotti (1988), and Safran and Segal (1990) have recently pointed out that these internal models influence relational style and the experience of connectedness with others. They become the programmes or operating rules for interpersonal relating. Like many theorists, it is early life that Safran and Segal believe sets the style of expectations, attributions, and models of self and others that individuals bring with them to their primary relationships.

Information Processing

Attachment theory also explores information processing. Bowlby (1980) suggests that there are different systems of information storage and organisation. He notes the important distinction between types of memory, especially episodic and semantic, and considers the possibility that information about attachment figures may be stored and organised in different systems. Thus there may be specific memories of actual parenting events (episodic), but there may also be more general semantic memories relating to generalised attributes of the parent(s). There is the possibility: (1) that either system may hold information which is discordant with information in the other system; (2) that information processed by each system may come up with different interpretations of actual events. In both instances the stage is set for potential conflict. The management and consequences of this conflict are central to Bowlby's model.

The idea that information is not stored and organised in some uniform way is important (see also Brewin, 1989; Dalgleish & Watts, 1990). It provides one framework to explain cognitive bias and distortion. It is also possible that a temporal conflict can exist between, and within, memory systems. Early (perhaps preverbal) memories of poor parenting may be stored at an affective level (Safran & Segal, 1990). Thus during the helpless stage of development, the child may experience his care-giver(s) as unrewarding, rejecting, hostile, etc. As the child grows, however, the interaction between the child and parent may change. The child becomes, and is experienced as, less helpless and demanding. The child–parent interaction may then be less rejecting, especially if the child complies with parental demands. Here again, however, a source of conflict may exist between early and later memories and types of (emotional versus cognitive) memory. It should be noted however that, at present, memory is still far from well understood. Loftus and Loftus (1980) point out that the view that memories are somehow permanently stored in the brain and remain potentially accessible and available throughout life is doubtful. Indeed, memories may actually fuse together or become distorted. It is possible that considerable distortion can occur in this actual fusion of memories. Memories are also highly susceptible to mood influences (Blaney, 1986).

Bowlby gives a different twist to the notion of unconscious processing. In this approach unconscious processing can arise from the activation of affective processes that were developed before conscious self-representation (Brewin, 1988; 1989). This is not an area we can explore here but certainly the days are now past when we had to assume that all processed information that has an affective consequence is conscious and well articulated (Power & Brewin, in press).

Defensive Exclusion

Bowlby (1980) suggests that conflict can exist over what the parents tell the child about themselves as parents, and what the child actually observes/experiences to be the case. The child may experience significant rejecting, demanding, or hostile behaviour from the parent, while at the same time the parent insists that they be seen in a positive light. As Bowlby (1980, p.71) says: "On threat of not being loved or even of being abandoned a child is led to understand that he is not supposed to notice his parents' adverse treatment of him or, if he does, that he should regard it as being no more than the justifiable reaction of a wronged parent to his (the child's) bad behaviour".

As a result of this learning history there will be a tendency to "defensively exclude" negative information about the parent. They become beyond reproach. If this style of information processing continues into adult life, not only will the person be prone to make poor choices of partners (because of the tendency to exclude negative information about the potential partner), but bereavement will be exceedingly difficult and painful. In these cases anger and ambivalence are not easily worked through since the lost attachment figure has become "untouchable". The extent to which this bears the hallmarks of more classical psychoanalytic concepts of repression and denial remains to be considered. However, when defensive exclusion is weakened, the patient finds a sense of disappointment and grief, not primary drives. Thus, as in self psychology, aggression and other affects are secondary products of thwarted needs.

Greenberg and Safran (1987) and Safran and Segal (1990) have also suggested that there may be inhibitions on the processing of information. Some sources of information (especially at the affective level) are not fully processed or articulated. It is not then so much distorted processing but processing failures that are at issue. These ideas also resonate with those of Ferster (1973; 1974; see Chapter 14).

ATTACHMENT THEORY AND DEPRESSION

Like Freud, who regarded mourning and melancholia as overlapping but different processes, Bowlby (1980) relates many psychological disorders to distorted processes of mourning (Pedder, 1982; Gut, 1989).

Also, like Freud, Bowlby believes loss of self-esteem is the way a sadness is turned into a depression. But gone are the concepts of id drives, libido energy, oral dependency, and aggression turned inward. Rather it is the lack of adequate care giving which sensitizes the individual to respond to subsequent loss (especially of attachment bonds) in a pathological way (especially by changes in self-evaluation) and/or to have difficulty in forming adaptive attachments. And the manner of the sensitivity lies in the cognitive-affective models of self and others.

In terms of the depressive disorders, Bowlby suggests that a perceived inability to obtain and/or maintain attachment relations becomes a crucial concern. Various processes significantly interfere with an individual's capacity to adjust to loss. Especially important is the predisposition towards feelings of helplessness (Seligman, 1975) and continuing perceptions of irretrievable loss. Predisposition to experience such profound helplessness can arise in at least three ways. Bowlby (1980, pp.247–248) suggests these as:

> (a) He is likely to have had the bitter experience of never having attained a stable and secure relationship with his parents despite having made repeated efforts to do so, including having done his utmost to fulfil their demands and perhaps also the unrealistic expectations they may have had of him. These childhood experiences result in his developing a strong bias to interpret any loss he may later suffer as yet another of his failures to make or maintain a stable affectional relationship.
>
> (b) He may have been told repeatedly how unlovable, and/or how inadequate, and/or how incompetent he is. Were he to have had these experiences they would result in his developing a model of himself as unlovable and unwanted, and a model of attachment figures as likely to be unavailable, or rejecting or punitive. Whenever such a person suffers adversity therefore, so far from expecting others to be helpful he expects them to be hostile and rejecting.
>
> (c) He is more likely than others to have experienced actual loss of a parent during childhood [. . .] with consequences to himself that, however disagreeable they might have been, he was impotent to change. Such experiences would confirm him in the belief that any effort he might make to remedy his situation would be doomed to failure.

Bowlby links these early learning experiences with the development of various predispositions for interpreting information in a negative way. Hence, depression arises from an experience of unwanted disconnectedness from others and the experience that adequate attachment relations are not available. The other key element as mentioned earlier, is that such a state of affairs lowers self-esteem and gives rise to the affects of emptiness and grief. In cognitive therapy this is seen as self-blaming (see Chapter 13).

In the third volume of his trilogy on attachment, Bowlby (1980) pays special attention to the work of Beck and his colleagues (Beck et al., 1979) and also to the sociological work of Brown and Harris (1978a) to explain the loss of self-esteem consequent to loss. Since Beck's cognitive theory of depression is discussed fully later, it will not be discussed here. The major differences between Bowlby and Beck, however, may be noted. Unlike Beck, Bowlby stresses vulnerability in terms of (1) distorted, early parental relations; (2) potential, unresolved mourning; (3) conflicts generated by information-processing strategies (e.g., memory systems) and also mechanisms, such as "defensive exclusion" which can operate at an unconscious level (see also Gut, 1989). As will be observed in Beck's work (Chapter 13) these factors are of only minimal importance, and Beck gives no major etiological role to unconscious information processing, or mourning, in the development of depression.

Appeasement Behaviour

There is a rather typical style which can be called an appeasement or accommodating style. In this case a person finds themselves in an unhelpful relationship but continues to appease the other. They feel guilty at trying to leave, in part because they think the other needs them (which boosts self-esteem and SAHP), but also because their emotional style is appeasement. They may also fear abandonment and aloneness. They may marry knowing in their heart it is a bad decision but are intent on appeasing the partner or even parents, or they marry to give a justifiable reason to escape from parental influence. They may dream of escape or of being rescued or that the partner will change (though they rarely do) and they harbour secret resentments. Sometimes these people are depicted as "loving too much", but this is rarely so. They are particularly prone to entrapment (see Chapter 15) from a sense of guilt and fear (see Chapter 8).

Comment

Bowlby has done much to advance our knowledge of how attachment behaviours may either facilitate or hinder successful adaptation to the social world. Undoubtedly, early disruptions of parental bonding are exceedingly stressful with various biological correlates (Reite, Short,

Seiler, & Pauley, 1981; Reite & Field, 1985; Gilbert, 1989). On the other hand, it appears that even gross disturbances in early attachment bonding do not automatically give rise to psychopathology (Clarke & Clarke, 1976) and the role of individual differences (e.g., Kagan, 1984) is played down in attachment theory. In regard to abuse, Kaufman and Zigler (1987) found that only about 30% of abused children will go on to provide inadequate care to their own offspring and that not all abused individuals become borderline personality disorders. New work is beginning to explore the nature of resilience to poor early life.

The presence of care-giving substitutes and the existence of rewarding peer-group or sibling relationships may do much to raise thresholds for subsequent emotional distress of inadequate care (Rutter, 1975; 1981). In regard to actual loss of a parent, it is the quality of parenting following loss that will affect long-term adjustment, not necessarily the loss itself. There are also other theories (e.g., Ferster, 1973; 1974) which suggest that the opportunity to have learned various adjustment behaviours in response to loss may desensitise an individual to depression.

Not all cultures follow the rule of a single attachment object as is implied to be necessary in attachment theory (Tronick, Winn,& Morelli, 1985). Further, as reviewed elsewhere (Gilbert, 1989), there are many types of attachment relationship (e.g. mother–infant, infant–mother, sibling, friend, sexual patterns, etc.). Dunn (1988) has outlined the importance of siblings to social development, and Sheldon and West (1989) and Hartup (1989) have raised the issue of the distinction between attachment and affiliation. The way early attachment relationships may set the stage for subsequent affiliative relations have been outlined by Heard and Lake (1986). In general poor early social experiences may make it more likely that affiliative relations (capacity to form and function in a network, see Chapter 7) will be disturbed by either efforts for over-closeness or withdrawal, submissiveness or aggressiveness.

Importantly, Bowlby's work points to a prepared basis for depression which revolves around the distortions of attachments and a reduction in care receiving (Henderson, 1974). It is, as we have seen, a needs-based theory. Bowlby's idea that poor early attachment relationships somehow block a more mature capacity to cope with loss has been increasingly advanced both in cognitive therapy (Safran & Segal, 1990) and more analytic-based therapy (Gut, 1989). How these blocks work and the issue of maturation of self-processes remain fundamental research questions.

SELF PSYCHOLOGY

Self psychology is another theory that is needs-based, but articulates these needs less in terms of attachment and more in terms of the needs for self-worth. Like Bowlby however, the focus is less on internal cognitive errors or drives and more on the environmental provision. There are various elements to this theory that are close to Cooley's concept of the looking glass effect (see Chapter 7).

Heinz Kohut was born in Vienna in 1913. He never met Freud but left Europe soon after Freud, taking up residence in Chicago in 1940. In 1971 he published *The Analysis of the Self*. This text began the movement that is now referred to as Self Psychology (although papers had been published in the 1960s). This was followed by other texts and modifications. He died in 1981. Self psychology has had a major influence in American psychotherapy especially during the 1980s but with less impact in Britain (possibly because of the work of the object relations theorists with which it is sometimes compared).

During the 1960s Kohut practised psychoanalysis in Chicago, working particularly with narcissistic and borderline individuals. He came to reject the traditional ideas that these personalities could not benefit from psychoanalysis. He argued, however, that empathic responding rather than the interpretation of unconscious material was the key to change. The shift of emphasis caused tension and opposition from traditional psychoanalysts (Basch, 1984; Eagle, 1987).

It is unclear what the sources of Kohut's ideas were. As Kahn (1985; 1989) has outlined, Kohut's emphasis on empathy as a key therapeutic ingredient bears careful comparison with Carl Rogers. It is unclear how influenced Kohut was by Rogers. However, they worked at the same university for ten years and Rogers himself questioned how much Kohut had been influenced by him (Kahn, 1989). Others (e.g., Greenberg & Mitchell, 1983) also draw attention to the similarities between Kohut and other theorists, especially the British object relations and ego analytic theory schools.

The Self

The central concept of self psychology is the "self and its inner experience", especially the experience of cohesion versus fragmentation. Although self psychology implies the centrality of the self, Kohut never fully defines it, believing that the essence of the self is undefinable. Hence most speak in terms of metaphors, "the centre of our psychological universe". Generally, Kohut speaks of the experiencing self (Wolf, 1988; Wolfe, 1989), the "I as" (e.g., I experience myself as competent, as able, or as incompetent, as weak, as cohesive, or fragmented). The self rather than drives were the central aspect of Kohut's position. In 1982 (p.401) he wrote: "Under normal circumstances we do not encounter drives via introspection and empathy. We always experience the not-further-reducible psychological unit of a loving self, a lusting self, an assertive self, a hostile destructive self. When drives achieve experiential primacy, we are dealing with disintegration products." Thus, drives are efforts to the restore cohesion of the self. Hence, Kohut is concerned with the experience of (a sense of cohesion of) self played out in roles, plans, aspirations, intentions, goals, and so on (for a further discussion see Wolfe, 1989).

The self "as experienced" evolves from interpersonal relations which become the internal, selfobject relations. For example, if others respond to me with empathy, approval, and so on, I come to experience myself as good and capable. If on the other hand others have responded to me with lack of empathy, hostility or denial of my needs then I may come to experience myself as bad or incompetent. Critical is the fact that how others respond to me influences my experience of myself, not just my experience of them. However, this idea is not new but was central to the ideas of people like George Herbert Mead writing in the 1930s (Gilbert, 1989).

In many respects self psychology is concerned with the origins and role of self-esteem in psychopathology and self psychologists frequently refer to self-esteem. However, they see self-esteem as a product of positive internal selfobject relations (or self-relations). Hence self psychology is a much richer theory of self "as experienced" than most self-esteem theories.

Selfobjects

As mentioned, influences on Kohut (but rarely mentioned by him) were the British school of object relations theory and especially the work of Winnicott, the ego psychologist Karen Horney and various others (Greenberg & Mitchell, 1983). It will be recalled that in object relations theory (see Chapter 9), there are three components of intrapsychic structure: representation of self, representation of other, and representation of interaction (i.e., experience of the interaction as loving, giving, fun, soothing, or hostile and withholding). It is the "experienced interaction" that is internally stored and important. This "stored representation of interaction" may or may not be an accurate reflection of actual characteristics of the other. Kohut adopts this basic approach and uses the term selfobject to define the internal representation of the other as experienced in interaction. But selfobjects are not representations of the others, rather they are representations of the self built up from interaction, a coming to experience self via interaction. Selfobjects form the basic mental structures of self-experience, linking experience with affective tone. As discussed later (Chapter 14) selfobjects have some similarities with the concept of conditioned emotional responses.

Wolf (1988) points out that proper selfobjects (remember these are internalised experiences of self in interaction, they are experienced as part of the self and not separate from it) facilitate the experience of self as cohesive and energic, to have vigour for life. Faulty selfobjects facilitate self-experiences (one's experience of oneself) as fragmented and empty. Fragmentation is a central notion and refers to the experience of falling apart, splitting up, being shattered or broken, losing that cohesiveness of self-experience that allows one to feel a sense of continuity with past, present, and future. We will have more to say about fragmentation later.

Development

Kohut offers a metaphysical theory of human nature which has within it a number of assumptions about developmental processes. Because the self develops via interaction (and the central role of selfobjects is their capacity to bring about a positive experience of self) it is during the development of an individual that subsequent vulnerabilities are laid down. Like all the psychoanalytic theorists (and unlike the cognitive theorists), Kohut suggests that the growing child has certain types of interpersonal needs and requires certain types of input. Failure to obtain these inputs results in vulnerability (or forms of hunger). This vulnerability arises because the individual does not have the selfobjects (internal mental representations) necessary to become a cohesive vigorous individual. For example, a parent who is constantly punitive and shaming, does not enable their child to develop an internal experience of self as being good, able, and competent. A positive internal self-relationship cannot develop autonomously. In this sense the human infant needs psychological inputs to be able to grow and function; the infant is not able to grow adaptively without them. Whereas the behaviourist would point to the role of positive reinforcement, Kohut might argue that it is an empathic awareness that allows the other to know what needs require positive responses and how these should be delivered. From an evolutionary point of view positive selfobjects create safety and positive affect. This facilitates the safety system to bring about an explorative and open orientation to the world and allow for an integration of psychological abilities. The defense system has the opposite effect (see Chapter 5).

This emphasis on empathy and introspection allowed Kohut to recognise that his patients required something from him and not, as in traditional analysis, wanted to do something to him (Wolfe, 1989). The patient was striving to obtain an input necessary for growth and not (as in traditional theory) struggling with conflicts of drives. The aggression and other affects that might be aroused in therapy where the result of failing to obtain what was felt to be needed from the therapist. Further, different patients have different needs. Some need approval, others need to be calmed and soothed (Kohut, 1977). Only by empathic introspection could these needs be identified.

Via his focus on empathy, Kohut identified three basic needs that should be fulfilled for the child to develop good internal selfobject relations (a positive sense of self). As far as I am aware no other therapy has outlined these needs in quite this way but they make much sense from an evolutionary point of view, as will be discussed shortly.

Mirroring Selfobjects

Mirroring refers to the "gleam in the mother's eye", the response of the other that approves, confirms, and rewards the exhibitionistic behaviours of the child. The response is empathic in that when the child displays (shows off) or demonstrates to others, the other (e.g., parent) not only recognises the need to praise, smile, and socially reward such behaviours but also does it with pleasure. In this sense we discover we are reinforcing to others (Gilbert, 1984), we are valued. Anyone with children can recognise these elements. For example children may direct the attention of the parent to their activities: "Watch this, mummy/daddy, look what I can do; look at what I am, how I appear, etc.". Sometimes in close contact, if the parent is looking away, the child will insist on being attended to, e.g., trying to turn the parent's head so that they look at the child. The rewarding response is both the directed, parental attention and the clear signal of pleasure in the display or "the being" of the child.

The exhibitionist aspects of early behaviour are part of grandiose aims (a grandiose self) in that they are often directed at the limits or beyond the limits of what the child can actually do. For example my six-year-old son watching me type this book said, "Let me have a go. I can write a book!" He sat on my knee for a while and slowly realised that maybe it is not quite as he imagined, or that much fun, got bored and went off to play but proudly telling his Mum that he had been writing a book. An empathic mirroring response (e.g., "that's very clever," giving a sense of pride) allows the child to discover that maybe things are not so easily achieved but it was a good try. This is without there being any sense of shame or major disappointment. A non-empathic response would be to inhibit the child from trying and focusing his attention on his/her limitations (see Schore, 1991). Yet at the same time the parent also sets the boundaries and protects from danger.

Thus, empathically given signs of approval and acceptance of the exhibitionist and grandiose actions of the child become internalised as self-esteem and vigour, a self open to possibilities and full of confidence. The vigour of this early enthusiasm, to exceed the actual limits, matures into healthy self-assertion and the pursuit of realistic goals and ambitions when handled by an empathic mirroring other. But ambitions may remain just at the limits of ability and are future directed. If they were not then we could never improve (hence self-deception, see Chapter 7). Thus there is, in healthy development, a tension arch between a healthy reaching for ambition—to improve, yet not to go so far beyond our abilities that it is either dangerous or that we are bound to fail. When grandiose tendencies have not matured (via failed mirroring) the individual becomes preoccupied with unrealistic ideals and may in some cases become reckless and not attend to limits and danger. Even in normal development, at times of excitement, we can become rather exhibitionist or reckless, thinking that we can do things we can't or briefly "go over the top". Alcohol can be a great releaser of our exhibitionism (as I know to my cost; thankfully I have passed the stage of table dancing).

However, by 1977 Kohut attributes more to mirroring than only approval of exhibitionistic actions. Mirroring "refers to all of the transactions characterizing the mother–child relationship, including not only reflections of grandiosity but also constancy, nurturance, a general empathy and respect" (Greenberg & Mitchell, 1983, p.355). By 1977, Bowlby's work on attachment theory was fairly widely known and Kohut would almost certainly have been aware of it. How far Kohut had expanded his views due to such an influence is unknown. Kahn (1985) also points out that, to Carl Rogers, positive unconditional regard is similar to mirroring. This internalised knowledge sets the psychic system towards an optimistic exploration of talent and creativity and their expression (display) in the social world (SAHP). It facilitates the development of the safety system (Gilbert, 1989). Problems arise not from occasional failures to validate self-experience but from chronic failures. This echoes Winnicott's concept of the good-enough mother.

Mirroring and the Attention of Others

Although Kohut does not speak in terms of social attention holding, to my mind this is what may be involved (see Chapter 7). Via the empathic awareness of the need to admire (and love) the child, the parent enables the child to internalise a positive representation of others and him/herself—that is he/she can hold and direct their attention in a positive way. In my view this is internalised as a kind of internal knowledge of self: "I live in the minds of another as a good, worthy, able, being. And if I live for them as this then I experience myself as this."

Let me offer an example that might make this a little clearer. A patient noted a hesitation in my making an appointment for her. She concluded that I was too busy to want to see her, that she was too difficult a case and had taken up too much time already. She felt I saw her as an irritant. She experienced herself being an irritant, a burden, and a nuisance to me and this resonated with earlier experiences. Hence what she thought was my experience of her became how she experienced herself—as an irritant to others, activating a negative/inferior selfobject experience. However, she wanted me to see her positively and not as an irritant. This generated anger and then fear that if that anger were known I would definitely see her as an irritant. She politely offered to terminate therapy and I nearly missed the injury that had been inadvertently caused.

This example gives a little insight into how cognitive therapy and self psychology can be used together and if the reader will excuse a slight digression let me point out how. Noting the subtle change in mood and using cognitive technique of questioning:

T. I noted a slight change in your mood just now. Can you tell me what was going through your mind?

P. (Showing the nonverbal signals of shame; head down, gaze avoidance and eyes darting about). I felt I was being a nuisance to you. Maybe you thought I should be better by now.

T. You felt I was irritated with you?

P. Yes.

T. How did that feel?

P. (pause, looking away again) I feel like a pain somehow. And am irritated with myself. May be I should be better.

T. You experienced yourself as a nuisance?

P. Yes very much so, that's why you seemed unsure if you wanted to make another appointment next week.

T. How come you were irritated with you and not me?

P. You're a very busy man.

T. Oh I see. Too busy to want to see you?

P. Yes.

T. Do these feelings remind you of anything?

P. (Pause). I guess it is like it has always been—like we spoke about before. Mother and father never had time. They smiled a lot but never had time to pay attention to me. Always felt I was getting in the way of other more important things.

Here the transference relationship activated underlying selfobject relations: the experience of being a nuisance and an irritant to others. At this point we were at the end of the therapy session so I summarised the interaction and checked it for shared meaning then said, " Look I am sorry you had that experience and I am grateful to you for giving us an opportunity to discuss this so we can both see how some of your hurts happen here in therapy and I can learn from you. I think this is a very important idea for you and maybe we can think about it in more detail later, like next week?" (Therapist smiles, patient smiles.)

Now there is much more to this short extract than we can discuss here. My main aim is to highlight how what she thought my experience of her was activated by her experience of herself. For me the empowering of the patient comes from the preparedness to engage the meaning in a non-judgemental way. At such a time I would not imply to a patient that their thinking is faulty or an erroneous cognitive distortion. I hope it can be seen that a direct labelling of her cognition could easily become another selfobject attack (e.g., I shouldn't have these feelings, I am just causing more problems by being so irrational). The therapist's reponse helps with the shame and acknowledges feelings, validates the experience and offers a recognition of the hurt as something to be understood. Later, she felt able to explore her anger at others.

But I have wandered from our central concept that to know/feel how we live in the minds of others is a key human concern. Again this is not a new idea—recall the quote of Pascal in Chapter 7. What is developed by Kohut is the idea that we can, as it were, walk on less solid ground (need less immediate reassurance) with the internalisation of positive selfobjects that have been developed from previous interactions. It is not surprising perhaps, that some self psychologists (e.g., Morrison, 1984) have again returned to the central role of shame in negative selfobject formation, a concern that was implicit if not explicit in Cooley's work (Scheff, 1988). What has been less articulated in self psychology (but is in the work on shame) is that mirroring depends in part on the valuing by the child; that is mirroring from another who is not valued will not be that helpful. Hence the perceived quality of the relationship is crucial. A patient's envy may get in the way of this (see Chapter 8).

Although Kohut speaks primarily of parent–child relationships, exhibitionist behaviour and mirroring needs are also common amongst children and their peers, and adults (Baker & Baker 1987; Hartup, 1989). As we grow we change the types of mirroring we require for self-validation, e.g., adults seek mirroring of their sexual indentity. The ways a female may wish to be mirrored may be different from those of the male. Males, for example, may use the preparedness of the female to desire sexual relationship as a positive mirroring response. Withdrawal of sexual interest acts as an injury to the sense of "valued, potent or attractive self". Problems in the way marital partners mirror each other and support their selfobject relations are often a significant area of conflict and anger (see Chapter 15).

Wolf (1988, p.73) points out that for some individuals there is mirror hunger (or what cognitive theorists would call approval addiction). The mirror hungry personalities "are impelled to display themselves to evoke the attention of others, who through their admiring responses will perhaps counteract the experience of worthlessness." Like our ethological analysis, the role of attention is crucial here. These individuals can become depressed as a result of failure to obtain sufficient approval (SAHP, see Chapter 7) to maintain self-esteem. In our ethological view, internal self-evaluation may switch to the experience of subordinate self-perception (e.g., in the above example "I am just a pain and the therapist is too busy/important to want to bother with me"). In other words the individual does not seem to have an internal sense of worth but requires constant support of worth. Beck (1983) might call such individuals sociotropic.

Idealising Needs

A second need is for idealisation. This also relates to valuing the other. By idealising another the child is able to internalise a sense of being loved, cared for, and esteemed by someone who is stronger, more able, etc. Idealising needs relate to "our need to merge with, or be close to, someone who we believe will make us safe, comfortable, and calm. The child who falls and bumps a knee runs to the parent for a kiss, which, through no known medical process, has profound healing powers—the pain disappears! Again an external object serves as internal function—calming and comforting—and so functions as a selfobject for the child" (Baker & Baker, 1987, p.4). (This of course is almost identical to Bowlby's ideas.) This allows the child to internalise a sense of what I would call safety provision or what Kohut calls soothing. The internal representation of a positive relationship with an idealised other allows the child to come to soothe him/herself under conditions of stress. (This may give a new insight into the issue of catastrophising in cognitive therapy. Catastrophisers have not internalised or have lost the capacity for self-soothing—possibly due to defense system activation.)

This aspect goes with the development of trust—that is, others can be trusted to be helpful. Because you can trust others there is no need to worry, help is at hand. But again it is the interaction that is important. If the child sees others as superior but believes that they are not prepared to put this superiority to help the child but rather keep it for themselves, or give it to someone else, or use it to exert controlling power over the child, then the calming elements and trust are not internalised and envy is more likely.

So this element of "looking up to others" is important for it carries the notion of being able to borrow, or call upon the abilities, talents or comfort provided by another. If envy or excessive competitiveness enters the relationship then it becomes difficult for the person to feel reassured by the presence of more powerful/able others. They may even refuse to acknowledge the talents or potential helpfulness of the other. Rather, the existence of superior others only confirms a sense of low self-esteem, of being less than others (see Chapter 8). This activates anger or withdrawal rather than a reaching out for support and help. If on the other hand the superior other uses their position to maintain a status imbalance the person might remain in an idealising state and not move on to develop their own talents and abilities to soothe themselves.

However, a certain degree of frustration of need is necessary to aid internalisation of control. Certainly parents who are fearful of not complying with the child and are over-controlled by the child's demands can lead to the "spoilt brat" syndrome as Alfred Adler noted many years ago. Hence internalised inhibition (because the parent sets boundaries) is part of healthy development. Without this we end up with a strong sense of narcissistic entitlement. As Coopersmith (1967) has pointed out there are differences between authoritarian and authorative parenting and these differ from over-permissive parenting. It is authorative parenting where rules and boundaries are understood, and there is a recognition of basic fairness and respect and warmth for parents, which leads to robust self-esteem.

There is another element in idealising that is akin to modelling. The idealised other acts as a model for development and over time helps to direct the course of development. It is this aspect that allows the child to become like, yet also separate from the "looked-up-to" other and in this way come to develop realistic goals about the kind of person they wish to become. The relationship between Kohut's concept of idealising and Jung's notion of the hero archetype is interesting. For Jung the hero archetype served both the function of looking up to and idealising others but also the function of moving the person along their own life course; to become the hero of their own lives (see Chapter 11). The journey of the hero nearly always begins with encouragement from an older, wiser type figure (as depicted in the Star Wars films which were very much influenced by Joseph Campbell's book, *The Hero with a Thousand Faces*). This theme is implicit rather than explicit in self psychology in that it is assumed that the therapist aims to help the patient become more self-sufficient and independent.

Wolf (1988, p.73) says that idealising hungry personalities "can experience themselves as worthwhile only by finding selfobjects to whom they can look up to and by whom they feel accepted". Such people have a great need to idealise others especially those they think will treat them as special in some way. Hence there is often a kind of contract, an unconscious trading of specialness: "You are a special type of therapist and I am your special patient." The unwary therapist can have their own narcissistic needs (to be seen as special and better than other therapists) activated in these kinds of relationships. The patient can be hurt either by the therapist doing or saying something that suggests that the therapist is but ordinary and fallible and/or by the therapist doing or saying something that suggests that the patient is but ordinary. For both therapist and patient there may be a fear of ordinariness.

Alter-ego Needs

Alter-ego needs reflect needs to feel the same as someone else. In evolutionary theory this may relate to ingroup–outgroup and network issues (see Chapter 7), or possibly the mentality of cooperation (Gilbert, 1989). At issue here is a sense of belonging, sharing, being like, having a common purpose, allies, and goal(s). In Hartup's (1989) terms they are horizontal relationships. These needs are secured with shared activity. Patients with excessive alter-ego needs may become upset if they find the therapist does not share their opinions (Wolf, 1988). This can produce feelings of being different and alone. These individuals have difficulty in tolerating differences of view in relationships and often present as disappointed loners (the outsider theme, see Chapter 11). A particular problem is that a sensitive therapist can be engaged in a very friendly relationship but the affiliative behaviour does not transfer outside of therapy and that patient maintains a view "I am different to others."

Overview

In general then these styles of relationship set the platform for an internal life or style of self-experience(s). Mirroring provides a sense of value in the eyes of others, leading to a non-defensive, optimistic and energic engagement in the social world. Mirroring is related to ideas about "how I exist for others". Idealising gives rise to an internal sense

TABLE 10.2
The Tripartite Self-System

		Healthy Development	
Child's Needs	Grandiose Exhibitionist	Idealising	Alter Ego
		Obtains Closeness	
Care giver (Selfobject) Response	Empathic Mirroring "Gleam in the mother's eye"	Soothing Accepting Modelling	Affiliative Cooperative Belongs with
Outcome	Healthy self-esteem, values, assertiveness	Healthy ideals, principles and self-soothing capacity	Talents and skills optimally utilised
Self-structure: Cohesive and integrated, able to achieve closeness with others and maintain contact with achievable goals and incentives and sense of internal vigour.			
		Unhealthy Development	
Child's Needs	Grandiose Exhibitionist	Idealising	Alter Ego
		Lacks Closeness	
Caregiver (selfobject) Response	Non-empathic, lacks mirroring or is shaming, neglectful	Unsoothing Non-accepting Lacks good model	Non-affiliative Non cooperative Outsider, Different
Outcome	Vulnerable self-esteem, lacks assertiveness or is aggressive	Unhealthy ideals, goals, unable, self-soothing	Talents and skills not developed or expressed
Self Structure: Lacks sense of cohesiveness; vulnerable to rage or withdrawal/shame, approval seeking, dependent, impulsive. Vulnerable to: feelings of depression, boredom lack of purpose, emptiness and fragmentation. (Adapted from Kahn, 1985)			

of safety and trust, together with models for behaviour: "I want to achieve this or be valued for that." Alter-ego needs allow for the sense of being like others and able to tolerate differences. These are depicted in Table 10.2.

FRAGMENTATION

Kohut speaks about the fears of self-fragmentation as loss of self-cohesion. Over the years I have been interested in this from an evolutionary view and there seem to me to be three types. The first is a kind of loss of control; conscious desires of self-presentation are swept aside on a tide of uncontrollable emotion and there is no way back

(Horowitz & Zilberg, 1983). It is the chaotic self. Various addictive behaviours such as eating are efforts to soothe the self and maintain control over inner feeling states. Associated here are fears of loss of self-identity. There is increasing evidence that a perceived inability to be able to control states is an important dimension to anxiety and depression (Barlow, 1991).

Another form of fragmentation is more associated with the existential concept of non-being. These patients talk less of becoming a chaotic entity of emotional outpourings and being out of control, and more in terms of becoming a nothingness. At first I was unsure what this "nothingness" was actually about, but as patients have struggled to articulate these feelings it has become my view that it is a fear of complete marginalisation, of subordinacy; that is, an individual can have no impact whatsoever on the feelings or actions of others. One patient said that "people may smile at you or even be kind but you know in your heart that to them you are a nothing. If there is a party or something needs to be done you know they will never think of you. To them you are out of sight out of mind and if you cause too much trouble, they will swat you like a fly." Here is expressed the fear of the omega, the lowest of the low, the nonentity and the outsider: "you have no real existence or importance in the minds or lives of others".

The third form of fragmentation is the disappearing act which is related to abandonment and isolation. One patient described her fear of spinning round and round disappearing down a plug-hole, simply disappearing. The closest I ever came to this was a dream. I was sleeping in a room on my own one night and dreamt that I had woken up. I looked around the room and everything seemed in order. I was about to go back to sleep when the window broke and I suddenly realised that outside had been created a vacuum, similar, I guess, to what might happen if an airline window broke in flight. For long minutes it seemed I was sucked steadily towards to window. In front of me and growing larger was a bright night sky with thousands of dancing blue stars. As I began to grab desperately for things to hold on to I realised that if I went out of the window I would be flung far out into the cosmos and there would be no way back again. The terror was of complete isolation for eternity. A certain unease stayed with me for some days.

I put this in since for me it brought alive the hidden terrors of fragmentation as total isolation. So terror inducing are the internal experiences of fragmentation and the sense of disconnectedness with self and others, that individuals will do almost anything to avoid it, mostly because they believe once fragmented (broken or lost) there is no repair, no way back. Whether or not this relates to an archetypal fear of being lost (e.g., away from the group) is unknown.

Compensation and Rage

There are various tactics to counteract fragmentation. Morrison (1984) notes Kohut's distinction of the "defensive self-structures" which mobilise efforts to conceal deficits in self and compensatory self-structures which mobilise efforts to make up for a weakness in self to, literally, compensate. Morrison offers a complex but interesting idea that depression often results from the experience of depletion of energy to maintain compensatory structures. The individual simply cannot achieve the ideals which are necessary (be it via a relationship or personal effort) which would lift self-esteem and restore a sense of cohesion. He notes similarities with Bibring's (1953) concepts but unlike Bibring he places shame as a central affect. Understanding shame helps us to understand narcissistic rage, especially in depression.

These are the experiences of the failed self, the worthless self: of Kohut's "tragic man". Also however, Wolf (1988) draws attention to the experiences of the empty self, the self without vigour or purpose. These people have not really failed since they have not really tried. Such people may be subject to low grade chronic depressive disturbances.

Rage. Wolf (1988) points out that Kohut distinguished two types of aggression. Competitive aggression relates to aggression aimed at objects and things that thwart our path to achievements and goals. Once the object is removed and the path is cleared, the self settles again. Aggression arises simply from not being able to get what one wants. This is very similar to notions of frustrative aggression and it would probably be better to use that term rather than competitive aggression. Narcissistic rage however is not just aggression directed at things that block a path but to things or people that can undermine self-esteem. Narcissistic rage arises from feelings of helplessness, inadequacy, and inferiority that are provoked. Hence this kind of rage is associated with the need for revenge (to regain power) and this can be long-lived even though the person on whom one seeks revenge can no longer hurt one.

Narcissistic rage can be thrown up whenever an event happens that damages the self—for example, when the therapist tells a patient that they are not entitled to special privileges or points out failings in the patient. In this sense the rage can be activated by shame (Morrison, 1984). The aggression of Hitler was pure narcissistic rage and he would blame everyone except himself. Thus Kohut does not see aggression as a drive but rather as a secondary consequence of some insult to the self. Needless to say the consequences of narcissistic rage are far more serious than frustrative aggression (e.g., desires for revenge). These aggressive feelings can be concealed for they may threaten an already vulnerable self and the patient may withdraw. The patient can be frightened by their own sadistic or vengeful feelings. The experience for patients who attempt to inhibit their narcissistic rage can be a sense of overwhelming helplessness and shame—a shame that threatens to reduce whatever mirroring they may have desired, a shame that reduces the ability to merge with an idealised other, a shame that separates self from others. But in my view narcissistic aggression can be expressed down the hierarchy. Whether a person suffers inhibited fury or attacks the other often depends on the power relationship between them.

SELF PSYCHOLOGY AND DEPRESSION

The self psychology theory of depression is very well summed up by Deitz (1988, p.605):

> The depressed patient has lost the ability to contact the affective tone of positive dimensions of his self-representation. The rage of the depressive is a narcissistic rage, resulting from his inability to autonomously activate important and positive self objects. Exogenous (e.g., loss of object relationships or attachments that activate positive dimensions of one's self-representation) as well as endogenous factors (e.g., loss of physical abilities that have been used to activate positive self-representations) can account for the decrease in ability to regulate mood and self-esteem.

The goal of therapy is to facilitate and develop contact with internal positive selfobjects that bring back or develop representations of self as having worth and being able, rather than those of being worthless and unable. Deitz (1988) notes these ideas are similar to cognitive therapists' notions of self schema.

In a way, the self psychology view of depression is that it is nearly always secondary to a painful sense of disappointment/frustration—disappointment that life has turned out the way it has, that others are not as loving or reliable as was hoped, that plans have not come to fruit, and so on. Somehow one has not made it—a position portrayed so brilliantly in Arthur Miller's play, *Death of a Salesman* (for a further discussion of this see Baker & Baker, 1988). In this sense it is important to help the person articulate their sense of disappointment and to reflect on the sources of this disappointment, often of unrealistic aspirations or unmet needs. Anger is secondary to feeling blocked and thwarted and not a primary drive.

Self psychology helps us understand a number of things about depression. First, it focuses attention on "needs" rather than deficits, repressed drives or cognitive errors. These needs include those of mirroring (Carl Rogers' positive unconditional regard) and so validate a sense of worth, the need to reawaken/develop healthy aspirations and goals and to counteract shame, the need to put people in touch with their vigour. In my view this is to turn off defensive styles of processing (Gilbert, 1989). Second, it articulates a theory of the rage and shame components of some depressives which at times can remain hidden. Third, it can be used to understand family relationships and how in these relationships vulnerabilities to the self are played out (see Chapter 15). Fourth, and perhaps most important, it points up a therapeutic attitude, one that is engaged with, and empathic to, the sense of a depressed self, its fragility. And it teaches us to walk gently but not distantly. Kohut was of the view that "the analyst employs his method for a specific purpose—in order to understand and then explain, thus enabling the patient to enlarge his knowledge of himself" (as quoted by Wolfe, 1989, p.561), indicting the role of education perhaps. However, unlike some cognitive therapies there is no emphasis on the idea of cognitive distortion or cognitive errors. (In fact I think that the depiction of cognitive errors is the worst thing that ever happened to cognitive therapy because this concept is so easily misunderstood and abused in therapy by the inexperienced, see Chapter 13).

AN EVOLUTIONARY PERSPECTIVE

Kohut was not concerned with understanding the biological basis of experience. His interest was with the internal world as experienced and the role of introspection. Further, he was not concerned, apparently, with the notion of the biological collective (species-typic) or universal elements of experience (Wolf, 1988; Wolfe, 1989). However, in arguing for common human needs (mirroring, idealising, and alter ego) his is, in fact, a theory of universal processes that are prominent in humankind. He had no desire to look for evolutionary roots to subjective experience or to consider that what we introspect on is not born from a tabula rasa. Yet our experience of ourselves is constrained by the themes of living that are part of our phylogeny.

It will come as no surprise that in my view self psychology is a kind of fleshing out of the complexities of the requirements for self-structures that have evolved from primate life styles—specifically, evaluations of attachments and rank being at the core. The desire to move up the rank to succeed in life, the need for reassurance from more dominant animals, and the need for allies are all part of primate social life. I would suggest for example, that in mirroring, the status relationship is often important, in that the higher the status of the approving other the more effective the response. This is often true in adult life where to be admired by those we value and regard as equal or of higher status is usually more mood elevating than to be admired by those we see as inferior or do not value. The importance of valuing the (potential) admiring other is crucial in therapy. A patient who does not value the therapist (for whatever reason) is unlikely to be influenced by the therapist.

Self psychology does not tell us why energy is lost only that with certain selfobject relations it is lost. Once we connect this to the issue of subordinate states as they have evolved and complexified, then their psychobiology and their energy controlling functions become clear. Idealising and mirroring are the means humans have evolved to stabilise and control the internal mechanisms for power and belonging. When we internalise a belief that we live in the minds of others as positive, worthy beings we are freed from the more primitive options of concealment and having to fight or involuntarily submit to others; we become less inhibited. This allows for greater internal cohesion and external affiliation.

Yet as Jung has made clear we must not become mechanical copies of others' wishes, but rather find our own individuality. Hence we must also address the issue of the blocked escape, the way we can be entrapped by a life style. We must at times be able to move away from others, to break free, and there is some doubt about how much self psychology addresses this issue.

There is nothing to be gained by denying our evolutionary history but rather on the contrary it shows us more clearly that the possibility of becoming a positive vigorous self in tune with others is a fantastic achievement of evolution requiring only that we follow certain rules, that we behave towards each other in certain kinds of way. Kohut, along with others, has articulated some of these rules and processes. Perhaps, like Bowlby, he has shown us how to avoid the path of the primitive possibilities that lie within and how to move us to a more fully human existence.

KOHUT AND BOWLBY COMPARED

They are alike in that:

1. Both emphasise that depression (and other pathologies) result from the failure of significant others to support maturation needs.
2. Both stress that via interaction individuals develop internal mechanisms (working models or selfobjects) that influence the experience of the self and self-esteem and guide interpersonal behaviour.

3. Both theories (and if not Kohut then certainly his followers) have drawn from research on child development.
4. Hence both stress that the patient needs something from the therapist, i.e., therapy is need orientated and the therapist's role is to understand that need rather than interpret deeply unconscious conflicts or only correct erroneous thoughts.
5. Both suggest that the anger associated with depression is secondary to thwarted interpersonal needs.

They are different in that:

1. Whereas Bowlby stresses what the parents do wrong (e.g., threats to abandon, reversal of child–parent roles) Kohut gives a greater emphasis to interaction of mirroring and idealising. Idealising is certainly part of Bowlby's theory (i.e., he believes attachments, in the first instance, develop to those seen as stronger and wiser) but this dimension is given less discussion. Indeed many followers of Bowlby hardly mention this rank aspect to attachment theory (Birtchnell, personal communication).
2. The concept of "selfobjects" is rather different to that of "internal working models". The former are viewed as part of the "self as experienced" and are emotional, whereas the internal working model is more cognitive and for this reason has appealed to cognitive therapists (e.g., Guidano & Liotti, 1983; Liotti, 1988), though this distinction is more one of degree. Selfobjects are closer to the behavioural idea of conditioned emotional response than internal working models.
3. For Bowlby it is loss of interpersonal bonds and disconnectedness from others that gives rise to depression, whereas for Kohut it is an internal experience of fragmentation, falling apart, and losing the cohesiveness of self-structures that provided the sense of self and vigour. This may or may not be triggered by actually losses.
4. Kohut's theory is much more therapy-focused with special importance placed on empathy and introspection. It is in fact comparatively recently that the therapeutic aspects of attachment theory have begun to be articulated (e.g., MacKie, 1982; Guidano & Liotti, 1983; Liotti, 1988; Safran & Segal, 1990). Furthermore, the focus of the therapy is rather different. For attachment theory it is focused on providing a safe base from which to explore and reconceptualise past experiences, whereas for Kohut it is the therapist's empathy

that cures by providing an opportunity to rework earlier, unmet needs.

5. Bowlby's model is strongly ethological and he draws on animal work to understand innate prepared mechanisms for attachment and their dysfunction. Kohut on the other hand had a rather negative view to such biologising and never drew ethological comparisons.
6. Bowlby's approach derives evidence from research psychology and the ideas of information processing systems and memory, whereas Kohut rarely engages the experimental literature (although his followers do), again primarily because of his insistence on empathy and introspection as the key method of knowing and understanding.

It would be unrealistic to compare in order to say which is better. Rather, attention is drawn to both their similarities and differences. Each addresses the subject in rather different ways. For me however I have found both Bowlby's and Kohut's work illuminating and helpful but, as I have tried to point out, the whole concept of our needing to "live positively in the minds of others" is not a new idea. The issue of idealising also is notable in other theories as is the need for kinship. It is more in how these concepts are articulated and used that makes the difference.

HISTORICAL EVIDENCE

Both theories suggest that early life is the prominent seed bed for later psychopathology, especially depression. In general most research work has been stimulated by attachment theory rather than self psychology. Hopefully, future research will focus more on the distinctions suggested by self psychology. The last decade has seen a vast increase in research on the early life of depressive and other forms of psychopathology. Much of this data is retrospective and requires the subject to rate their recall of their early life with parents. Lewinsohn and Rosenbaum (1987) used various measures of parent–child relationships, in depressed, recovered depressed, people who become depressed at follow-up, and controls. Their results indicate a possible state-dependency effect for negative memories of early life. As subjects recovered they tended to become more like normals in recall of their early family relationships.

However, Perris et al. (1986) investigated the experience of rearing in groups of unipolar, bipolar, and neurotic depressives, and controls. They collected various data on recovery (or discharge). Their results confirm that various measures of lack of emotional caring may be an important risk factor to depression. Unlike Lewinsohn and Rosenbaum

(1987), these researchers used trained interviewers to gather their data. Gotlib, Mount, Cordby, and Whiffen (1988) explored groups of depressed, remitted depressives, and non-depressed subjects in a longitudinal follow-up design and found that perceptions of parenting were remarkably stable over time. It was also found that only those subjects who reported both low maternal caring and over-protectiveness were still depressed at follow-up. In a major review using a meta analysis of studies, Gerlsma et al. (1990) found that for anxiety/phobic disorders there was consistent evidence of early, less parental affection and more control compared to healthy subjects. However, findings for depression were less consistent and there seemed to be a difference between bipolars and neurotics, with the former more like controls. Nevertheless, the largest distinction with controls remained on less parental affection and more control.

The importance of this research area is matched by its difficulty. There are obvious concerns about accuracy of recall and state-dependency. Also, as mentioned elsewhere (Gilbert, 1989), depressives are often very concerned with self-presentation. For example, a patient changed her story on recovery with drugs, because she thought is was "not nice to criticise her mother". Hence researchers using certain methods can only study what a patient is prepared to admit and shame, concealment, and defensive exclusion can surround this area. Also, Brewin (1990) has noted that there are different types of memory. Personal memory (e.g., picture of scenes and events); generic personal memory (memory of themes over time); autobiographical facts (e.g., grades in an exam); and self-schema memory of self-characteristics (e.g., shyness). It seems that time sequences become blurred and lost. Also, personal, specific, positive memories in depression may suffer various processing blocks (Moore, Watts, & Williams, 1988). In Chapter 6 we argued that this may be part of (general) internal inhibition to reduce challenge and general "go getting" behaviour. Memory for themes may be more reliable. In some therapies the question, "What are your earliest memories?" is illuminating. Social memory may differ from non-social memory since different kinds of processing may be occurring for social as opposed to non-social events. Another factor is that attachment problems may have their major impact before maturation of either language or memory systems (e.g., hippocampal structures, Jacobs & Nadel, 1985). Hence this area of memory for parental style is complex.

Finally, recall that there is evidence that depression runs in families and also that depressed mothers can have a significant impact on child development (Gelfand & Teti, 1990; Gotlib & Lee, 1990). Hence a mother may be depressed for the early years of a child's life which affects C.N.S. development but later she may recover. What effect would this have on self-organisation and memory? At the present time researchers debate the methods and design of studies, but generally affectionless parenting and control appear to be important. In the next decade we are likely to see further major developments in this area including studies of resilience and the role of sibling relationships (Dunn, 1988) and the importance of non-shared environments of siblings (Reiss et al., 1991). (For a review of the complexities of developmental psychopathology see Sroufe & Rutter, 1984.)

SUMMARY

1. Attachment theory focuses on the innate attachment needs of the infant. According to how these needs are met various internal representations of self and others are built up.
2. These internal maps or working models guide the person in their subsequent attachment relationships. Vulnerability to depression is the result of early life experiences.
3. Depression results when a person confronts later losses and feels helpless to overcome them. These experiences of helplessness, or even self-blame for the loss, relate to early attachment styles.
4. Kohut developed the concepts of self-cohesion for healthy development and outlined a set of special needs: mirroring; idealising and alter-ego—being like others.
5. Satisfactory provision of these needs results in the maturation of a cohesive sense of self that is able to follow healthy and realistic ambitions and goals, feel calm in the presence of others and develop mature relationships.
6. Unsatisfactory provision of these needs results in a constant searching to fulfil these needs, e.g., high approval-seeking, seeking others to idealise, or unrealistic aspirations.
7. Depression occurs when internal selfobject relationships begin to fragment, leading to a loss of cohesiveness and vigour. Therapy is aimed at provision of a relationship that helps to reinstate the sense of cohesion.

CONCLUDING COMMENTS

Whereas Freud talked mostly about the agonic system (of aggression, sexuality, envy, and fear) Bowlby and Kohut are much more focused on the hedonic system (attachment, need for SAHP, and sense of value) and the mental mechanisms that are essential for us to move forward in life as optimistic, loving, and socially able beings. It is understandable, therefore, why in Kohut's work, aggression, envy, shame, and rage are seen as secondary disintegration products. As we have argued earlier (Chapters 6 and 7) the hedonic possibilities sit on top of, or evolved later than, the more primitive agonic system. Whereas the Freudians suggest that there is, in all of us, an agonic personality trying to get out, but it is constrained, the self psychologists suggest that humans are trying to fulfil or reach their higher level functions/possibilities and will do so if conditions are right (Gilbert, 1989). Hence the more aggressive and automatic, defensive options are in some sense regressive responses to various threats (Bailey, 1987). Further the agonic system will have a different set of affects, motives (need to exert control), images, and symbolic representations linked with it, compared to the hedonic system (valuing, love searching). It can be noted that the old and new testaments of the bible also reflect this split (God as vengeful, jealous, and punitive, versus God as loving and forgiving).

The idea that a certain dependency carries vulnerability to depression has been with us since Freud's 1917 paper. However, in Freud's theory there was less emphasis on what a child needs from his/her care-givers and more focus on internal development. Consequently, there was little in psychoanalytic therapy that emphasised the role of the therapist as a provider of needs. Indeed the passivity of the therapist was aimed very specifically to interpret but not to satisfy needs. In a way both Bowlby and Kohut have turned that idea on its head. Both focus on the unfulfilled needs of the patient and see it as the therapist's role to support those needs and facilitate healthy development and maturation. In my view an understanding of attachment theory and self psychology gives a therapist a way of conceptualising very difficult processes in therapy. Both theories focus on human needs and this helps counteract the idea that we are nothing but information processing systems. Kohut's theory (which is actually very difficult to understand from his own writings) gives a depth of understanding of the depressive experience of dread (see Chapter 8). However, on the down side he rarely acknowledged his sources and his therapy tends to be very long. Some accuse it of being too cosy. Although self psychology can be used in a cognitive way, Kohut would have seen thought monitoring, recording, and evidence testing as an anathema.

If the reader has felt in tune with the evolutionary arguments put forward in Chapters 5–8, then they will realise, I suspect, why self psychology has appeal. The idea of the mind as a mixed structure of different elements that can conflict resonates with notions of fragmentation and a sense of powerlessness. The idea that we have evolved to live in the minds of others resonates with mirroring; the idea of needing to idealise others resonates with the importance of rank and our accommodation to it; and the idea of alter-ego needs resonates with the idea of the need for networks and allies, ingroups and outgroups. Whether self psychologists will feel able to extend their theory into a more evolutionary context is yet to be seen. I obviously hope so.

As far as therapy goes, an understanding of the evolved needs of internal psychic life requires us to orientate ourselves to the social life and the importance of valuing each other. In the next chapter we shall explore Jung's theories, and some have seen Jung as having covered some of the same ground as Kohut (Samuels, 1985). So I would like to leave you with a favourite story on Jung told by van der Post (1976, p.59).

Jung was presented with a depressed, simple soul whose main problem was that her community had:

> poured scorn on all her simple beliefs, ideas, customs and interests. Accordingly, he got her to talk to him at length about all the things she had enjoyed and loved as a child. As she talked, almost at once he saw a flicker of interest glow. He found himself so excited by this quickening of the spirit of a despised self, that he joined in the singing of her nursery songs, and her renderings of simple mountain ballads. He even danced with her in his library, and at times, took her on his knee and rocked her in his arms, undeterred by any thought of how ridiculous, if not preposterous, would be the picture of him in the eyes of orthodox medical and psychiatric practioners.

After a few days, the girl was restored to health never to relapse. When a local doctor asked how he had achieved this miraculous outcome, van der Post says, Jung replied, "I did nothing much, I listened to her fairy tales, danced with her a little, sang with her a little, took her on my knee a little, and the job was done." But the local doctor never did believe him.

NOTES

1. At the time of going to press we have heard of the sad death of John Bowlby. This section is a small reflection on his enormous contribution to human understanding.
2. Kin altruism (see Chapter 5) is supposed to organise things such that relatives benefit from interactions and are given an advantage. However what is an advantage? In many families the patterns of relationships appear more like reciprocal altruism and than kin altruism (Gilbert, 1989). What I mean by this is that in our clinics we constantly find people who are trying to prove to their parents that they are worthy of love, respect, and being seen as an agent of value. The misery that they may have disappointed their parents is tragic and the desperate desire to be recognised causes intense

suffering. A patient who had obtained a good degree told me in sobs how she had "looked for any small signal that my parents now noticed me and felt I was someone to be proud of". The human need for sociocultural success has brought with it distortions in attachment relations not seen in other primates. In humans we can acquire various internal models of self that place on us burdens and conditions that (we believe) must be met to elicit parental investment in the form of love, approval, support, and SAHP.

CHAPTER 11

Archetypes, Biosocial Goals, Mentalities, and Depressive Themes

In the preceding chapter we explored depression from the point of view of the thwarting of needs. In this chapter we shall widen our focus and consider the idea that humans have evolved predispositions to form internal reprsentations of various forms of social behaviour and roles. To explore this aspect from an evolutionary angle requires consideration of how these social dispositions are laid down in gene-neural structures. To put this a different way, we are interested in pursuing the idea that the mind is a mixed system containing various policies (Ornstein, 1986) or special purpose processing modules (see Chapter 5), or archetypes.

ARCHETYPES

Carl Gustav Jung (1875-1961) first met Freud (who was nineteen years his senior) in Vienna in the winter of 1907. Very shortly after, he joined the inner circle and became one of Freud's favourites. But by 1913 serious differences of view emerged and they parted company. The reasons for the break were various (Ellenberger, 1970) but one was Jung's rejection of libido theory and his growing belief that the psychic was not made up of competing drives but rather of various, internal meaning-making and action-directed systems. These systems, which he called archetypes, influenced the unfolding of development—e.g., to seek care, to become a member of a group, to find a sexual partner and become a parent, to find meaning and wisdom, and to come to terms with death (Stevens, 1982). These themes are enacted in the rituals and myths of all societies.

Jung's work has sometimes been dismissed as too mystical and obscure for serious study. Certainly he was concerned with the spiritual aspects of life but it would be wrong to dismiss his ideas on this score. Although his ideas on the inheritance of archetypal forms, via repeated experience over generations, are false, Hall and Nordby (1973) suggest the concept of "archetypes" remains valid and appropriate from the Darwinian perspective. Wenegrat (1984) also sees merit in the concept of archetype (for a further discussion see Gilbert, 1989). Jung postulated that humans, as an evolved species, inherit specific predispositions for thought and action. These predispositions exist as foci within the collective unconscious capable of guiding behaviour, thoughts, and emotions. He distinguished the collective unconscious from the personal by suggesting that the personal unconscious represented those aspects of personal experience that were rooted in real events. They had at one time been conscious but were either forgotten or repressed. The collective unconscious, however, was the realm of the inherited universal predispositions; the internal motivating systems that form the bedrock of species typical behaviours. As Ellenberger (1970) suggests, Jung's (1972, pp.13–19) theories on the archetypes have often been misunderstood, but his own definition seems reasonably clear.

> The archetype in itself is empty and purely formal, nothing but a *facultas praeformandi*, a possibility of representation which is given a priori. The representations themselves are not inherited, only the forms, and in that respect they correspond in every way to the instincts, which are also determined in form only. The existence of instincts can no more be proved than the existence of the archetypes, so long as they do not manifest themselves concretely. With regard to the definiteness of the form, our comparison with the crystal is illuminating inasmuch as the axial system determines only the stereometric structure but not the concrete form of the individual crystal. This may be either large or small, and it may vary endlessly by reason of the different size of its planes or by the growing together of two crystals. The only thing that remains constant is the axial system, or rather, the invariable geometric proportions underlying it. The same is true of the archetype. In principle, it can be named and has an invariable nucleus of meaning but always only in principle, never as regards its concrete manifestation.

Hence archetypes represent a possibility, a preparedness for meaning and purpose. Today we speak in terms of modules or policies or social algorithms, but although these are reaching after a similar idea the concept of archetype is broader. Archetypes are seen as motivators, and fantasy generators and they are actualised in roles and self-identity. Jung followed the philosophers Kant and Plato. Both suggested that meaning is given by the mind to things and events, not the other way around. So Jung was first and foremost concerned with those universals common to humanity and attempted to articulate the internal psychic mechanisms that (across various cultures and time) brought into existence (into relationship) various life themes, myths, rituals, and stories. One can therefore consider Jung both in terms of an articulation of underlying psychic structures and in terms of socio-cultural themes. Archetypes are ways of knowing, making sense of, and responding to the world and are also internal generators of fantasy (e.g., fantasising being a very famous rock star relates to the hero archetype; fantasies of one's ideal woman or ideal man to the anima and animus, etc.).

Archetypes and Depression

Jung never fully articulated a clear theory of depression. He believed that it could have many roots. However the most common was that the self become divorced from important archetypal potentials, or an archetype could function negatively. We may dream of how we wish things were but feel unable to achieve them. Like Kohut and others there was a concern with fragmentation of the psyche and a lack of wholeness and integration. Jung believed that in our dreams and paintings we could begin to see recovery of the self when circular forms began to appear (Jacobi, 1968).

The archetypes relate to depression in different ways and each individual depression represents both a collective (archetypal) aspect and a personal aspect. Among the most central archetypes relating to depression are the following.

The Persona. The persona represents the predisposition to form a social role model for self which finds acceptability in the eyes of others. In Chapter 7 we called this "living in the minds of others". As Hall and Nordby (1973) make clear, the persona is an inherited predisposition to behave in a way which facilitates conformity, social acceptance, and social integration. It is the archetype which motivates us to be accepted by others. More specifically, it is the mask which is exhibited to one's fellows "with the intention of presenting a favourable impression so that society will accept him" (p.44). Although individuals may play different roles with different groups, these are all part of the same need to conform, that is, they have the same function. Since the persona is only one aspect of the self, too little or too much development of the persona can have unfortunate consequences.

A malfunctioning of the persona is a common causes of depression. In cases of "persona inflation", the individual over-identifies with his mask. He becomes too involved with conformity and too reliant on external sources of reinforcement secured from others with the use of his persona. Hall and Nordby (1973, p.45) suggest that:

> a persona-ridden person becomes alienated from his nature, and lives in a state of tension because of the conflict between his overdeveloped persona and the underdeveloped parts of his personality.
>
> On the other hand the victim of inflation can also suffer feelings of inferiority and self-reproach when he is incapable of living up to the standards expected of him. He may, as a result, feel alienated from the community and experience feelings of loneliness and estrangement.

The persona dominated person says, "I am nothing but my role. Others must approve of me." The person can only be happy if the part he is playing (parent, lover, academic, sportsman, etc.) is acceptable and is reinforced by others. In other words, the individual seeks to play his part to the full and failure must be avoided, for without the reinforcement of others self-esteem is dealt a catastrophic blow. For Kohut (1977) this is a mirroring need dominated personality; for cognitive therapists (Beck et al., 1979; Burns, 1980) it is the approval addict and for others it is the person who is out of tune with their own needs, their own individuality. Unlike these other theorists, Jung saw these difficulties coming about through the underdevelopment of other aspects of the personality. Clearly, the persona is linked to issues of shame (see Chapter 8).

In Jung's view, depression results when the persona act fails and a sense of emotional isolation can appear as the individual begins to realise that no matter how successful the persona, happiness and contentment are short-lived and empty. This may occur when the "shadow" archetype intrudes into persona functioning. In this case individuals become aware that their act is false, it is not a true or complete reflection of the person they are or wish to be.

The Hero. The hero archetype represents a number of aspects. It can be involved in idealising and hero worship but it is also the predisposition to follow one's own path, to take on the challenges of life, break away from parents and security. In many myths the hero cycle is depicted by the person who leaves behind the familiar, has various adventures and in this way is changed, gains new insight and knowledge and then returns. In mythology the hero is depicted as the slayer of dragons which is symbolic for the overcoming of one's own fear.

If the hero is "that which propels us outwards" then it is also that which sets us on course to find our individuality. For various reasons of fear this outward (and sometimes inward) journey may never be undertaken and leads to a self preoccupied with his/her unlived or unfulfilled plans. At times the hero archetype may break through as is depicted in H.G., Wells' wonderful novel, *The History of Mr Polly*. This tells the story of a chronically, mildly depressed man who one day burns down his tailors shop and sets out for a new life. Many archetypal themes are in this story.

Depression can arise from a failure of the hero archetype to mature. At times the hero archetype operates only in fantasy. The person dreams of success and achievement but (perhaps because of the persona) feels too inhibited to "go for it" and remains, "at home", as it were. At other times the fantasies can be so grandiose, they are themselves frightening. As for Kohut (1977), the cure of depression involves re-engaging a person's sense of vigour and helping them through the various anxieties and life difficulties that inhibit individuation. At times failure to engage the internal hero leads to the person who does not grow up or who cannot accept leadership roles or take the initiative. It is the security dominated personality.

The Shadow. The shadow represents the predisposition to conceal (sometimes even from oneself) the less pro-social or persona-threatening qualities of the personality. It is the archetype of the hidden aspects of the self. The shadow is reminiscent of Nietzsche's comment that we should beware, that in throwing out our devils we throw out the best part of ourselves. The story of Dr Jekyll and Mr Hyde tells of the split between persona and shadow. However, the shadow also contains the energy and vitality of the person. An inhibition of the shadow can lead to a shallow and bland life.

Jung suggested that the shadow related to the more instinctual qualities of the mind. There seems to have been some tendency for the concept of the shadow to overlap Freud's idea of id function. But a simple equation of shadow with id is incorrect. Jung (1940, p.20) suggested that the shadow consisted of "the inferior or less commendable part of the person". Looked at in cognitive terms, the shadow reflects those attributes of self which are "judged to be", by individuals themselves, less commendable or inferior. Since such judgements are usually culturally determined, it is not surprising that shadow qualities are often considered more primitive and immoral. However, while this may be true, it is also the case that qualities of shadow are negative attributes based on the "person's own judgement" of good and bad. Thus, for a man with a strong male persona, qualities of self which are seen as weak, tender, or sentimental may take on shadow function. Thus the strong male seeks to repress those attributes of self which he judges to be bad, overly emotional, useless, or weak. As Jung (1940) says, the anima and shadow may become largely identical. In Leary's (1957) theory the shadow may be the realm of the "not me".

The Anima/Animus. The anima (female characteristics of the male) and the animus (male characteristics of the female) relate to the predisposition to be capable of behaviours typical of the opposite gender. Hence men, via the mobilisation of their anima, would be capable of nurturing and compassionate behaviour, and women, via the mobilisation of the animus, would be capable of competitive and dominant behaviour. In fact Jung used these terms in two different ways. The first as described above, the second referred to the ideal images that individuals have of the opposite sex (i.e., the characteristics of one's ideal man or woman). This latter usage may fit with the findings that suggest there are indeed innate aspects to mate selection (Buss, 1989).

The idea that each personality has both a feminine and a masculine aspect is an old idea and can be found in various religious teachings especially Hinduism. These archetypes are nurtured by the parent, giving rise in the child to the internal representations of male and female. Problems in relating to the opposite sex arise from distortion of the anima and animus. A patient married a rather introvert lady and treated her as a subordinate when under stress. Although, consciously, he recognised her strengths and limitations he couldn't help blaming her for some of his problems. The relationship between his parents had been the same. His father was autocratic and the patient had craved a strong mother who could defend him from his father's put-downs. This "disappointment in the feminine" was played out again in his marriage. On the other hand women that displayed more masculine traits of initiative and competitiveness he found a "turn off" and rather threatening.

In some depressions there is an idealising of some fantasy partner—the desirable, all loving, sexually active, male or female. When ideals are not met the patient may become depressed. In Jungian therapy these would be seen as anima and animus projections. One patient would fall madly in love with a woman, live with her for a while only to become disappointed, feel trapped, seek out another, and repeat the cycle. Rejection by an idealised sexual partner is a more common trigger for depression than recognised and I have seen a couple of bipolar men in whom sexual rejection seemed to be a major triggering event.

The Ego. To Jung the ego belongs to the conscious mind. It appears similar to Freud's notion of the ego (Hall & Nordby, 1973), although others disagree (Samuels, 1985). The ego acts as the foci/screen for conscious experience. Hence the ego is concerned with things like self-awareness. In Chapter 12 we will see that various theories of depression stress the importance of the ego and therefore we will give less space to it here. (For a further discussion see Samuels, 1985.)

The Self. The ego and the self are quite separate concepts in Jung's psychology. The self represents a special kind of archetype, one that is responsible for integrating the personality and bringing elements together. Here Jung has the idea of a recipe model as opposed to a lego model of development (see Chapters 4 and 8 for a discussion of these two models of development). The self, in Jung's theory, is the totality of the personality, and the type of self one becomes depends on how the other archetypal functions are blended together. In this sense it is similar to Kohut's notion of a need for cohesiveness. Jung also argued, however, that the psyche was made up of opposites and that maturation of the self came from integrating and resolving (to a degree at least) opposites (e.g., love–hate, controlling others versus enabling them, distance–closeness).

Hence, as a number of theorists have noted, Jung's concept of fragmentation and being split up (Greenberg, 1979; Gilbert, 1989), or if you like unblended, is a major component of his theory of both wholeness and psychopathology. Indeed, most personality theorists agree that a personality contains elements and opposites that may come into conflict with each other. For various reasons the components of the system may grate together and cause unpleasant reactions. Usually this is because one archetype inhibits another and interferes with integration. To put it another way, our internal polices (Ornstein, 1986) or innate social strategies (Wenegrat, 1984) may conflict. It has not gone unnoticed that Jung's ideas emerge again in Kohut (Samuels, 1985; Jacoby, 1989). Horowitz and Zilberg (1983) take an almost identical view but do not acknowledge Jung. Cognitive therapists work with the attitudinal level and while they are well aware of the role of conflicts of beliefs, illogicalities, and inconsistencies, they have no views on the integration of a personality and tend to treat cognitions and attitudes in a piecemeal fashion.

Overview

This approach to psychopathology is now quite diverse with different schools within Jungian psychology having grown up. Also there is a move towards integration of ideas with other theories. The interested reader is referred to Stevens (1982) and Samuels (1985) for more detailed exposition.

There are also many other archetypal forms such as the great mother, the saviour, the martyr, the trickster, the wise old man, and so on. The writer Hermann Hesse, a friend of Jung, felt that Jung was not actually saying anything that had not been known (at least intuitively) to good storytellers over the ages—namely that most of the archetypes Jung depicted were clearly visible in the crafting of plot and relationships of the novel. Like authors, Jung believed that each archetype had a positive and a negative pole. That is, it could function positively and creatively in a system of social relationships or it could function negatively and be destructive. Hence the hero archetype, for example, functioning positively facilitates growth and development and is ultimately helpful to self and others. When this archetype functions negatively (attached to the shadow), we may end up with a Hitler figure whose need to be a hero and be recognised causes intense destruction. The hero ideal may also cause suffering in that it sets too high standards and floods the psyche with desires of ultimate success, the situation of the narcissistic personality who, in a sense, is set on being a hero to others, outstanding and special in some way. Often patients have identified with a hero ideal or an over-idealized perfect image for so long that with its departure they find themselves unsure of their real self and frightened in case parts of them are less than acceptable. This archetypal theme appears in many theories of depression.

A conflict between archetypes can also be a source of depression. As individuals begin to realise that their persona act is false and life is meaningless, they are forced to acknowledge all those aspects of themselves which have been hidden by their mask. They may become aware that there is aggression behind their mask, which they have hidden both from themselves and others. Thus shadow–persona conflict can exist within many depressive disturbances. Also, as for the existentialists (Yalom, 1980), there may come a time in life when a person looks back with regret and becomes aware of all the unlived possibilities and missed opportunities. This also can be a source of depression. A fifty-year-old man with moderate chronic depression came to therapy complaining that his life was unfulfilled. He had had to give up a degree course early in his life because of the health of his mother.

He had had the opportunity to go and finish the degree but for various reasons did not do so. The hero in him had died and he refused point blank to take risks or see that there was anything he could do to help himself. In a way his life of regret and having missed out was such a key part of his self-definition and self-organisation that he was extremely resistant to intervention. Anything that brought him in touch with anger was met with bland denial.

Jung in Retrospect

Jung's notion of psychic energy can be criticised in much the same manner as Freud's concept of energy. He had little idea how such energy might operate in the central nervous system. His tendency to work and write "at breakneck speed" and his rather free association of ideas, overlaid with religious connotations, resulted in much that was oddly written and obscure. This has probably done much to confuse issues. When synthesising his ideas he could write with clarity (Jung, 1933/1984). In some ways Jung (1984, p.21) followed a cognitive approach, stressing the importance of a person's attitude(s) to life and to internal experience:

> The unconscious itself does not harbour explosive materials, but it may become explosive owing to the repressions exercised by a self-sufficient, or cowardly, conscious outlook. All the more reason, then, for giving heed to that side! It should now be clear why I have made it a practical rule always to ask, before trying to interpret a dream: What conscious attitude does it compensate?

Although, like others, Jung believed that early childhood played an enormous role in psychopathology, a major distinction between Jung and other psychoanalysts was his view that neurosis could be produced in the present, not the past (Storr, 1973). A life event may cause a disturbance in functioning of the collective unconscious. The event calls on the individual to access some part of their nature they may not be prepared for (war is a typical, although extreme example). In therapy, a major concern was to keep the patient in touch with reality by focusing on the here and now and to focus on the challenges that the person should attempt to meet. These challenges might be dealing with various events or coming to terms with their inner life, the shadow, the hero, and so forth. Jung was among the first to outline how personality types influence the form and nature of the individual's neurosis. His view that different personality types had different biological make-ups has been proved by Eysenck and others.

Jung was also responsible for the idea of the life process (Staude, 1981; Stevens, 1982) and for noting that many depressions commence later in life. In his spiritual approach he was in total opposition to Freud. But this concern was mostly with the nature of individuation, or what Maslow called self-realisation. On the idea of God Jung certainly believed there was an archetype for a God, an innate tendency to create Gods, worship them and so on but whether any God actually exists outside of ourselves, this he regarded as unanswerable.

We should note that the biggest criticism of Jung came from his studies in alchemy but again it is easy to misunderstand what attracted to him to this. Basically it is the issue of transformation: the phoenix from the ashes. Jung was concerned with the means and symbols of transformation, how it is that individuals change and seem to blend different archetypes together. Like others he was concerned with the idea of containment (symbolised as the alchemist's crucible) that held forces in check while transformation went on. This idea is to appear again in Winnicot's notion of the "holding environment", Kegan's (1982) notion of the supporting environment and Kohut's (1977) soothing selfobject relationship. All these ideas have in common the idea of some kind of protection being given while an individual is growing, developing and new possibilities are being worked out in the psyche.

For many reasons Jung has been an easy target for the scientific community, with his writing style and occasional flight of ideas. Yet, with today's recognition of our human Multimind (Ornstein, 1986) and the importance of innate social algorithms, was he really so far out? Personality theory too is being given a kind of archetypal treatment with ideas of basic traits such as dominance, sociability, nurturance, and so forth (Buss, 1988; MacDonald, 1988). And is not self-deception vaguely reminiscent of shadow? So we may like to divide and label the constituent elements of the psyche in different ways, but Jung recognised this would happen. The key point however is the returning and returning again to some concept of an inner archetypal life as prepared and laid down in our gene-neural structures and the transformation, development, and inhibition of these inner aspects via experience.

BIOSOCIAL GOALS AND MENTALITY THEORY

Mentality theory is derived from the idea that we are biologically predisposed to seek certain goals and play certain roles. It shares with archetype theory the idea that there exists in the mind, underlying dispositions for human social behaviour.[1] Another way of considering this aspect is via the study of human traits (Buss, 1988; MacDonald,

1988). These have been important for social success over the long term (Gilbert, 1989, and Chapter 5 this volume). In other words animals that followed certain types of biosocial goal increased their reproductive fitness. For example, eliciting care from parents and caring for offspring increased reproductive success under K-selective conditions. Consequently, over time animals became motivated to elicit care when young and provide care when a parent. Also, if forming groups, cooperating with others, and seeking alliances carried reproductive advantage, then these will have become established as basic biosocial goals and become laid down in gene-neural structures.

Mentalities are the psychological apparatus necessary to pursue goals. Mentalities involve the co-assembly of motives, affects, behavioural repertoires, attention structures, and basic algorithms that enable us to pursue goals. Hence when pursuing a biosocial goal we attend to the environment in a certain way, look for certain kinds of stimuli, may plan out certain behaviours, feel good if the goal is reached, but experience negative affect if the goal is blocked or thwarted (Nesse, 1990). For example, when a child is hurt the biosocial goal of care eliciting is activated, and the mentality involves the arousal of affects to energise behaviour and accesses actions plans—e.g., crying and running indoors in search of mother. Specific stimuli (e.g., comfort from mother) which satisfies the goal, gradually calms activity in the mentality, or deactivates the psychological components of the goal-seeking system. The child feels better after a time, stops eliciting care and returns to playing in the garden. If, for example, on the other hand, a child repeatedly finds that there is no-one available when he/she is hurt, the care eliciting biosocial goal and associated mentality is inhibited. The goal or motive system and algorithms of care eliciting however cannot disappear since they are wired into gene-neural structures. Consequently, each time the child is hurt the mentality (affects and action plans) will be inhibited (e.g., the child hides away until he/she feels better). However, at times of stress this inhibition may break down, disinhibiting the mentality and allowing the biosocial goal to be activated. In these situations the person experiences the arousal of the mentality (the desire for comfort) but memory informs them that this is not available. Hence they also experience strong negative affect.

The basic assumptions of mentality theory are:

1. Core structures and predispositions for social intercourse are inherited. As such they are part of a human collective set of potentials for social behaviour and experience. They are also subject to genetic variation, but are shaped and integrated in a personality via social experience.

2. Biosocial goals (like personality traits) represent various orientations to social life (to seek care, to give care, to lead, etc). Hence *a biosocial goal is actualised via the enactment of a role(s).*
3. Mentalities represent the various co-assemblies of affects, action tendencies, cognitive styles (and innate social algorithms) that are necessary to pursue biosocial goals and to operate successfully in given roles. They provide for our inherent meaning-making abilities or competencies. At any point in time these co-assemblies will be patterned by conditioned responses, memory systems, internal self–other models, and so on.
4. Mentalities also act as signal detectors that allow the individual to track the environment and analysis information to see whether a role is being successfully enacted. For example, the crying of a child may activate (in the parent) the care-giving mentality, leading to a searching for the infant and a preparedness to comfort and soothe, or protect. The successful enactment of a role produces positive affect. Unsuccessful enactment produces negative affect.
5. Negative affect can then be seen as information that a goal has not been achieved or a role is not being enacted successfully, or is thwarted.
6. Like Jung's concept of the archetype, biosocial goals and mentalities represent no more than a potential and their exact articulation and their interaction with each other depends on both genetics and learning (experience).

Social mentalities help us orientate to role relationships in certain ways. At least five basic ways appear to exist, called: care eliciting, care giving, cooperating, competing, and gender (the latter was mentioned only in passing in Gilbert [1989]; it is a goal in so far as an individual is motivated to be like members of his/her own gender and form images, ideas, and attitudes about his/her own gender and the opposite gender). The core social mentalities reflect the characteristic ways an individual construes and experiences self in interaction. The self is seen in one position or role and the other in a complimentary position and role. A brief review of this system was given in Table 5.2, but is given again here to help exposition. In Table 11.1 SELF is shorthand for self as seen/experienced, and OTHER is shorthand for other as seen/experienced.

The pursuance of each goal/role is coordinated via the self-protective defense system or safety system (Gilbert, 1989; see Chapter 5). The defense system can be activated if a person(s) to whom a role is targeted

TABLE 11.1
Core Social Mentalities

	Self As	*Other As*
Care Eliciting	Needing inputs from other(s): care, protection, safety, reassurance.	Source of: care, nurturance, protection, safety, reassurance.
Care Giving	Provider of: care, protection, safety, nurturance.	Recipient of: care, protection, safety, nurturance.
Cooperation	Of value to other, sharing, appreciating, contributing, affiliative.	Valuing, contribution sharing, appreciating, contributing, affiliative.
Competition	Contestant, inferior–superior.	Contestant, inferior–superior.

does not respond as desired. For example, if someone initiates a suggestion in an effort to be cooperative and affiliative but others put them down, this will activate the defense system. (In Gray's 1982 model of the behavioural inhibition system, this would result from either signals of frustrative non-reward or punishment—see Chapter 6). The individual may switch to aggressive competing (if they think this will be successful) or back down (shut up), feel resentful, inhibited/controlled, and/or inferior. If on the other hand the signal back is appreciation (reward) of the suggestion then the safety system is maintained and the person continues to work/explore with others and think up other suggestions. Things are a little more complex (e.g., to a put-down, a person may inhibit themselves from offering further suggestions, may plan an even more major suggestion to ensure appreciation, or check on allies first, or plan a counter put-down revenge, and so forth). But the next time it comes to making a suggestion the person is more wary and aroused. In the extreme, we may have social anxiety (Trower & Gilbert, 1989; Gilbert & Trower, 1990).

To understand mentality theory it is necessary to link it with the concepts in Chapters 5–8—that is, many of our social roles are designed to elicit reassurance from others (hence maintaining low defensive arousal); to elicit investment from others, and/or to secure access or control over resources and positive reinforcers. Hence we can ask: (1) What kind of impression is a person trying to create in the minds of others? What are they trying to elicit from others? (2) What kinds of behaviours raise (or lower) their estimates of SAHP and self-worth? (3) What is the image they have of themselves?

PATTERNS AND DEPRESSIVE THEMES

So then, we have argued that there are various social mentalities that help structure our social experience and orientate us to the social world. However, each mentality has various options of strategies to achieve the biosocial goal being pursued. Also, different affective and conceptual patterns are associated with failure to achieve the goal. The novelist knows these different aspects of our inner mental life well and these are the repetitive themes noted in cultures throughout the world (the love relationship, self-sacrifice, deception, power, belonging, etc.). In ancient religions different Gods were seen as responsible for guiding the different themes of our personal lives. Hence for love one would pray to the love goddess, in war and for victory over enemies to Zeus, etc. Mythology is replete with the importance of understanding the basic themes of human life and this was why Jung was so attracted to it.

To aid understanding of how these different mentalities are organised and related to social success or lack of it, I have outlined some typical social interpersonal themes that are related to each mentality and biosocial goal. They are themes that are related primarily to depression, but here are just called themes, to avoid the cumbersome term, depressive themes. All of us have these potentials but in depression and other states of psychopathology they are often highly aroused, are associated with negative affect and are often sources of repetitive fantasies. Different themes may be in conflict with each other and produce response competition (Horowitz, 1988).

It is not sufficient, however, to note what the patient brings but also what they do not. What themes are missing, what is underdeveloped? Thus, as in Jungian theory and more recently cognitive theory (Beck et al., 1990), consideration is given to underdeveloped and overdeveloped aspects—and equally to expressed and unexpressed themes. It may be that it is not "needing" that is the problem but the inhibition of self-assertiveness and the trait of dominance (Buss, 1988). On the other hand, an individual may have functioned well until a certain stress (re)activates a more defensive way of relating. The self-organisation takes up a new (archetypal) pattern or theme as a way to elicit other peoples' investment or to protect self. Below we will talk of individuals, but this is shorthand for *individuals in whom these themes are (or have become) prominent.*

Care Eliciting

As suggested in Table 11.1, the care-eliciting mentality is focused on the need for others. The impression to be created in the minds of others is one of need, the desired elicited response is some aspect of care flowing from others and the internal self-image is of needing or needful.

The abandonment theme is represented in individuals who are preoccupied with being left/deserted and (as in a child) being unable to function alone. Small signals of rejection may trigger care-eliciting action tendencies (e.g., seeking reassurance, crying, and so forth). These individuals can become clinging and highly dependent, making excessive demands on the therapist and others. They may be prepared to put up with appalling relationships in order not to be alone. Separation anxieties are common. In Bowlby's theory (see Chapter 10) these may be anxious attachers. Depressive responses follow from a perception of loneliness, or following loss of significant relationships. This is a common theme in various theories of depression (e.g., Arieti & Bemporad, 1980a,b; Blatt et al., 1982; Beck, 1983).

The protection theme occurs when it is less aloneness and more danger that is the focus. They fear disaster may strike in the form of illness (e.g., hypochondriasis) or other events and require some dominant/wise other as a constant source of reassurance. They may also become over protective of others, e.g., of their children. A fifty-two-year-old man lost his father and within six months his best friend dropped dead. He developed severe hypochondriacal symptoms and major depression. He was convinced he had cancer and sought constant reassurance. Illness is also a way of signalling need for investment (protection) from others as well as signalling "out of action" and no-threat (i.e., "I am unable to enter the competitive arena of life"; but see Kellner, 1990).

The emptiness theme arises from feelings that no one can actually give to the self a sense of being okay. This theme is often associated with a history of emotional neglect and gives rise to the inner experience of the empty self, a self needing to be in a loving relationship before they can feel alive and "full". Sometimes physical touching and/or hugging are sought out. "Without love I'm nothing. I don't feel I exist without love." Sometimes these individuals can be fearful that there is nothing to them, that behind the "social face" or persona there is emptiness. A secondary fear arises therefore that "if others get to know me they will discover I am all hot air, boring and of no substance". This produces approach–avoidance conflict.

The victim theme arises in individuals who feel they have suffered more than most and, having suffered, attempt to elicit others' caring attentions and investments almost as a way to make up for past injuries. To portray oneself as a victim achieves two things: it is a cry for help and a signal that one is "no challenge" and out of the arenas of competitive life. However, victims can compete to be seen as the most needy and deserving; the most injured. The role of victim can also hide a sense of injustice and desires for revenge (see page 346). A problem is that to acknowledge help and give up this strategy/role carries the cost of losing later opportunities to elicit care and also the possibility of revenge (e.g., a patient may say, "My depression is living testament of how others treated me."). In the extreme these individuals may have no clear self-identity and removal of the sense of having been thwarted or harmed through life by others leaves them with a sense of emptiness. Sometimes they inhibit themselves from feeling happy in case others think that they are now okay. If their glumness is used to punish others then this can be difficult to change in therapy.

A patient had always been regarded as the unhappy one in the family. The family had a taboo on anger and the only way she could (as the youngest) express her displeasure with the way things were in the family was by "being glum and catastrophising". Gradually, in therapy she recognised how her self-identity was focused on the need to see herself as "hard done by", and how she used this to get at her husband and also to elicit attention. She knew it was irrational but found it difficult to change. At times she recognised that she would force herself not to show happiness, because she did not want to send this signal. Some therapists talk of this as the self-pitying theme.

Overview: In the above themes the biosocial goal of care eliciting is active (the patient feels needy) but it is felt to be threatened, blocked, thwarted or used maladaptively. The patient's orientation to the therapist may be one of "you must make me better, I can't do it". If the patient has had much disappointment in care-receiving relationships then as depression sets in, the self-image is one of needing, but the other is seen as deficient: "My needs are too great, I'm beyond rescue; I feel no-one can get in my head, you can't reach me, or no-one can help me." If anger is also aroused then the patient may say, "you could help me more, do more for me, give me more time, etc, but you refuse to do so"; or "you can't understand me; you are not able to help me or refuse to do so; you are bored with me". The therapist counter-transference can be guilt ("I'm not good enough or the patient's needs are overwhelming, a bottomless pit"), or anger ("how ungrateful, after all I've done for you, why don't you grow up you sod"). These kinds of reactions in others maintain a self-defeating cycle. At first people may try to get close, but then feel overwhelmed by a person's needs and withdraw. If the victim theme is strongly operative the therapist may get exasperated.

The compulsive self-reliance theme arises in individuals who are defensively avoidant of any need for care or recognition of need for others. Whereas the above types have highly amplified care-eliciting biosocial goals, these types keep this goal strictly inhibited. Sometimes these patients can be experienced as stealers in that they rarely acknowledge the help of others but may internalise it and claim it as their own. Here there is avoidance of the biosocial goal of care eliciting.

The burdener theme arises in people who are fearful of being cared for and is a subtle variant of self-reliance. A rather more common fear, that I personally share, is that of growing senile and being kept alive. If my brain wears out, I want out. In depression the fear of being a burden is common and, especially in the elderly, can signal a suicide risk. A mother felt that the only reason to live was to care for her children. A year earlier she had the idea that, because of her depression and irritability, her children would be better off in a home, and she overdosed. In therapy this theme can show up as a fear of being a nuisance. However, this sets up powerful conflicts because the person may actually feel quite needy.

Attachment theory has focused on the care-eliciting system and has described these themes in detail (e.g., Bowlby, 1980; Liotti, 1988; Safran & Segal, 1990; see Chapter 10 of this volume). However, in my view there are many other themes that are not directly related (at a phylogenetic level) to attachment. It may, none the less, be true that failure to form adequate early attachments can distort the maturation of other mentalities.

Care Giving

In care giving, attention is focused on the other and not directly on the self. The other is seen as needing something that the self should provide. The self-image is of being a good provider/helper, curer of souls and miseries, etc.

Fogel, Melson, and Mistry (1986) define nurturance as " the provision of guidance, protection and care for the purpose of fostering developmental change congruent with the expected potential for change of the object of nurturance." This not only requires a preparedness to respond to signals of need but also to evaluate and plan to satisfy the needs of others.

The theme of the nurturer derives a sense of worth from nurturing others. The role of nurturing is associated with a positive self-image and they may have problems when either others reject their nurturing or have no need for it. I had one patient who could only feel love for her children if they were sick or injured and she could look after them. As they grew up she became depressed feeling she had no role in life and life was empty. These kinds of depression can arise when children leave home and the role of parent is no longer active.

The theme of the rescuer arises in the individual whose self-worth is linked with the wish to save others, or to cure them, or in someway lead them out of difficulty. In its hero forms it can lead to efforts to take on major feats, or a vocation, or missionary zeal. In the extreme it can lead to over-controlling and feelings of guilt or anger when in spite of their best efforts people aren't saved, patients don't get better. Sometimes, if patients don't recover, they lose their interest for the rescuer-therapists. This is a common problem in training therapists, especially if their sense of worth is tied up with being a good rescuer/healer. Others would call this a narcissistic theme.

The theme of the martyr arises when an individual derives their sense of self-worth from caring for others, putting other people first. However, the martyr wants others to know how much they sacrifice for this, how special they are, how wonderful they are—like the parent who says to the child, "Look how much we have sacrificed for you; everything we did was for you—your education, etc." A parent may constantly inform their children what they have given up for them. In the extreme they can be tyrants and very controlling, giving others a sense of intrusiveness and expecting their gratitude/reciprocation. Jung's concept was related to that of the devouring mother. To feel good, these folk like others to be dependent on them and to see themselves in the needed role: "If I don't do it nobody else can or will." The efforts of others are often undermined in order to foster a certain dependency. The thing about martyrs is that they let others know (or tell themselves) how much they are giving up in order to be caring. "How on earth would people manage without me!"

There is another theme of the martyr that accords with more religious ideas of self-sacrifice and self-mutilation. For a fascinating discussion of this theme and its role in depression and suicide see Bradford (1990).

Caring guilt theme arises when, to put self first, the person feels guilty and inhibited. Guilt is a common motivator of caring (Eisenberg, 1986). The individual feels bad/selfish about themselves if they do not behave in a giving/nurturing way. This theme can arise in many contexts (e.g., caring for elderly parents, or staying in a poor marriage) and can lead to a sense of entrapment (see Chapter 8). Some novice therapists seem preoccupied with this theme. If their patients do not get better the therapist must work harder or is doing something wrong. To avoid guilt, low self-esteem, and feelings of letting others down, the patients must recover and prosper. Failing others is the common source of bad feelings and is often linked with moral judgements (Gilbert, 1989). Some analysts (e.g., Bowlby, 1980) argued that care-giving mentalities can be amplified in persons who have experienced their parents as demanding. The person puts aside their own needs in order to try to heal the parent. In consequence their own needs remain undeveloped and they obtain their sense of self-worth from giving rather than "being/living for oneself ". Often they are hoping to be *cared for* in return.

The protector theme arises in individuals who feel unduly responsible for others' protection. It can be associated with a certain kind of obessionalism. The early history often shows that a parent has turned to the child for protection. In one case, a patient as the oldest sibling, was given responsibility for her six siblings. Mother would often panic about where the children were and the patient had to go and find them. The patient was punished, if anything happened to her siblings, for not having looked after them properly. In adult life she had panic attacks whenever the phone rang, thinking it was bad news. She feared letting her own children grow up and explore in the world. If she enjoyed herself and forgot about her protection role, she believed that something bad was going to happen (various forms of magical thinking were also present; happy thoughts could lead to disaster). An obsessional toucher and checker had to look after her mother who was always threatening suicide. From an early age she developed various rituals to stop bad things happening. Later in life, she had to go through various rituals before her children went to bed. Behind both themes was a certain rage, which was also feared.

All these themes have in common a particular orientation to self–other relationships. Individuals can shift from one theme to another. For example, a person with a strong rescuer theme became angry and dysphoric and played the martyr role when others around him refused to acknowledge his talent and abilities. He required a certain kind of signal from others to support his sense of self-worth.

Cooperation

The themes of cooperation are on sharing, a sense of kinship, belonging, being like others, a member of a team or network; concern is with affiliation and being valued as an equal (Brown, 1986; Haviland, 1990). In Chapter 7 we put this as "feeling part of a network". Heard and Lake (1986, p.431) discuss this in terms of the companionable relationship.

> The goal of companionable relating is reached whenever an individual construes from the emotive messages sent by companions, that they are taking interest in and showing appreciation of his contribution and the way he his making it; and at the same time, realises that the interest he is taking in the contribution of his companions is also appreciated.

The cooperation mentality also enables individuals to make judgements about ingroup or outgroup membership. Hence, failures in cooperation can lead an individual to feel an outgroup member.

The theme of the outsider arises when an individual has not made a satisfactory adjustment to their peer group, or even society at large. They may become over reliant on family for friendship and something of a loner. These patients often express the themes of being different from others, an outsider looking in, standing on the sidelines. There are various sub-themes here—for example, the theme of having being left behind, or the themes of being inferior and passed by. These themes are not focused on a specific person but rather on a general sense of being different. In some cases, fear of being an outsider leads to ideas that others can control them in some way and they may become suspicious or paranoid. Often this is directed towards organisations (e.g., groups, the police, the mafia, etc.). For example, a patient lost her role on a local committee. Out of this role, she no longer felt part of the group and thought others where ganging up on her and might come to her house to steal things. Patients with basic mistrust nearly always have a general view of "them" rather than specific individuals, suggesting it is the ingroup–outgroup algorithm that is involved.

Sometimes, those with a strong sense of being outsiders may try to turn therapy into a companionable relationship as a subsitute for outside affiliative relationships and have problems of separation. Sometimes they are actually quite competitive (or dominance orientated, Buss, 1988) but too shame prone to compete or take on leadership roles. At other times they have difficulty valuing others and although they long for comradeship never find anyone good enough or "like them" to share with. These patients can have narcissistic problems although the feelings engendered in the therapist is of their loneliness. We have indicated in earlier parts of this book how this is often associated with depression. On the other hand some individuals enjoy being outsiders because it gives them a sense of individuality.

The theme of the insider arises in a person who is so concerned to belong to some group that they will be quite prepared to lose their individuality to the group. Drug addiction, particularly, is a problem when the person does not want (or feels unable) to move away from the group which provides their sense of self via identification with group values and rituals. It is common also in cults. In the group they identify with, they are highly conformist. The positive affects of belonging and security maintain their conformist behaviours and make withdrawing from (say) an addiction difficult. This is because it is not only the physical symptoms of withdrawal from the addiction that is diffcult but because without the habit and social rituals, they feel like aliens in the world, without a sense of belonging or social place. In cults, group leaders may activate primitive fears of outgroup members (common in religion). These individuals can suffer depression when the group no longer supports their sense of self-worth and belonging, or they become disillusioned; i.e., they begin to feel outsiders.

The theme of the rebel arises in individuals who wish to break free from group constraint and values. In some sense it is also a competitive theme, but the rebel may not be trying to gain status or rise in rank, at least not with those they are rebelling against. In some adolescents this theme is strongly aroused, but the main concern is individuality and breaking free, pushing against authority and non-conforming. In some families there can be a fight for the control over who decides how each will behave. Being forced to submit or comply can produce depression and sometimes a sense of failure/isolation. In some culture clashes, when children rebel against traditional values, much strife occurs. In this kind of depression the person tends to withdraw.

All of us like to think we are a little bit of a rebel. To be told that we are rather ordinary, conformist, and without any originality is not rewarding. If the rebel strategy or theme is strongly aroused, however, relationships may be fraught and the person may not come to feel part of a group—hence leading again to a sense of being an outsider and alone. Sometimes an individual may rebel against one set of standards in order to be accepted by another group. For example, a patient told me that she was very rebellious and cheeky at school, but this was in order to win peer approval. She now deeply regrets not having taken the opportunity to learn. Also, previous rebellions may later lead to depression and self-blame. A patient had had a very difficult relationship with her mother and had been rebellious. When she was twenty-two and was just beginning to develop a strong positive relationship with mother, mother died of a heart attack. The patient was full of self-recriminations for not "having grown up sooner", having given her mother a hard time and that her early rebelliousness may even have contributed to her mother's death.

The theme of the moralist arises in people who are preoccupied with equal give and take (defined by them) and the moral virtues. They have very clear ideas of how others should behave and often complain of others' injustice or selfishness, and how others are morally weak or take advantage. The moralist often has narcissistic problems and can be rigid and unforgiving. In their language they talk often about fairness and lack of reciprocation. Their sense of self-worth derives from living up to their strict moral codes. These types are common in certain autocratic religions. I tend to find them rather joyless, lacking in warmth and bogged down. This may say more about me than them however.

There is also the theme of the immoralist arising in those who are exploitative of others and blatantly engage in self-interest, and are cheaters. On the other hand we can sometimes behave immorally because of wanting to belong (insider theme) and we turn immoral behaviour (group violence) into an appeal to virtue (e.g., to defend our interests, cleanse the system, etc.). If we have serious doubts about our behaviour and recognise it as an act of cowardice, then depression might follow ("How could I have done that?"). Coping with the demands of war may be one such situation. A person had to sack half his work force and his own job was on the line. He complied to avoid loss of his job but suffered internal guilt and deep resentment as a consequence.

Competition

The competitive/ranking mentality is focused on there being a winner and loser, a one up and a one down, and an acute awareness of where one is in the rank. The competitive mentality has a number of strategies: (1) straight aggression; (2) seeking to gain some advantage, to be special or excel in some attribute; (3) taking the initiative and attempting to lead, or (4) their opposites, submitting. The competitive mentality alerts the individual to the ranking implications of all other roles. The competitive themes are concerned with exerting social control over others or having to submit.

The aggressor theme arises in individuals who are focused on their needs for power via strength and aggression, to avoid the one down position and maintain a sense of superiority over others. Some Type As fit this pattern as do some psychopaths. Under threat, their first response is counter-aggression (Gilbert, 1989). When they become depressed there is often a history of conflicts which they have lost. Their aggression can be blatant or more subtle and autocratic with threats of withdrawal of support and expulsion from the relationship. Hence their basic tactics of social control are threats of one form or another. One patient told me, "I don't really care what people think about me as long as they respect me and know not to fuck with me." This theme is (unfortunately) all too common in many films nowadays.

The theme of the avenger arises in people who feel they have been wronged in some way and are preoccupied with turning the tables and seeking revenge. This can work at both a personal and cultural level. The self-organisation is orientated around a sense of having been harmed and put down which mobilises efforts to avenge. A motto is: "They must not be allowed to get away with it". At times these individuals may bear grudges for long periods and snipe at others and they can live in a world of secret resentments. This theme is sometimes associated with the victim theme. It relates to competitiveness and rank since these themes are often associated with having been humiliated and desires for power over others. Sometimes people only engage in fantasies and ruminations of sadistic themes of revenge ("I know what I would like to do to them"). My experience of these individuals is that they can be difficult to engage, are often withdrawn when depressed and can feel prickly. For others, when a good relationship exists an outpouring of desires for revenge emerges. Sometimes people are attracted to certain types of work from their own sense of moral outrage and desires for revenge.

Sometimes a need for revenge protects against a depression, but having to recognise that maybe people will "get away with it", and that one is helpless, can lead to depression. When this theme of helplessness arises depression is more likely (see Chapter 8 for a discussion of shame and envy). Sometimes these feelings remain hidden in depression and a person doubts their right to feel vengeful. Self-blame may protect from vengeful feelings towards others. One is reminded of Nietzsche's claim that no one will accuse themselves without a secret wish for vengeance (see Chapter 9). In many modern approaches to depression this theme is woefully neglected.

The theme of inhibiting others arises in individuals who wish to control others primarily to stop others controlling them. They may take on a role or aspire to high status, but if they get there they do not have any clear plan of what they want to do, partly because they are not motivated to pursue some vision. This is also a bureaucratic style. These individuals tend to see the world in a fragmented way. They tend to take on tasks in a piecemeal fashion and are not very explorative or creative and lack overall vision. They are preoccupied with where the next attack might come from, and are very rank sensitive. Thus they are very stress prone. These individuals often have histories of being dominated in childhood by parents and/or siblings. Passive aggressive aspects can be present.

The theme of the special arises from heroic-type concerns to be special or outstanding in some way. Ideals are less in exerting control via aggression and power and more of eliciting it from positive attention from others. The desired response is admiration (rather than appreciation). This is classic narcissistic behaviour described so well by Yalom (1980). If they achieve status they expect others to be beholden to them, they feel superior and entitled. These individuals are well represented in professions like law and medicine. The person may have sought out these professions precisely because of the admiring attentions of others. These individuals can become depressed if they "fall from grace" or others block them. Sometimes under threat they take up the aggressor theme.

There are of course many ways in which we like to feel special. For example, we may feel more caring than others, more intelligent, a special kind of therapist, etc. Self-esteem can be dealt a blow when we discover that maybe we are not so special but rather ordinary, experience affects or thoughts that show us that our sense of specialness has been invalidated.

The theme of excessive standards arises in individuals who seem never satisfied with their achievements, but always want to go "higher" or further. They can be preoccupied with possible attacks from others if performance is not faultless. Their obsessional traits do not endear them to others. This theme is well described by Blatt et al. (1982) as the self-critical types. It bears on the competitive mentality, because the evaluation that flows in the wake of failure is inferiority. This can also lead to the "driven personality".

The theme of the subordinate arises in individuals who feel easily overwhelmed by others. They see the social world primarily in terms of rank (others are stronger or more able) and their way of coping is with submissive behaviour. They may need much reassurance before they feel safe with others. They can be unassuming characters and are highly represented in avoidant personality disorder, who in turn are highly represented in hospitalised depressives (Pilkonis & Frank, 1988).

If the theme of revenge is associated with the theme of the subordinate then we have elements of passive aggressive personality. Jung pointed out that the highly ordinary, conforming, bland individual can in fact become a tyrant if put into a role, as noted in Hitler's regime. Also, in the extreme, those that often commit the worse crimes of violence have premorbid personalities that are highly submissive and withdrawn. Their fantasy life can be rich in themes of power over others. Obviously, this only applies to a minority. Equally, such individuals can become self-sacrificing heroes in certain contexts (e.g., war). As Leary (1957) pointed out, the subordinate/submissive positions may be docile or hostile.

The defeated theme arises in most depressed individuals in one form or another. It can be expressed as running out of steam, being at the end of one's tether, at the end of the road, finished. In this there is the expression of coming to an end in someway and having no energy left to struggle. Another variant is of being beaten or pushed down, overwhelmed, things piling in on one. The image is of some weight or force bearing down from above. Another theme is that of entrapment, being caught in a black hole or pit. This image can be associated with feeling that the sides of the pit are smooth and one can't get a grip. However it is expressed, it conveys the sense of lacking the resources or energy to change, or that demands (which may be internally or externally generated) exceed resources (e.g., see Hobfoll, 1989). This is often linked with the experience of hopelessness and anxiety. In Kohut's

(1977) terms, it can relate to the experience of fragmentation, loss of vigour and self-cohesion. Shame may be part of the experience.

Using Socratic questioning (see Chapter 13) the focus of these defeat themes can be ascertained. It may be in interpersonal relationships—others making excessive demands, or treating one as subordinate, or in feeling that one's group does not accept one (e.g., a professor had worked for a year on a project, but at the first conference presentation his ideas were slated and rejected). It can relate to some reversal of rank. Or it can relate to not being able to reach goals/ standards or enact roles that have been the focus of a sense of self-worth and meaning. The defeated theme is almost always associated with other themes (e.g., outsider, or empty self theme).

Gender

The gender mentalities relate to the themes of belonging to a particular gender. How we perceive ourselves as an example of our gender can have a major influence on feelings of self-worth. Cultural stereotyping plays on this fact. While we may chose one set of gender-typic values over another the fact of our gender means that we have to make some kind of identification: "I want to be this kind of man or woman". When we make social comparisons we often have in mind our own gender. If you ask people, "Who would you most like to be like?" they usually pick someone of their own gender, even though the attributes they may wish to have are not particularly gender related, e.g., intelligence, artistic talent, etc. Dysfunctional themes to gender often relate to early life, feeling that parents wanted self to be of the opposite gender (as depicted in the film *On Golden Pond*). Many of these themes are discussed elsewhere (Gilbert, 1989). However, it sometimes arises in therapy that attitudes and feelings about gender are important. Gender themes also relate to internal images of sexual partners.

Overview

The above themes, about when people are depressed, are no more than rule of thumb guides for how the basic mentalities are operating. They are derived from the theory of biosocial goals (Gilbert, 1989) and clinical experience. Themes may be viewed as "sort of" tactics for the elicitation of others' investment, or efforts to promote self in some way, (see Chapters 6 and 7). Table 11.2 offers and overview of concepts discussed.

I am sure the reader can think of other themes, such as the theme of being unlovable or inwardly bad (we met shame and envy in Chapter 8) or that others are basically bad. There are also themes of the magical

TABLE 11.2
Relationship between Mentalities and Themes

				MENTALITY			
Care Eliciting		Care Giving		Cooperating		Competing	
Self	*Other*	*Self*	*Other*	*Self*	*Other*	*Self*	*Other*
Need	Provider	Provider	Need	Share	Share	Winner	Loser
				Exchange			
				BASIC DEPRESSIVE THEMES			
abandonment		nurturer		outsider		aggressor	
protection		rescuer		insider		avenger	
emptiness		martyr		rebel		inhibitor	
victim		guilt		moralist		special	
compulsive self-reliance		protector		immoralist		excessive standards	
burdener						subordinate	
						defeated	
				shame		shame	
				envy		envy	

rebirth: "I always hoped someone would wave a wand, or find a drug that would change/cure me." There may be idealised images of what the person would be like (or do) if they were well. Failure to achieve the ideals ignites self-downing. Also there are the themes of shame, guilt, and envy which we have explored in Chapter 8.

This chapter has focused mainly on depression themes of self–other interactions. Although these ideas may seem new, actually they are not. Nearly all theories of psychotherapy speak in terms of patterns of adjustment (Leary, 1957; see Appendix B). Gardner (1988) has classified a number of evolved forms of social communications serving various roles (e.g., dominance and nurturance, ingroup–outgroup). Personality theorists speak in terms of underlying traits (Buss 1988; Ewen, 1988). In this sense all of us are searching after the same basic concerns and hopefully research will help us iron out fundamental errors.

However, we should stress that at this time, these are but the crudest of approximations. They may be useful to the therapist who is interested in a social and evolutionary approach to psychopathology, but I emphasise that there is nothing concrete about these themes and each individual will manifest depressive themes in slightly different ways, and the same is true for personality traits. Most patients have various complex mixtures of different themes and these can change from session to session and even within a session. Often they may conflict. Thus we could also regard them as types of interpersonal problems. New themes crop up as therapy progresses. Some themes are up front and others are not. Safran and Segal (1990) talk about meta-cognition and meta-communication. For example, while a patient was talking of his need to protect others he became more animated and his nonverbal behaviour was aggressive. Directing his attention to his nonverbal behaviour brought his focus to unrecognised anger at having to carry this responsibility (now and in the past) and this linked with his anxiety. A patient may express one theme verbally, but another nonverbally. By understanding people in terms of "moving patterns" we are helped to engage this complexity.

We have also noted that many of these themes are related to the problem of narcissism. However, mentality theory suggests that narcissism is a broad concept which misses important differences between people, especially on the specific roles that carry the potential for narcissistic injury and sense of self-worth. Very narcissistic individuals can be friendly or aggressive, active or shame prone and inhibited. Most depressions are associated with some kind of narcissistic injury, hence, a more detailed exploration of themes is needed.

In some sense we expect, scan for, seek out or try to elicit a particular response from the environment according to which biosocial goal is active. Hence mentalities are complex co-assemblies of cognition, affect, and behaviour. They are ways of conceptualising, feeling about, and behaving towards self and to others. They provide a bedrock for that illusive of all qualities, experiencing. When we go to see a Shakespearean play or other art forms, we are interested in becoming part of the interaction of different themes.

I am not, however, saying that all is innate but, rather like Jung, I am talking in terms of potential for meaning, a potential that is articulated by life events. All of us (mostly) have these archetypal themes in our personality and they are not in themselves pathogenic. It is their pattern of organisation or extremity which may be dysfunctional. It is, as Paulhus and Martin (1987) suggest, a balanced self that is able, according to context, to play out a number of these themes (see concluding comments).

We should also note that we have tended to pick on the more negative pole of each theme but, as in archetype theory, they can have positive functions also, which we have not the space to discuss here (but see Gilbert, 1989). Perhaps the novelist understands the issue of 'patterns of themes' better than the psychologist. Unlike the psychologist the novelist must take us through time, point up relationships and how they change via their ongoing interactional forms. The novelist must also hold our attention by resonating something within us. Although not much of this would be new to the novelist we are a long way from systematic research on these themes and how the themes influence the expression of the depression.

Mentality Theory and Depression

Any of the themes we have discussed may have ranking or network (social success) implications. I may feel inferior because nobody seems to care for me or take much interest in me, they care for others, but not me; I may feel inferior as a care-giver, because I don't have the same wonderful relations with my children that the books say I should, or if they leave home, I have no other role that gives me a sense of purpose and self-worth; I may feel inferior because I don't seem to get the therapeutic results that others get; I may feel inferior because I have always felt an outsider and never accepted by a group, and so forth. Whether or not I will get depressed depends on how much this is a basic goal, a basic way I evaluate self-worth. If our themes are associated with lack of social success (e.g., SAHP) then depression is more likely.

Changing

Helping patients change with this approach involves understanding their basic themes and why they enact them. It follows a cognitve behavioural orientation but is constructivist rather than rationalist (Mahoney & Gabriel, 1987). Unlike the rationalist cognitive approach, theme work focuses on self-organisation and the difficulty that some individuals may have in coming to new self-organisations and developing new themes that can be enacted in the world. Outside of the therapy one is interested in how the patient begins to enact new themes and their cognitive and affective experience of these enactments. Thus behavioural aspects (exposure and skill development) are important. Unlike the behavioural approaches, this approach recognises the role of the loss of ideals and a sense of self-definition that may go with change. Hence therapy becomes more of a journey which follows stages (Katakis, 1989) and in this sense is in tune with Jungian ideas.

SUMMARY

1. Jung introduced the idea that the human mind contains various archetypal potentials or possibilities and that these unfold over the life cycle.
2. Depression could have many sources, but the central idea was the person was in some way blocked from progressing in life. He spoke in terms of transformation as a process by which internal archetypes blended together. The therapist should help the person remain in contact with their self-organisation without fragmenting. Therapy concerns this transformation.

3. Today we are perhaps less aware of archetype theory or feel it is too mystical and unscientific. Nevertheless, in all kinds of areas, and especially with regard to personality, we are beginning to recognise that there are basic traits for sociability, nurturance, attachment, self-deception, altruism, cooperation, dominance, and so on. These traits have a powerful influence on how a person engages life and what their basic incentives, plans, aspirations, and fantasies will be about. Consequently, they will influence the expression of depression.
4. Mentality theory is a kind of bridge between archetype theory and personality theory. It offers a classification of basic internal mechanisms for understanding special types of interaction between self and others. These are care eliciting, care giving (evolved probably from attachment), cooperating, and competing.
5. Social themes are the types of self–other relationships that are part of our meaning-making experience. Each mentality has a variety of possible themes.

CONCLUDING COMMENTS

In 1988, at the World Conference in Cognitive Therapy at Oxford, I attended a workshop by Jeffery Young in cognitive schema therapy (Young, 1988). To my surprise I found a very similar set of ideas to those of mentality theory (which I had been working with for some years). These were called basic schema. Schema for abandonment, mistrust, entitlement, guilt, and so on were presented. These schema are seen as basic unconditional beliefs. This is all very exciting work. However I am aware that my ideas have been built up from others and are not that original. Moreover, I prefer to work with evolutionary theory and try to think in terms of underlying social algorithms, or archetypal mechanisms. Mentality theory does not focus purely on the cognitive domain but tries to get at the idea of co-assembled patterns of appraisal, conceptualisation, feelings, and behaviour. Themes are ways of being in the world—acting in it and trying to elicit certain responses from it, often some kind of investment from others, to exert personal power or stay out of action if these two options aren't working. As argued before (Chapters 8 and 16) I prefer the view of self-organisation in terms of patterns rather than those of the more lego model of schema.

One further big difference is that I tend to follow Jung and Kohut and think in terms of how these are put together to avoid self-fragmentation. Schema therapy has no clear notion of fragmentation of the self or the loss of coherence. But if our new theories of mind are correct (e.g.,

Ornstein, 1986; see Chapter 5 this volume) that we are made up of different modular processing systems, algorithms and the like, then clearly a sense of internal cohesion is important. For example, Horowitz and Zilberg (1983) talk in terms of regressive alterations of the self and states of mind. This kind of understanding is absent from many schema theories. Mentality theory also considers the teleological issue of how individuation grows from within (Mahoney & Gabriel, 1987). This developmental aspect is more noted in work on personality disorder (Beck, et al., 1990). Themes are emergent patterns that tend, on average, to take a special form but with much individual variation and blending. This brings us back again to the issue of transformation. Very few theories have offered us much insight into this aspect of psychological functioning though it is implicit in many developmental theories (Gilbert, 1989).

It is rare indeed that one will find only one type of theme to be addressed in depression. As suggested elsewhere (Gilbert, 1989), our attention is directed to the pattern. I am really unsure how working on one of them (e.g., to increase assertive behaviour) does, as a consequence, sometimes lead to a more friendly personality or a more competitive personality. Why do certain powerful experiences sometimes lead to an apparently complete transformation of a person? In common language we say, "I was changed by that experience", or "that experience had a deep effect on me", but we are not here saying that a single theme or schema has changed. We feel that the very "I" has changed—that is our inner pattern.

A man who recently loss his job got depressed and came for therapy. After a year he was not only better but was spending more time with his family. When he looked back he thought that over the years his job had "slowly devoured him". He could not fully understand how it had happened. My question is: how was it that the therapy (possibly) or the experience of the depression made him a different father and changed a whole set of values, incentives, and goals that were not the focus of the therapy? Therapy sometimes brings about a complete transformation of values and incentives. I do not think we really understand how these emergent patterns can be (sometimes) so radically altered. We are too busy dividing up the system into schema, conditioned responses, or whatever and then forget to put it back together again.

NOTES

1. As A'level students in a technical college we had the choice of doing various subsidiary subjects called (in those latter days of the sixties) liberal studies.

I signed up for psychology. For reasons now forgotten the tutor turned it into a year's course on the influence of Jung and others on contemporary society. The tutor fitted my personality with his keenness and passion and within a couple of months I was activated and never missed a lecture. Hence, unlike many students today, I came to psychology with various preconceived ideas about our internal innate structures and how these themes were played out in our everyday relationships and various cultures. I was surprised to find how little impact Jung had had on academic psychology and I guess a motivating influence has been to bring the concept of archetypes into a more scientific form.

CHAPTER 12

Aspirations, Incentives, and Hopelessness

In the preceding three chapters we explored depression with theories that have some basic overview of human psychic life. All of them (except Kohut) are based strongly in evolution theory of one form or another. In the next three chapters we explore theories that have moved away from or ignored questions of evolutionary heritage, basic human dispositions, and social needs. In my view something is lost in this avoidance of our "basic nature". We lose a certain richness and complexity in understanding the basic biological infrastructure of human life. We also lose the issue of integration of the personality and the concepts of internal teleological transformation. Nevertheless, as we shall see we can greatly advance our understanding of depression by placing issues of human nature in the background. The theories reviewed in the next three chapters articulate different aspects of the processes of depression not necessarily alternative ones to those expressed previously. I will let the reader judge for themselves whether they are easily integrated with our evolutionary theories or not.

EGO ANALYTIC

Ego analytic theories arose from the work of Alfred Adler (1870–1937). Some, like Karen Horney (1885–1952), working in the 1930s and 1940s were influenced by the existential theorists (see Ewen, 1988). Others like Bibring (1953) worked closely within the psychoanalytic tradition and were influenced by people like Rado and Jacobson. It was probably Bibring, however, who with his classic 1953 paper, set the stage for a new conceptualisation of depression that would lead to the cognitive approach.

Like so many breakaways from Freudian orthodoxy, Bibring rejected the notion of conflict of drives and gave scant regard to Freud's theory of personality development. He abandoned energy concepts, instincts, and inherited psychobiological response patterns. He stressed instead the importance of ego states and ego ideals. Freud recognised ego ideals but did not see them as central to depression. In Bibring's conceptualisation, depression exists as one ego state with three others, which he considered to be:

1. The state of balanced narcissism (normal self-esteem).
2. The state of excited or exhilarated self-esteem, the triumphant or elated ego.
3. The state of threatened narcissism, the anxious ego.
4. The state of broken-down self-regard, the inhibited or paralysed, the depressed ego.

This latter ego state was seen as the mechanism for depression.

In today's terms, Bibring's approach is one which emphasises social learning and the perception of personal control, that is, the ego's ability to control the pursuit and securing of individually acquired aspirations. When these aspirations are perceived to be beyond the person's best efforts, a sense of helplessness and depression results. Thus depression is conceived of as an ego state, that is, the ego becomes chronically aware of its inability to live up to its own internalised aspirations or standards. Bibring suggested that it was partly the nature of these aspirations that made them unobtainable. Horney, and later Beck (1976), also placed emphasis on the individual who attempts to strive for aspirations which are absolute and in reality unobtainable. Bibring (1953) suggested three types of aspirations which the (pre)depressive may seek:

1. The wish to be worthy and loved, and to avoid inferiority and unworthiness.
2. The wish to be strong, superior, secure, and to avoid being weak and insecure.
3. The wish to be loving and good and not aggressive, hateful, or destructive.

We see aspects of archetype and mentality theory here in the sense that these are believed to be more or less universal. In the latter case,

Bibring suggests that the awareness of internal aggressive impulses deals a blow to self-esteem. This is a kind of shadow–persona conflict. Bibring (1953, pp.25–26) suggests:

> depression is primarily not determined by a conflict between the ego on the one hand and the id, or the super-ego, or environment on the other hand, but stems primarily from a tension within the ego itself, from an inner-systemic "conflict." Thus depression can be defined as the emotional correlate of a partial or complete collapse of the self-esteem of the ego, since it feels unable to live up to its aspirations (ego ideal, super-ego) while they are strongly maintained.

Becker (1979, p.324) points out that vulnerability to depression, according to this model, has a number of causes. These include: "constitutional intolerance of persistent frustration, severe and prolonged helplessness, and developmental deficiencies in skill acquisition. These deficiencies are enhanced by the ego ideals which tend to be high and rigidly adhered to by depressives."

Bibring opened the door to the exploration of how beliefs and attitudes, incentives, aspirations, and goals are the key elements in the origin of psychopathology. The mode of transmission, from parent to child, group to group, or individual to individual, was subject to speculation and research. Within this atmosphere Cohen, Baker, Cohen, Fromm-Reichman, and Weigert (1954) suggested that high achievement strivings, learned and acquired in response to family pressure, resulted in depression when failure was confronted later in life. Cohen et al.'s suggestions encapsulated well the idea of learned beliefs and attitudes, producing vulnerability to depression.

There is no basic conflict between Bibring's view and those of mentality theory except that we would say it is the way self-worth is defined that sets the style of aspirations, the choice of various social themes and strategies, and that social comparisons are importantly involved in whether a person feels they have failed or not (see Chapter 7).

DOMINANT OTHER, DOMINANT GOAL

Arieti and Bemporad (1980a,b) developed ego analytic theory in an interesting way. Like Bibring they also abandoned Freud's notions of id and aggressive impulses turned inward. They do not engage object relations theory but rather suggest that depression results from the failure to achieve important incentives upon which self-esteem is based. Unlike Bibring they retain Freud's concept of dependency but analyse dependency in a completely different way. Their theory moves towards mentality theory but is not quite so broad. This theory of depression distinguishes two types of depressive vulnerability. These are labelled dominant other and dominant goal.

Dominant Other

They suggest that individuals whose vulnerability is based on the pursuit of a dominant other are excessively reliant on the other as a source of meaning and self-esteem. In talking about these individuals, Arieti and Bemporad (1980a, pp. 1360–1361) say:

> They do not experience satisfaction directly from effort but only through an intermediary, who gives or withholds rewards. They have formed an imagined agreement with the important other that may be called a bargain relationship ..., in which the individual forgoes the independent derivation of gratification in return for the continuance of nurturance and support of the esteemed other. This pattern of relating was initiated by the parent during the childhood of the predepressive individual but in later life the individual will reinstate similar relationships in a transferential manner. Other characteristics of this type of depressive personality are clingingness, passivity, manipulativeness and avoidance of anger. These character traits may be seen as the means by which the individual attempts to extract support from the needed other as well as to ensure continuation of the relationship.

Beck (1983) calls these types sociotropic and Blatt et al. (1982) refers to them as anaclitic. As with existential theorists (e.g., Yalom, 1980) Arieti and Bemporad emphasise the failure to individuate and develop autonomy. They suggest that this style is more common in women. Arieti and Bemporad (1980b) offer helpful cases to illustrate this approach. Discussing a case of postnatal depression, they outlined how the mother–daughter relationship was one where the mother dominated and was over-intrusive into her daughter's life style such that the daughter was not able to come to see herself as "grown up". Hence the daughter arrived at her own time to be a mother completely ill-equipped to have the confidence to function in this role, seeing herself as inadequate and unable to be a mother. There may also be cultural reasons why women are more vulnerable to this "dominant other" type of depression but in my view these arise from power and dominance– submission issues such that dominant others are sought out to compensate for a view of self as weak and unable. But not only may this arise from parent–child interactions but also from the limited roles and social validation of roles that are necessary for female individuation and status. This may be why postnatal depression varies across cultures (see Cox, 1988).

Dominant Goals

Those who attempt to ward off depression by obtaining lofty goals may have a more chronic form of personality difficulty characterised by many taboos (e.g., on pleasure). Arieti and Bemporad (1980a, p.1361) outline the characteristics of these individuals in the following way:

> These individuals invest their self-esteem in the achievement of some lofty goal and shun any other activities as possibly diverting them from this quest. Originally, achievement was rewarded by the parents, and so high marks for some outstanding performance was sought as a way to ensure support and acceptance. In time, the individual selects some fantastic goal for himself which he then pursues frantically, apparently for its own sake. However, closer scrutiny reveals that the achievement of this goal is burdened with surplus meaning. The individual believes that the goal will transform his life and, possibly, himself. Attaining his desired objective will mean that others will *treat him in a special way* or that he will finally be *valued by others* (my italics). Just as the dominant other type of depressive individual uses fantasies of the relationship to derive a feeling of worth, the dominant goal type of depressive individual obtains meaning and esteem from fantasies about obtaining his objective. Both types also use these fantasies to eschew ratification or meaning from other activities in everyday life. In contrast to the "dominant other" type, this form of depressive personality is usually seclusive, arrogant and often obsessive. In addition, this form of personality organization is commonly found in men.

In other types of theory these would be seen as narcissistic vulnerabilities. They are aimed at following a strategy of dominance (gaining high SAHP) via achievement. Although they may deny they wish to be dominant, the fantasies of such people show that this is the issue. In one of my own cases the person felt that, as the second child, his parents would rather he had been a girl. His older brother did well at school and in a subsequent career, whereas he felt he was a disappointment to his parents. Much of his striving had been to try to do something his family and others would recognise and bestow high respect and value on.

Comment

The idea that individuals come to invest in others' or their own efforts has a long history in psychoanalytic thinking (Macdiarmid, 1989). In Chapters 5–8 we discussed this distinction in terms of different strategies for investment and linked it with ideas on the evolution of mental mechanisms. Arieti and Bemporad (1980a,b), however, give a clear perspective on this issue and link choice of strategy (which will influence how the self will become organised) with early childhood. They argue that on reviewing the childhood of depressed adults one does not find the disorganization of families of schizophrenic or psychopathic adults. Rather, the family structure may have been too stable, with little tolerance for individual deviation from an expected norm. One parent was usually dominant and the rest of the family accepted a submissive role. Hence control is a central concern (see also Chapter 10).

Note the use of the term the submissive role, the importance of being constantly confronted with powerful others to whom compliance is expected. This compliance may be enforced by threats of punishment or the withdrawal of approval or love. However, the role of submissiveness in children who go on to become pathology prone requires more research. A retrospective study by McCraine and Buss (1984) suggests that control, demands for submissiveness, and inconsistent affection were high in the back-grounds of both dominant-other and dominant-goal types. However, dominant-goal types also experienced their parents as requiring more achievement and achievement was used to regulate self-esteem. It may also be that if a child experiences lack of control in their early care-giving relationships, as they grow up they may find that they can obtain control (e.g., direct the attention of significant others including parents, teachers, and peers) by accomplishments, be these academic, athletic or whatever. Since status is about the capacity to direct social attention towards the self, then this may be a good tactic. However, they may find themselves in significant difficulty when they are unable to interpose their achievements (role) between themselves and another, e.g., during intimacy. The experience of intimacy may again arouse the fears of being controlled, abandoned or shamed.

Arieti and Bemporad (1980a,b) also identify a chronic form of depressive predisposition. Such individuals suffer a constant feeling of depression which they are unable to ward off, either by the pursuit of goals or with a meaningful relationship. Personality characteristics of this group include hypochondriasis, harsh attitudes to self and others, and pettiness (this may be our moralist types). The pursuit of pleasure is inhibited because of strong taboos instilled by family and culture. All three types share a difficulty in obtaining pleasure from spontaneous activity, overvalue the opinions of others, overvalue social approval, and underestimate their effects on other people.

INCENTIVE DISENGAGEMENT THEORY

Another theory of depression that bears very much on mentality theory, but stresses a slightly different angle, is incentive disengagement theory (Klinger, 1975; 1977). One only has to substitute the word role for the word incentive and the theory is extremely relevant to mentality theory and one that could be integrated with it. I will leave the readers to make this substitution and derive their own ideas.

Klinger (1977) maintains that humans organise many aspects of their lives (plans, intentions, efforts, behaviours, thoughts, fantasies, and so on) around the pursuit of valued incentives. While social events (being liked, having friends, obtaining support, etc.) are incentives valued by the majority, incentives are largely personally determined. The commitment to, and pursuit of, incentives give meaning to life. The major personal upheavals and life's crises centre around disappointments, frustrations, and obstacles which interrupt the pursuit of incentives or render them unobtainable. When life's circumstances force us to give up, abandon, or lose our major incentives, depression can be an inevitable consequence.

Incentive disengagement theory rests on a number of central concepts. Klinger suggests that incentives or goals obtain value because they are associated with potential sources of reinforcement, or the avoidance of aversive outcomes. In other words, they are acquired. The degree of positive reinforcement and the expectancy of final obtainment are important factors in determining the value of an incentive and the degree of commitment to it. Klinger points out that, in the process of becoming committed to goals or incentives, there must be some internal process(es) that enables the individual to pursue the valued goal in its absence, or in the absence of cues signalling its presence. Thus, according to Klinger (1977, p.36), people will work for years to obtain certain things, "overcoming repeated obstacles and improvising a long succession of tactics". In this way individuals move nearer their incentives and goals. The process by which they become set to pursue a goal is a *commitment*. They will remain committed to this goal until either they achieve it or, for one reason or another, it is abandoned. Klinger suggests that during the committed stage the incentive is a *current concern*. Current concern is a hypothetical state which refers to the process of being committed to a goal. It is present all the time even when the person is not actively engaged in pursuing his goal directly.[1]

Commitments and current concerns exert significant influences over behavioural and cognitive processes. Plans are laid, considered, carried out, and changed in the light of information which helps or hinders the approach path to the incentive. Attention to cues signalling opportunities to reach a goal is heightened. Individuals will have more than one incentive, of course, and the processes of commitment and current concern apply to an infinite variety of anticipated outcomes. Moreover, the relation between valued incentives or goals, and therefore commitments and current concerns about them, shift and change in relationship to a variety of factors (Klinger, 1977). Klinger suggests that, as we grow older, different incentives become important as our external and internal worlds change. Extinction, habituation, and satiation are all processes which change the arrangement of valued incentives for the individual. Depression is one of the consequences of abandonment and disengagement from incentives that are still highly valued.

Not all incentives have equal value. Many acquire value by their association with higher incentives, e.g., studying and forgoing pleasure promise to bring the valued rewards of respect, money, or prestige associated with some qualification. The perception of failure or a reduction in the value of the qualification may reduce behaviours associated with it (e.g., studying). Furthermore, some potentially positive reinforcing behaviours may not develop because they are associated with a high negative outcome (e.g., drinking with mates may be associated with failure of the qualification). The aversiveness of loss of a sub-incentive (e.g., the opportunity for study) will depend on the perception to which this threatens the end-point incentive. Hence, behaviours and incentives share complex facilitatory and inhibitory interactions. Some behaviours may fail to develop. For example, the student who overvalues academic qualifications and spends all his time studying may become depressed when he finds he has no friends. Instead of bringing him happiness, studying has led to alienation. He may now face conflict between presenting himself as competent, worthy of respect, and developing social relationships which require the investment of time and energy, all of which might detract from his ability to "become competent". Klinger (1977, p.161) puts the matter clearly when he suggests:

> there are ways in which extinction can spread beyond the lost object. If a complicated chain of actions is required to achieve a goal, then there are likely to be many subgoals whose value depends on the ultimate goal. For instance if a child has learned to organize much of its behaviour around a parent's approval, then losing the parent may make all of the actions learned to please him or her meaningless and unattractive.

Klinger goes on to suggest that this does not explain the depressive's pervasive sense of loss. Incidentally, it does not offer any mechanism by which these forms of extinction can produce the varied and intense symptoms of a depressed person (e.g., loss of appetite, loss of sexual interest, sleep disturbance, diurnal variation, and so on). But behaviours may vanish from a repertoire for many reasons and not all the behaviours that appear to be extinguished in the depressed state need to be under the control of the same process. A number of sub-processes might be involved which, though interactive, can nevertheless be studied individually. Vulnerability to extinction of certain behaviours seems one such process. However, we still do not yet understand how certain behaviours, which were not directly related to an incentive, appear to become so when that incentive is removed. Thus a bereaved person may have enjoyed diverse activities ranging from playing weekend football to business lunches, none of which maintained the marital relationship which is broken in bereavement. Nevertheless, the person may feel no pleasure or purpose in engaging in these activities following the death of the spouse. This suggests there can be a general shift in the capacity to experience pleasure following the loss of a loved person.

To help understand this more generalised process Klinger's model stresses disengagement, rather than commitment, as the key process in depression. Since commitments and current concerns exert a powerful organising influence on behavioural, emotional cognitive, and biological processes, the failure to attain and/or maintain a valued incentive or goal can be expected to produce significant upheaval in all three systems. These upheavals, Klinger suggests, follow a predictable cycle. First, there are attempts to rescue the incentive (invigoration). When these attempts fail the incentive needs to be abandoned and the abandonment produces depression.

Invigoration

Klinger (1975; 1977) suggests that the first thing that happens when incentives become more difficult to obtain, or are blocked, is an invigoration of behaviour. To support this he reviews a large body of research evidence including Amsel's (1958; 1962) frustration effect experiments. It is widely known that animals will demonstrate greatly invigorated behaviours, if previously learned avoidance responses are blocked. Mandler (1975) also suggests that interruption of ongoing behaviour causes significant increases in behaviour and arousal. This arousal is often associated with negative affectivity such as aggression and irritability and gives a different explanation to the increased aggressiveness of the depressive noted in Chapter 8. In the early stages of invigoration, it seems that the valued incentive moves up the hierarchy of incentives, that is, it becomes more important. This increased importance may have both behavioural and cognitive consequences. Cognitively, more activity is geared toward thinking about the incentive, looking for incentive cues, and so on. In the studies of infant separation, the first behaviours to be seen are intense searching behaviours. In humans, the loss of a loved one causes cognitive activity to focus very sharply on the missing person (Parkes, 1972).

The fact that the incentive becomes more important when it is threatened or removed has implications for cognitive theory. Individuals who, when depressed, appear to have highly idealised views of how they should behave may be demonstrating invigoration. In other words, the ability to be a good, lovable person (say) takes on increased importance if the ability to behave in a "good" way is threatened (e.g., loss of the opportunity to be a care-giver). As the person recovers from the depression we would expect this incentive to lose some of its importance or value. This does seem to happen.

Incentive disengagement theory strengthens various theories by indicating mechanisms whereby key themes, cognitive or social incentives, become dominant in the individual's cognitive processing at certain times. A concept of invigoration may help to explain why certain negative constructs become dominant at certain points in time. In other words, under the threat of not achieving important incentives (be this to be loved, be a good care-giver, or whatever) they become invigorated concerns.

Klinger argues that in the process of invigoration, anger and aggression are also increased. Again, there is evidence that this is so. In rats, aggressive behaviour increases following frustrative nonreward. Klinger points out, however, that there are different types of aggression, including territorial, defensive, rage, and so on. These are mediated by different brain areas and we should not regard increased aggressive behaviour as being relevant to all these. He proposes that it is "irritable aggression" which is increased by blocking incentives. In depression it is indeed noted that depressives often show increased irritable anger and aggression (see Chapter 8). Self psychologists (see Chapter 10), however, would draw a major distinction between frustrative aggression and narcissistic rage. Klinger's theory does not deal with shame or envy or the role of rank and power in the expression of anger.

Depression

Eventually, if invigorated behaviour fails to secure the incentive, the individual must give up pursuing the now unattainable incentive. The downswing into depression commences as the expectation of success in maintaining or obtaining the valued incentive falls. The actual processes involved in this downswing are complex. Generally, it is marked by an increase in hopelessness about obtaining the incentive. Klinger points to separation studies to demonstrate this aspect of the cycle. As depression ensues, behavioural output falls. But this does not mean that cognitive activity, centred on the incentive, diminishes. Rather, it may change its form. In the invigorated phase, cognitive activity may centre on how to overcome the obstacles in the path to the incentive. In the disengagement (depressed) phase, cognitive activity centres on the dire consequences of having lost. Depending on the value of the incentive this cognitive activity may be painful and intense. Preoccupations and ruminations on the consequences of the loss may appear. Although behavioural activity may significantly fall (e.g., because of a collapse of a behavioural network), cognitive processes do not necessarily decline, for invigorated cognitive activity (e.g., ruminations) on the consequences of the loss may be present. The processes which terminate preoccupations and ruminations on these consequences require further investigation.

Klinger suggests that individuals can be at various points in various incentive disengagement cycles, and that the depression produced by final incentive disengagement may vary from mild depression to intense clinical depression. Much would seem to depend on the pursuit of alternative incentives. He also suggests that there is a natural tendency to recover. The intensity and duration of the depressive phase will vary according to a host of factors, some cognitive, some behavioural, but some biochemical. Indeed, one of the strengths of Klinger's model is that he attempts to show how various elements of the incentive disengagement cycle are biochemically mediated. Thus, the idea that some severe depressions are biochemically driven is not at all at variance with Klinger's theory.

Comment

Klinger's theory has a number of strengths. It highlights what clinicians have been aware of for a long time. Although some behaviours are lost to the depressive, there are also, paradoxically, invigorated components. These centre on agitated states and painful, often constant, internal ruminations. Moreover, it is often noted that obsessional states wax and wane with depressions. The invigoration component offers some insight into this aspect of depression.

Klinger also offers some interesting ideas on mania, though these will not be discussed here. Klinger's important contribution is to focus attention on the idea that there is a cycle of events which can include both invigoration and disengagement in depression. In pathological cases, the biological mediators of this cycle may be significantly disturbed. He also draws attention to the need to take up new incentives as part of recovery. In mentality we would also stress the development of new themes and consider what adjustment behaviours are underdeveloped.

There is an aspect to Klinger's theory which needs special concern. He suggests that depression, be it mild or severe, is an almost inevitable result of disengaging from valued incentives. Moreover, there is a natural tendency to recover. If this is so, then we should not ask why depressed, but why so severe or long, and why no recovery? Here one may turn to either biological factors, the arousal of negative self-cognitions and/or the role of social relationships (see Chapter 15).

There is a possible confusing factor in Klinger's model. This is the implicit idea that disengagement is relevant to both mild and severe depression. One problem for some depressives is their failure to disengage (which we called blocked escape and entrapment, see Chapters 6–8 and 15). Actually, disengagement can be a normal and good coping behaviour. For some depressives, however, there is a failure to disengage and seek new incentives. The cost of doing so seems just too high. Gut (1989) makes a similar case. Thus they are trapped in remaining committed to incentives which are unrealistic and are not obtainable. Biologically, their systems may have moved beyond the invigoration point, yet still at a cognitive–emotive level no disengagement is made. The level of stress is, therefore, "pathological", because it cannot be resolved.

LEARNED HELPLESSNESS AND HOPELESSNESS

We first met learned helplessness theory (Seligman, 1975) in Chapter 6 and outlined the basic early axioms. The key issue was lack of control. Since then learned helplessness theory has undergone two major revisions.

Learned Helplessness Theory: The First Formulation (1948-1978)

As we saw in Chapter 6, Mowrer and Viek (1948) were probably the first to observe the effects of subjecting animals to uncontrollable shock. During the 1960s further work was conducted by Seligman and his colleagues, and in 1975 Seligman published his important book called,

Helplessness: On Depression Development and Death. Depression was only one of the applications of the theory.

During the 1970s much human (mostly student) experimental work was published on the effects of lack of control examining: (1) the degree of generalisation of the disruptive influence on subsequent behaviour (e.g., problem solving) following experience with uncontrollable trauma or unsolvable problems; (2) the similarities between experimentally induced learning disruption and learning deficits observable in depressed individuals; (3) the depressant effect of uncontrollable situations. Most of these studies have been well reviewed by others (e.g., Blaney, 1977; Costello, 1978). In general, the findings suggested that the disruption in learning produced by uncontrollable events does, to a degree, generalise to other learning situations; that there are similarities in persistence measures and expectation of success in skilled situations between pretreated (with uncontrollable events) individuals and depressed students (i.e., both give up more quickly); and that experience with uncontrollable events can have a dysphoric impact (Miller & Seligman, 1973; 1975; Hiroto & Seligman, 1975; Klein, Fencil-Morse, & Seligman, 1976; Klein & Seligman, 1976).

Blaney (1977) suggested, however, that much of these data are open to alternative explanations. For example, manipulations of self-esteem often had contaminating effects in some of these experiments and may also have generated unfavourable social comparison. Moreover, Forrest and Hokanson (1975) demonstrated that for some forms of learning (e.g., self-punitive responding following assertive behaviour from others) depressives actually show superior learning, while Thornton and Jacobs (1971) failed to observe significant differences between a control and an inescapable shock-treated group. Klinger (1977) indicated that the type of goal/incentive over which control was lost was important.

The Journal of Abnormal Psychology (February, 1978) dedicated a special edition to the learned helplessness model. In this edition arguments for and against Seligman's theory were put forward. Depue and Monroe (1978a) suggested that the parallels drawn between learned helplessness and depression make it appear more in keeping with endogenous rather than reactive depression. Costello (1978) critically examined a number of papers relevant to the learned helplessness model of depression and points up possible alternative explanations. Moreover, whether one believes in the dimensional or categorical approach to depression, there is dispute over the value of using students as experimental subjects for a theory of pathological states.

In addition to the possible contaminating influences of self-esteem manipulations, it was noted that the learned helplessness theory and Beck's (1967) cognitive theory made opposite predictions about self-attributions. In Beck's theory (see Chapter 13), depressives are seen to blame themselves (internal attribution) for negative outcomes (called, personalisation). In Seligman's theory, however, negative outcomes are themselves seen as uncontrollable (external attribution). Despite Klein's (1974) claim that neurotic depressives actually blame others, and Harrow, Colbert, Detre, and Bakeman's (1966) finding that many depressives blame their illness, learned helplessness theory was reformulated to agree with Beck's theory, and turned to attribution theory.

Learned Helplessness Theory: The Second Formulation (1978-1989)

Attribution theory rests on the philosophical positions of Hume and Kant, who asserted that causes cannot be observed, but are constructed by the perceiver to render the environment more meaningful. In this sense they are psychologically construed. Attribution theorists have addressed themselves to the question of how causes are attributed to different events. The general events most studied by attribution theorists have been success and failure in achievement-related tasks (Weiner, 1972).

Weiner and his colleagues (Weiner, 1972; 1974; Weiner, Heckhausen, Meyer, & Cook, 1972) argued that causal perceptions require two dimensions of explanation. One of these comes from the social learning theory of Rotter (Rotter, 1966; Rotter, Seeman, & Liverant, 1962). This dimension is the locus of control, or internal–external dimension. According to this theory, causality is attributed either to internal factors (self) or external factors (the world). Those that adhere to the locus of control dimension of causality argue that expectancy and the persistence of behaviour depend on whether the individual perceives an event as being internally controlled (by self) or externally controlled (by others or the world). Perceptions of internal control produce high persistence; perceptions of external control produce low persistence.

Attribution theory, on the other hand, argued that it is the stable–unstable dimension that best explains expectancy change and behavioural persistence. If the individual perceives the cause of success or failure as due to stable factors, then the same outcome can be expected in the future, and persistence is determined accordingly. If the person perceives the causes of success or failure as due to unstable factors, then persistence may be high in the case of failure (tries harder, effort attribution), or low in the face of success (e.g., slot machine, luck attribution). The stable factors most investigated by attribution theorists have been ability and task difficulty. The unstable factors are

TABLE 12.1
Interaction of the Dimension of Internal–External and Stable–Unstable Attributions

	Internal	*External*
STABLE	Ability (a)	Task difficulty (b)
UNSTABLE	Effort (c)	Luck (d)

effort and luck. The interaction between these two dimensions of perceived causality is shown in Table 12.1 .

Although these issues are not straightforward, there is some evidence that the stable–unstable dimension is a better predictor of behaviour persistence and expectancy change than the internal–external dimension (Dweck, 1975; Weiner, 1972; Weiner, Nierenberg, & Goldstein, 1976). In regard to depression, research demonstrated that attributions are important variables, influencing mood changes and performance decrements (Douglas & Anisman, 1975; Dweck, 1975; Klein et al., 1976; Roth & Kubal, 1975; Tennen & Eller, 1977; Weiner, Russell, & Lerman, 1978; 1979).[2]

In 1978 the reformulated theory of learned helplessness was published by Abramson, Seligman, and Teasdale (1978). These researchers stressed three dimensions of attributions: internal–external, stable–unstable, and global–specific. They suggested that when individuals find they are unable to control desired outcomes, they seek causes for this state of affairs. The severity and chronicity of depression are in part the result of the perceived cause for not being able to control desired outcomes. Internal, personal, stable attributions will lead the individual to believe that the failure to control an outcome is due to deficits within themselves and that (because of a stability attribution) the same state of affairs will remain in the future. In this way the chosen dimension of attribution will lead to both a fall in self-esteem and a hopeless view of the future. This model is outlined in Table 12.2.

This reformulated model is thus a two-stage model. First, individuals must become aware of a response–outcome incongruence; depression will then result if the individual blames him/herself for their helplessness and sees the situation as unchangeable (stable). It is suggested that depressed individuals make more global, stable, internal attributions.

TABLE 12.2
Interactions of the Dimensions of Stable–Unstable and the Global–Specific Attributions

	INTERNAL ATTRIBUTIONS FOR NEGATIVE EVENTS	
	STABLE	*UNSTABLE*
GLOBAL	I am a boring person	I am sometimes boring
	I am a weak person	I am sometimes weak
	I am a stupid person	I am sometimes stupid
SPECIFIC	My conversations are uninteresting to him/her	She/he is sometimes not interested in what I say
	My conversations with her/him are not as assertive as I would like	My conversations with him/her are sometimes not as assertive as I would like
	My conversations with him/her are not as clear as I would like	My conversations with him/her are sometimes not as clear as I would like

Seligman, Abramson, Semmel, and Baeyer (1979) demonstrated that depressed college students do tend to attribute negative outcomes to more internal, stable, and global causes than nondepressed students. Garber and Hollon (1980) further demonstrated that the attributions of depressed college students relate to personally relevant variables rather than universal variables. In other words, depressed students tend to see themselves as less able to control outcomes, but do not view the outcomes themselves as uncontrollable. This is important for, in the original learned helplessness theory (Seligman, 1975), it was the perceived uncontrollability of events themselves that produced depression. Now, however (though this view accounted for the animal data), it is abandoned in favour of personal attributions, which animals do not have. Garber and Hollon (1980) suggest that their data support both Abramson et al.'s (1978) reformulation model and Bandura's (1977) distinction of personal efficacy expectations and outcome expectations. The main problem with much of this work, especially with students, is the issue of personality (see Chapter 4). It is unclear whether these results apply to dysthymic, borderline, avoidant personality or other traits, or have specific relevance for major depressive episodes.

Hammen, Adrian, and Hiroto (1988), in one of the few studies of its kind, used a longitudinal design with children and adolescents to explore the attributional theory as a predictor of depression. They did not find much support for the attribution theory but rather future depression was predicted by initial symptoms and life events. Beck

(1967) suggests that children may learn to blame self for failure in response to being labelled as having attributes for failure. Such learning may also take place in response to rigid efforts to obtain social approval and reinforcement.

Self-blame may also start off as a strategy for self-protection (and not a real evaluation of cause). Self-blame may protect the agents of reinforcement from criticism and reduce the chances of rejection (Bowlby, 1980; Gut, 1989). Self-blame signals "no threat" and an absence of anger with another and therefore does not invite (counter) attack. It is quite unclear how self-blame as a self-protective defensive strategy differs from other forms of self-blame, but clinical work attests to the fact that for some patients self-blame is self-protective. I have seen various patients over the years who, once in a trusting relationship, give quite a different account of events than when they first entered therapy. Self-blame can also be used to try to elicit sympathy from others, especially in dependent types of personality. However, Driscoll (1989) has outlined twelve different types of self-blame serving different functions—most seen to be self-protective. Clinicians should be aware of these differences (see also page 397).

Recently Parry and Brewin (1988) explored attribution style and self-esteem in regard to three models relevant to the attribution model: (1) negative cognitions are a symptoms of depression; (2) negative cognitions plus life events lead to depression; (3) negative life events or negative cognitive style can be causal of depression. Their data support the third formulation with some support also for the symptom model. Brewin (1985; 1988) reviewed much of the evidence concerning attribution style (in association with life events) as a causal model of depression and found that there was only weak supporting evidence. There is more evidence for negative attributions acting to maintain depression.

Lewinsohn et al. (1981) studied a community population of 998 over one year. Three hypotheses were investigated: (l) depressive cognitions are antecedent to depression; (2) depressive cognitions are a consequence of depression; (3) recovery from depression leaves residual negative cognitions. In general, their evidence suggests that it is impossible to detect a depressive style, prior to becoming depressed, but negative cognitions certainly accompany depression. Although not necessarily related to etiology, depressive cognitions may make recovery more difficult.

It is unclear whether depression is related to the failure to achieve the desired outcome (the event) or to the attribution as such. After all I may be depressed because I have no money and can't achieve my goals (e,g., buying a house, supporting my family) but I may recover by winning a state lottery which is entirely luck. Hence how concerned are people about the way they come to achieve their goals?

The Third Formulation: Hopelessness

The reformulated attribution theory of depression has now been called the "hopelessness theory" of depression (Alloy et al., 1988; Abramson et al., 1989; Abramson & Alloy, 1990). These researchers review much of the current evidence for the role of attributions in depression and make a plea that perhaps hopelessness depression is a special/particular type of depression. They suggest that understanding causality from a psychological domain may come to influence current nosologies. I doubt that this is a change that is close at hand since psychiatric nosology is dominated by phenomenology and not causal theory. At some point psychologists may have to develop their own systems rather than tampering with the phenomenological approach.

Abramson et al. (1989) make the surprising point that the original (1978) reformulation was primarily related to helplessness and made only passing reference to depression. Surprising because so much research on depression followed the 1978 paper. In any event the second reformulation is a more comprehensive model. It focuses on the role of hopelessness and "deemphasizes causal attributions" especially the internality dimension. Thus it is less important whether an individual judges themselves to blame or not.

In the new theory, they outline a pathway of processes that produce hopelessness depression. The most distal cause in the chain, are negative life events (or stress). Situational cues and certain inferential styles increase the depressive effects of negative life events. At the next stage, the life event is seen to have major importance to long-term plans and goals and there is a stable and global attribution style; and/or the person derives negative judgements about themselves. An individual may not see themselves as having caused the bad event but coping with the event may show up personal deficits. These two links (e.g., negative events and perceived implications) give rise to hopelessness. Hopelessness may be increased by low social support (see also Chapter 15). As a result of extreme hopelessness various symptoms emerge. These include, retarded initiation, lack of energy, psychomotor retardation and so forth. Hence depression arises from a perception of hopelessness to achieve desired outcomes. Bibring's ego analytic theory is not discussed although the overlaps with this 40-year-old theory are striking. There are also similarities with Klinger's (1977) theory.

Abramson et al. (1989) compare their theory with that of Beck (see Chapter 13) and Brown and Harris (1978a). Personally I found these comparisons unconvincing since Brown has always stressed the role of hopelessness. And recent work of fresh start events are believed to work precisely because they offer hope of change (e.g., Brown, Adler, & Bifulco, 1988; Brown, 1989). It is true however that, unlike Brown, they do not place special emphasis on social events. Other problems with the theory are that hopelessness has always been associated with suicidal intent, regardless of diagnostic category rather than a special type of depression, and to suggest a subtype of hopelessness depression may be difficult to prove since hopelessness is nearly always associated with depression. Some patients become more hopeless as they lose energy, experience anxiety difficulties and other symptoms persist and they feel that they won't get better (Teasdale, 1988).

As they point out it is too early to judge the evidence for this new theory. There is little doubt that hopelessness is always going to be part of the depressive experience and I have yet to met a patient with moderate or severe depression, who does not feel hopeless, or to put it another way, feels optimistic. This reformulation is at present an interesting development and one looks forward to seeing how it works out. But with the rising tide of young suicides and increasing levels of depression one may look to cultural changes to see if there are social factors that are increasing a sense of hopelessness in the population at large (see Chapter 3). Recent documentary programmes on the effects of East Germany's unification suggest that there is increasing widespread hopelessness and possible increasing depression but we must await research to confirm this. In many cases it may be the "dashing of hope" that produces the collapse into depression.

Pessimism

Seligman (1989) has turned the attribution model into a personality theory and discusses the styles of pessimists and optimists. He asks, "Is the word in your heart yes or no?" This idea does have a certain appeal. It turns out that pessimists (whose word in the heart is "no") are not only vulnerable to depression but also to other forms of (physical) illness, may vary in terms of immune functioning and also can be underachievers. Pessimism however is a much wider concept than attribution style and individuals can become pessimistic and hopeless through a whole range of factors, including biological differences, thwarting life events, the dominance behaviour of others and so on. There is however not much doubt that when people are depressed they are indeed pessimistic. What is exciting however is that early identification of pessimism in childhood coupled with attribution retraining may have protective effects to subsequent disorder

(Seligman, 1989). However, it is going to be some time before we have the evidence for this.

Also there is some reason to be doubtful (e.g., Hammen et al., 1988; see page 372 this volume). We also know that many children are abused or subject to authoritarian parenting and it is difficult to see how attribution retraining, which does not address these social factors, is going to be helpful. As it stands, the learned helplessness model pays little regard to attitudes, e.g., "I should be hard-working", "I must be loved", "I must be successful", etc. As with Beck's model, the role of anger in depression is also not discussed, yet for some theories (e.g., psychoanalytic) anger is a central component of certain depressions. As mentioned in previous chapters (e.g., Chapter 7) depressives may not only be generally pessimistic but have had hopes "dashed", hopes of a marriage or career that don't come to fruit. Indeed, some depressives may be grossly idealistic and reality turns out to be rather more "tatty". Thus, as mentioned earlier, disappointment is a common source of some depressions (see Chapter 10).

Many of the distinctions between the reformulated theories of learned helplessness/hopelessness and ranking theory are similar to those that apply also to cognitive theory. So these will be held over until the next chapter.

SUMMARY

1. Ego analytic theory focused on goals and aspirations. The two most important relate to forming dependent/subordinate/protective relationships, and individual achievement. These dispositions mirror later ideas of sociotropic and autonomous personality (e.g., Beck, 1983). Blocking of these basic aspirations results in ego collapse. When the ego feels unable to live up to, or achieve, basic aspirations, depression results.
2. Incentive theory takes us into the mechanics of the pursuit of incentives and goals, outlines how an individual becomes committed to incentives and goals and how depression is a form of disengagement from valued incentives.
3. Learned helplessness theory has undergone some radical transformations. From the original theory of lack of control the first reformulation stressed attributions, especially those of self-blame and stability.
4. The most recent reformulation has been in terms of hopelessness to achieve desired outcomes and the various cognitive factors that result in hopelessness. The role of internal attributions has been played down, though it remains

part of the theory. Here we seem to have returned to Bibring's basic ideas on depression.

5. Seligman has focused on an attribution style which he calls pessimism. Pessimism relates not only to depression but also achievement and physical illness.

CONCLUDING COMMENTS

Bibring is a major source of many of the recent cognitive ideas on depression, although critics have pointed out that ego ideals were always part of Freud's theory. Although Bibring did not focus on it, many of his basic aspirations are social. Arieti and Bemporad developed the social dimension further. For reasons that are not entirely clear to me, many of the developments in learned helplessness theory have not followed the social path. Perhaps this is because the roots of the theory are in laboratory shock experiments. An evolutionary approach, however, will never move far from the social domain, not only because social success may be a prime mover in evolution (Vining, 1986; Nesse, 1990), but also because social success is coassembled with many affect, cognitive, and behavioural systems. Thus it is social success that has been selected for and why many of our affects are linked to it (see Chapter 5).

The way hopelessness is related to social comparison, a sense of being different, of being an outsider and having a low "social place" (see Chapters 6 and 7) and so forth remain for the future. Somewhere in our different theories we are all touching parts of a complex, evolved, potential self-organisation or brain state. Hopelessness is involved somehow, but we need more work, with a much broader focus, to illuminate it.

NOTES

1. Current concerns exist at different levels. For example, a central current concern may be to achieve rank, status, and admiration. This will lead to sub-concerns such as passing exams, maintaining a positive self-presentation, choosing a particular type of spouse, and so on. Some concerns will be closer to the central concern than others and be more attended to, thought about, and have greater affective consequences.
2. Caution should be exercised in the consideration that these two dimensions are independent. For example, effort probably depends on the perception that the individual does have the basic ability but needs to try harder. If the individual perceives that he does not have any ability then there is really not much point in trying. Furthermore, to what extent is effort simply a

measure of behavioural persistence? Similarly, for luck and task difficulty: luck attributions are more likely if the task is first perceived as being either unpredictable or difficult. Outcomes of tasks judged to be predictable and simple probably do not lend themselves to luck attributions.

CHAPTER 13

Cognitive Theories of Depression

We are what we are
All that we are arises with our thoughts
With our thoughts we make the world.—Buddha

The 1970s saw the cognitive approach establish itself as the major alternative to both psychoanalytic theory and behaviour theory of psychopathology (Mahoney, 1974; Mahoney & Arnkoff, 1978; Marzillier, 1980). The enthusiasm for the cognitive approach became a tidal wave in the 1980s and was applied to almost all forms of psychopathology including, anxiety disorders (Beck et al., 1985), personality disorder (Beck et al., 1990), and just about all forms of neurosis. The reader can find excellent reviews on these developments in Hawton, Salkovskis, Kirk, and Clark (1989), Freeman et al. (1989) and Scott, Williams, and Beck (1989). But in this era, cognitive approaches began to diversify and vary such that various debates between different schools have emerged (Dryden & Golden 1986). A major distinction is between the rationalists and constructivists (Mahoney & Gabriel, 1987; Carmin & Dowd, 1988).

There are a number of reasons why cognitive theories became so successful. First, the refusal of behaviourism to involve itself with internal mental phenomena meant that it would eventually collapse under the weight of evidence that people think about things, form theories about themselves and their lives, and that these internal events mediate stimulus-response outcomes. Second, throughout history, ideas, beliefs, and attitudes have always been regarded as sources of distress (Ellenberger, 1970; Zilboorg & Henry, 1941). Albert Ellis, one of the founders of the cognitive approach, tells us how the Greek philosopher, Epictetus, over 2000 years ago, argued that it is the view we take of things and not things in themselves which disturbs us. Kant believed that mental illness resulted when private sense and common sense drifted too far apart. Charot (1825-1893) believed that certain dissociated ideas could cause symptoms of hysteria. Jung (1963; 1964) argued that complexes, which are integrated sets of ideas, attitudes, and emotions, often caused mental distress, especially when there was a conflict between unconscious predispositions and maladaptive conscious attitudes. And Weiner (1972) and Erdelyi (1985) suggest that many of Freud's theories pay particular attention to memories and fantasies and in that respect are cognitive. Thus, there is little new in the idea that meaning and beliefs are important in suffering. However, the more recent forerunners of cognitive therapy are to be found in Alfred Adler, Karen Horney and Bibring. Third, unlike earlier attempts to work with beliefs, the cognitive therapy of Beck was simply formulated, clearly structured, and easily taught. Fourth, Beck's preparedness to expose cognitive therapy to control trials (something that even now psychoanalytic theories are reluctant to do) gave cognitive therapy a scientific advantage. Fifth, during the eighties increasing efforts were made to link cognitive therapy with experimental cognitive psychology (see Power & Brewin, in press).

All in all the cognitive approach offered a new paradigm that: (a) could deal with past observations; (b) make testable predictions; (c) was easy to teach and comprehend (at least compared to psychoanalysis); (d) promised and demonstrated fast effects—carefully selected patients got better quickly; (e) integrated behavioural practice and exposure into its treatment packages; (f) became linked to academic, experimental cognitive psychology on the one hand (e.g., studies of attention and memory) and social psychology on the other (e.g., attribution theory).

The major axiom of the cognitive theories is that cognitive processes (e.g., ideas, beliefs, and schema) translate external events into meaningful internal representations (Beck, 1976; Kelly, 1955; Lazarus, 1966; Safran & Segal, 1990). It is these "internal representations", and not the events themselves, which were seen as the pathogenic agents. However, this view has changed recently (Beck, 1987) and cognitions are given less of a causal role than previously. Learning contributes to pathology not because of a direct relationship with behaviour, but via the development of maladaptive internal mechanisms for the organisation, storage, and retrieval of information. Lazarus (1966) made the important distinction between primary appraisal (the evaluation of the meaning of an event) and secondary appraisal (the evaluation of coping abilities/options for dealing with it). The most researched cognitive approach to depression has been Beck et al.'s (1979) approach. This cognitive therapy has three main explanatory concepts: automatic thoughts, rules, and self-other schema.

Below we will spend a little time looking at the basic structure of cognitive therapy. This is because cognitive therapy can be used as a basic set of core concepts and procedures that can be adapted to various theoretical positions, especially those that have been advanced throughout this book. Not all would agree with this but I hope to give a flavour of how this is possible.

AUTOMATIC THOUGHTS

Beck was trained in traditional psychoanalysis and began developing cognitive therapy in the late 1950s, just five years or so after Bibring published his famous paper on depression and shortly after Kelly (1955) published personal construct theory. Beck's (1976) description of how he became aware of the powerful effects of automatic thoughts is illuminating. During an analysis of a patient who was relating sexual material, he noted an increase in her anxiety. At first he thought her anxiety related to the material being presented. Later, however, Beck discovered that while talking to him, she also had a series of self-evaluative thoughts; about how she thought Beck regarded her. The more she thought Beck did not like her, was bored, and wanted to terminate therapy with her, the more anxious she became. Thus, Beck reasoned, her anxiety in therapy was not related to the sexual material itself, but to her automatic negative thoughts about how the interaction was going.

Automatic thoughts, as the name implies are those interpretations/ideas/thoughts that seem to come automatically to mind. They are the immediate, consciously available thoughts. Often they have an important self-evaluative component. Automatic thoughts are not necessarily in clear/syntactic language and can be poorly formulated, using fragments of grammar. Their most salient aspect is their core of meaning.

Automatic thoughts can be represented in mental images. These images may either flash in and out of consciousness (in which case the patient may need to be trained to sharpen their focus so that they can be subject to more detailed analysis, communication, and challenge). At other times these images can be intrusive and present for long periods of time. Personally, I prefer the term automatic fantasies (see Chapter 9) because there is an important distinction between a thought like "it's raining today" and automatic thoughts related to affective disturbance. In the latter case automatic thoughts have themes (see Chapter 11) and represent various scenarios of self–other interactions; they are like mini films/plays within the mind, linked with affect, and they often involve some underlying (innate) social algorithm or mentality. For example, the lover who does not phone as expected may lead a person to fantasise about the possibility that the lover is out with someone else. They may construct scenarios of seeing the lover in some particular place (e.g., a pub) and imagine him/her having a good time, laughing, drinking, etc. We may enter into (internal) dialogue as a result of our automatic thoughts and fantasies. For example, having decided that the lover is out having a good time we may start to rehearse in our minds an argument or what we intend to say the next time they do phone. We may even rehearse something that we know in reality we would not carry out due to fear of being rejected/disliked or to moral concerns.

Daydreaming is another area where we engage in fantasy. Sometimes asking people to note the content and repetitive themes of their daydreams reveals important aspirations, concerns or fears. The internal constructive process of meaning-making is rich, varied, and powerful. It is the understanding of these processes for the construction of meaning that is the key to cognitive exploration. (Orthodox cognitive therapists however are more circumspect and are not entirely happy with the idea of internal fantasies, in part because it sounds too analytic).

A very important procedure of therapy is to explore the immediate thought, teach how to recognise these thoughts and how to challenge them (e.g., Beck et al., 1979; Fennell, 1989; Blackburn & Davidson, 1990). There is also another aspect which involves the search for some underlying, deeper meaning. Hence, the search for hidden meaning, as in psychoanalytic theory, remains but in cognitive therapy it is not repressed motivations that are explored but rules and schema. One of the most common forms of exploration is called inference chaining or laddering. This technique is one of *guided discovery* and not interpretation.

Inference Chains

An inference chain follows an "if A then B" form of reasoning. In other words the patient associates one idea or outcome with another. Usually a subsequent inference is more global and emotionally laden.

Examples:

1. If my friend ignores me then it means he/she does not like me. This is because I am a boring person. If I am a boring person then I am unlovable. If I am unlovable I will never find a loving relationship and will be alone and depressed forever.
2. If I go to town I may start to get anxious. If I get anxious then my heart rate goes up. If my heart rate goes up then I might have a heart attack. If I have a heart attack then I will die.

An inference chain seeks to explore the relationship between: (a) automatic thought(s); (b) more general assumptions/rules of living; (c) schema of self and schema of others.

In the first example, the rules might relate to needs for approval, and the schema of self, to ideas about being boring and uninteresting. In the second example there is a concern with physical safety. Beck suggests that there are particular types of error in the reasoning and automatic thoughts of depressed patients:

1. Arbitrary inference—drawing a negative conclusion in the absence of supporting data.
2. Selective abstraction—focusing on a detail out of context, often at the expense of more salient information.
3. Overgeneralisation—drawing conclusions over a wide variety of things on the basis of single events.
4. Magnification and minimisation—making errors in evaluating the importance and implications of events.
5. Personalisation—relating external (often negative) events to the self when there is little reason for doing so.
6. Absolutistic, dichotomous thinking—thinking in polar opposites (black and white). Something is all good, or totally bad and a disaster.

Others have added egocentric thinking, "people must think the same way I do", and the telepathy error, "people should know how I feel without my having to tell them". Some of these "errors" are not original to cognitive theory. For example, black and white thinking is what object relations theorists call splitting. Also it has become apparent that human reasoning in general often involves these kinds of errors (Hollon & Kriss, 1984) and that depressed patients are not untypical in this. Content is more important. Moreover, we evolved to think adaptively rather than with logical inference (see Chapter 5). When we teach evidence gathering this may not be a natural thing to do and we have to work at it.

In my view the use of the word "error" to describe these cognitive styles is unfortunate and has led to debate about whether or not patients are erroneous in their thinking. There are many reasons a patient may fall into a certain style of evaluation: life events, or as a result of previous history and so forth. Also to suggest error is to suggest a correct way of thinking. These debates cloud the key issue of understanding meaning. Others have tried to overcome this problem with terms like dysfunctional versus functional/adaptive or goal-securing thinking.

Exploring Inference Chains

Cognitive therapy is not derived from new principles. Rather, as Albert Ellis is fond of telling us, it has an important relationship with the stoic philosophers. They were interested in the nature of subjective meaning. What is beauty? what is honour? what is justice? what is evil? etc. They believed that subjective meaning had to be open to discourse and discussion and derived what became called the Socratic Method of Dialogue. Basically this involved a style of questioning that seeks to help identify the criteria people use to make subjective judgements.

Much of cognitive therapy should be understood from this perspective. It is not about "retraining" in the sense that one might teach a dog new tricks. It is rather engaging with a person's internal constructions and meaning-making processes and helping them to explore alternatives, to treat beliefs as hypothesises and to test out ideas; to understand the relationship between thoughts (inner constructions and feelings and behaviour); and to acquire new skills.

To begin to explore an inference chain two things are important. First a person should be instructed in the basic premises of the cognitive approach. After a period of general discussion around the type of problems a patient may have or examination of the history, the therapist may say: "Okay, could we look in more detail at your own personal meanings about things. In order to do this I would like to show you how we might work together to explore this." The therapist then writes down three columns A B C. A stands for an Activating event, B stands for Beliefs, and C stands for Consequences.

A	B	C
Activating Event	Beliefs/appraisals Interpretations	Emotions Behaviour Biology

The therapist may then use the example of hearing a sound in one's kitchen at 2 a.m. First the therapist discusses various possibilities for the consequences, e.g., fear, anger, relief, etc. These are then written down together with the beliefs that would lead to the different emotions.

A	B	C
Sound in kitchen at 2 a.m.	It may be a thief	Anxiety fear
	It is my drunken spouse who has forgotten the key	Anger
	It is my cat	Calm
	It is my child home safely after a party	Relief

The therapist may use this type of example to indicate how the interpretation of an event is associated with the emotional, behavioural, and biological changes. This should be done in a friendly way, and the use of gentle humour during the example sometimes helps to relax a patient. It is important to check with the person that they see the validity of this approach. When this has been agreed the therapist can then say, "Okay now let's use the same kind of approach to the kinds of problems you seem to be having. Can you give me an example of an event that has upset you in the past week. Right now, we are mainly interested to understand what this event meant for you." This is then written down under A. The affects and behaviours elicited are written in column C. Then the therapist says, "Now let's look at what was going through your mind at B, to see if we can understand what leads to those feelings and behaviours at C." When exploring an inference chain it should be conducted in the manner of a collaborative-friendly venture; it is not an interrogation. The style of the interaction should be one of caring interest (Gilbert, 1989). One tries to foster in the person a desire to explore and discover (called guided discovery), yet also convey a sense of safety.

When one decides to introduce the model of cognitive therapy, this part of a session, at least in the early days, should be clearly described so the patient can follow what is going on. This enables the person to be clear that the style of the session at this point is going to follow a certain procedure which involves explorative questioning. At all times the therapist checks with the patient that they understand and agree with the procedure. If the patient has a desire to share painful feelings and be understood, has serious shame problems or is very inhibited then there is little point in doing a highly focused work, and the therapist must be sensitive to these issues. Sometimes behavioural work may be a more early form of intervention (Beck et al., 1979).

Eliciting an inference chain is a kind of directed (as opposed to free) association. Unlike the psychoanalytic approach, which simply asks the patient to relate any thoughts (to which the therapist may then offer an interpretation), the cognitive therapist is active and directive in the use of questions and does not go beyond what has been said. To explore an inference chain requires a preparedness to suspend any effort to modify thoughts as the exploration unfolds. Some therapists tend to jump in too quickly with their own interpretations or ideas, e.g., "Do you think you are thinking this because.....?" or, "Isn't this because.....?", etc. In cognitive exploration the therapist tries not to suggest ideas but let the person discover them for themselves. Cognitive therapists believe that self-discovery works better than interpretation. Hence the importance of the Socratic "what" question. The most basic questions are: " What went through your mind?" or "What is going through your mind?"

Other common questions are:

What would happen if..... ?
What would happen then/next?
What does that lead you to think/believe?
What conclusions do you draw from that?
What do you think this means?

To get at more specific self–other schema:

What do you think other people thought?
What do you think was going through their minds?
What do you conclude about yourself?
What were you thinking about yourself
What do you think they were thinking about you?
What were you feeling about you?

To work with historical data:

When was the first time you thought/felt this way and what was happening? (elicit images and memories)
Do you often have that view?
How often have you felt/thought this way?

As a rule of thumb "what" questions encourage the person to explore the "implications" of their thoughts/interpretations. The implications the therapist is particularly interested in are those related to the pursuit of long-term goals and rules for living, idealisations, hopes and fears, and schema of self and significant others. In other words, what does this thought or idea imply? In my approach I am also interested in the underlying themes, issues of shame and blocks to exploration.

Another form of questioning seeks to explore a more causal form of thinking. In this case the questions follows a "why" set of questions, or less often a "how" set of questions.

Why do you think that?
Why do you think that happened?
How do/did you reach that conclusion?
How do you think other people would see you because of that?
How do you think other people will react to you?

Often patients only require prompts, such as "ah-ha", etc. Subtle prompts may call forth different types of information than more direct questions which can be controlling or directive. Sometimes it is useful to encourage exploration with simple words like, "because?", or "and?", "so?". This is short for, "this happened because....?", "You see that as important because....?" (Nonverbal behaviour and voice intonation are important. A "so" can sound hostile rather than indicating a position of interest.) This helps the person to link ideas and allows the discussion to flow more naturally. At other times the therapist can encourage exploration with "Can we look at this more closely?", "Can you say more about that?" Also if the therapist does not understand what the person is saying or meaning then it is often helpful to say so, e.g., "I'm not sure I understand that, could you help me by explaining further", or "Can we go into that a little", etc.

The Fantasy Journey. In some cases people find difficulty in working with real or actual events. In these cases it can be helpful to suggest a fantasy journey/scenario. For example, a person was having difficulty finding the source of his social anxiety and depression. Hence we explored something that tended to lead to anxiety. "I want you to imagine that you have to go on a crowded train. We will call this our A. Let that image come into your mind and explore with me what is going through your mind as you fantasise this." You may increase the imagery with, "Can you smell the train and hear the closing of doors?" As the person explores the image one may use the "what would happen then?" question.

Example:
T] Okay, so here you are on the train and you feel it start to move. What is going through your mind?
P] I might get anxious.
T] Okay, you get anxious. What would happen then?
P] I start to sweat.
T] And that bothers you because?
P] Other people might see this.
T] I see. So you are worried that you may become anxious and this might lead you to start sweating. If this happened other people might see it. Is that how it seems to you?
P] Yes.
T] Okay, can we explore the meaning of sweating and other people being able to see this? Let's just focus on that for a moment and see what is the most worrying thing about that?
P] Well, they may think there is something wrong with me, like I'm ill or something.
T] Like you are ill or something?
P] Yes, they may feel I'm contagious and be repelled by me.
T] Repelled by you?
P] Yes, repelled by the way I look. Later I think if I can't control this I will always be alone.

In the above case a short exploration brought the belief that other people would find the patient repellent in some way. This is what I have previously called shame/disgust (see Chapter 8). This in turn led later in the therapy to an exploration of self-concepts and (in this case) ideas that he was ashamed of his physical appearance. This turned out to be linked with his masculine identity and a long-lived fear of others seeing his body. He would not go abroad because he would have to take his shirt off in the sun and refrained from sexual activity for fear of being seen as "a poor specimen".

In other cases one might say: "Let's explore the worst. Let us for the moment fantasise that X has happened. Now what is going through your mind?"

Speaking In Pictures. This is an under-utilised technique but can be quite powerful. As we have said, automatic thoughts, especially those surrounding deep schema, are not well coded in spoken language. If the person is having particular difficulty in translating his/her ideas into language, then the therapist may ask: "What pictures come into your mind?" or "Can you describe a picture of this for me?" One person, who was having difficulty expressing his thoughts about his depression in language, was asked to describe a picture. After some thought he said: "It's like I can see this party going on and I'm standing in the garden or somewhere. It's very cold, maybe snowing and very dark. I know that no matter what I do I will not be allowed in, but must stay outside just looking in and being on my own."

In mentality theory this is close to the "outsider theme". Asked to explore this in more detail, he added that he felt a mixture of great loneliness and also anger/envy at being different from other people. This in fact was a central concern for him. Sometimes it can be helpful to ask the person to actually paint/draw a picture and then discuss the meaning of the picture with the patient. In one case the person did a clay sculpture. In describing the meaning of the sculpture he was able to articulate a sense of personal meaning that had escaped him when working with language. The sculpture acted as a kind of gestalt of meaning. Where appropriate, it is useful to use a medium of communication that makes sense and has value to the person. Paintings and sculptures however are taken as hypothesises or approximations that can be changed in the light of new information. Some patients really enjoy working with paintings and drawings and, as Jung indicated, one can see changes in the themes of the pictures over time. All the time however one is working on the meaning.

Role Play. Role play is also a very powerful technique for eliciting various forms of meaning. There are a number of ways this can be done. For example, a person who is frightened of behaving assertively may be asked to role-play an assertive sequence of behaviour.

The therapist then explores the beliefs about this (e.g., I am being unkind, other people will think I am being selfish and I must maintain other people's approval; or, I will be embarrassed and go blank). Other forms of role play can involve the re-enactment of previous painful events, e.g., arguments. Again the therapist can check the meanings that the person constructs about these episodes. As a rule of thumb, role play works best when the patient and therapist have developed a good working alliance. Without this the patient may not really get into the role play but just mimic it and not really be in touch with the powerful emotions that need to be understood and worked with. Other techniques for exploring internal dialogues and affects within the self are those of the two-chair techniques (Greenberg, 1979; Greenberg & Safran, 1987; Greenberg et al., 1990; Safran & Segal, 1990). Some cognitive therapists will even use role play in more abusive experiences. However, I am not sure about this and I think there may be a problem with therapist trust here and this may produce transference confusions. In my own case I stay in the role of therapist and use the patient's own experiences and dialogues or an empty chair.

Complex Chains

Dryden (1989) has recently articulated the importance of complex chains, that is, how one set of ideas and conclusions set off another set of ideas and conclusions (or in my view how one theme triggers another). For example, a person may become angry because they thought that someone was deliberately doing something to hurt them or was neglectful. However, the experience of anger led to fear, with the thought "If I get angry I may get out of control. If I get out of control I will look silly and be humiliated." If a person gets into a high state of arousal it is important to recognise that it may be very difficult to get out of this cycle with cognitive restructuring. Typical here is the person who says, "I understand the ideas but when I get into this state I can't get out of it." Sometimes physical activity can be helpful like running or digging the garden. Relaxation is rarely helpful in depression if this increases focus on self and rumination on thoughts. Hence distraction can be more helpful. The therapist identifies complex chains (or interacting themes) and teaches early identification. Here it is preventive measures that must be taken.

Summarising and Challenging

Summarising is used in many different ways. It is often used in taking a history and can be a form of crystallisation, to help a patient and therapist to focus on recurrent patterns/themes of behaviour, events and styles of explanation for events. As the therapist proceeds with an inference chain it is important to summarise frequently, starting at the top of the chain and working down. It is in fact an important skill to use. Often the therapist is attempting to help the person reveal, usually in language, but not always, the (sometimes hidden) meanings that tend to control their behaviour and affect automatically and most novice therapists do not summarise enough. The person may never have done this kind of exploration before and can sometimes find putting their meanings into language difficult.

Recursive Feedback. Cognitive therapists often like to draw or diagram out their summaries with a patient to give a visual overview. This is especially helpful to show positive recursive feedback, which can be drawn as a circle. For example, "I feel depressed—when depressed I can't do anything—when I can't do anything I feel useless—when I feel useless I get more depressed—when I get more depressed I do less, etc." Types of feedback circle are shown in Fig. 13.1(a).

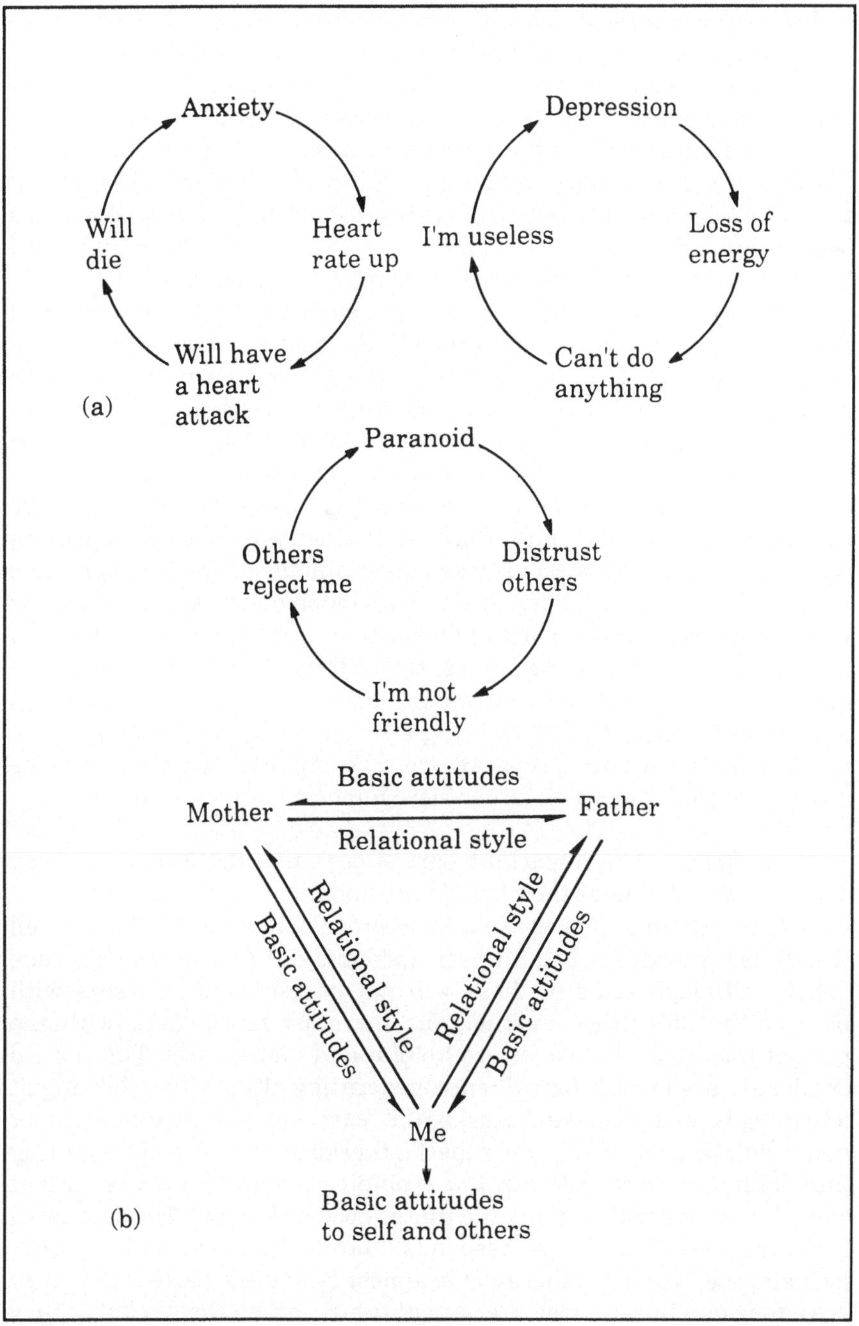

FIG. 13.1. Examples of recursive feedback

Discussion can centre on where best to intervene and helping make predictions—e.g., "If you could stop putting yourself down when you feel unable to do things would this be helpful? What would be the advantages and disadvantages of giving up putting yourself down"?

Some therapists also find it useful to link with the past by asking "When was the first time you thought of things like this?" This may reveal that the explanation the person offers was picked up in childhood and has been used as the standard explanation in the face of certain undesired life events. This can be drawn out more fully as shown in Fig. 13.1(b).

A patient's father had left home when she was eight. She explained this as due to her mother being moody. Subsequently not only did she believe she was like her mother (moody) but also, in intimate relationships, she feared that if she were not constantly happy her boyfriend(s) would leave her. In fact she had much evidence to discount this view but therapy revealed that when she became unhappy she was also very rejecting. As she said later this was "to reject them first before they could reject me." In other words in complex ways she was repeating patterns of behaviour she had picked up in childhood. The key cognitions were, "If I show I'm unhappy they will abandon me; if they abandon me I am worthless. However if I abandon them first then at least I'm in control." This led to a sense of resentment ("why do I always have to be happy to loved"). She had not come to understand her experiences as individual to her, rather than being a rerun of mother. Helping her to re-label her experiences, separate from her mother, and deal with the anger and grief over a lost father were important therapeutic steps.

Challenging. The important part of cognitive therapy is teaching clients how to challenge their beliefs and meanings. This can be achieved by helping patients to keep thought records (Beck et al., 1979). Fennell (1989) has provided a helpful patients' hand-out for how to challenge beliefs, although some of these will not be useful for patients with personality difficulties. Further, the therapist must check with the patient that such challenges are helpful and make sense. The central challenges are looking for evidence, generating alternatives, looking at advantages and disadvantages, and carrying out experiments or homework (Burns, 1980). One aspect a therapist should avoid is getting into arguments with patients. For example, a common one is a patient says, "There is nothing in my life that is good or I enjoy." The therapist, hit by this overall blackness, responds, "Surely there is something. Let's look and see." Here the therapist is almost telling the patient that they are wrong and this can lead the patient to strengthen their belief as they battle with the therapist to have their experience of blackness understood. Second, homework or experiments can lead to a patient feeling worse. Again the therapist must avoid implying that the patient has done something wrong but rather show interest to understand what happened.

Flash cards can be helpful. On one side the patients works out with the therapist their thoughts, e.g., "I am never able to do as good a job as I'd like. I always seem to fail. I am a really useless person. What's the point of trying." Rather than having to write out these thoughts for themselves they can put a tick on the card as a thought happens. On the back, therapist and patient work out some challenges that the patient feels are helpful. For example: "These are pretty unkind things to be saying to myself when I'm feeling down; I would not speak to a friend like this; I don't HAVE to do everything perfectly; just because my mother called me these things doesn't make it true; I can take it in stages and learn to focus on what I can do; I can define a half-full glass as half empty or half full", and so forth. Different patients find different forms of challenge helpful. In one, an appeal to reason is helpful; in another, the appeal to self-nurturing is helpful. Sometimes patients say, "When I looked on the back of my card I heard your voice and that was helpful". This helps the internalisation of selfobject relationships and cues memory. Gradually patients learn to challenge for themselves.

RULES, ASSUMPTIONS, AND ATTITUDES

Rules are operating instructions for life. In general they can be regarded as the instructions or beliefs that relate to happiness and the avoidance of pain and unpleasantness (I must be loved, or I must be successful, to be happy, and so forth). In fact many of the rules suggested by Beck (1976) are very similar to Bibring's concepts of aspirations and ego ideals. Certain rules and attitudes have been developed into the dysfunctional attitude scale (DAS) (see Blackburn & Davidson, 1990, pages 209–214, for a copy of this scale). Here are some typical dysfunctional attitudes from the DAS, as suggested by Beck:

4) If I do not do well all the time, people will not respect me.
11) If I can't do something well there is no point in trying.
16) I am nothing if a person I love doesn't love me.
23) I should be upset if I make a mistake.
25) To be a good, moral, worthwhile person I must always put the needs of others first.

Dysfunctional attitudes measure various domains and social themes, e.g., perfectionism and approval (e.g., People will probably think less of me if I make a mistake; if a person asks for help it is a sign of weakness).

Much work has now been conducted with the dysfunctional attitude scale (Blackburn & Davidson, 1990). It has been found that depressed patients score significantly higher on the DAS than nondepressed people. However, so do many patient groups and dysfunctional attitudes are not specific to depression. DAS scores correlate with neuroticism (Teasdale & Dent, 1987). It has also been found that the DAS is mood sensitive and subject to changes in state. However, high levels of dysfunctional attitudes may predict poor response to treatment, and endogenous patients tend to score lower than nonendogenous patients (Peselow, Robins, Block, Barouche & Fieve, 1990). For a review of the research and issues surrounding the whole area of cognitive assessment in depression see Clark and Beck (1989) and Goldberg and Shaw, (1989).

Different attitudes are prominent in different personalities (Beck, 1983). Sociotropic (socially dependent) individuals follow rules that say, "I must maintain my relationships, I must be close to people who can support me." Autonomous people have rules like, "I must succeed. I must be in control." Beck's concepts of sociotropic and autonomous types are so similar to Arieti and Bemporad's (1980a,b) ideas of dominant other and dominant goal types (see pages 359–362 this volume) that we will not explore them again here (see also Chapter 4). Research has shown that high needs for approval and sociotropic traits are associated with depression, although the evidence is less clear for autonomy (see Chapter 4 and Nietzel & Harris, 1990). Sociotropy shows a high correlation with neuroticism (Gilbert & Reynolds, 1990).

Personality disorders also have different rules and self–other schema (Beck et al., 1990). Different types of cognitive therapists have come up with different types of rules and dysfunctional attitudes and some, like Albert Ellis (Ellis & Whiteley, 1979; Ellis, 1977a,b,c,), believe that there are about ten or so basic rules that are nearly always associated with distress. These are things like "I can't stand it if....." (called awfullising), or, "I must have or be....." (called musturbation), or, "I demand that....." (called demanding). Sometimes people will deny they are "musturbating" or demanding, etc, but if this is so it is usually possible to show that the strength of their affective reactions to events suggests otherwise.

SELF–OTHER SCHEMA

By now the reader will be familiar with the fact that self–other schema are core ideas in object relations theory, attachment theory, and self psychology, and are not original to cognitive therapy. Such theories see self–other schema as originating from early experience. However,

TABLE 13.1
Self–Other Schema

	HISTORY (A) parents (B) siblings (C) peers	
	Self	*Other*
Positive	good, friendly, strong, able etc.	good, friendly, strong, able etc.
Negative	bad, unfriendly, weak, unable, etc.	bad, unfriendly, weak, unable, etc

cognitive therapist give them a cognitive treatment, i.e., they are interested in their core of meaning. A useful way to consider them is given in Table 13.1.

However there are other domains such as, "how I think others see me" (e.g., as able, kind, etc) and another of "how I want others to see me", etc. Cognitive therapists also make a distinction between conditional and unconditional self–other schema. A conditional view is "I am good if..." whereas an unconditional view is "I am bad regardless", i.e., there is nothing I can do to make me into a good person (Beck et al., 1990).

In depression it is believed that there is a switch from previous (usually) positive schema of self and others to the activation of negative schema. This is important for therapy because it is believed that, stored in long-term memory, are a set of positive schema and that working at the level of automatic thoughts and rules, gaining and testing hypothesis, will help to reactivate these positive schema which do exist, but have become latent in the depression (Beck et al., 1979; Fennell, 1989; Blackburn & Davidson, 1990).

In personality disorder, however, positive schema of self and others may not exist or at least be very fragile even at the best of times. Hence techniques to reactivate and tap into a person's premorbid level of functioning are ineffective because there is rather little (in long-term memory) to tap into. The therapy with personality disorders then becomes much more one of developing something "anew" and this takes much longer, requiring a different focus of the therapy especially the importance of the therapeutic relationship (Beck et al., 1990). As discussed in Chapter 4, it is important to gain some idea of the person's premorbid level of functioning. Often novice therapists attempt to use techniques designed for non-personality-disorder folk with personality disordered folk, to the disappointment and frustration of all concerned.

Self-schema have become a source of research in their own right (e.g., Kuiper, 1988; Kuiper et al., 1990). And there is growing evidence that self-perception is focused on negative information, possibly as the result of the activation of negative self-schema. Interpersonal schema have also been suggested (Safran & Segal, 1990). These developments greatly enrich the cognitive model and in the latter case offer up new ways of working therapeutically.

Self-schema or Selfobject?

The concept of schema is focused on knowledge, beliefs, styles of information processing, and attention. The concept of selfobject is focused on self "as experienced" and therefore has a more direct relationship with affect (see Chapter 10). In my view both concepts are valid and necessary. However, selfobject relations are more easily related to the idea of conditioned emotional responses (see Chapter 14). There are however some elements crucial to the selfobject idea that are not obvious in self-schema. First is the view that selfobject experiences also indicate types of need. Second the concept of selfobject points to the importance of the therapist acting as a soothing selfobject and not in such a way as to activate negative selfobject experience. This does not mean avoidance of negative affect, but rather the avoidance of the therapist acting as a source of (internal) attack. Indeed it is common for patients to fear the therapist getting too close in case the therapist discovers that they are really no good, bad, evil, etc. One patient felt like "a turd with a hat on. I don't want you to get too close because while I let most people see only my hat you may see I'm all shit underneath." With some patients this needs to be explored very early in the therapy. Any shame selfobject experience motivates concealment and avoidance.

Third, certain experiences in the therapy will be avoided if the patient experiences these as possibly fragmenting. At these times the patient can retreat into their own internal fantasy world, not revealed to the therapist, and so not allow for new learning and experiences to take place. Hence self psychology is more concerned with the therapeutic relationship and how the therapist should set about the process of healing with a clear "feel" and empathy for the patient's internal experience. As I have indicated in Chapter 7, so much of our lives are spent "living in the minds of others" that this aspect of therapy is crucial. Also to some extent it may be common that we are not able to experience ourselves positively until we have had some experience of reflected positiveness from others. Our earliest experience of ourselves is to some extent secondhand, for as children we may not be able to generate our own self-experiences. Rather, they are created by others from positive rewards given and pleasure in self that others provide.

It–Me

Most cognitive therapists suggest that many of us have a basic it–me problem. There is a certain fuzziness in the boundary between evaluations of performance and evaluations (experiences) of self. The problem here is that we can become puppet or yoyo people. If I do (it) well then I feel good about myself. If I do poorly then I experience myself negatively. In my view this separation of performance and self is crucial to successful therapy, but it is never absolute. This boundary is helped by cognitive and role complexity (see Chapter 4). But sometimes a focus on the concept of self-worth is necessary to help patients separate experiences of performance from evaluations of worth. Using the advantages–disadvantages techniques the therapist may find that the patient wants to maintain a belief in self-worth = performance for it carries a certain hope of meeting ideals (if I succeed then others will love, respect me). Or a patient may believe that if they do not continually attack themselves they may become lazy and useless. Also there is the good–bad paradox (see Chapter 4).

In ranking therapy I spend some time exploring the switch from an internal competitive (self-downing, performance-focused) relationship to an internal caring (nurturing) relationship—in other words to change the main mentality that seems to be the source of self-experience. Another way to think of this is as a switch from an agonic internal style (punishing, unforgiving, shaming) to a hedonic internal style (forgiving, caring, encouraging) style. One can use the friend technique, or two chairs to help this develop.

Unfortunately our culture is competitive rather than cooperative. Hence the performance-based evaluations of self are constantly reinforced. But like the Buddhists (Crook, 1980) we can nevertheless attempt to help people see that their attachment to success is a source of suffering. In cognitive therapy we talk of this as the "musts". "I must succeed or be loved otherwise I am useless, valueless, no good, etc." What is being attempted here is a gradual withdrawal from the world such that the person begins to be more in touch with an internal sense of self or the core of one's experiencing self: one's "isness." In this way the person becomes more able to set their own goals, enjoy things for their own instrinsic properties, rather than succeed only to please others and for secondary rewards.

TABLE 13.2
Overview of Cognitive Therapy Concepts

COGNITIVE THERAPY CONCEPTS

1. Automatic Thoughts
   (a) Personalisation (attributions)
   (b) Overgeneralisation (global thinking)
   (c) Attention
   (d) Black and white thinking, etc.

2. Rules/Assumptions
   (Musts, Have to's, Shoulds and Oughts)
   (a) I must be successful
   (b) I must have a loving relationship
   (c) I should never make mistakes
   (d) I must be approved of, etc.

3. SELF–OTHER SCHEMA

	Conditional	*Unconditional*
(a)	I am good/bad if ...	I am good/bad regardless
(b)	I am competent/incompetent if ...	I am competent/incompetent regardless
(c)	I am lovable/unlovable if ...	I am lovable/unlovable regardless
(a)	They are /good/bad if ...	They are good/bad regardless

(etc).

Automatic thoughts are the rapid images and ideas that come to mind, elicited by specific events. Rules and assumptions are the constantly present, basic concepts for attaining goals (e.g to be happy I must, etc). Self-schema are the core internal focusing constructs that are at the centre of experience. The strongest affects are aroused by events and cognitions that have personal meaning.

Overview

An overview of the main elements of cognitive theory is given in Table 13.2. Having given a flavour of the basic principles of this approach we now turn to the assumptions of the theory.

BASIC THEORY AND ASSUMPTIONS OF THE COGNITIVE MODEL

Beck (1974b) points out that there are those who believe that for normal subjects the conceptualisation and appraisal of events determine the affective state, but in psychopathology the affective state is believed to determine cognitive content. This complete reversal of cause and effect, between normal and abnormal emotion, is, in Beck's view, erroneous and constitutes a major source of confusion. In Beck's (1974b, pp.128–129) model of depression the difference between abnormal and normal emotional states:

> ... lies in the degree of correspondence between the conceptualization and the veridical stimulus configuration. In psychopathological states perseverative faulty conceptualization leads to excessive or inappropriate affective disturbance.
>
> The typical conceptualizations leading to specific affects appear to be the same in both "normal" and "abnormal" responses. In abnormal conditions, however, conceptualizations are determined to a greater extent by internal processes which distort the stimulus situation.

The concept that the theme of the appraisal is the same for both normal and pathological mood states is a crucial element of Beck's theory and leads directly to two basic assumptions: (1) that normal and abnormal states exist on a continuum and are determined by the same processes; and (2) that the factors (conceptualisations) which determine normal emotion (anger, sadness, joy) also determine abnormal emotion. For abnormal emotion, however, the congruence between the external event and its cognitive appraisal (meaning and implications) is low and the affective disturbance is a consequence of this low congruence.

These two assumptions need careful consideration. In regard to the first assumption, it is possible that discontinuities are manifest in abnormal emotional states but are not observable in the cognitive domain—that is, they may be present in biological or behavioural response systems only. In this sense we can hear again Zilboorg and Henry's (1941) warning that an overconcern with how things appear from the outside may lead us to derive unwarranted conclusions about how things work inside. In regard to the second assumption, sociological models of depression (Brown & Harris, 1978a) have some grounds for argument. These researchers have shown that depression is not so much a problem of cognitive incongruence (or distortion) but is related to real life events.

Beck suggests that the general content of the depressive appraisal system is much the same throughout the spectrum of the depressive disorders and that cognitive distortions are ubiquitous among persons suffering from depression. The major theme of the depressed person's cognitive appraisal system centres on the appraisal of loss. He suggests that loss is "the clue" to understanding depression, whereas threat and danger relate to anxiety (for a comparison see Beck et al., 1985). He proposes that a lowering of mood occurs when individuals appraise or evaluate that a reduction in their domain has taken place. Moreover, the attribute or object that is perceived as being lost must have had some positive value. For the depressed person the appraisal of loss pervades evaluations concerning *the self*, *the world*, and *the future*. As a result depressives perceive their world as full of obstacles; they see themselves as losers, having experienced some significant loss(es) in their personal domain and lacking the necessary skills and opportunities to make up the perceived deficits and inadequacies; they see the future as unchanging and empty and that they are doomed to be this way forever. The light has gone out on life. These powerful negative attitudes all contain significant loss implications. Together, the negative views of the self, the world, and the future are referred to as the *negative cognitive triad*.

Beck's theory also outlines the processes which bring the negative cognitive triad into being and maintain its prominence, distorting information processing. There are a number of influences involved in these processes. Thus, as Beck et al. (1979, pp.14–51) describe:

> As is apparent, depressed persons are prone to structure their experiences in relatively primitive ways. They tend to make global judgments regarding events that impinge on their lives. The meanings that flood their consciousness are likely to be negative and extreme. In contrast to this primitive type of thinking, more mature thinking automatically integrates life situations into many dimensions or qualities (instead of a single category), in quantitative rather than qualitative terms and according to relative rather than absolutistic standards. In primitive thinking the complexity, variability, and diversity of human experiences and behaviour are reduced into a few crude categories.

They suggest an analog between the primitive thinking of the depressive and the childlike styles of thinking outlined by Piaget. This is an important comparison because it raises a number of questions. First, to what degree have depressives learned adult (mature) styles of thinking? Beck himself is unclear on this. Sometimes he seems to suggest that depressives have, by nature, a tendency toward primitive thinking. At other times primitive thinking only emerges as the person begins to become depressed. It would be untenable to suggest that all depressives (when well) have a tendency toward primitive thinking, though this may be true for a subgroup (e.g., those with personality difficulties). Some depressives make very good adjustments when their illness is treated, and there is no evidence, as yet, to suggest that they are any more primitive in thinking when well than non-depressives. Moreover, if this style of thinking were present all the time would the individual ever be free of depression? Why do some depressions not appear until comparatively later in life? If Beck is correct in his primitive thinking argument, then we must be observing a fluctuating picture.

The second question, then, is what triggers this style of thinking? Is it incidents which invoke latent, evaluative schema (Beck's view), biological shifts associated with mood change, and/or real events in the world?

Vulnerability. Beck suggests that various internal constructions of the world are learned in childhood. Later experiences may displace these learned constructions (or schema) so that more adaptive ones are normally used, but the early constructions remain, ready to become dominant again when situations similar to those existing at their initial developmental period are present. Beck (1967, p.277) argues thus:

> The vulnerability of the depression-prone person is attributable to the constellation of enduring negative attitudes about himself, about the world and about his future. Even though these attitudes (or concepts) may not be prominent or even discernible at a given time, they persist in a latent state like an explosive charge ready to be detonated by an appropriate set of conditions. Once activated, these concepts dominate the person's thinking and lead to typical depressive symptomatology.

Thus, Beck's theory of predisposition suggests that the negative cognitive triad already exists in the depression-prone adult, but in a latent state. The development of this triad, the place of origin, can be found in the early learning history of the individual. Beck (1974a, p.7) comments:

> In the course of his development, the depression-prone person may become sensitized by certain unfavourable types of life situations such as the loss of a parent or chronic rejection by his peers. Other unfavourable conditions of a more insidious nature may similarly produce vulnerability to depression. These traumatic experiences predispose the individual to overreact to analogous conditions later in life. He has a tendency to make extreme, absolute judgments when such situations occur.

Beck (1967) also argues that the depression-prone individual attaches negative attitudes to certain attributes, such as "It's terrible to be stupid", or "It's disgusting to be weak". The tendency to label the self as having these "bad attributes" again appears to occur in the early learning history of the individual. Beck (1967, pp.275–276) believes that failure may be labelled as evidence of being inept or inadequate. For example:

> ... a child who gets the notion that he is inept, as a result of either a failure or of being called inept by someone else, may interpret subsequent experiences according to this notion. Each time thereafter that he encounters difficulties in manual tasks he may have a tendency to judge himself as inept. Each negative judgment tends to reinforce the negative concept or self-image. Thus a cycle is set up: each negative judgment fortifies the negative self-image which in turn facilitates a negative interpretation of subsequent experiences which further consolidates the negative self-concept. Unless this negative image is extinguished, it becomes structuralized, i.e., it becomes a permanent formation in the cognitive organization. Once a concept is structuralized, it remains permanently with the individual, even though it may be dormant; it becomes a cognitive structure, or schema.

Thus Beck's model of depression suggests that the depression-prone individual, early on in life, develops particular negative cognitive schema relating to the world, the self, and the future. Although these negative schema may not be discernible at any given time, they are easily invoked by life events which are similar to those that were responsible for their formation. Thus, for example, the individual who has been labelled as inept or inadequate by others in failing at a certain task will tend to respond to failure with this concept (of being inadequate or inept) when he confronts failure in the future. The result of this is the activation of the negative view of the self. This is not that dissimilar to selfobject relations, except that selfobjects operate at a more affective level and are important for the integration of the personality and its cohesiveness. Beck gives no role to the process of mourning previous (perhaps early) losses or ideals but this is sometimes important.

As negative schema come to dominate the individual's cognitive processes, the individual will interpret all failures, trivial or otherwise, as evidence that they are inadequate. This shift toward a negative appraisal of other events outside the invoking situation is a cognitive distortion which results from the activation of the (previously dormant) negative view of the self. The cognitive distortion, however, confirms the correctness of the invoked negative schema and leads to a further increase in its dominance in cognitive processing. Thus the more dominant the negative cognitive schema becomes, the more cognitive distortions occur and the greater the disturbance of affect and depth of depression. Hence Beck argues for positive recursive feedback system in depression.

Who Benefits?

Beck (1963; 1967; 1970; 1974a; 1974b; 1976; 1987; Beck et al., 1979; Clark & Beck, 1989) and others (e.g., Fennell, 1989; Blackburn & Davidson, 1990) have published many accounts of the cognitive therapy of depression. A number of studies have shown that this is an effective treatment of many forms of depression (see Free & Oei, 1989; Blackburn & Davidson, 1990; Hollon, Shelton & Loosen, 1991, for a review). There is also preliminary evidence that cognitive therapy may reduce relapse (Hollon & Najavits, 1988; Hollon et al., 1991). The relationship of endogenous symptoms to response is complex and may relate to severity. Persons et al. (1988, p.572) found that four variables were related to outcome with cognitive therapy: endogenous symptoms; initial level of depression as measured by BDI; compliance with homework, and interaction between initial BDI level and homework. In regard to drop-out from therapy, lack of endogenous symptoms, presence of personality disorder, and high BDI scores, and possibly education level were associated with drop-out.

The model is primarily relevant to the unipolar, non-psychotic depressions, at least as regards its current therapeutic implications (Beck et al., 1979). However, I have used the approach with bipolar depressed patients as they move out of their acute phase. I personally do not think these patients should be excluded from possible help in trying to restore their self-structures just because their disorders are bipolar. Also, helping new bipolars to manage their illness, deal with shame and fear of the future, identify early warning signals, slow down, and decatastrophise the illness (i.e., give social information about successful bipolars like Winston Churchill) can be helpful. My experience is that patients have found this useful and my psychiatrist colleagues and I certainly feel that adding the kinds of approach I have discussed here to drug treatment has reduced relapse. I am quite unclear why no research trials have been conducted with this group. May be it shows again the over-medicalisation and false assumptions that go with disease theories. Indeed, recently, Beck (1987) also notes that biological factors may be important in some unipolar depressions and has moved away from a causal theory of depression. The focus is more on the recursive thought patterns that amplify dysphoric responses to life events and maintain depression.

Comments

Beck's model of depression suggests that predisposition is laid early in life. Sensitising experiences which produce negative views of the self, world, and future become dormant cognitive schema. Under certain types of stress these schema become invoked again as organising cognitive systems and produce a variety of distortions in sampling (attending to) information and deriving conclusions from that information. Cognitive errors and distortions confirm these negative schema and lead to a vicious circle. In this situation the negative schema produce cognitive distortions and the cognitive distortions produce greater dominance of the negative schema which in turn produce still greater distortions and so on. In other words our thoughts and fantasies can have recursive, amplifying effects that lead us into one state of mind or another. Hence our thoughts and appraisals shape patterns of self-organisation. This recursive element is not articulated in other theories quite so clearly. Trying to nail down schema like lego pieces runs the risk of loosing this sense of fluidity. As the person enters into a downward spiral the style of thinking becomes less differentiated and the probability that accurate conceptualisations of external events can be made is reduced. Also explorative behaviour is reduced. In my view this style of thinking emerges as the pattern of depression begins to crystallise and internal defensiveness and inhibition begin to exert an effect.

There have been many recent developments to the cognitive view of vulnerability (Brewin, 1988; 1989). Among the most important has been the linkage with attachment theory (e.g., Guidano & Liotti, 1983) and the development of interpersonal schema theory (Safran & Segal, 1990). In terms of the therapy, the emphasis on the role of collaborative empiricism, gaining data and testing out ideas and the introduction of homework and important behaviour components, role play, and so forth into treatment, make cognitive therapy a watershed in psychological treatment. What all cognitive based theorists share is a concern with what has been called meaning-making (Gilbert, 1989), the construction of subjective internal meaning. As with other therapies, the cognitive therapist realises that no one can live easily with others until they can live with themselves. For me the growth of positive self-organisations and the alleviation of the bad/weak/subordinate self-organisation is at the heart of treatment.

SOME CONTROVERSIES OF THE COGNITIVE MODEL

Because of its attempt to offer a scientific theory, the cognitive approach has generated much research and debate. Many of the controversies discussed below are not specific to cognitive approaches but are introduced here because it has been in the cognitive arena that they have been most frequently debated.

1. *Cognition–emotion interaction*: Zajonc (1980; 1984) suggested that stimulus events can be appraised by emotional systems and cognitive systems relatively independently. Affective judgments are precognitive, automatic, holistic, and irrevocable, and to a considerable degree occur independently of cognitive processes. These suggestions seriously challenged the cognitive axiom that abnormal emotions are "nothing but" the products of specific, cognitive conceptualisations. Lazarus (1982) disagreed. This area is controversial, but potentially embarrassing to cognitive therapy (although see Kuiper et al., 1990). However, this interface is now regarded as extremely complex (Rachman, 1981; Leventhal & Scherer, 1987; Bradley & Power, 1988) and a new journal devoted to this issue, called *Cognition and Emotion*, is now established. Emotional processing and blocks to emotional awareness often need to be tackled directly (Greenberg & Safran, 1987; Safran & Segal, 1990).

2. *The role of unconscious processes*: In 1976 Beck more or less ruled out the importance of unconscious motivations or inferential processes. But Shevrin and Dickman (1980) suggest that unconscious processes clearly exist and may operate with rules that are different to those of conscious ones, and conscious awareness may occur at a relatively late stage in information processing (see also Dixon & Henley, 1980; Nisbitt & Wilson, 1977; Brewin, 1988; 1989). The extent to which latent schema, rules, and some automatic thoughts (fantasies) operate at levels below awareness is not clear from Beck's theory. But they are certainly processes which are not always in the forefront of consciousness. Ellis (1977c), on the other hand, does not rule out the role of the unconscious as does Beck (1976). Ellis (1977c) suggests individuals may be unaware of the ideas and attitudes which predispose to distress, but this does not mean they are deeply hidden or repressed. However, new work shows that certain types of judgement may not be accessible to conscious processing and information processing is extremely complex (see for example, Safran & Segal, 1990; Barnard & Teasdale, 1990).

Power and Brewin (in press) have compared early analytic theories of unconscious processing with modern cognitive models derived from research. They argue that conscious processes tend to be sequential, slow, flexible, effortful, and are easy to modify compared to unconscious processes which tend to be in parallel, fast, inflexible, effortless, and more difficult to modify. They explore the research that suggests that much unconscious processing is modular and that modules can be encapsulated from each other. As in evolution theory modular processes evolved for speed and their adaptiveness, not rationality (see Chapter 5). Also, affect can have a powerful encapsulating effect, i.e., the more highly aroused an affect the more difficult it is to switch from one theme of module to another (Gilbert , 1989).

3. *Brain state*: Healy and Williams (1988) have drawn attention to the importance of internal, biological states to our experience and evaluations. Gilbert (1984; 1989) pointed out that brain states have important modulating effects on cognitive processes and that brain states could be changed by various means, endogenous hormonal changes, head injury, viral infection and so forth. A very skilled cognitive therapist told me how surprised she had been by the dysphoria and loss of energy she had felt following a hysterectomy and how much better/well she had felt on hormone replacement therapy. In Chapter 4 we explored seasonal affective disorder and in Chapter 6 (and Gilbert, 1984) we saw how loss of control exerted direct biological effects. Breier et al. (1987) have demonstrated that even laboratory induced lack of control over noise in humans can have an effect on activation of the hypothalamic–pituitary–adrenal axis. Hence brain states are important mediators of experience and changes of brain state occur for many reasons other than just cognitive-evaluative reasons.

4. *Specificity*: Some of the cognitive variables held responsible for depression are not specific to depression. Anorexia nervosa, alcoholism, personality disorder, and some schizophrenias are often associated with dysfunctional automatic thoughts and attitudes, low self-esteem and negative views of the world. Hopelessness occurs across diagnostic subtypes (Melges & Bowlby, 1969) and is more highly correlated with suicidal intent than depression per se (Minkoff, Bergman, Beck, & Beck, 1973; Wetzel, 1976). Blackburn and Eunson (1989) found that of the three elements of the negative cognitive triad (negative views of self, world, and future), negative view of the self and the world occurred significantly more frequently than negative view of the future. This data was gained from a sampling of depressive thoughts as they underwent cognitive therapy. A psychiatric control group is required for further study. It is unclear what the implications are for those theories that focus on hopelessness (e.g., Abramson et al., 1989) but such data support the evolutionary theory.

5. *Subjects*: There is considerable doubt as to the value of work using students as subjects, and mood induction procedures in nondepressives. While such investigations point up important cognitive–mood interactions, they may show little more than the fact that cognitive appraisal is "one of" the variables which influence affect (see Chapter 16). Very few, if any, of the studies using unhappy students have controlled for personality or background levels of stress. Further, real

life events are related to depression (Brown & Harris, 1978a; Brown, 1989), may provoke depression independently (Parry & Brewin, 1988), and are associated with recovery (Tennant, Bebbington & Hurry, 1981a; Brown et al ., 1988; Brown, 1989; Chapter 15).

6. *Cognitive distortion*: The idea that depressed patients are in some sense distorted in their thinking and are making errors is troublesome. In some depressions, cognitive bias and distortion may be gross and across the board. In other cases, cognitive distortion of the real world may be relatively minor. This suggests that cognitive distortion may be dimensionally represented and not equally relevant for all cases. Whether or not the degree of cognitive distortion correlates with severity, or type of disorder, is unknown. More serious perhaps has been the growing conclusion that depressives may not be distorted in their thinking but rather more realistic (Krebs et al., 1988; Taylor & Brown, 1988).

7. *The social domain*: Although Beck et al. (1979) acknowledge the importance of social comparison, early experience with care-givers (Beck, 1967) and other social phenomena such as sociotropy, cognitive therapy is not really a social cognition theory. The role of envy, shame, and anger is not given any special prominence in the theory. Yet, as stressed in this book, social evaluation has been at the centre of the evolution of mind. Also, these cognitive processes did not evolve for rational thinking but to facilitate social success. It is social success that is most associated with positive affect, and the lack of it with negative affect (see Chapters 5–8).

8. *The therapeutic relationships*: In cognitive therapy the therapeutic relationship is one of collaboration. The problem is that cognitive therapy (like psychoanalysis) tends to be a very intra-psychic theory and although the role of empathy and positive regard are recognised they are not given special importance but are in the background. Yet the capacity to mobilise hope and counteract demoralisation may depend crucially on the therapist–patient interaction, and some therapist personalities are almost certainly more likely to be able to mobilise these than others (Gilbert et al., 1989). Ranking theory would predict that any therapy that enables a patient to feel valued by another (especially one seen perhaps to have higher status or skill) could be helpful. Therapies would also be effective that enable a patient to explore, as opening up exploration is a shift towards the safety system that allows for the integration of new information (Gilbert, 1989; Chapters 5 and 6). Ranking theory would therefore predict that therapy would fail if (amongst other reasons) the patient saw the therapist as of lower status than themselves, if this led to lack of respect for the skills of the therapist, if they had significant problems with envy that went unaddressed, or felt unvalued by the therapist.

9. *Philosophical differences and the issue of development*: Important philosophical differences are beginning to emerge within the cognitive camp (Carmin & Dowd, 1988; Dowd & Pace 1989). A key issue centres on whether humans are simply accessible to a re-educative and a logical positivist approach or whether they are maturing growing beings—the teleological approach (e.g., Mahoney & Gabriel, 1987). The role of maturation until recently (Rosen, 1989; Beck et al., 1990) has been ignored and humans have been treated as scientists who simply test theories and correct false assumptions (given the right education).

10. *Segregation*: Cognitive theory suffers from a tendency to select one aspect of phenomenology at the expense of others. When we do this we are confronted with the problem of how cognitive processes give rise to other aspects of depression (e.g., the vegetative changes, sleep disturbance, and so on, see Chapter 16). Also the issues of individuation and transformation are not discussed in cognitive theory. But a key concern is how do people mature, become able to integrate information over different domains, and from different processing modules (Power & Brewin, in press)? A highly defensive psychology that is threat sensitive and non-explorative may never integrate other aspects of their potential, may close out choices and so forth.

11. *Therapeutic specificity*: Does cognitive therapy have mode-specific effects? Well, at the present time this is unknown. However, one recent, large collaborative study (Imber et al., 1990) of interpersonal therapy, cognitive behaviour therapy, and clinical management plus drug or placebo found that there were very few substantive differences in mode of effect except, possibly, need for approval. In ranking theory this would be an important finding (especially if it linked with social comparison). The absence of other, mode-specific effects lead these researchers to agree with Frank (1982) who suggested that most therapies work in similar ways. However, we still await work on relapse and prevention of new episodes.

Space does not allow us to enter further into the discussion of the fascinating debates over the controversies but I hope the reader has a general grasp of the main points. Those interested in more detailed discussion of the controversies within the cognitive theory of depression might consult Bradley and Power, (1988); Alloy (1988); Freeman et al. (1989); Kuiper et al. (1990); Mahoney and Gabriel (1987).

Evolution Theory and Cognitive Therapy

Cognitive therapy has had an enormous impact on the treatment of not only depression but other disorders as well. Furthermore, many therapists who do not endorse all the tenets of cognitive therapy (e.g., Bowlby, 1980; Greenberg & Safran, 1987) have, nevertheless, been greatly influenced by it and have modified various aspects to their ideas (Safran & Segal, 1990). My own practice is centred around a core of concepts derived from cognitive therapy. But in terms of a theory for the explanation of depressive phenomenology, ranking theory parts company with cognitive theory in some important ways.

1. Evolution theory places much greater emphasis on innate (modular) mechanisms of mind and social predispositions and needs. Evolution theory suggests that social relationships and the way we treat each other can play an important role in depression (see Chapters 6, 7, and 15). Evolution theory places less emphasis on the person as responsible for their own distress though it endorses the role of recursive feedback (called the internal referee, Chapter 6). It also recognises that learning new ways of coping is often paramount to treatment. However, evolution theory sides with the theories of human needs (Chapter 10) and suggests that understanding human needs (which are subject to individual variation) are important for a *theory* of depression. The concept of innate needs is absent from cognitive theory (although see Safran & Segal, 1990).

2. Evolution theory is a more environmental (or at least interactional) theory than cognitive theory. The environment can be thwarting through no fault of the person; others' needs for power and dominance may turn a perfectly reasonable individual into a depressed person. Cultural changes and styles may also have negative consequences for some people in terms of devaluing their roles or abilities or decontextualising them. The sad state of aborigine culture is a case in point. We are not as socially decontextualised and autonomous as cognitive therapy implies and this aspect of the theory may represent an American cultural/value aspect. It appears that our notions of selfhood are both historical and culturally influenced (Baumeister, 1986).

3. Evolution theory plays particular regard to the various forms of internal inhibition in depression, especially when linked with social comparison. It suggests that these are associated with the activation of an internal mechanism that evolved with group living such that subordinates reduce their assertion, exploration, and other goal-seeking behaviours (see Chapter 6). In many cases, hopelessness is part of the activation of this involuntary subordinate/defeat routine. Changing a person's preparedness to explore (often with the support of a dominant other) reduces this internal inhibition and allows for a more positive orientation.

4. Although cognitive theory often talks about "musts" (e.g., I must succeed) this is seen as a cognitive error when in fact they speak of the term as if it is a drive. It is clear that some patients talk in terms of "musts" but don't feel compelled and suffer less. It is the affect of the "must" that causes the problem. To talk about the strength of a belief as if this was not related to emotional/motivational factors is misleading since "certainty" or strength of belief is probably related to limbic system activity (MacLean, 1985). Evolution theory would argue, therefore, that some of the "musts" represent the activation of underlying innate motivating systems. Hence individuals feel compelled, not simply as the result of a cognitive error, but as the result of something more primitive driving a person. Our experience of ourselves should not be biologically or evolutionarily decontextualised. However, again this does not imply that changing cognitive variables are ineffective in reducing depression.

5. Evolution theory focuses more on interaction, on power struggles, on self-worth, the human need to be valued, to find an accepted place/role in life, shame and envy and so forth as part of our human nature (Chapter 7; Oatley & Boulton, 1985; Gilbert, 1989). Long-term prevention has both economic and political implications (which as yet cognitive theorists rarely discuss). We cannot accept that changes in economic policy (for example) that may involve massive increases in unemployment are neutral in regard to mental health or only affect those who are somehow vulnerable by virtue of being pessimists. Especially important is the effect of such changes on family life and child development (see for example, the Special issue of the *American Psychologist,* Feb., 1989, "Children and their development").

SUMMARY

1. Cognitive therapy has three main explanatory variables: automatic thoughts, rules/assumptions, and self–other schema.

2. These cognitive elements form recursive patterns in the mind that lead to spirals into depression—e.g. a person is not invited to a party and thinks this is because the host does not like them. They then think this is because they are not much fun to be with. This leads to the idea that if they are not much fun to be with, nobody will like them. They may look for evidence of rejection and, being focused on evidence for rejection rather than acceptance, they may well find it. They then conclude that they will never be happy.

3. These recursive patterns lead to a negative view of self, world, and future (hopelessness). This saps energy and produces further evidence of failure.

4. In the early days, the cognitive theory of depression was focused on easily accessible information, but it has become more complex in the last ten years. Important refinements in the areas of vulnerability, self-schema, and interpersonal schema have appeared. Even the role for unconscious processing has now began to appear (e.g., Brewin 1989; Power & Brewin, in press) and new ways of working with depressed people derived from a cognitive perspective are appearing constantly. In a sense cognitive therapy provided a major arena for new thinking and research and it has been its research potential, both for therapy and underlying psychological processes, that in part accounts for its success.

5. Cognitive therapy always included some notion of the role of life events, especially those that were thwarting to life rules and eliciting of (latent) schema. However, these were not seen to be inherently depressing but only becoming so via cognitions. Researchers differ in their view of whether cognitive vulnerability necessarily predates the first episode, or if there is a subgroup for whom this so.

6. There is now convincing evidence that cognitive therapy is effective for many forms of depression. Future research is aimed at investigating those patients who do not respond and those who respond but relapse.

7. The role of personality as a major complication for our understanding and treatment of depression with cognitive therapy is now well accepted (Beck et al., 1990).

CONCLUDING COMMENTS

The cognitive approach to depression was one of the main developments that enabled psychologists to move out of a predominately anxiety-focused behavioural approach to the exploration of mood and other forms of psychopathology. There can be no doubt that its impact on treatment has been revolutionary. There is, however, one problem in this area which needs to be considered. In the hands of less skilled therapists a "cognitive errors therapy" can be easily turned into an "it's your fault" approach. Recent public debate on alternative/complimentary medicine has revealed this to be a serious problem. If people are led to believe that there is something about them that has caused their illness, or that they can control their illness, then, if they struggle to do so and fail, they are left with increased guilt and shame. I have called this unintentional shame (see Chapter 8). It is obvious that most of us do not intend this to happen. Also it is true that there may be ideas and behaviours about the person that contribute to depression. But as Murphy (1978) points out, ours is a culture that stresses personal responsibility for success, pain, and suffering and this can increase rather than reduce our sense of inferiority. So cognitive models are a double-edged sword. On the one hand it helps a person gain control, learn new coping behaviours, and so on, but on the other it can imply that it is the person themselves that are (in part at least) responsible, by virtue of having erroneous beliefs. Messages can be implicit as much as explicit. At all times evolution-based theory works against involuntary subordinate (inferiority) self-perception.

A too liberal use of the dictum, 'It is not things in themselves that disturb us but the view that we take of them.' is plainly wrong. What little we do know about the development of the nervous system suggests that (in the main some) negative life events and early experience that deviate from innate needs nearly always cause subsequent disturbance and this is true whether we look at animals or humans. Furthermore, sufficient cross-cultural work exists to suggest that as a culture fragments there are many casualties (e.g., the Australian aborigines). The consequences of a loss of roles and sense of belonging are not just about "views we take".

As we enter the 1990s we are becoming more cautious of the role of cognitions in depression. One of the clearest statements of our current understanding has been given by Hammen (1988, pp.102–103) and I will end this chapter with her review of the evidence.

> There are few specific cognitive contributions to understanding depression that have universal applicability. Beliefs about the causes of negative events seem inconsistently or only weakly related to depression. Perceived uncontrollability may be as linked with non-depression as with depression, while the self-blame that may exacerbate depression for some might be adaptive for others. In any case the self-blame may be accurate, at least it must be considered that qualities of persons may contribute to the occurrence of events. The construct of loss that is so central to traditional formulations of depression seems so elusive as not to be a useful predicator of depression at present. On the other hand, the cognitive constructs of meaning and self-efficacy recur in the literature in many forms, and the available data are consistent with their potential mediating role in depressive responses to stress. The mere occurrence of undesirable events, or the mere presence or lack of coping resources predicts depression far less adequately than does consideration of the meaning of the event for the person and the person's sense of personal efficacy. It continues to be the challenge for depression researchers to clarify the determinants and modes of operation of such self-related cognitive processes.

CHAPTER 14

Behavioural Theories of Depression

Psychoanalytic perspectives regard various behaviours as symptoms of psychopathology, as indicators of a deep, underlying, often unconscious, conflict. If the behaviours are changed without resolving this conflict, symptoms will change their form (due to a diversion of energy), but the individual will not be restored to healthy functioning. Behaviourists, on the other hand, regard behavioural symptoms either as a sample of the disturbance or as the actual disturbance itself. They do not, it is said, look for underlying conflicts. This polarisation of perspectives is unhelpful and misleading. In fact, behaviourists also regard much neurotic behavior as originating from inner conflict. These conflicts, however, are not unconscious, but relate to approach-avoidance conflicts, problems of conditioned anxiety, and perceived response-outcome contingencies.

Behaviourists believe that enabling a patient to change their behaviour directly (rather than by insight) is the best way of alleviating dysphoric mood states. In this sense they share much with family therapy (see Chapter 15). It is suggested that changing behaviour directly also changes various cognitive parameters, including beliefs and expectations of self-efficacy (Bandura, 1977). It is recognised that generalisation of change outside of the therapy session requires behavioural change. An analogy might be that one can read all there is to read about cars (have insight) but never be able to drive and remain fearful of doing so. Thus one needs experience.

Behaviourists try to understand their patients' problems in terms of specific learning histories and environmental responses or stimuli maintaining maladaptive behaviours (e.g., see Rehm, 1981). Their therapeutic approach attempts to provide structured opportunities for new, more adaptive learning. Most behaviourists accept that this opportunity cannot be taken if it is not conducted within an atmosphere of concern, understanding, and support (Wachtel, 1977).

There are two basic paradigms in behaviour theory, classical conditioning and operant conditioning, although much discussion revolves around their relationship (Mackintosh, 1974; 1978).

WOLPE'S CONDITIONED ANXIETY MODEL OF DEPRESSION

In 1971 Wolpe presented a classical conditioning theory of depression, suggesting that depression was a consequence of conditioned anxiety. At this time he largely favoured Seligman's learned helplessness model. But Wolpe (1979) later challenged the learned helplessness model on a number of grounds and now believes it to be inadequate as a model of depression. Unlike many of the behavioural models, Wolpe's draws sharp dividing lines between normal, neurotic, and endogenous depression. He suggests that symptom profiles, sedation thresholds, and evoked potentials point to the existence of qualitative differences between neurotic and endogenous depression. (Some of these issues are discussed in Chapter 2.) Wolpe tends to equate endogenous with psychotic depression and this is an error (see Akiskal et al., 1978). Although the biological states of psychotic and neurotic depression are obviously different, whether this suggests different etiologies is questionable. Further, Wolpe's (1979, p.556) idea that "biological depressions fade and disappear as a function of remission of the relevant biological process" is also questionable and is dualistic.

Wolpe (1979) limits his analysis to the neurotic depressions. He maintains that depressive neurosis should be regarded like other neuroses, which are fuelled by conditioned anxiety. He defines neurosis as a "persistent unadaptive habit acquired by learning in an anxiety-generating situation or succession of situations." Thus, rather than examining uncontrollability as in Seligman's (1975) learned helplessness model of depression, Wolpe suggests we should turn our attention to the older forms of experimentally induced anxiety which, as he correctly maintains, tend to get forgotten these days.

To cause neurotic behaviour experimentally it is necessary to produce anxiety in an animal repeatedly, in a constant situation, or to induce strong emotional conflict. This can be done by presenting food in a cage which has been associated with shock. In a situation where anxiety has been conditioned there is no tendency for anxiety to diminish unless adequate counter-conditioning trials are conducted (Gray, 1971 and 1979, offers a good review of these situations.) The explanations of why anxiety reduces with counter-conditioning include notions of reciprocal inhibition, habituation, and extinction. Wolpe argues that animals placed in cages that have been previously associated with shock will show significant reduction (cessation) of normal positive behaviour, e.g., exploration, eating, copulation, etc. This, in my view, is because of activation of the defensive-protect system (Chapter 5 and Gilbert, 1989). It appears that it is this general inhibition of positive reinforceable behaviour that Wolpe equates with depression.

However, these behaviours are under stimulus control and removal from the cage will (depending on other factors) reinstate positive behavioural responses. Thus, the question of stimulus specificity is important here, since depressives often show a general inhibition of positively reinforceable behaviour and explorative behaviour which is not stimulus (situation) specific. This concern might be overcome by suggesting that it is social stimuli that are the controlling stimuli. Wolpe's observation of the relationship between conditioned anxiety and cessation of positive reinforceable behaviours is an important one. Indeed, although Ferster's model (pp.421–426) does not explicitly state anxiety as an intervening process in the reduction of positively emitted behaviour of the depressive, there is no reason why this could not be adapted to do so. What Wolpe is pointing out here is the emotional and behavioural consequences of strong approach–avoidance conflicts.

Wolpe (1979) offers a neat subclassification of neurotic depression along the lines of differently acquired conditioned anxiety responses. He suggests four subtypes of depression:

1. Depression as a consequence of severe and prolonged anxiety that is directly conditioned.
2. Depression as a consequence of anxiety based on erroneous self-devaluative cognitions.
3. Depression as a consequence of anxiety based on an inability to control interpersonal behaviour.
4. Depression as a consequence of severe or prolonged responses to bereavement.

Wolpe suggests that in the absence of counter-conditioning of these habits of responding, they will not dissipate over time. He suggests that this explains why neurotic depressions are relatively enduring and contrasts it with the dissipation effect (Miller & Weiss, 1969) often noted in learned helplessness experiments.

Wolpe (1981a) has outlined important concepts on how various fears can be acquired, either by direct autonomic conditioning, or via new cognitive associations to the feared stimulus. Wolpe (1981b) claims that pure exposure to strong anxiety-arousing stimuli for any length of time, without an interposing competitive anxiety response, is completely ineffective as a treatment. This area is complex because some behaviourists now question the need for relaxation in the treatment of anxiety. Although it is a crucial question, we cannot examine it here.

There is clinical evidence which has some bearing on this model. For example, Kendell (1974) found that a high percentage of anxiety states go on to be diagnosed as depressive states at some subsequent period. Moreover, we now know that anxiety and depression are often related (see Chapter 2). In regard to depression, Wolpe's model is the only model that clearly outlines a classical conditioning model for this disorder. Although Gray's (1971) reworking of Eysenck's model offers a possible foundation for a classical conditioning theory of depression, as far as I am aware this has not been developed. However, the model has difficulty with the findings that tranquillisers are ineffective for the treatment of depression. Also our whole understanding of classical conditioning is changing. Rescorla (1988), for example, points out that conditioning is a way an animal acquires information about its environment and that many of the ways clinical psychologists think about and use the concept of classical conditioning is simply wrong.

CLASSICAL CONDITIONING, SELFOBJECTS, AND FRAGMENTATION

You may recall from Chapter 10 that we discussed the nature of selfobjects as internalised experiences gained from interaction with others and how these became experienced as part of oneself. Let me put this question: How far is a selfobject a conditioned emotional response? I do not think it unreasonable to suggest that there is much in the nature of selfobject experience that could be explored by conditioning theory. The child displays to her/his parent and others and they reward with (evolutionary expected) positive responses, i.e., pleasure, pride. The experience of parental responses could well become a conditioned emotional response for pride and pleasure such that on subsequent occasions the conditioned emotional response is accessed under conditions of display and exhibitionism. Equally, shaming responses may come to work as conditioned aversive emotional responses. In so far as the therapist uses empathy to recognise the inner experience of the patient, they are also attempting to explore the emotional reactions that have been internalised (conditioned to certain forms of self-experience and action).

When I first came across Kohut I was struck by how similar some aspects of the concept of selfobjects (e.g., mirroring) were to those of a conditioned emotional response. The affective quality and automaticity of both selfobject and conditioned responses is especially interesting. Of course behaviourists have no theory of innate or developmentally related social needs, which is unfortunate in my view. However, here I simply share my "hunch" and leave it to the reader to draw their own conclusions.

Fragmentation

Wolpe is helpful in directing our attention to experimental neurosis, which no other behavioural model does (see also Gray, 1979). It works thus: Suppose a red light signals a reward to an animal and cues running to the maze for food, but a blue light signals shock in the maze. If both lights are presented simultaneously then we see increased arousal and a disorganisation in the animal's behaviour as different motive (approach–avoidance) and actions tendencies are cued and compete. In some respects certain aspects of fragmentation (see pages 312—313) can be understood as a kind of disorganisation produced by conflict. The patient wants closeness and comfort yet also fears it (e.g., fear of shame, see Chapter 8). Fragmentation is experienced at an affective level and being with patients that have this experience (e.g., of wanting to stay in the room with me but also wanting to run away, reminds me of the power of experimental neurosis conditioning). Also these competing action tendencies can be seen as basic splits (Greenberg, 1979), e.g., "I'd like to but I can't".

In evolution theory attention is focused on the fact that stimuli/signals have both an arousal and information component and how stimuli/signals cue emotive-action tendencies. Fragmentation can also be understood as the activation of defensive responses which are automatic, rapid, and involuntary (see Chapter 5). Under these conditions a "cohesive sense of self" (Kohut, 1977) maybe lost due to the disruption and increased arousal caused by these 'emergency' defensive responses. In some cases it is the therapist that acts as a safety signal, and helping patients stay with the therapist and experience soothing can have a powerful counter-conditioning effect (they are literally internalising a safety signal/experience or a soothing selfobject). Gradually over sessions they talk more and feel more relaxed, become more explorative and less shame prone (at least in the therapy). This increase in exploration allows integration and reconstruing of information (e.g., memories and current beliefs) and the therapy progresses.

Although I see various complexities to this integration of theory, I cannot see any major problem in principle. Also I have no problem with the idea of some kind of classical conditioning of various emotional experiences (e.g., shame) and how recursive self-evaluation may amplify the shame response. The cognitive point is that the therapist must address the self-organisation and meaning-making aspect of the person's experience. And the therapeutic relationship must not increase defensiveness but reduce it.

SELF-CONTROL MODEL OF DEPRESSION

The self-control model is both a classical conditioning and an operant model. Rehm (1977; 1981; 1988) considers depression as a problem of self-control. The development of self-control theories of psychopathology has been reviewed by Mahoney (1974) and Mahoney and Arnkoff (1978). The self-control model of depression suggests that depressives show deficits in self-monitoring, self-evaluation, and self-reinforcement.

Self-monitoring. Rehm suggests that depressives attend selectively to negative outcomes. In this regard the model fits the idea of a cognitive distortion as suggested by Beck (1967; 1976) and others. It is, however, unclear whether extinction events, or punishment events, are equally relevant in this self-monitoring deficit. The suggestion is that negative events are attended to at the expense of positive events. Additionally, depressives attend selectively to immediate, rather than delayed, reinforcement outcomes. They lose a future perspective and are trapped by immediate consequences and outcomes.

Self-monitoring has also been called self-consciousness of which there are at least three aspects: private self-consciousness—a focus on internal covert events; public self-consciousness—a focus on aspects of oneself as they may "exist for others" (i.e., self-presentation) and social anxiety—a focus on the reactions of others. There are now various theories suggesting that self-consciousness (e.g., Pyszczynski & Greenberg, 1987) is related to depression and if not causal then certainly sets up a positive recursive feedback cycle. As yet, whether self-focused attention is a symptom of mood change or a cause, or even related to a personality trait (e.g., narcissistic personalities are reported to be highly self-focused) is unknown. Also, the role of rumination on the self might be considered. Negative self-focused attention is high in shame (Chapter 8).

Self-evaluation. This aspect of the theory is derived from the attribution model. As reviewed in the last chapter depressives in general are more negative in their self-evaluations (Rehm, 1988), although they can also blame others and are extrapunitive (Blackburn, 1974). Depression may vary according to whether a patient blames their actions (behavioural self-blame) or their character (characterological self-blame) the latter being more depressogenic (Janoff-Bulman & Hecker, 1988, and Chapter 8). Also, depressives make more negative social comparisons (Swallow & Kuiper, 1988). Rehm also suggests that depressives set high standards for self-evaluation. This is similar to the ego-analytic concepts and the idea that depressives evaluate themselves more negatively because they have unrealistic aspirations (see also Moretti et al., 1990). It is suggested that "all or nothing" thinking significantly interferes with self-monitoring skills. Kleinians would call this a paranoid–schizoid mechanism.

Self-reinforcement. Rehm suggests that lower response initiations, longer latencies, and less persistence, may be accounted for by low self-reinforcement. There is evidence that depressives self-reward less and self-punish more than normal controls. Whether or not this is a function of self-reward per se, or whether there are "greater rewards" from punishment (e.g., secondary gains, avoidance of aversive responses from others) is unclear. Also guilt is strongly associated with notions of entitlement (Gilbert, 1989) and it may be guilt, irrespective of depressive affect, that reduces self-reward. In general, the concept of low self-reward implies an excessive concern with external reinforcers, and the depressed person is heavily "dependent" on others for reinforcement. This idea crops up in a variety of forms—for example, in ego-analytic theory (Arieti & Bemporad, 1980b) and in Beck's (1983) concept of sociotropy, in Freud's concept of dependency, and in Kleinian concepts of a projected good object, to name a few. It is one of the most common elements of many theories of depression (Birtchnell, 1988a). Perhaps describing these processes as those of self-reinforcement makes them more manageable and open to investigation. Fuchs and Rehm (1977) and Rehm, Fuchs, Roth, Kornblith, and Romano (1979) have evaluated a behavioural programme for depression based on the self-control model and found it to be effective with mildly depressed patients.

LOSS OF REINFORCER EFFECTIVENESS

Costello (1972) addresses the problem of how it is that depression brings about a loss of behaviours, for which the reinforcement contingencies have not actually changed. It is not the loss of reinforcers themselves that Costello sees as important, but their inability to maintain established behaviours; they have become ineffective for the depressed person. He notes that discriminative stimuli (e.g., a loved person) may cue many forms of behaviour which may be extinguished with the removal of that discriminative stimulus—self psychologists might argue because these reinforcers/stimuli functioned as selfobjects relationships.

Costello (1972, p.241) considers two processes which may account for the general loss of reinforcer effectiveness of the depressive: (1) biochemical-neurophysiological change; and (2) disruption of a chain of behaviour. He suggests that: ". . . the reinforcer effectiveness of all the components of the chain of behavior is contingent upon the completion of the chain at either an overt or covert level; that this is a characteristic of complex organisms particularly humans, and that it is of functional significance in evolutionary terms". This is similar to Klinger's (1975, 1977 view (see Chapter 12)

While there is a good case to be made for the importance of behavioural chains, or complex network of behaviours, Costello's argument that evolutionary pressure produces a need for complexity, and when cohesiveness is lost depression results, requires validation. It is possible, however, to suggest that "certain types of behaviour" do have evolutionary importance and disruption of these behaviours in a chain will have more "pathogenic effects" than other behaviours. Thus, disruptions in socially cohesive behaviour may have great power to produce a general loss of reinforcer effectiveness—primarily because much activity is now diverted to attempting to reinstate the individual's social integration. It seems to me, therefore, that Costello's model would be considerably strengthened by considering the notion of certain reinforcers being (evolutionarily) more important than others. The idea of equipotentiality may be relevant here in a similar fashion to that now investigated in anxiety neurosis (Eysenck 1979; Rachman, 1978; Seligman, 1971).

Costello considers the experimental evidence which suggests that reinforcing properties are passed backwards from an unconditioned stimulus (UCS), that is, only antecedent stimuli and not stimuli subsequent to a UCS are endowed with reinforcing properties. There is reason to be cautious of this view, however, since humans generate new goal-directed behaviours without their ever having appeared previously. In this sense forward planning does allow for the possibility that behaviours in a complex chain develop for other reasons than being antecedent UCS associations.

The problems for behaviour theories are well observed. For example, Costello (1972, p.244) says: "there is no obvious reason why an emigrant who has not maintained contact with his father loses his appetite for food, sex and things in general on hearing of the death of his father. There is no obvious reason why a man, on failing to be promoted or on reaching retirement age, may react in the same way." Ranking and attachment theory would however be able to explain these effects by virtue of a loss of role and SAHP.

Generally, this model has not generated much research. It has not been developed to a degree of specificity which would allow, say, discrimination between depression and schizophrenia. At a descriptive level, loss of reinforcer effectiveness seems sensible. However, some behaviours may actually increase (e.g., passive avoidance, submissive behaviour), which suggests that some reinforcers (avoidance of punishment) actually became more powerful during depression. Moreover, the concept that secondary gain behaviours are maintained by their reinforcing (short-term) properties is difficult to fit with Costello's ideas. Nevertheless, at least Costello recognises that behavioural data needs to be linked with evolutionary and biological considerations.

FERSTER'S MODEL

In 1973 and 1974 Ferster published two important papers on depression outlining the applicability of an operant model of conditioning to this disorder. Ferster's functional analysis approach has a number of strengths. First, it outlines in a clear way how investigations of ongoing behaviour may provide many insights into depression. Especially important is the emission of positively reinforced behaviour, passive avoidance responses, and the degree to which some depressive behaviours are under aversive control. Second, it offers potential areas of overlap with Bowlby's work, in that Ferster places special emphasis on the opportunity of an individual to have learned the necessary skills to adjust to life's crises (e.g., losses of reinforcement). These skills are learned in childhood as a function of exploration. Factors which inhibit learning through exploration can produce developmental arrests and behaviours that are easily extinguished. Third, Ferster suggests important processes which cast light on phenomena that psychoanalytic writers have discussed, e.g., anger turned inward and fixation.

Ferster suggests that like infantile autism, depression is especially appropriate for a behavioural approach because of the poverty and missing elements of certain behaviours. It would not be wise to push the comparison too far however, since depression can be a fluctuating disorder with returns to normal functioning, whereas this is not true for autism. Moreover, depression from an operant viewpoint is an adjustment disorder, that is, there appears to be maladaptive or reduced adjustment behaviour to changes in reinforcement schedules. From this point, causes rather than symptoms require detailed investigation.

Ferster makes the important distinction between functional and topographical behavioural analysis. The difference arises from the outcomes that the behaviour is emitted to produce. Two individuals may take an overdose of sleeping tablets (similar topographic behaviours) but one may intend to die, the other may have been drunk and made a mistake. Hence the "function" of the two behaviours is different. In the case of depression it is the functional analysis of behaviour which has relevance. Critics of behavioural approaches often overlook this important distinction.

Ferster's approach, then, highlights the need to look very closely at the functional behaviours of the depressed person. From this, two important observations become apparent. First, the depressed person demonstrates significant passivity in the presence of aversive events. Complying with demands from significant others is a passive attempt to avoid the aversive consequences of refusal. This is especially important when the behaviour requested is against the wishes of the passive person. Thus, as Ferster (1974) points out, one connotation of a passive response is that it becomes negatively reinforced (i.e., it is reinforced because it succeeds in avoiding aversive interactions with others). The second component of passivity is associated with failure to deal with aversive (social) events. In this situation Ferster has in mind a passive tendency to assume responsibility for negative events. Though Ferster does not state it as an attribution as might Beck (1976), this it clearly is. However, for Ferster it is not so much the attribution that is the problem, but the failure to tackle the problem directly and seek confirmatory or other data for passive acceptance.

The second prominent observation, in addition to passivity, is the reduction in the frequency of positively reinforced behaviours. Activities that may have been enjoyed previously, such as socialising, sex, games, hobbies, work, etc., significantly decline. They appear to be on an extinction schedule, where there is insufficient reinforcement to maintain them in the person's repertoire. The less the behaviours are engaged in, the less opportunity there is for positive reinforcement and so the less they are engaged in. In discussing these issues, Ferster notes the well known behavioural finding that continuous, predictable reinforcement schedules produce behaviour that is fragile compared to variable reinforcement. In other words, behaviours that are maintained on variable reinforcement schedules show a greater resistance to extinction than those maintained on continuous reinforcement. The relevance of this distinction (a major axiom of operant laws of learning) is that, under situations where reinforcement contingencies change rapidly, the continuously reinforced behaviour is much more vulnerable to extinction than the variably reinforced behaviour. Thus, the schedule of reinforcement that maintains a behaviour will have a significant bearing on how long that behaviour will be maintained in the presence of reduced or total reinforcement withdrawal. This view is echoed in many analytic theories in that they point out that frustration (or frustrative non-reward) is an inevitable consequence of development and that the child must develop strategies for coping with it.

The operant approach regards depression as a maladaptive adjustment response or set of responses. Not surprisingly, the changes that require adjustment(s) are changes in the levels (schedules) of reinforcement. Thus adjustment behaviour is required in the presence of significant life events which reduce reinforcement. These may include loss of a loved one, loss of a job or friends, movement away from a community, children leaving home, etc. If the individual is to adjust to these significant changes, there must be some degree of in-built resistance to extinction of certain behaviours and the capacity to generate new, reinforceable behaviour. Unfortunately, for the depression-prone individual, there seems to be an incapacity to achieve this satisfactorily. The previous schedules of the reinforced behaviour are of variable of importance. However, the capacity to adapt to the changed situation and to maintain behaviour, perhaps in the face of little immediate reinforcement, is also important. We could also view this in terms of reinforceable social roles.

Turning to this latter problem (the ability to initiate new, potentially reinforceable behaviours or enact social roles), Ferster suggests that failures in adjustment behaviour may be related to distorted perceptions of reinforcement contingencies. He highlights three such distortions:

1. A limited view of the world; in this situation the person may be unable to see which behaviours are appropriate for reinstating adequate levels of reinforcement. They may sulk and complain but have little insight into what behaviour on their part would bring the required reinforcement.

2. A lousy view of the world; in this situation the patient may be aware of what behaviours are required but fears the aversive consequences of such behaviour. In other words, their passivity is under aversive control by its potential negative-reinforcing properties. This view is very similar to a ranking theory of depression (see Chapter 6).

3. An unchanging view of the world; in this situation it is not so much a lack of perception, or a fear of aversive consequences, but a lack of skills. In other words, the behavioural repertoire is not sufficiently

developed or comprehensive to be able to adjust to significant changes in reinforcement. Ferster likens this view to a kind of development arrest (similar to, but not identical with, psychoanalytic concepts of fixation).

These three views of the world freeze the individual in a set of behaviours which are not positively reinforcing and may elicit aversive outcomes (e.g., depressed patients are unattractive). Compensatory behaviours—clinging, demanding, self-blame—may have some immediate reinforcement value, but their reinforcement may be highly variable, making them difficult behaviours to extinguish and blocking the development of the more adaptive behaviours necessary for the individual to make a satisfactory adjustment. Thus, Ferster views the maladaptive behaviours of the depressed individual as crucial etiological factors.

Among the behavioural parameters Ferster calls upon to help us to understand why a limited repertoire of adjustment behaviours exist is the notion of stimulus discrimination learning. Discrimination learning is a complex and important field of instrumental (operant) learning. Generally, it depends on accurate, predictable responses to specific events (emitted responses). Discrimination learning is likely to be poor if reinforcement is unpredictable and is response variable. To enable children to predict the outcomes of their own behaviour (environmental responses to them), the socialising agent must be sensitive to the subtleties of the child's behaviour. If the socialising agent is insensitive and responds arbitrarily to the child, the environment is rendered unpredictable. In consequence, unpredictable or insensitively applied reinforcement can block accurate discrimination learning. Most importantly, not only does the child fail to show subtle discrimination learning in interpersonal situations, but also exploratory behaviour may be inhibited. If the child does not know whether he will be shouted at, smacked, ignored, or smiled at for exploring, then exploring becomes an extremely hazardous venture.

For those interested in similarities between theories, then the idea that the inhibition of exploratory behaviour significantly limits the development of a behavioural repertoire has a clear overlap with some of Bowlby's ideas and ranking theory. Ferster would, perhaps, put less stress on the importance of mothering per se, but lay emphasis on the predictability of reinforcement, comprehensive discrimination learning, encouragement of exploration, and the development of complex response repertoires. Poor mothering may indeed fail on all accounts.

Those most prone to depression are individuals who have developed a limited response repertoire and have failed to learn to generate alternative, adaptive, reinforceable behaviours when adjustments in responding are required. In consequence, there is a limit to the amount of behaviour which can be emitted for positive reinforcement, and aversive consequences to maladaptive, inappropriate responding are inevitable.

Anger

Ferster makes a major contribution to the role and analysis of anger in depression. The psychoanalytic concept of "anger turned inward" is not discussed by most of the newer behavioural models of depression, and in this regard Ferster offers a refreshing approach. He suggests that inadequate reinforcement not only interferes with discrimination learning and the acquisition of a complex response repertoire, but also produces emotional arousal which further interferes with such learning and produces considerable conflicts. In early learning, primitive or atavistic rage may be aroused in the child by inappropriate positive reinforcement, punishment, or a failure of positive rewards from the parent. The expression of this anger may itself produce a withdrawal of positive reinforcement or punishment (i.e., the parent punishes the child for showing it—this we might call shame).

The expression of anger may serve to reduce the flow of positive reinforcement. In the young infant for example, an irritable or aggressive style may lead the mother to turn away from the infant or put it back in its cot, thus depriving it of a soothing selfobject (to use Kohut's term). In this way the mother attempts to control the child's expression of negative affect especially towards her. If the environmental response is to remove the source of food or comfort (the Kleinian good breast), subsequent anger may become associated with a reduction in positive reinforcement. In other words, anger may come to act as a "pre-aversive" internal stimulus, that is, the associated, preceding event for the loss (withdrawal) of positive reinforcement. Hence felt anger becomes associated with a negative outcome. If such associative learning becomes established then situations which would normally produce anger may cue anger suppression. This is a similar view to that suggested by Greenberg and Safran (1987). Also one can get secondary effects. If I am angry I expect others to withdraw and this expectation makes me more angry. Hence part of my anger relates to the anticpation of the response.

On the other hand a child may later come to model the aggressive behaviour of the parent since they learn that control over others is the key to obtaining reinforcers. This can lead to increased aggressive and less cooperative behaviour especially in peer relationships. The orientation is less explorative and more controlling. Ferster does not make the distinction between assertiveness and anger control but such a distinction is important (see Chapter 8).

Overview

Ferster's theory highlights a very important set of phenomena in depression. It points out the need to examine the antecedents of behaviour and to consider behaviour functionally. Second, Ferster suggests, there is a fear of loss of positive reinforcement contingent on anger expression. Third, there is an overdependence on these certain sources of reinforcement (many psychoanalytic writers may call this high dependency needs). The reason for the high dependency is the failure to develop: an independent repertoire (in our model this would be healthy assertiveness); the ability to work through frustration; the ability to maintain independent behaviour in the face of little reward and to seek out alternative sources of positive reinforcement if and when reinforcers are lost, be these people or activities. In ranking theory these may be consequences of the inhibitory effects of involuntary, subordinate self-perception.

LEWINSOHN'S SOCIAL REINFORCEMENT THEORY

Lewinsohn's model of depression is, like Ferster's, based on operant learning principles. The main differences between the two is Lewinsohn's emphasis on social behaviours, and the comparative absence of discussion concerning childhood vulnerability or conditioned anger suppression.

Lewinsohn, Youngren, and Grosscup (1979) acknowledge the multi-component nature of depression (including the role of cognitive, genetic, and biochemical processes) and point out that reinforcement depression relationships are but one aspect of depression. His research has been particularly concerned with interpersonal behavioural interactions.

In Lewinsohn's early work (1974; 1975) depression was related to a low rate of response-contingent positive reinforcement (RCPR). Lewinsohn stresses the point that it is not positive reinforcement per se that is crucial, but its response contingency. He suggested that a low rate of RCPR could arise from: (1) few reinforcing events in the environment; or (2) a lack of social skills; thus the individual is unable to emit potential, reinforceable behaviour.

Low rates of RCPR, it is assumed, produce states that elicit unhappiness, fatigue, and various symptoms of depression. However, there is no clear mechanism, as yet, which shows how low rates of RCPR actually produce these specific symptoms. Becker (1977) points out, for example, that many pathological groups may experience RCPR but do not necessarily have depressive disorders.

Coyne (1976a) demonstrated that conversations (on the telephone in this case) with depressives could make recipients themselves feel more depressed, hostile, and rejecting. This evidence does support a second assumption of Lewinsohn's, that the interpersonal behaviour of the depressive alienates potential (social) sources of reinforcement. Hammen and Peters (1978) noted that Coyne used females. In their study of mixed sexes, rejections were much higher for the opposite sex. That is, depressed behaviour in opposite sexed persons were viewed as much less attractive than depressed behaviour in same sexed persons. Such data point to a high degree of subtlety in interpersonal verbal interactions which may have evolutionary significance. Further, although depression may, in the short term, elicit care it does not in the long term and depressives tend to be rejected (see Chapter 15). Once again this points to a ranking explanation in that depressives give off signals of submissiveness, being defeated and being "out of action" and this is unattractive to potential allies and mates, resulting in less investment by others. Also, subordinates are often ignored by dominants (Crook, 1980).

Lewinsohn suggests that the interpersonal behaviour of depressives is an important modulator of the type and frequency of reinforcement they will obtain from others, but does not link this to the fact that it may be an issue of a preparedness to invest in others (see Chapter 7). Evolution theory would argue that individuals will only invest in others if there is some chance of gain reciprocally (e.g., mutual support of self-esteem) and depressives may signal an inability to do this. However, because humans are moral and caring to some degree, maladaptive behaviours are likely to achieve partial, inconsistent reinforcement, which makes them difficult to extinguish. Much of the evidence for and against Lewinsohn's theory has been well reviewed (Becker, 1977; Blaney, 1977, and more recently Rehm, 1989). In general, much of the evidence is correlational, which can at best offer only weak support.

Lewinsohn et al. (1979) point out that, behaviourally, two hypotheses of depression are possible:

1. Depressives engage in fewer pleasant activities and experience greater aversiveness in regard to all events.
2. Reduced engagement in positive events and increased aversiveness are related to a specific subset of events. If such a subset does exist, then it has major importance.

Lewinsohn and his colleagues investigated these questions with specially designed schedules: the interpersonal events schedule (IES), the pleasant events schedule (PES), and the unpleasant events schedule (UES). By examining the correlation matrices produced by the use of these schedules with measures of dysphoria, Lewinsohn et al. (1979) investigated the possibility of subsets of events being important in depression. Their evidence does suggest that it is social reinforcements that are the crucial controlling reinforcers of depressive behaviour. Positive mood states seem related to feelings of being loved, socializing, being with liked people, and so on, while aversive social reinforcement such as arguments, marital discord, and being overworked are associated with lowering of mood. Negative interpersonal interactions, especially those associated with aversiveness or feelings of reduced self-worth, are associated with low mood. Lewinsohn et al. (1979, p.313) suggest that:

> these are the types of events bearing a critical relationship to the occurrence of depression. When the good ones (PES) occur at low rates and the negative ones (UES, IES) occur at high rates, the individual is likely to feel depressed. We also hypothesize that these are the major types of events that act as reinforcers for people; occurrence of the ones that are negatively associated with dysphoria serve to maintain our behavior, and the occurrence of events that are positively associated with dysphoria reduces our rates of behavior.

These findings are highly consistent with ranking and network theory (see Chapters 6 and 7). Lewinsohn et al. (1979) suggest that these are the important reinforcement parameters governing depressed behaviour. They do not suggest that they are the crucial etiological determinants of pathological depression. As they discuss later in the same paper, the "causes" of depression are probably multi-component.

Youngren and Lewinsohn (1980) provide further support for the findings outlined above. They point out, however, that differences between depressed and non-depressed patients are largely at a self-report level; the former reporting a lower frequency of pleasant social and interpersonal events and a greater frequency of aversive events. Although the depressives were rated as less socially skilled, behavioural deficits are of a subtle kind and difficult to identify objectively.

In a further study Lewinsohn et al. (1980) examined the problem of perceived self-competence. Many writers on depression have noted that depressives rate themselves low on social competence. However, this study attempted to investigate whether this perception was a cognitive distortion, or a realistic appraisal, of poor social skills. Using self and observer ratings following group interactions, the data suggest that depressed patients have a fairly accurate picture of themselves; that is, they see themselves as others see them. Of course, this does not mean that these people are less socially skilled since, when their depression recedes, various behaviours may again become part of their repertoire. However, it does suggest that at that point in time (when depressed), perceptions of low competency were accurate perceptions since they corresponded fairly closely with how others saw them. Hence when ill, depressives may not only exhibit less socially reinforcing behaviour, but may be all too painfully aware of it. The most interesting finding, perhaps was that normals had illusionary self-perceptions and saw themselves more positively than others saw them (i.e., are self-deceptive, see Chapter 7). Moreover, depressives also tended to become more positively self-illusionary as they recovered. These researchers discuss their findings in terms of the "warm glow" hypothesis of Mischel, Ebbesen, and Zeiss (1973; 1976) (see also Chapter 7, pages 205–207).

Lewinsohn believes that the social reinforcing elements of behaviour are the central elements of changes in behaviour associated with depression. However, it might also be suggested that these pleasant and unpleasant events, which Lewinsohn and his colleagues highlight, have evolutionary significance. The behaviours which threaten social cohesion and signal lack of social success may be innately set up to produce dysphoric states (e.g., Nesse, 1990). The events that Lewinsohn outlines as being important in depression may be important for other reasons apart from simply reducing positive reinforcement.[1]

SOCIAL SKILLS AND/OR STATUS ENHANCEMENT

Much of the operant approach to depression focuses on how skilled a person is to manipulate their interpersonal environment and elicit positive reinforcers. Williams (1986) has recently given an overview of social skills in depression, exploring both the theory and evidence in favour of social skills training as a treatment for depression. He points out that social skills deficits can be assessed in a number of ways, namely by: self-reports of difficulty in interpersonal situations; structured interview; self-monitoring; observer ratings of interactions; and observer ratings of specific elements of social behaviour. Williams notes that it is the global ratings of interpersonal behaviour that best discriminate the depressed from the non-depressed and that the micro skills analysis (eye gaze, speech duration, Ellgring, 1989) provide less consistent findings. Further, speech content is also an important communication style. These facts point to more complex interactional sequences as a problem in depression. For example, the speech content of the depressive may be self-focused and uninteresting to others (see also Chapter 6).

Social skills training can be understood as both attractiveness training and assertiveness training. One encourages the person to take on the postures of a more open and dominant stance, e.g., to stand upright rather than slouch, to meet eye gaze, and so forth, that is, not to behave like an involuntary subordinate. One also teaches how to be reinforcing to others, show interest, and so forth.

Bergner (1988) has drawn attention to the fact that patients need to get back into touch with status and esteem-maintaining roles and behaviour. The basic goal of status dynamic therapy is "status enhancement". This may include changing internal status, reducing self-esteem attacking (e.g., I am a failure, useless, etc.) or developing roles and behaviours that are status enhancing. Also a more social orientation may be necessary. For example, Gilboa, Levav, Gilboa, and Ruiz (1990) found that in a kibbutz, ratings of demoralisation were correlated with occupational prestige. Hence as Bergner points out, loss of an esteem-maintaining role or lack of a role can lead to depression. Throughout this book we have stressed the importance of a sense of internal value and how this evolved from ranking and group living behaviour. However one looks at the data the issue of social success (Vining, 1986; Nesse, 1990) appears to be a significant factor in depression.

Evolution Theory and Behaviour Theory

Like so many other theories in psychology, behaviour theory is not grounded in any good theory of basic social-biological infrastructures. Hence it tends to be correlational and simply able to note how one event correlates with another. When it comes to suggesting why particular events are associated with particular outcomes it is struggling (although see Staats & Eifert, 1990, for a theory of social behavioursim that may go a long way towards advancing behaviour theory).

In many respects ranking and network theory are also social behavioural theories. At their core they view social success not only as the driving force in evolution but view affective states as informational systems for facilitating social success (see Chapter 5; we emphasise social success not economic success, which is very different). Moreover, certain kinds of signal are necessary to help the individual track social success.

Hence an evolutionary theory argues that we are innately social animals, that certain types of social signals and responses are associated with positive affect (exerting control over social outcomes such as: finding a lover, making friends, feeling supported, gaining respect) while other social signals (losing a lover, losing or not having friends, losing or not having respect or status) are associated with negative affect. We have also stressed the importance of our ability to be attractive to each other to gain SAHP or mirroring and feel valued. Further we have argued that there are inhibitory and social communication styles that switch in when signals arrive that tell us we are socially unsuccessful or we are trapped in undesirable relationships and situations. These may be external (e.g., uncontrollable stress, losses or put-downs) or internal, i.e., internal self-devaluations. Hence there is very little in the behavioural approach that is contradictory to the evolutionary view but its theoretical basis needs to be broadened. Moreover ranking theory would see the therapeutic relationship as providing powerful signals that can be soothing and deactivate the defense system. One reason interpretation is a poor choice of treatment is that it does not deactivate the defense system and may actually amplify it (i.e., literally put the patient on the defensive).

SUMMARY

1. Depression can be explored with two different behavioural paradigms: (a) classical conditioning and (b) operant learning.

2. The classical conditioning paradigm focuses on depression as secondary to anxiety and views much of the depressed person's behaviours as controlled by various forms of anxiety. However, classical conditioning may also provide helpful insight into the self psychology concepts of selfobjects and fragmentation.

3. Self-control uses both an operant and classical conditioning paradigm. It focuses on the internal (self-delivered) contingencies, especially self-monitoring, self-focused attention, self-evaluation, and self-rewards and punishments.

4. The operant approach offers a functional analysis of the behaviour of the depressed person. Ferster's theory notes various predictions a depressed person makes (e.g., a limited view of the world, a lousy view of the world, and an unchanging view of the world). Ferster also draws attention to the role of previous learning that inhibits: (a) explorative behaviour, (b) learning adjustment behaviour to loss, and (c) the expression of anger. Such constructs are used to explain depressive passivity.

5. The social theory of Lewinsohn explores the social behavioural repertoire of the depressed person. Depression is related to a low rate

of response-contingent positive reinforcement (RCPR). Lewinsohn stresses the point that it is not positive reinforcement per se that is crucial, but its response contingency. He suggested that a low rate of RCPR could arise from: (1) few reinforcing events in the environment; or (2) a lack of social skills; thus the individual is unable to emit potential, reinforceable behaviour.

6. Ranking and social network theory highlight the evolutionary importance of social success and the innateness of social reinforcement negative affect relationships. It also highlights the importance of certain types of signal in the environment.

CONCLUDING COMMENTS

The behavioural theories of depression have, in their short history, provided fascinating insights and testable hypotheses. In general terms there is one area which will need careful consideration—the question of equipotentiality. The study of anxiety has shown that different classes of stimuli are more easily fear-conditioned than others. Thus various conditioned stimuli (CS) differ in their propensity to acquire fear-arousing properties from an association with an unconditioned stimulus (UCS). (See Eysenck, 1979, for a good review of these issues.) In the study of anxiety, early conditioning theories failed in their ability to explain adequately the acquisition of anxiety conditions and their resistance to extinction (Rachman, 1978). In the case of depression certain types of social signal or stimuli may fall into this case.

One of the oddities of behavioural theory of depression has been the almost total ignoring of the therapeutic relationship. I am not entirely clear about why this is. One reason may be that behaviourists have a kind of conditioned aversive response to anything vaguely psychoanalytic. The second is that behaviourists have been reluctant to come to terms with the internal workings of the mind. I have to say that this leaves our science the poorer. I am fairly convinced that the concept of "selfobject" is a major concept and that it has so many hallmarks of an emotional conditioned response that it is surprising behaviourists have not taken to it. Rescorla's (1988) model of classical conditioning seems particularly suited to a social behaviourism that focuses on social relationships as the key controllers of affective state.

I was once called a social behaviourist. My immediate response was to reject the label. (I personally dislike labels and the clichés and theoretical dogmas in psychology which reduce scholarship.) However, on reflection there is much in behavioursim that I would endorse. First, I tend to focus on the social signals a person is receiving and sending and I may use the transference and counter-transference relationship to do this. Second, I focus on the social signals a person would like (their fantasies), "How would you like others to behave towards you? and "How do you behave towards them"? Third, I tend to explore how behaviour tends to track the enactment of various themes. Fourth, I focus attention on recursive feedback and how this links with internal models of self and others. I don't know if this fits social behavioursim, but maybe it does.

However, my guiding light is indeed social behaviour. I try to help in my small way to enable a person not to behave towards themselves or others as an involuntary subordinate, to deactivate defensive and agonic styles and to exert more control over life. Sometimes external contingencies make this a painful struggle.

NOTE

1. While such theorising has its place, it should be remembered that interpersonal behaviour is of considerable importance for the prognosis of schizophrenia (Leff, 1978; Vaughn & Leff, 1976). Relapse rates are much higher for those schizophrenics whose environments provide aversive interactions (e.g., high expressed emotion families). In low expressed emotion families schizophrenics do much better and drugs may make only a marginal difference to relapse. Moreover, drug effects and psychophysiological responses have been shown to be responsive to aversive social interactions in schizophrenics (Tarrier et al., 1979). Thus, while Lewinsohn's work is of considerable importance, the question of specificity of some of the variables to depression requires validation. Moreover, an increase in positive social interactions has a significant impact on the interpersonal behaviour of retarded psychiatric patients (Matson & Zeiss, 1979). Thus, positive social interactions are important in both schizophrenia and depression. We need to know whether there are qualitative differences in the reduction of positive (and increase in aversive) interpersonal events between schizophrenia and depressives. Such data would have a bearing on ethological and evolutionary theories of psychopathology.

CHAPTER 15

Life Events, Interpersonal Theories, and the Family

INTRODUCTION

The evolution of K-selected attachment mechanisms means that babies are born with the expectation of, and need for, attachment objects. Not only this, but attachment objects must respond in certain ways (e.g., with mirroring and nurturance) in order for the child to survive and prosper. But what about other aspects of the social environment? Can we, as humans, say that we evolved such that there is now an expectation of a certain kind of environment that would allow us to live our lives in a relatively secure (non-defensive) way. Throughout this book we have answered this question affirmatively. Two major domains have been suggested: (a) the dimension of social control, relating to a freedom from domination, and various factors that elicit involuntary, subordinate self-perception; (b) the dimension of belonging, relating to a sense of shared social identity (being like others), reassurance, acceptance and support of one's self presentation and validation of social roles, such that one feels valued by others (e.g., Heard & Lake, 1986). We have seen how these needs evolved (Chapters 5–8 and 10) and how they are related to social success on the one hand, and our affective experience on the other (Chapter 5). Before exploring the interpersonal theories in more detail some preliminary observations of early human life styles can be made.

Like chimpanzees, early humanoid bands were marked by consistent, face to face contact and where there was division of labour (Power, 1988; Glantz & Pearce, 1989; Haviland, 1990; Itzkoff, 1990). Bands were often formed from genetically related individuals (Wenegrat, 1984). These groups flourished and evolved over millions of years because of the social organisation of the small group. It is this type of social life we are adapted to. Although we now know that hunter-gatherer groups can take various forms (Hill & Hurtado, 1989) many (but not all) were basically cooperative, hedonic groups. Sharing and the recognition of mutual dependency was a key to survival (Power, 1988). For example, in the Ache in Paraguay, women who share food are praised and hunters nearly always hand over their kill to the group to disseminate (Hill & Hurtado, 1989). In various hunter-gatherer groups, children learn from an early age that meanness and possessiveness are unacceptable. Also, it is adaptive to facilitate each individual to explore and develop their talents because it will benefit others. Inhibited subordinates waiting for commands from above were not adaptive (except in war situations perhaps). At the same time individuals are not encouraged to behave as individualists. For example, blowing one's own trumpet would be seen negatively. In some hunter-gatherer bands there is a positive fear of resource differences emerging and various rituals exist to reduce the difference in any accumulated wealth such as parties and potlashes to use up excess. This was also adaptive since possessions were difficult to carry around. What work has been done suggests that self-awareness is very much linked to group values and identity; a sense of belonging is crucial (Haviland, 1990).

The issue of leadership in hunter-gatherer groups is also salient. Leaders come from within the group and in general arise from respect, although they have little power (Haviland, 1990). Hence leaders tend to be the elders and/or people who have demonstrated to the band some particular qualities to others, such as hunting or healing ability. Leaders have played a consistent part in the life of the band, are well known to everyone, and have high face to face contact and accessibility. Leadership is derived from the possession of knowledge gained over the life span and depends on consensus validation of the role. Leaders are the conveyers of the myths and stories of the group, helping to define belonging, tradition, and the identity of the group.

In brief then, the hedonic groups of the hunter-gatherers are marked by the following characteristics:

1. Consistent face to face contacts in small bands.
2. Focus on sharing resources and responsibilities.
3. Inhibition of gross individualism and possessiveness.

4. Awareness of group dependency (all in the same boat).
5. High levels of cooperative behaviour.
6. Shared values, goals, traditions.
7. Mutual recognition and valuing of roles.
8. Relevance of affiliative enhancing rituals.
9. Social structure predominately affectionate and relaxed.

As far as we can tell, many early hunter-gatherer bands were marked by high levels of cooperation and early humans probably spent over 2 million years evolving in these kinds of social structure. During hominoid evolution, the brain was to undergo radical transformations. For example, primitive prehuman primates (e.g., *homo habilis*) had a brain capacity estimated at less than 1000 cubic centimetres, while in modern humans this is 1600. Not only did it increase in cubic capacity, with the increasing role for higher level cortical, cognitive processes, such as conceptual and symbolic thinking, but also the social emotive structures in the limbic system, so necessary for our highly social and cooperative life styles, were significantly expanded and modified. These adaptations were related to facilitating social success. The brain did not evolve as an organ of rationality but as an organ of adaptive, social competencies. Indeed, many of our social behaviours are far from rational. Even simple programmes like Star Trek recognise this fact and have used it in plot and character to good effect.

One does not want to paint a too ideal picture of hunter-gatherer life styles (Hill & Hurtado, 1989). Some may have been rather warlike (Itzkoff, 1990) and punitive (see MacDonald's [1988] comparison of the Gussii and Kung!). Rather, we should emphasise the importance of interaction and ingroup mutual dependency, the consistency of social relationships and sense of community, and the role and inhibition of individualism. Some possessions remained important such as bows and arrows, but these were usually things that were easily transportable. Those that felt very disgruntled were free to move off to another group (Haviland, 1990), as also happens in primates (Dunbar, 1988).

Research on life events, social support and other interpersonal processes should be seen against this evolutionary background. The marginalisation of many groups of individuals and the loss of value for basic human roles, such as child-rearing in today's society, arise from the brisk pace at which culture and economic structures have imposed a life style that, in many respects, our biological evolution is not adapted to. For example, if, as Cox (1988) suggests, there are cultural differences in rates of postnatal depression, this may relate to the acceptance and support of women at these times and the process of reintegration into group life. In no hunter-gatherer society do men play any role in childbirth (unlike our current hospital-based procedures). The event of a mother becoming socially decontextualised and living in small living spaces, having to cope alone for long periods of the day with her young children, is a gross abnormality to all primate and hunter-gatherer life styles. In hunter-gatherer bands, females work and travel together, while their children associate/play with peers in the mother's vicinity. Watching families shop with children straining to get out of push chairs and explore, and being shouted at or even hit for being irritable and restless, can only be seen as a tragic distortion of our biologically adaptive patterns. On a different level, aspirations on the one hand, and same–different comparisons on the other were all constrained by the consistency of living in a small band. Many of the enormous stresses of self-identity, forged by continually having to interact with strangers, and our over-developed sense of competitiveness and autonomy (e.g., Lasch, 1985) were not part of early hunter-gatherer life. At every turn we see that our economic structures (the lure of resources, more is better) exert a fragmenting and decontextualising power over our lives (Gilbert, 1989).

Research into life events (e.g., see Smith & Allred, 1989; Brown, 1989) and social support (e.g., see Stokes & McKirnan, 1989) have proliferated in the last ten years. Although many methodological problems have been overcome and new ones have emerged, there has been little attempt to ground these findings in evolution and an understanding of our innate needs.

LIFE EVENTS

To answer the question, "Do life events ever produce symptoms?," the answer is clearly, "Yes, they do." At the extreme, severe life events and major crises produce symptoms in the vast majority of subjects exposed to them. Tennant, Bebbington, and Hurry (1981b) suggest that: "When subjects are exposed to the horrific sequelae of a disaster involving personal threat to life, death or serious injury of friends and relatives, loss of personal effects, and disruption of social bonds, the risk of psychological morbidity may approach 100% in the short term." Seligman (1975) also reviews evidence which demonstrates that major disasters can produce significant disturbances in functioning. He attributes this to helplessness. Generally, major disasters ignite symptoms by their capacity to threaten, or actually disrupt or destroy, the social, integrative fabric of people.

Less extreme, but still major events which focus on the individual, also produce disturbances in functioning. Grief is one example (Averill, 1968; Parkes, 1972: Parker et al., 1988). Horowitz, Wilner, Kaltreider and Alvarez (1980b) provided important data on the sort of symptoms that emerge following traumatic stress. They demonstrated that various symptoms of depression, anxiety, obsessive–compulsive, anger–hostility, and somatization—are consequent to traumatic stress. Often these symptoms appeared in over 90% of cases. Again it turns out that the most serious stresses invoking these symptoms are "the loss of a relationship with another, the loss of self-esteem, or the loss of a physical aspect of the self" (p.91). Horowitz et al. (1980b) note particularly the intrusive and avoidance episodes that characterise these syndromes. They point out that the engagement of psychological processes necessary for adapting to these aversive events plays an important part in these syndromes.

During the 1980s the new syndrome of post traumatic stress disorder has evolved. Its relationship to depression is obscure and here we simply note the fact that this new diagnostic "entity" is in part recognition of the enormous importance of life events.

It is clear that major life crises do provoke symptoms. More specifically, severe disturbances in social (interpersonal) life and attachments produce symptoms for the vast majority of people. Armed with this general finding we can now ask the question, "Can life stress, occurring within certain social contexts, produce (what we often call) depressive illness?" Now here the sociologist and psychologist enter into conflict with the more organic theorist. While there has never been any doubt that depression involves biological changes or that for some depressions genes play a major role, as soon as one starts to show connections between life events and depression the organic psychiatrist says: "Well yes, but that is not depressive illness" (e.g., see Brown, 1989). By and large the organic theorist has lost the debate since we now know that the timing of onset and recovery are related to life events for the majority of cases (although again I stress not all). Even mania seems related to life events (e.g., Ambelas, 1987; Ellicott et al., 1990). Our theories are (slowly) becoming more sophisticated, biopsychosocial and less categorical (illness versus not-illness).

In a recent study, Ganzini, McFarland, and Cutler (1990) investigated the consequence of severe financial loss (retirement savings in a bank fraud). Over the 20-month follow up, 29% of the group (n=72) developed major depressive disorder (compared to 2% in matched controls). Twenty-seven percent also met criteria for generalised anxiety disorder (compared to 10% in controls). Somatic symptoms where common. Only 4 of 21 with major depression sought help. Ganzini et al. (1990) agree with Brown (1989; and pp.440–443 this volume) that life events which have long-term implications can cause major depression. Also of note, this study found that controls and ill subjects did not vary in their use of social support or coping strategies. Hence it was the long-term implications of the event itself that had the pathogenic impact.

In an effort to overcome data gathering difficulties, which are not easily handled by life event inventories, Brown and Harris (1978a) developed a measure of contextual threat. This was derived by the use of trained interviewers allowing any event to be considered potentially stressful and then rated blind by other workers. Tennant et al. (1979) have evaluated this procedure and found it to be "highly satisfactory". Clearly, it is not possible here to go into detail about the adequacy of research design, but there are several papers that the interested reader may consult (Bebbington, 1980; Brown & Harris, 1978b; 1980; Cooke, 1980b; Harre, 1980; Paykel, 1978; 1979; Tennant & Bebbington, 1978; Tennant et al., 1981b; Tennant & Thompson, 1980).

Brown and Harris (1978a) provided a comprehensive investigation of the role of life events in depression. They investigated the relationship of life events to depression in two populations—a depressed female patient group and identified cases from a female working-class population in London. Importantly, Brown and Harris made major efforts to identify true cases of depression, using generally accepted descriptive psychiatric phenomenology. This was achieved with trained interviewers using a structured interview, based on the Present State Examination (PSE; Wing, Cooper, & Sartorius, 1974). As Brown (1979a) makes clear, it was the symptom cluster and not simply depressed mood, no matter how severe, that identified cases as true cases of depression (bipolar patients were excluded). Furthermore, for cases identified from the non-patient population, it was generally agreed that had those individuals presented themselves to medical agencies they would have been regarded and treated as depressed.

In general, then, it seems fair to conclude that Brown and his colleagues did identify true cases of depression and did develop a measure of contextual threat which is highly satisfactory. We can now consider the findings of this major study. These are presented as findings concerning the events themselves, and findings concerning vulnerability factors.

The Events

Provoking agents. It is only long-term, threatening events which play any role in depression (see also Ganzini et al., 1990). Short-term threatening events play no role in depression onset. The long-term threatening events were generally those that involved disturbances in the socially integrative relations of the person. These were threats or actual losses, and included: loss of a significant other (e.g., separation from husband), an unpleasant discovery forcing a reassessment of major relationships, a threatening illness to someone close, material loss and disappointment, and miscellaneous stresses concerning redundancy following a period of secure employment (Brown, 1979a, p. 270). Brown, Bifulco, and Harris (1987) draw a distinction between ongoing difficulties, strong commitments, and role conflict, but again stress that it is their long-term implications for the person that is most strongly associated with depression.

The stresses and major difficulties outlined by Brown and his colleagues are labelled "provoking agents". However, Brown makes it clear that the social context within which these events occur has a significant bearing on the probability of developing a depression. Thus provoking agents themselves need to be considered against a background of ongoing vulnerability. Provoking agents affect depression onset, but it is the combination of vulnerability factors and provoking agents that is most associated with depression.

There is evidence that depressives tend to appraise life events as more threatening than non-depressed subjects, and perceive them as requiring significantly greater readjustment (Schless, Schwartz, Goetz, & Mendels, 1974). Paykel (1978; 1979) confirmed Brown's findings, that the quality of life events is related to depression. Exit events, especially those that threaten or involve real, important, interpersonal losses, are the most significant events associated with depression.

Tennant and Bebbington (1978) raised technical and statistical arguments against the idea that vulnerability factors and provoking agents can be regarded separately. More recently, Champion (1990) re-analysed a number of published studies and found that the lack of an intimate relationship was related to more adverse life events. As we shall discuss in Chapter 16 however, there is no clear way of understanding how these might be related—e.g., both could be independent but have a shared relationship with a third or other variable(s). Brown outlines two types of vulnerability factors and the relationship between them is also complex and a matter for further research. To make our exposition clear, I have labelled these "social vulnerability factors" and "psychological vulnerability factors". Brown does not discriminate between these factors in quite this way.

Vulnerability Factors

Social vulnerability factors. The probability of becoming depressed in the presence of provoking agents is increased if a woman does not have, within her social network, a close, confiding relationship. The most important relationship, which looking at it positively confers some protection, is a confiding relationship with her husband. Other vulnerability factors include: having no full- or part-time employment, having three or more children at home, and having lost her own mother (especially by death) before the age of 11. This last factor, Brown believes, may also have a significant bearing on the form the depression takes. He relates this factor to symptom formation.

Brown (1979b; 1989) suggests that these vulnerabilities in themselves do not trigger depression, but do significantly increase risk in the presence of a provoking agent. The combination of provoking agents and vulnerability factors goes some way to explaining major social class differences in the prevalence of depression. Working-class women are more likely to have severe life events and difficulties, and to have significant social vulnerability as described by the factors outlined.

Psychological vulnerability factors. Brown (1979b, p.253) says: "I believe that present evidence suggests that clinical depression is essentially a social phenomenon in the sense of being usually the result of a person's 'thoughts' about his or her world." He goes on to say that he would not make the same claim for schizophrenia. In view of the arguments put forward earlier, concerning the social and evolutionary aspects of depression, it is possible to see a considerable degree of agreement between those ideas and Brown's, although each set of ideas was reached via different paths.

Brown suggests that the two most important perceptions that provoking agents and vulnerability combine to produce are low self-esteem (we might prefer the term, involuntary, subordinate self-perception) and hopelessness. He suggests that if there is a tendency toward generalized perceptions of hopelessness and low self-esteem, then depressive symptoms manifest. The relationship between the causes of low self-esteem and vulnerability factors is obscure, however. Sometimes Brown suggests that self-esteem might be low before a depression occurs, at other times the provoking agents and vulnerability factors appear to bring about low self-esteem. Both might be true. This is an important point, I suspect, since ongoing, low self-esteem may significantly influence the type of relationship a woman chooses, together with the style of interaction. Low self-esteem women may pick low self-esteem husbands, who may be less capable of providing a confiding, secure, and good selfobject relationship. I have seen some cases which might support this view. Recent work has shown that there is certainly a relationship between social support, self-esteem, and depression (Brown, Bifulco, Harris, & Bridge, 1986) although their relationship is complex (Crammer, 1990). Also, whether or not a depressive cognitive style is necessary to turn a provoking agent into a depression is doubtful, although it may occur in some cases (Parry & Brewin, 1988).

Subsequent work has confirmed the findings of the pre-1979 studies (see Brown, 1989; Smith & Allred, 1989). Concepts have been refined (Brown et al., 1987), such as the importance of a person's role relationship and incentive structure, but the major distinction of provoking agents and vulnerability factors has been supported by further research. The symptom formation factor of maternal loss remains more controversial. One of the new findings relates to recovery. It has been found that recovery from "caseness" is often associated with "fresh start" events. These events are not without risk or threat, but in Brown's (1989; Brown et al., 1988) view they carry the hope that things can change.

The distinction between endogenous and neurotic depression does not seem to be related to life events (Akiskal et al., 1978; Brugha & Conroy, 1985, Grove et al., 1987). Even mania may be ignited by life events (Ambelas, 1987) and its course related to life events (Ellicott et al., 1990).

Life Events and Evolution Theory

From an evolution theory perspective, provoking agents can be divided into three types: Direct attacks, loss of SAHP (indirect attacks), and entrapments.

1. *Direct attacks.* There are those who are in critical or abusive relationships. Here there is a direct attack on self-esteem and the forcing of the person into a subordinate position from which they cannot retaliate (Price & Sloman, 1987). Pre-existent low self-esteem may mean that one either accepts these attacks as valid or has no way to counteract them. Events may reinforce a sense of helplessness and subordinacy. Andrews and Brewin (1990) found that, while females are in an abusive relationship, they tend to blame themselves, but when they move out, they become more blaming of the partner. This supports ranking theory, in that in conditions of forced subordinacy, attacks up hierarchy are inhibited (because it would be dangerous) and self-blame is a way of reducing aspirations to attack back (see Chapters 7 and 8). Andrews and Brewin also found that characterological self-blame (see Chapter 8) was associated with previous (childhood) history of abuse (i.e., previous history of intense subordination from a powerful, aggressive, dominant other) and was associated with depression (see Chapter 10).

2. *Loss of SAHP.* These events are those that would undermine SAHP and a person's sense of rank/attractiveness/value (see Chapter 7). Many of the life events discussed above seem to rob a person of their roles that have functioned as a source of self-esteem. It is unclear from Brown's

work how much social comparison and shame are involved here. For example, a patient lost her potential husband to another women. She had prided herself on being a loving person. In therapy she constantly asked "What do you think he saw in her? What did she have that I didn't? I must have done something wrong." It was her resentment and sense inferiority to the other woman that caused much distress. The event of children getting into trouble with the police (Brown, 1989) may also be an event that provokes shame and loss of SAHP. In any event the sense of personal failure that these events seem to convey is in accord with ranking theory.

Loss of a confident or close relationship, who has acted as a mirroring selfobject (see Chapter 10), might also reduce SAHP. Hence, this kind of loss might be crucial for some. Loss of SAHP and a sense of self-worth may also come from failing to achieve certain goals (e.g Areiti & Bemporad's [1980a,b] dominant goal types; see Chapter 12). A different kind of event is that of entrapment.

3. *Entrapments.* In some cases a person is trapped in a poor relationship that she/he cannot get free from (feeling too guilty at leaving, or too fearful) or is trapped by economic circumstances (e.g., a single mother's dependency on parents, or inability to give up one's job because of economic responsibilities—this is more common in men than is recognised and can lead to anger at the family). This is the equivalent of blocked escape. It is associated with the idea of "caging", being confined and limited in actual movement (especially away from an aversive situation). Helplessness does not convey the sense of being caged and trapped although at another level they are probably equivalent. Entrapments focus more on the theme of "freedom of movement" and blocked escape. Events can occur that make one acutely aware not only of how little one can do, but also of how "confined one is". Fresh start events would probably reduce the sense of being trapped/caged (Brown et al., 1988). It is unknown how far these events tap into self-esteem. The most extreme example would be the depression associated with becoming a hostage or captive of some kind.

Entrapment can also be internalised. For example, a patient found her marriage extremely boring. However, her moral/religious beliefs (which in part seemed a cover for her fear) prohibited her from leaving (see Chapter 8 and the relation of guilt to entrapment). Other forms of entrapment may relate to helplessness and loss of control (e.g., Ganzini et al., 1990) and hope (Abramson et al., 1989). Long-term goals and plans cannot be pursued and in this sense the person's movement and capacity to explore the environment, gather resources and exert control over a desired life style is seriously reduced. None of these ranking concepts are mutually exclusive.

SOCIAL SUPPORT

It is becoming increasingly clear that the impact of life events in relationship to social support is complex (Stokes & McKirnan, 1989). Hong, Wirt, Yellin, and Hopwood (1979) point out that individuals are not simply passive recipients of life events, but to some degree actively shape their environments (see also Bebbington et al., 1989). Recent models, describing the mechanisms that translate life events into illness behaviour, usually outline social support and resource availability, psychological and biological processes. Rahe and Arthur (1978) offer an interesting model for understanding the intervening processes between life change and illness. Andrews, Tennant, Hewson, and Vaillant (1978) point out that coping style and social support influence risk of psychological impairment. But they suggest that coping and social support are independently related to neurosis and do not primarily exert their effect by detoxifying the effects of high stress. Nevertheless, their data suggest that: "In those without stress, with good coping and good support, the risk of psychological impairment was 6 per cent, while in those under stress, without support and with poor coping, the risk was raised 5-fold to 30 per cent" (p. 313). As mentioned above, Champion (1990) re-analysed a number of published studies and found that the lack of an intimate relationship was related to more adverse life events.

Paykel, Weissman, and Prusoff (1978) examined the relationship between social adjustment and severity of symptoms. Social maladjustment did not correlate well with severity of symptoms during an acute disturbance. The reasons for this are obscure, but suggest that illness severity and interpersonal coping should be regarded as separate processes. Also much depends on what one means by social maladjustment. Would Type A and autocratic behaviour be classed as social maladjustment? Paykel et al. (1978) point out that mild depressives may have significant social maladjustment. Life events also adversely affect relapse (Paykel & Tanner, 1976). Indeed, the importance of social and interpersonal variables on relapse is clinically well noted (Hooley & Teasdale, 1989; Beach, Sandeen, & O'Leary, 1990). It is not uncommon for recovering hospitalised patients to return from a weekend leave with an intensification of their symptoms or even outright relapse.

Warheit (1979) investigated complex interactions between life stress, coping, and depressive symptoms. A large sample were interviewed, of which 517 cases were re-interviewed three years later. His general finding was that symptoms at first interview had a better predictive capacity of symptoms at second interview than life stress or losses. However, he also found important associations between depression and social-psychological processes. Amongst the findings were: (l) the presence of a spouse was significantly correlated with level of depression regardless of (other) losses; (2) life-event losses were higher for the higher depression scoring subjects; (3) for the high-loss individuals, having friendships was associated with lower depression scores; (4) losses and the absence of resources were significant variables when used to predict depression scores. Warheit suggests, therefore, that the effects of life-event losses are mitigated somewhat by the availability of personal, familial, interpersonal, and other resources. Hence depression proneness and life events seem to go together (see also Bebbington et al., 1989).

Such data again suggest important interactions between life events, social support, and psychological processes. McC.Miller and Ingham (1976) confirmed the importance of social support, especially that of a confidant, in the manifestation of various symptoms. Moreover, as in Warheit's study, friendship was found to be important. In an edited volume, Hojat and Crandall (1989) have brought together many of the main themes relating social functioning (socioemotive bonds) to various forms of pathology and unhappiness. There is no doubt now that social relationships are vital to health for the vast majority of people and have major psychobiological regulatory effects (e.g., Hofer, 1984). Pre-existent relational style, developed perhaps in childhood, may increase risk of a number of interrelated phenomena: (a)low and/or vulnerable self-esteem and negative attributional style; (b) encountering aversive life events; (c) becoming poorly integrated in a network and poor formation of supportive emotional bonds; and (d) depression and negative affectivity.

The few studies outlined here represent the tip of an ever-growing iceberg of research which demonstrates important associations between life events, social support, and coping. Bebbington, Hurry, Tennant, Sturt, & Wing (1981) offer further support to these associations and a good review of findings. Although methodologies can be criticised, and the relationship between distress reactions and illness is uncertain (Tennant et al., 1981b), the results are in the main consistent enough to safely conclude that the environment does play a significant role in many depressions.

Types of Effect

Brugha et al. (1987) investigated personal relationships and social support in neurotic and endogenous cases to see if these variables identified differences. They did not find any difference between personal relationships and social support for each type of depression. However, for endogenous cases, availability of a close confidant related to outcome, whereas in neurotic depression a number of social support variables related to outcome. More recently, Brugha et al. (1990) found possible gender differences in regard to various elements of social support. In men recovery seemed associated with negative social interaction and being married whereas in women satisfaction with social support and a number of supportive relationships in a primary group were related to recovery. Many explanations are possible, e.g., gender differences in preparedness to acknowldge negative social interaction (though this may also reflect a rank effect; women who are the dominant partner may be more likely to acknowledge negative social interaction especially if they blame the partner, whereas those who feel more subordinate may be less likely to do so). There may be biological differences in the way networks function for males and females (Kevles, 1986). In any event more research is needed in this area.

It has been common in social support research to argue in favour of two hypotheses. The first is the "stress buffering hypothesis" which suggests that support protects against the harmful effects of stress. The second is the "main effects hypothesis" which argues that social support is health promoting. Although these two hypotheses have sometimes been presented as alternatives of how social support works, in fact they are not mutually exclusive and both are valid. In their review of the research evidence, Stokes and McKirnan (1989, pp.277–278) caution against simple notions of causality and social support. They say:

> any one of several causal relations between depression or anxiety and social support is possible. Low levels of support or sudden losses of supportive relationships may lead to depression or anxiety, or may fail to buffer one from the stressors that induce these states. Second, anxiety or depression may render one undesirable as a companion or confident, or might be associated with a lack of social skills needed to develop relationships and initiate supportive interactions. Finally, where social support is conceptualised as a subjective state it may relate to adjustment because both constructs reflect NA [negative affectivity, see Chapter 2, this volume]. Of course, all these processes may operate simultaneously or may compliment each other in a complex fashion.

These researchers also point out that there are developmental factors that can work against being able to either elicit or use social support even if available. Various attitudes—such as "it is demeaning to ask or need; one should conceal one's true feelings; others should help me without my having to ask; no one can help me or give me what I need"—can mitigate against social support (even if available) functioning as a helpful mechanism. Basic mistrust may make support receiving difficult (especially those with a strong sense of being an outsider). Also, social support can be used to maintain dependency and a sense of inferiority/weakness. Hence where support ends and overprotection and intrusiveness begins is uncertain. In a case of postnatal depression, a mother was all too ready to "support her daughter", but she was highly controlling and intrusive. The daughter couldn't tell her about this for fear of hurting her mother's feelings (and mother might withdraw completely), and fear that she could not cope without some degree of mother's support. However, she felt entrapped by the intrusiveness and compared to mother felt much less able (mother would constantly tell her how things had been so much harder in her day, etc.). Consequently, she became more depressed, setting up a vicious circle of mother "offering" more support (taking over) and the daughter gradually "disappearing". Some patients do not seek support for fear of intrusiveness and obligation. Recent work suggests that there maybe genetic factors that influence coping behaviours such as turning to others for support (Kendler et al., 1991).

Types of Support

Different types of social support may have different effects for different individuals. For example, we can distinguish between social support and emotional support (e.g., see Hojat & Crandall, 1989). Coyne, Aldwyn, and Lazarus (1981) distinguished between problem-solving behaviour and emotional support seeking. They found that depressives did little of the former but much of the latter. Weiss (1986) suggests six forms of what he calls "social bonds". These are: (1) attachment based on the development of affection and related to Bowlby's idea of attachment systems; (2) affiliation derived from the sharing of interests, mutuality of feelings, affection, and respect; (3) nurturance which relates to a sense of commitment and investment of responsibility for someone; (4) collaboration which relates to the relationship based on shared commitment to achieve a goal; (5) persisting alliances which, again, are strongly associated with feelings of obligation to help the other and are related particularly to kinship ties; and (6) help-obtaining which relates to relationships in which someone is perceived to be more knowledgeable and wiser, and looked to as a source of guidance.

Hill (1987) found that people seek out others for various reasons. He identified four major dimensions: (a) emotional support; (b) attention; (c) positive stimulation; and (d) social comparison. It is unclear how far these different aspects are related to depression and support seeking. An individual who needs financial help, or contact with a supportive solicitor, may not benefit from a therapist who focuses on feelings. What the social support literature does imply is that we need to separate more clearly affiliative relationships from intimate relationships. Rook (1987) has drawn attention to the role of friends and suggests these are more important to well-being than has been recognised.

Shame and Social Support

Shame complicates the social support literature because shame is associated with concealment (see Chapter 8). Depressed women have been found to be less self-disclosing than non-depressed women in their families (Keitner & Miller, 1990). Brewin, MacCarthy, and Furnham (1989) found there was a significant interaction between social comparison, shame, self-blame, and support seeking. In shame, there may be things that one would not want all one's family or friends to know about (e.g., that one had been or was being abused). This relates to the ideas on social presentation (see Chapters 7 and 8). In therapy an issue can sometimes arise as to what to tell a spouse. And this issue can be quite delicate even if the spouse is loved. A patient had had an affair early in her marriage. Some years later the man turned up again and threatened to tell the husband unless she resumed the affair. At first she agreed, but then became depressed. It was quite unclear if the husband could have coped with this knowledge. She was forced into this dilemma by her ex-lover. Although she had a supportive close friend, she knew that only she could solve the dilemma. Further, because of shame she never fully confided in her friend.

Also we need to separate relationships in which a person hopes to share goals (as suggested by Weiss, 1986). A man had agreed to set up business with a friend whom he had known for some years. Slowly, however, the friend started to dominate the partnership, taking decisions without consultation and leaving my patient (by his account) to sort out the resulting problems (in effect treating him as a subordinate). Although the friend agreed to change and be more cooperative he never actually changed his behaviour. The patient thought that success had "gone to his head". Arguments followed and the working atmosphere "became just terrible". The patient gradually became moody and obsessional. His wife and friends were very supportive, but it put a great strain on the marriage, especially his irritability. This went on for sometime, the patient became suicidal (especially in the early hours) and had to have time off work and take antidepressants. This angered him even more because he felt it made him look in the wrong and weak. Not until he had decided to terminate the business and start again did the depression recede. (There was something of a revenge theme here). While he felt trapped (to maintain his life style and all the effort he had put into the business) he remained depressed. In another case a women felt so envious of her friends that she would never seek their help as this would put her in a one down position. These examples show that social support works in complex ways in individual cases. Many of these individual traumas are lost in large studies that pool data.

Hence shame and envy can be reasons that support, even if available, is not taken or cannot be used. Some find needing help a sign of weakness and it reduces rather than lifts self-esteem (Fisher, Nadler, & Whitcher-Alagna, 1982). A psychiatrist colleague mentioned to me that one of the reasons mental health problems are rife in the medical profession is because these individuals (due to their perceived status and ideas that they should be able to cope) do not seek help, either because they think they shouldn't suffer like the rest of us or because of the shame of revealing.

The Psychobiology of Relationships

It is important to recognise that our interpersonal lives do not simply work at some abstract cognitive level, but actually influence biological state (Hofer, 1984). Let me give just a few examples. On the negative side the effects of separation and abandonment result in serious changes of biological state (e.g., see Reite & Field, 1985). Coe et al. (1985) found that hormonal and immune function changes arising from separation were significantly influenced according to whether separation resulted in isolation or occurred in the presence of familiar others. It was familiar others that were crucial, because separation in the presence of unfamiliars did not exert any protective effect. Hojat and Vogel (1989) have reviewed some of the evidence outlining the links between social bonds and biological processes.

Montagu (1986) has written extensively on the role of touch and how touch can be translated symbolically. Symbolic signals of approval act like physical touch offering reassurance and lowering defensive arousal (assuming people are receptive to these signals, i.e. trust these signals). We speak of being "touched" by another's kindness. Touch in various (physical or symbolic) forms has psychobiological effects and these are direct stimulus response connections. In some states of depression, patients have strong desires to be held and stroked. In my view these are not regressive child-like needs, nor disguised sexuality, but arise from needs for reassurance. And in these states, nonverbal forms of reassurance are sought.[1] Chimpanzees use touch, stroking, and holding at a high level. In some respects (as argued in Chapter 7) the social signals of acceptance we obtain from others are a form of reassurance that relaxes us and promotes changes in psychobiological state. Social relationships, then, that offer reassurance provide biologically meaningful stimuli and their effects are widespread. They influence directly the self-defensive system (Chapter 5 and Gilbert, 1989).

THE INTERPERSONAL APPROACH TO DEPRESSION

In many ways much of this book has been about interpersonal processes and social cognitions and therefore it is somewhat artificial to select out all those factors that have been discussed through preceding chapters. However, there is a treatment approach that is directed specifically at changing interpersonal behaviour (Klerman, Weissman, Rounsaville, & Chevron, 1984; Gotlib & Colby, 1987). It has been this therapeutic model (Klerman et al., 1984) that has recently been compared to cognitive therapy, drug plus clinical management and clinical management plus placebo (Elkin et al., 1989; Imber et al., 1990). Frank et al. (1989) found that interpersonal therapy, given only once a month at follow-up, was a better predictor (preventer) of relapse than drugs.

The interpersonal approach emphasises the role of (social) life events, the nature of significant relationships (mostly in the present, but also with some consideration of early relationships), the interpersonal tactics a person uses to gain and maintain relationships and resolve conflicts. This model proposes various specific causes of depression: grief and loss, interpersonal role transitions, role conflicts, and social skills deficits. The model outlines various therapeutic interventions for dealing with each source of difficulty. Needless to say much of this formulation is consistent with ranking and network theory, but as yet lacks the focus on the issue of social comparison (Swallow & Kuiper, 1988), the nature of internal inhibition and the role of a loss of a sense of value; involuntary, subordinate self-perception.

Coyne (1976a,b) presented a model of depression that suggested that the depressed person is unattractive to others and therefore tends to elicit aversive responses. In this way a depression can be maintained. But depression is not a form of care eliciting. Care eliciting behaviour may be a "strategy" for dealing/coping with depression (Rippere, 1981). It is usually direct and effortful. According to the theory outlined in this book, depression originally evolved to signal "no threat", it's an "I am out of action" signal. Indeed Biglan et al., (1985) found that depression temporarily reduces aggression from the spouse but may increase resentment.

Depressed people are not good at acting as mirroring selfobjects (see Chapter 10). They withdraw sexually, and engage in less positive, reciprocal interactions. They initiate fewer positive interactions (e.g., going to a film, out to see friends, or sex, in part because they see it as too much effort). Not surprisingly, then, many marriages involving a depressed person are marked by a good deal of hostility (Coyne, Kahn, & Gotlib, 1987; Gotlib & Colby, 1987, Beach et al., 1990). For both partners marriage can be seen as a trap as much as a source of support.

Coyne (1982, 1989) has been a critic of the cognitive view that distorted cognitions cause depression and has emphasised instead the role of the social environment. Hooley and Teasdale (1989) found that spouse criticism was associated with relapse. Vaughn and Leff (1985) found that few depressives who had chronic low self-esteem and lack of confidence lived with a supportive or sympathetic spouse. Those who did were well at follow-up. Hence it is unlikely that depression evolved as a care eliciting tactic. More likely, depression is a primitive avoidance of aggression response that does not work because of the evolved changes in our life styles (see Chapters 6 and 7). Even if care eliciting is targeted at a spouse, the spouse may not be able to respond appropriately, find it unattractive and withdraw, or denounce it as further evidence of the elicitor's inferiority. There is much in the growing literature on expressed emotion (Vaughn & Leff, 1976; 1985; Falloon, 1988) that could be explored from a ranking theory perspective (i.e., the dominance relationship of who expresses criticism to whom and how—e.g., sustained negativity and hostility versus temper tantrum outbursts with returns to a more submissive state, etc., see Chapter 8).

MARRIAGE AND THE FAMILY

The family in both its narrow and extended forms is often a major source of both stress and support (see Clarkin et al., 1988; Keitner & Miller, 1990; Beach et al., 1990, for reviews of both theory and a family therapies approach to treatment). In today's culture, families and marriages are under extensive stress and function in a very different way to those of other primates. It is worth reminding ourselves that non-human primates (especially chimpanzees) are highly promiscuous and for them nothing resembling a marriage or monogamy exists. Young are brought up by the mothers, and males play a role in protection of mothers and offspring. As current figures on divorce rates suggest, marriage is often a difficult relational style to sustain over the long term and requires a set of beliefs and cultural practices to sustain it. Nevertheless the issue of sexual possessiveness and control of mates are major concerns throughout the animal kingdom.

Families produce the minor (and sometimes not so minor) and chronic hassles of life. It is now commonly accepted that families who have a hostile (agonic) structure are more prone to depression. The hedonic style of interacting (see Chapter 7) depends on a constant flow and exchange of good, friendly relationships. In self psychology terms, this is a constant exchange of selfobject mirroring (see Chapter 10). There is now much evidence on the adverse role marital relations can play on the onset and maintenance of depression (Coyne, 1988; Coyne et al., 1987; Beach et al., 1990). Families that have poor cohesiveness and express high levels of criticism report more depressive symptoms. Birtchnell (1988b) found that, compared to non-depressed married women (aged 25-35), depressed married women rated their marriages as much poorer. The depressed women were also found to have poor relationships with their own mothers (both currently and in the past) but not their fathers. They were also found to have a much poorer relationships with their parents-in-law. I am unaware of much work on in-laws but I have found that in various cases they can be helpful (e.g., a person may develop a better relationship with the in-laws than with their own parents) or on the other hand in-law relationships can have a very detrimental effect. I have the feeling that in-law relationships may be more important for women than men but know of no evidence.

Keitner and Miller (1990) report evidence that women who have disputes with their husbands and divorce, have disputes with their new husbands also. It is unknown whether this reflects poor selection of a spouse (assortive mating), whether at remarriage they remain mildly depressed and the new marriage is engaged as a coping response for mild depression, or whether the tendency to take a certain style of relating from one relationship to another reflects personality and/or early attachment style (or various combinations). Keitner and Miller (1990) also report that marriage may be less protective for women than men (see also Brugha et al., 1990). This may be because of the dominance relationships in the marriage (i.e., women are more likely to be treated as subordinates). From their review of the evidence they offer an interesting interactive model but again there is little attention given to the issues of dominance–submission. The nature of dominance relationship (i.e., which partner is dominant) may have a bearing on depressive type (Price, in press).

Gotlib and Colby (1987), Clarkin, Haas, and Glick (1988) and Beach et al. (1990) give an overview of the kinds of family interactions that may be associated with depression. First, they point out that research on associative mating suggest that depressives tend to marry similarly disposed individuals at greater than chance levels. What each is selecting for, however, is unclear. Almost certainly it is not depression but it may be similarity with parents (who may have depressive traits), i.e., there is something in the potential partner that reminds them of mother/father (adoption studies might control for this). Relationships that follow a predictable style, even if this stye is agonic or lacking in warmth, may be preferable to unpredictable styles. (For example, a rather submissive man married a woman who was domineering. His mother had been domineering. A woman married a harsh autocrat, her father had been a harsh autocrat). Hence some marriages may start out on a bad keel for selection reasons. Alternatively people might not select partners where there is too high a self-esteem gap. I have one patient who joined a dating agency. She is attractive and found a number of suitors. However she turned some away because they "felt too above her" and she felt anxious and inferior with them. You can guess the kind of man she would go out with.

Individuals may come into a marriage with various expectations and needs but may marry someone who is not actually able to fulfil these. There may be various attitudinal difficulties in forming intimate relationship: "I should be loved come what may. If he/she does not constantly show they love me then they dislike me" (Beck, 1989). For those wishing to study more about the family approach to treatment Gotlib and Colby (1987) and Beach et al. (1990) provide very helpful overviews. There is increasing evidence (Hickie, Parker, Wilhelm & Tennant, 1991), that some forms of depression are related to issues of control and warmth in intimate relationships.

Reconciliation

How is it that some marriages can have high levels of conflict, but survive? Remember the song, "You always hurt the one you love." One area where marriages containing a depressed person seem to function poorly is skills for resolving conflicts. Indeed, in ranking theory one looks very closely not only at the degree of conflict but how it is resolved. Marriage partners who have high levels of conflict but good reconciling repertoires and who are basically valuing of each other tend not to suffer depression. If chimpanzees provide any kind of model for us (see Chapter 7) then one thing stands out: their reconciling behaviour (de Waal, 1988). In many cases we find that marriages of depressed people have very poor reconciling repertoires. Furthermore, it is not uncommon to hear that in their early life (for at least one of the partners) reconciliation following conflict was notably absent. Without reconciliation the individual remains in a high state of defensive arousal and resentment continues.

The reasons that reconciliation does not take place are complex. One is that people don't know how to do it, or feel too embarrassed/awkward. Another is that a spouse will never reconcile unless they are given the dominant position. Sulking may go on as a way to punish. All kinds of inhibition may linger under the surface so that even if reconciliation apparently occurs, it is not genuine but glitters with resentment. Alternatively, if an individual wants to reconcile there may be poor skills for expressing emotion/affection. As far as we know reconciliation in intimate relationships probably works best via hugs and physical contact. An expressed feeling of "even when he/she is trying to be nice I can't bear them to touch me" suggests much unresolved resentment and failure of reconciliation. Reconciliation may act on the safety system (Gilbert, 1989).

In ranking theory it would be relationships that either directly of indirectly undermine a person's sense of value that will have the most dysphoric effects. Competition to be noticed or exert control can result in various members at various times "picking up" the role of subordinate. In some families there appears to be a kind of passing around the position of subordinate. Family therapists have informed me that it is not uncommon to find that as one member overcomes depression another member sinks into it. In some families the one that shows the most pathology is the one that has been forced into the subordinate role or is trying to exert control in maladaptive ways.

OVERVIEW

In Chapter 5 we pointed out that evolution has brought about a structuralisation of our affect systems such that social success tends to elicit positive affect, while lack of social success tends to elicit negative affect. When we look back in time to our non-human primate ancestors and our early hunter-gatherer beginnings we see how both culture and the relationships of "the family" have undergone radical recent change. It is unclear to me whether these are biologically sustainable without many casualties.

Many theorists now believe, as Freud and Nietzsche did, that mental suffering arises because our evolution is running up against the brisk pace of cultural change. But, unlike Nietzsche and Freud, they believe it is not aggressiveness that is caught in the friction of this change but rather a sense of security, belonging, and self-value. In this sense I follow Kohut (see Chapter 10) and suspect that much of our aggression in relationships is secondary to the failure of mirroring selfobjects. When such failure occurs it signals to the brain a lack of social success. By now I hope the reader will have a sense of the role of social power and belonging in depression.

SUMMARY

1. To understand the role of various life events and social support in depression, it is useful to have a sense of evolutionary history. To remember, especially, that humans evolved to live in stable hunter-gatherer bands. These bands provided predictability and continuity of relationships and roles.

2. There is ample evidence that life events are associated with both the onset and termination of symptoms.

3. Events that have long-term adverse consequences to goals, plans, aspirations, and role relationships are particularly depressogenic. Events that undermine self-esteem or act as entrapments are also important. In various ways these signal detriments to social success.

4. In many cases depression is ignited with a combination of vulnerability factors, such as quality of personal and social relationships, low self-esteem and hopelessness. The interaction between these variables is complex and subject to individual variation. The relationship between depression and loneliness is still to be fully explored.

5. Interpersonal psychotherapy explores depression specifically from the point of view of the patient's social life and outlines various psychosocial factors related to onset, maintenance, and recovery. Various psychotherapy procedures have been developed.

6. The marriages of depressed people often show higher levels of disturbance than those of non-depressed people. Often there are various fights for power and control. Families can be both a source of help but also a source of great distress. Dominant members in a family may undermine self-esteem and limit control of other members.

7. Much work in the social area of depression has little contact with either evolutionary or ethological thinking. But our needs for social relationships are evolved phenomena and our understanding of these processes would be greatly advantaged with such a perspective. We should also not decontextualise the family and social factors from the wider issue of culture.

CONCLUDING COMMENTS

To state it once again: we need a social life by virtue of our evolution; our brains are wired up for it. Hence, we can imagine that the social world and our orientation to it relate in very important ways to biological processes. As is common in research, the work on depression is running parallel with another area, but is not well integrated with it; this is loneliness (Hojat & Crandall, 1989). There is much in the loneliness literature that may help research in depression and vice versa. On the other hand, as Storr (1989) suggests, we need space for solitude and the ability to "live with ourselves" is an important aspect of health also. As we noted in Chapter 13, few can live with others if they cannot live with themselves. The fear of abandonment haunts many and yet without facing this fear we may become trapped and held to ransom, and from fear of losing the other, may never live as ourselves (Yalom, 1980). Without a sense of self-value this is a difficult risk to take.

If we look back, say, twenty years, it is astounding how many in-roads the sociological approach has made into disease theories of depression. I think that now all but the most rampant bio-die-hards recognise that the world we live in can be responsible for eliciting distress and that depression in only a small percentage "comes out of the blue". The claims of the early writers, whose ideas were submerged by the Kraepelinian revolution and Plato's return in medicine, have resurfaced. And it is not only in depression but in many other disorders that we find a combination of person–environment interactions playing major roles in illness onset, expression, and recovery (or lack of it). But there is much still to do. Methodologies continue to be refined. This is not an easy research area with so many variables and individual differences in biological processes, personality, coping, and so on. Still progress has been swift and the next decade looks fascinating. Perhaps the social approach holds out the best hope for prevention.

As we move into the next decade it is likely that further evidence will come through on how social relationships are extremely important to the functioning brain and various vulnerabilities to illness. We are still only just getting around to these vital research areas because we have been so influenced by macho images of the self-sufficient, not-needy person as the mark of health, the technique and technologically dominated culture, and the Platonic disease entity perspective. Why, we should ask, has it been self- help groups that have pushed medicine to recognise the role of support, comfort, kindness, and sense of belonging, in recovery and outcome, instead of simply believing in technology? (e.g., in cancer treatments). Our culture has removed us so far from our evolved style that we no longer recognise ourselves. The social constructionists point to the major role of the social environment, but have got it wrong in de-biologising humans.

NOTE

1. Therapists who misunderstand these needs, deny them, label them child-like, or sexualise them, are not only unethical, but misinformed. The correct response is to help patients be in "touch" with these needs and not label them as evidence of inferiority or weakness and to be able to make connections with others such that adult affectional styles can be formed.

CHAPTER 16

Conclusions: Complexities, Therapies, and Loose Ends

INTRODUCTION

In this last chapter I will try to bring out some of the main themes we have been following. Our first task is draw distinctions between vulnerability, onset, maintenance, and recovery, relapse, protection/resistance. As we have progressed through this book the reader will have become aware that these aspects share complex relations. Below is but a brief summary.

1. Vulnerability

(a) Genes: For some the greatest vulnerability is, in the main, genetic. But this percentage is likely to be small. Also it is extremely unlikely that there is a gene or genes for depression. The genetic contribution will probably arise from ranking, ingroup–outgroup algorithms (or possibly attachment), i.e., the gene(s) will have some role in the social domain and relate to social functioning rather than depression as a mood state per se. Depression is a human construct of the dysfunction. A key question is threshold (McGuffin et al., 1991).

(b) Personality: Some personalities seem more at risk than others. Again genes may play some role here but these may be different from those of depression where there is not a personality aspect. To put this more crudely, genes for introversion, which may convey risk, may be different from genes for bipolar depression. More important is that personality can also be affected by perinatal factors and of course by development factors.

(c) Development: We now know that early life not only influences psychological processes but also influences the way the nervous system matures. Animal work suggests that very early distortion in development may be difficult to compensate. Personality represents the combined effect of experience interacting with biological endowment. A vulnerability may be biologically altered via early life or wired in, when none may have existed had the person had a different early experience. In any event the notion of latent self–other internal representations and the experience of an affectionless childhood, and over-control in early life seem involved. But not all those who experience an affectionless early life will come to suffer depression.

(d) Compensation: A child who has a rough time early in life may find some goal or ability that allows some compensation to developing a depression. For example, a person was poorly treated early in life but had a talent for music. His commitment and the appreciation of his talent by others seemed to protect him. How far/long this compensation would work no-one knows. But the point is that there may be things within a person—or relationships or opportunities—that compensate for a potential vulnerability (see also pp.313–314).

(e) Social factors: Lack of close relations may set the psychobiological environment for the activation of depression as suggested by Brown (see Chapter 15). Included here might be poor marriages that do not function as supporting selfobjects or have chipped away at self-esteem; also entrapments. More positively, social factors may protect against depression even in the face of some underlying biological or personality, vulnerability factors.

2. Onset

(a) Genes: There are cases where onset is related to some underlying genetic aspect that determines the time of the first and subsequent episode. Those depressions that seem to have regular cycles may be a case in point. The relationship of life events to timing is unknown, but recent evidence suggests a connection.

(b) Biological: Many biological changes can produce an onset. Head injury, hormonal change, the menopause, thyroid dysfunction, steroid and other substance abuses, various physical (viral) illnesses, and so forth. Their interaction with social and psychological factors is still to be researched.

(c) Season: There is now growing evidence that some depressions are light triggered.

(d) Life events: There seem to be various life events that can cause depression for most people, e.g., loss of a child, and those that have long-term implication for roles and plans as discussed by Brown and his colleagues (see Chapter 15). In some cases the coping style may be compromised because the event itself (loss of a confidant) removes the main source of coping. Brown's work suggests that a majority of depressions are associated with life events. Abuse and entrapments and family pressures also play a role.

(e) A Combination: Interactions between personality, incentive structure, coping or cognitive style, self-esteem, latent memories, and life events are probably involved at the point of onset. Events that have particular meaning to a person's sense of self, or selfobject relationships which no longer function, and a reduced sense of self-efficacy come together to produce onset. In our view a change in how a person feels valued by self and others is a crucial variable. Hopelessness may be another.

(f) Spirals: Various factors in biopsychosocial functioning may act in a recursive feedback pattern to produce a spiral downwards into depression.

3. Maintenance

(a) Biological: Once a person has entered a severe state of depression their biology may be so disturbed that the depression remains until a biological shift takes place. Whether genes play a role in maintenance as opposed to onset is unknown. Is it possible to get depressed because of a life event (and one would not have become depressed without this life event) and then be trapped in it because of a genetic inflexibility in some way? Are those genes controlling onset or personality different from genes controlling maintenance? We don't know. Inappropriate medications or other substances with depressogenic side effects should also be considered.

(b) Cognitions: There is some general agreement that, if not involved in cause, then cognitions are almost certainly involved in the maintenance of many depressions. The automatic thoughts outlined by Beck et al. (1979) act as positive, recursive feedback systems to maintaining depressive self-organisational patterns. Also, Teasdale (1988) has suggested that we can be depressed about being depressed. Shame about depression is also common. Entrapments at an internal level (e.g., guilt or having to 'achieve') may block changes in life style.

(c) Unresolved issues: A person may have functioned well until a certain point and then get depressed. Once depressed, a number of latent self-organisational patterns (e.g., of not being loved as a child, loss of a parent, abuse) may re-emerge. In this sense the person begins to live through the depressive experiences that had been blocked off in some way earlier in life (e.g., Gut, 1989). Until the issues, arising from earlier in life, are resolved the depression remains. This is much more common than is currently recognised. Another way to think of this is as a breakdown in compensation mechanisms (see pp. 313–314).

(d) Events: A person may get depressed for any number of reasons. As a result of the depression they may lose their spouse or job, or the marriage may turn sour. These subsequent events and losses also act as recursive feedback and maintain the depression. Lack of opportunities to change one's life style may also be involved (entrapments).

(e) Interpersonal: Various (often family) interpersonal factors such as poor reconciling behaviours, increased hostility, abuse, and so forth may lead to a cycle of put-down and the undermining of a person's sense of value and efficacy. Depression-maintaining feedback can be elicited from the environment.

(f) Social skills: A person may become depressed because of the death of a spouse. However, their introverted personality or low social skills may make it difficult to find other supporting relationships. In other cases the low rate of emission of positively rewarding behaviour can act to maintain low levels of behaviour and depression.

4. Recovery

(a) Biological: In the presence of some specific biological disturbance (e.g., thyroid, hormonal) much depends on the skill of the psychiatrist in diagnosis, and the preparedness of the psychiatrist to explore possibilities. In other cases directly changing brain state may be helpful with drugs or ECT, light therapy for SAD. Diet and exercise can also be helpful in some cases, as might sleep deprivation, though these are controversial.

(b) Drugs: Why does a drug work for one person and not another? There are various psychological reasons, since drugs do not re-train or re-educate and do not address any of the social problems or previous historical problems a person may have. But a biological reason can be in the different ways individuals metabolise drugs. The same dose may not result in equal amounts getting to the brain in different individuals. Also of course non-compliance can be a problem. Some patients do better with MAOI's rather that tricyclics (e.g., Stewart et al., 1989).

(c) Psychological: Much depends on the person's ability to work psychologically and the skill of the therapist. Those who dogmatically follow only one approach are likely to have failures. At the very least therapists should be skilled in basic counselling techniques. Nevertheless, it is important to identify positive feedback, such as:

"When I'm depressed I can't do anything, if I can't do anything I'm a failure, as a failure I feel more depressed", etc. Psychological interventions come to the rescue of the self and attempt to reduce internal self-downing, shame, and guilt, and increase explorative behaviour. New themes in life style may be necessary and new self-organisations may need to evolve.

(d) Life events: Some depressions remit in the presence of life events. A set of events labelled "fresh start events" by Brown et al. (1988) are associated with recovery.

(e) Social support: Many patients attest to the importance of having supporting, loving relationships whilst going through their depression and feel these played a large role in their recovery. Current evidence suggests that, for some at least, social/emotional support is crucial in the recovery process. Social support is a complex variable with different aspects however. In a few cases, some can feel smothered by too much support, or the marriage is the source of the problem. So the therapist should be cautious if and how family members are brought into therapy.

(f) Spontaneous remission: There is an old saying, "It's nice to be in the vicinity of a spontaneous remission". This is a controversial area: some argue that there must be some reason (life event or change in relationships, etc.) that brought recovery; on the other hand, for some cases, spontaneous remission does seem to occur and we remain perplexed by it. However, over the decade research has suggested that often spontaneous remission is not spontaneous and the label owes much to lack of awareness on the clinician's part.

(g) Personal resources: Some patients have enormous resources for recovery (or what is called ego strength) and recover without professional help. Probably the vast majority of depressed people get themselves out of it by talking to friends or working through it or they experience fresh-start events. Certainly only a minority of depressed people come for treatment. Some radical theorists have even suggested that therapy of any kind is counter-productive. At the same time we should recognise that some depressions (up to 20%) may be chronic and drag on for years to such an extent that the person comes to think "This is just the way I am". These will have serious effects on family life.

5. Relapse

(a) Biological: One cause of relapse may be feeling better and stopping medication. Most believe that a period of six to nine months on medication is necessary, post-episode, in the majority but not all cases. In other cases failure to spot a cyclical depression and use lithium may increase the chance of relapse. The problem of relapse following withdrawal of medication may suggest that drugs (in some cases) actually produce artificial or unstable recovery as depicted by catastrophe theory (Gilbert, 1984).

(b) Flight into health: In some cases patients make a flight into health that rarely lasts and therapists should be aware of this. Hence there is a premature termination of treatment. Careful follow-up is advisable. Cognitive therapists are now trying to identify those who recover but remain vulnerable. Providing small stresses and seeing if the negative cognitive style re-emerges is one paradigm. However, how long patients should be in therapy is controversial. The distinction between relapse and new episode is also controversial as researchers follow different criteria (e.g., BDI of less that 9 may not be an adequate measure of full recovery).

(c) Failure to resolve: Some depressives do not reveal their key themes out of shame, or the therapist does not work on early life experience and unresolved early grief/abuse. Alternatively, even if a patient is prepared to reveal, a therapist may not be prepared to work on historical data for various (usually dogmatic theoretical) reasons.

(d) Life events: Life events may happen at a crucial time during convalescence. For example, a patient had recovered and was doing well when his mother died and he became depressed again. Any of the events that can cause depression can be involved in relapse.

(e) Social support: Increasing evidence is coming through that spouse criticism is a key variable in relapse. Also, living alone and other social factors can contribute to relapse.

6. Protection/resistance

(a) Biological: Some individuals may be extraordinarily resistant to major depression for biological reasons. Recently, some attention has turned to explore this area rather than focus on depression. As Bebbington et al. (1989) have pointed out, in some areas of social deprivation, resistance is as intriguing as depression.

(b) Personality: Since the time of the Hippocrates it has been known that some people are extremely resilient to depression. These individuals are often social and non-aggressive and have high self-esteem.

(c) Development: Some individuals may have been able to internalise very good selfobject relations and self-esteem as a result of early life. The self-organisation is so strong that it is difficult to switch into depression. It reminds me of the toys that you turn on their side and they immediately flip upright again. They have the capacity for self-soothing, or do not catastrophise or self-down. The issue of brain state switching (Gilbert, 1984) is still to be researched.

(d) Cognitive style: In Seligman's (1989) view, optimists are less prone to depression. However, it is unclear yet if when they fall they fall into more serious depressions.

(e) Social Life: In some cases a person may be so well integrated with a way of life that provides their sense of self, sense of belonging and purpose that they are never exposed to those events noted for cause. Recent work on cults (e.g., Galanter, 1990) have suggested that this may be one of their positive functions.

The above outlines just some of the complexities that we have met on our journey. I am sure the reader can think of many other kinds of interaction between the above. Different theories speak to different aspects of depression. At the present time it is unclear how different factors operate in different cases. Not only this, but depression is not one thing, it is quite heterogenous, and can shift its pattern over time (e.g., Akiskal et al., 1978).

Interactions

Any theory that suggests causal factors, will have to come to terms with these complexities. To help understand how tricky this can be for researchers let us suppose that we have a theory that Factor X (this could be negative cognitions, genes or life events) causes depression. Now we know that depression is associated with a number of changes in biological functioning (e.g., cortisol and biogenic amines), thinking, feeling, sleeping, social behaviour, and so forth. Let us call all these other aspects the Syndrome D.

Fig. 16.1 offers some of the ways that Factor X might relate to Syndrome D. Add to this the fact that Syndrome D is heterogenous and unstable over time and you get a feel of the difficulty.

Re-biologising Mind

If our evolution had been different then our experience of life and we ourselves would be different. Equally of course, if our culture were different the same could be said, but culture is in some measure constrained by the underlying mechanisms (archetypes/biosocial goals) that all humans share. The themes and myths of all cultures have a timelessness that transcends cultural differences, as Jung often noted. One of the reasons why we suffer the complexities noted above, is that we divide up the psyche arbitrarily, into thinking, feeling, and behaviour. Yet the mind simply does not work this way. As we saw in Chapter 5, there are module systems that are concerned with processing

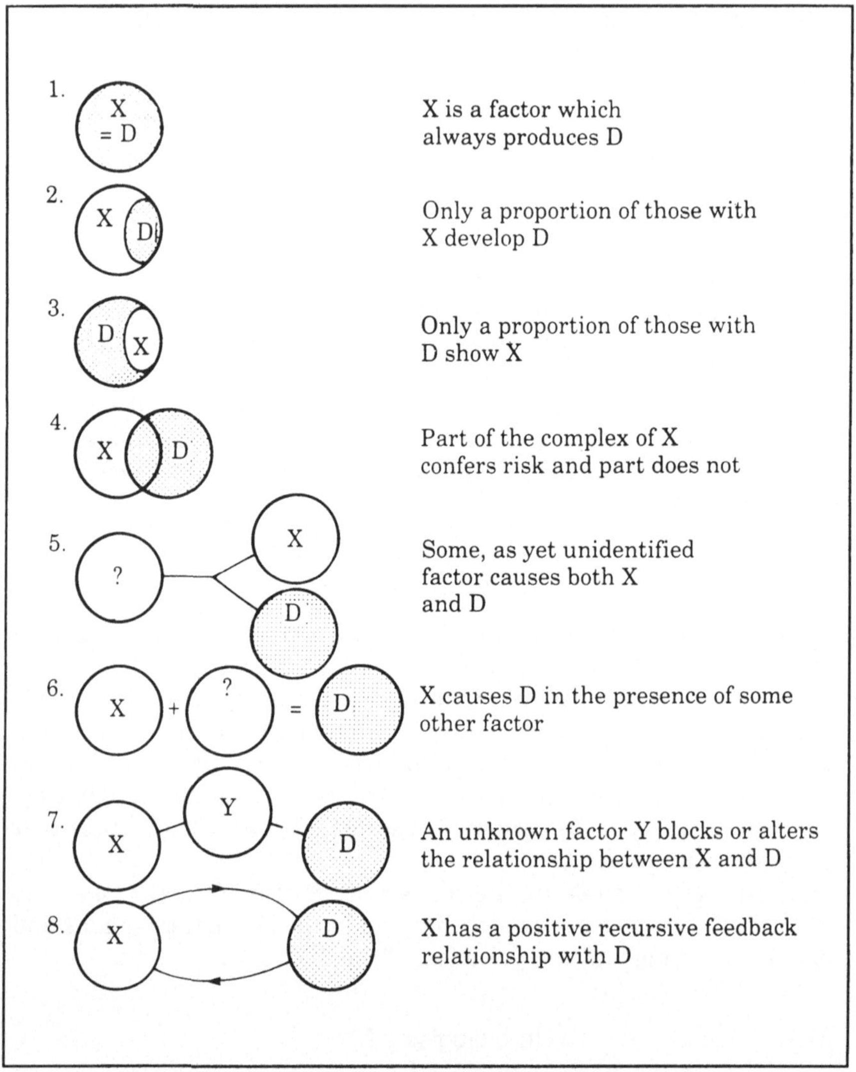

FIG. 16.1. Possible relationship between Factor X and the Syndrome of Depression D (adapted from V. Price, 1982)

different types of information. Hence it may be more helpful to think in terms of patterns of organisation of brain processes, or potential self-organisational states (see Chapter 8).

Throughout this book we have had recourse to talk often about the self; selfobjects, self-schema; self-esteem and so forth. At the present time many of these concepts are biologically decontextualised. We don't know how they are represented in brain patterns. To a struggling evolutionary theorist like myself this is a problem. It opens the door to rampant organic theorists that are socially and psychologically decontextualised. This means that they can approach their subject with little thought of how our brains, as meaning-creating devices, operate and are orientated to our social worlds (Gilbert, 1989). This, in Eisenberg's (1986) view, is mindless science. On the other hand, the psychologically minded can relegate our bodies to (at worst) irrelevancies. At every turn we are confronted with the cold metaphors of the computer. We draw boxes with arrows pointing this way and that, we talk about schema as if they were lego blocks that float about, become latent, come to the surface, and so on, when in fact the brain probably works as a pattern generator and it is through the patterns of its organisation that the emergence of states of experience come into being (Iran-Nejad & Ontony, 1984; Greenberg et al., 1990).

One of the fundamental tenets of my approach is that our way and content of our meaning-creating faculties operates on and through biologically prepared, archetypal patterns. Let me give an example. Suppose you break from reading this book and go and lie on you bed for ten minutes and engage your own sexual fantasy. What happens? Well, after a while you may note various stirrings in your body and you may begin to feel sexual. If we could drop in on you and take a few biological measures we would find various changes in your body—not too surprising. You would not accept, I think, that these feelings are only your imaginations. You would talk more about you internal experience, and this might include a mixture of feelings (in the loins), impulses, desires, memories and images, thoughts about who might fancy you, and so on.

Suppose, however, we gave you a drug that blocked all biological responses associated with sexual arousal, or maybe you are extremely tired. After a while you would find your sexual fantasies doing nothing to you and would (maybe) come back to reading this book. There would be no desires, urges or thoughts about later tonight. What is the point of the story? Well, to certain kinds of imagination our body or biological self responds in certain kinds of ways because it is preparing for certain kinds of action. So our imagination has access to biology.

Our internal imaginations, our appraisals, and so on, produce "felt-experience" by virtue of the internal patterns they evoke. We cannot pretend these are similar to a computer without a body. Let us move the imagination closer to depression. Suppose you imagine (maybe because of early experience) that basically you are no good, a rather inferior specimen and one who should conceal from others your true feelings. Following the same reasoning, do you think your body will be neutral to this? Well, of course not. And once your body has responded to this (preparing you to live as a subordinate) it will take you into states that at one time were biologically adaptive perhaps but not now. You will not only think of yourself as inferior, but experience yourself as inferior, as blocked to pursue your life goals, your initiative and explorative, free-expressive self will also be blocked and energy gone. And this experience may be with you even when you are not dwelling on how inferior (you think) you are. As a human, you'll have a further problem because, unlike other animals, you can imagine a future too and you can introspect on your state; your experiencing self can draw further conclusions that, because you have no energy and are fearful of asserting yourself, you really must be a pretty low sort of being. Imagination gives us the unfortunate (in this case) opportunity for positive, recursive feedback. On the other hand, it is our imagination and fantasy life that makes us the species we are. In our imaginations we can create things, for we can model and map the world. Sometimes, if we feel subordinate our fantasises are the only place where our explorative side is active.

Rossi (1989) has articulated a fascinating psychobiological model of what he calls "the mind-gene connection". This is the kind of model we need to be able to cope with the complexities of a disorder like depression. As here, Rossi's model stresses the role of internal patterns of activity and how our internal models affect the biological self.

This kind of analysis is okay as far as it goes and is often missing in most of our theories. But it is still dualistic and quite unsatisfactory. It assumes a starting place and a series of interactions. In reality there are no clear starting places and our division of thinking, imagination, and feeling are arbitrary divisions, necessary only because understanding the components of experience and meaning is so complex. It is also socially decontextualised and needs to account for how our internal meanings and imaginations are shaped via social interaction. Nevertheless, it perhaps offers us an approach to begin to consider what kinds of changes in our conceptual processing abilities have emerged on our journey from reptile to human.

Our complexities of symbolic thought and our capacity for introspection on experience do not magically remove us from the realm of our biological heritage. Our biological structures are both the creators of, and responders to, the world we inhabit. Our biosocial goals and social reasoning algorithms are biologically plumbed in, not in a fixed manner, but as potentials. When we begin to address the issue of self-experience we need to recognise that our meanings are not created out of some symbolic thin air. They are resonating with something within us. We are as much captured by them as their creators. Our art, rituals, and religions home in on the archetypal.

FLIPPING IN AND OUT OF STATES

If the basic social mentalities that offer us our sense of depressive experience are those to do with power and belonging then is it possible to flip from one inner self-organisation state to another? Patients suggest that this flipping (or sometimes sliding) from one state to another is common. There are various ways that one can understand this. Classical conditioning is one model that works quite well. Animals can be flipped into anxious states by the presentation of particular (conditioned and unconditioned) stimuli. Although behaviourists often concentrate on behavioural responses, in fact it is more accurate to think of state changes, since so many aspects of the animal can be recruited to various stimuli.

In 1984 I used catastrophe theory to show how state switches might be modelled. Today the theory is called Chaos theory (Gleick, 1987). We know that small changes can, if conditions are right, produce major changes in the behaviour/organisation of the whole system. At present, biological theorists approach their subject as if searching for gold at the end of the rainbow—that they will, one day, be able to identify the key chemical or the gene(s) that is/are responsible for depression. Unfortunately, we now know that many illness are multifactorial and that small changes in one variable, can, depending on the "state" of other variables it interacts with, produce major dysfunction. Susceptibility to infection is like this also—hence, Chaos theory. We know that interactions in one type of system (person) maybe different in another. And we already suspect that many who might have a genetic vulnerability to depression never actually manifest it. We also suspect that once a depressed state is turned on and actualised it may be more easily recruited in the future (possibly via some form of conditioning). Unfortunately, Chaos theory is not yet of interest to depression researchers although I am sure it will soon become so. Brain modelling on Chaos theory is some years away and yet I believe that a model like Chaos theory will one day bear great fruits to researchers.

Although I have not included catastrophe theory here (see Postle, 1980; Gilbert, 1984) some additional comments can be made. One issue that catastrophe theory draws attention to is the activation of two (or more) conflicting motives (Gilbert, 1984). This can be understood in different ways. One is by a bipolar tension produced by strong motivation. For example, if I have a strong need to succeed then I may also have a strong fear of failure. The approach–avoidance situation is that as I work hard to succeed I also work hard to avoid failure. The strength of one motive tendency increases the strength of another (see also Solomon 1980, for an opponent–process theory of motivation that bears centrally on this argument). Or to put it another way the strength of one self-organisation (successful and proud) may increase the likelihood of shifting into an alternative (a failure and ashamed). If I have a strong need to be loved, I may also increase the possibility of flipping into an unlovable or unloved state. Following Kelly (1955/1963), Jung (1964), and Solomon (1980), flipping from one self-organisational state to another depends on the bipolarity of these underlying self-organisational patterns. Kohut (1977) has a similar view.

A different example, and one we met in Chapter 4, has been put forward to explain borderlines. Now borderlines are well known for their tendency to shift states of self-organisation rather rapidly. Hence, Melges and Swartz (1989) suggested that borderlines have both a fear of abandonment and fear of domination. As they move close to others they fear domination and control. Various memories may be recruited of abuse and so forth. This activates efforts to pull away and repel possible dominators. As they pull away this activates fear of abandonment. Hence, they oscillate between two high arousal self-organisational states, and can flip between them. In people with self-organisational structures that are very split and not well integrated, this flipping of self-organisational states, especially when under stress, is common.

One more example. A patient told me that she often felt weak and unable but, a couple of times, she had noticed that in a crisis she "flips" into her coping mode, takes charge and sorts things out, even though others appear to be "flapping about" around her.

It seems then that we can have various internal states of self-organisation and can flip between them. Horowitz (1988) has called these self-organisational states, "states of mind". There is much similarity between his views and those proposed here, except that his is not an archetype or evolutionary theory. He also highlights, as we have done throughout this book, the importance of social roles. In therapy it is sometimes helpful if patients can be in touch with two (or more) alternative self-organisational states, at the same time. Different self-organisational states are often associated with different memories and styles of cognitive processing (Morey, personal communication). Somehow, in ways that are mysterious, this "holding" of alternative self-organisational states allows a certain reduction in their extreme and split-off effects. This may be because they become blended in the way that affects can become blended (Lane & Schwartz, 1987) or because they somehow produce something new, be it insight or a new, not previously existent, self-organisational pattern (Jung, 1964).

In general then, following the idea of the brain as a modular system (see Chapter 5), these internal dynamic aspects can be studied from various perspectives. I tend to favour Chaos theory and ponder how states switch, given both the internal dynamic relations of different self–other representations or self-organisational states, and how background state (e.g., elevated stress hormones) can activate this switching. Arousal is almost certainly a necessity to "flip". From my own experience, I have found that under stress my internal patterns become unstable and I can become more easily irritated, anxious or dysphoric. Things I would take no notice of when calm can become real frustrations.

I think all of us have the potential internal states of self-organisation of the triumphant versus the inferior, the accepted versus the rejected outsider. Most of the time we don't shift into the extremes or if we do others are around (acting as soothing selfobjects) to flip us back again. Moreover, we may not have memories of disturbed early life to recruit.

POWER AND BELONGING

Flipping into different states is interesting and important therapeutically. But are there special kinds of events that switch us into depressed states? In my view depression relates to two, basic, social outcomes. The first is power. Depressed people often feel powerless. This powerlessness takes various forms.

1. *Powerlessness to achieve major goals*: Goals may seem beyond the person's efforts, or ability, in which case the person feels defeated. Our ideals can be filled with the power of success and achievement. To have a sense of social success we may have set (or had set for us by parents) unrealistic goals. We crave for pride and the avoidance of shame and inferiority by achievement. The environment may simply block our aspirations.

2. *Powerlessness in social interactions*: A person may be subject to put-down or abuse in relationships and is rendered subordinate. Their own self-development is not nurtured but purposefully blocked by the desires of the dominant to maintain submissive signals and compliance. When even these stop coming, because the person is too depressed, or becomes a hostile subordinate, agonic interactions rather than hedonic ones escalate.

3. *Power to escape*: Escape behaviour may be blocked from fear or guilt of leaving. Economic restrictions are common difficulties. A mother may worry about being able to support children on her own. Men worry that if they leave a marriage they will not be able to take their children with them, and about all the emotional complications that will ensue. As the spouse or family are seen as potential trappers, further resentment builds up and internal struggles to break free increase,

especially in fantasy. People in an unhappy work situation worry about finding another job and so forth. These kinds of difficulties block opportunities for change. This kind of dependency may make us limit our assertiveness (can't complain too much in case the boss sacks us). This is the theme of freedom of movement. The great thing about money is the freedom it buys. But I emphasise freedom is often blocked by guilt.

4. *Powerlessness to attract others*: Many times our powerlessness is about feeling we have no internal power, that others regard us as marginal, that we are not talented, beautiful or able; we do not match the cultural stereotypes; that we have no SAHP. We live in the minds of others as a non-entity to be passed by. Our opinions don't matter; our needs and values don't count. When these become internalised we have little attraction to ourselves and live within ourselves as a failure and ashamed.

In all these there is a loss of control over one's (desires) destiny and life style. Our internal models of ourselves, gained perhaps in childhood, exert a powerful influence, leading to various forms of self-blame and self-downing and various ideas that we are incompetent or unlovable, and so forth. The self-organisational state of depression is activated.

But power is not the only dimension. Interacting with power and control is a sense of belonging, being part of a relationship, network, group or gang and valuing the groups we do belong to. Hence we can see various themes of belonging.

1. *Ingroup-outgroup*: We can relate to groups as if they are single bodies and we search for a place within them. We can see ourselves as different from others and subject to ridicule or scorn, and being made an outsider, or not fitting in. The sense of being cut off from fellow humans beings, that they can't understand us, is common in depression, and for archetypal reasons, we may fear our position as an outsider and become paranoid. Our envy can be another obstacle to feeling like others.

2. *Shared values*: Sometimes we may find that it is difficult to share values and goals with others. Too much nonconformity threatens being made an outsider. Too much success threatens with envious attacks from others. The pressure to conform limits our individuality (Brown, 1986). For example, a nurse moved to a new job and found that his colleagues were "far behind the times". When he tried to instigate new practices he was marginalised. A feminist confided that she had "real cravings" to be married and have a normal family life. However, she was frightened of being rejected by her anti-family lesbian friends.

3. *Reassurance*: Humans are often very ambivalent to the giving and receiving of reassurance signals. In marriage, some do not recognise how

dependent they may be on the partner for reassurance of their identity (e.g., Bird et al., 1983). I have frequently heard in the media that men and women shouldn't need reassurance from their partners about their sexuality or attractiveness, that they should be able to do it for themselves. But this is precisely what they can't do because so much of our lives involve living in the minds of others. The reason why men fail to elicit reassurance from wives is often because they treat them as subordinates, rather than equals, reciprocally giving reassurance and help and accepting each other's needs. Also, in our society the motto for men is, "Show us your strengths but keep your wimpish vulnerabilities to yourself".

4. *The loss of value*: Our sense of belonging is, in part, acquired by feeling that we play a useful role in social relationships; we have value for others, we have a useful place. The sense of not having value is common in depression and if the person sees themselves as a burden to others, this can be a real suicidal risk, especially in the elderly.

5. *Vested interests*: Vested interests of one group selectively operate to force some other group into outsider roles. Women in male-dominated occupations are particularly subject to vested interests and are not offered reassurance or help as might be necessary. Even needing it is seen as weak.[1] Vested interests are powerful reasons for marginalising people, closing ranks, and rendering them outsiders.

Treatment Considerations

These are only some of the themes that are involved in power and belonging. Table 16.1 outlines the typical issues that a therapist wishing to work in this way may focus on.

In depression the inner experience is of being unable or dis-abled. This loss of energy effectively removes the person from the social arena and signals to self and others "I am out of action". As we have moved through this book, we have seen that this loss of energy may be the result of internal inhibitory processes that switch in when a person senses that they will fail, are inferior and/or an outsider. Internal and/or external selfobject relationships fail to support a cohesive and vigorous sense of self. Maybe, in earlier evolutionary times depression was a self-protective response, but today when so much depends on self-presentation and the ability to maintain a flow in positively rewarding interactions and exchanges of reassurance signals, the depressed position of being "out of action" often leads to further loss of support and help. At what point we can see depression as maladaptive or an illness, or view it as a self-protective state that can lead to growth, is a difficult issue (Gut, 1989). Certainly, depression can in some cases

TABLE 16.1
Salient Issues of Power and Belonging

1. Social comparisons.
2. The role of shame (self-dislike or blame), envy and needs for approval/reassurance.
3. Inferiority beliefs; origins and current maintaining influences/relationships/events.
4. Premorbid functioning–e.g. as dominant and up hierarchy orientated, or chronic submissiveness and/or fear of being outsider/abandoned.
5. The nature of ideal self-future fantasies (power, success, love, sense of belonging or finding one's place).
6. The themes and roles of self-organisation; repetitive themes in fantasy, conflicting themes and their underlying affect. (e.g., for care, social control/power, fear of being an outsider). Unresolved early difficulties; are themes compensations? (e.g., if I succeed everyone will love me and I will turn out good and be redeemed, etc.).
7. The inhibition of explorative behaviour and assertiveness. What blocks free expression of self? Exploration is necessary for development, and depressives are non-explorative
8. Biological states of defeat (withdrawal) and submission; need for drugs? Type of illness (e.g., bipolar?)

Cases vary as to the importance of these issues. In one case it may be a marriage and chronic put down by a partner, in another it may be chronic inferiority beliefs associated with hostile early parenting, or failing to live up to parental ideals. The above are no more than points for consideration.

be followed by radical changes in a person's self-organisation, or (to use Jung's term) individuation. Be this as it may, depression should not be glorified. Its consequences can often be serious not only to self but also to other family members (e.g., children).

All psychotherapists who work with depressed people try to come to the rescue of this self-experience. This may be by re-engaging explorative or positively rewardable behaviour; problem solving; challenging self-downing and other negative cognitions; working on maladaptive styles of social relating or unblocking emotional disturbance from the past; acting as a valuing and supportive selfobject. In all therapies (apart from some suspect practices in classical psychoanalysis) one helps the patient to become more self-secure and future directed; to begin to engage life again. In so far as we loosen the grip on need for social approval, we see that this need was in part to counteract internal self-downing and sense of inferiority/weakness/badness. Table 16.2 gives a thumbnail sketch of some of the similarities and difference of therapies.

For a more comprehensive treatment see Dryden (1984; 1990; his 1984 edition is rather better at comparing and contrasting different approaches). Karasu (1990, p.276) has also given a wide ranging overview of the many problems of treating depression and the need to respond to the depression on a multitude of levels. He says:

TABLE 16.2
A Brief Comparison—a Theory and Therapy Focus

Theory	*Treatment*
Biological state	Various interventions aimed at changing biological state directly, e.g., drugs (MAOIs, Tricyclics) ECT, light therapy, sleep deprivation, exercise; stabilising mood switching, e.g., lithium.
Unconscious Conflict	Relationship is based on transference, interpretation of "hidden" unconscious motivations, repressed affect-laden memories. Unacknowledged anger, hostility, or grief. Historical data primary (e.g., Freud 1917).
Ontogenetic	Therapeutic relationship is holding and supportive or re-parenting. Re-activate developmental arrests; work with early memories or through early grief; importance of interpersonal schema derived from childhood. Focus on unmet needs (e.g., Bowlby, 1980; Kohut, 1977; Safran & Segal, 1990).
Affect	Therapeutic relationship supportive: Focus on blocked affective processing. Getting in touch with unacknowledged or poorly processed affect (e.g, Greenberg & Safran, 1987; Greenberg et al., 1990).
Cognitive	Therapeutic relationship is collaborative (no or little interpretation, nor emphasis on holding, mirroring), guided discovery. Re-education central; teaching thought monitoring, identifying negative recursive feedback (e.g., self-downing), direct involvement in teaching to test alternatives, avoid/correct cognitive errors (overgeneralisation and dysfunctional attitudes) coping skills training. Little concern with developmental process, or historical reworking (e.g. Beck et al., 1979).
Behavioural	Therapeutic relationship not empathised. Functional analysis of behaviour, teaching how to increase positive rewarding behaviour; social skills training; deconditioning anxiety which blocks social behaviour and exploration. Little concern with dysfunctional rules, cognitive or interpersonal schema. Little concern with historical data (e.g., Ferster, 1974, Lewinsohn, 1975, Wolpe, 1979)
Interpersonal	Therapeutic relationship supportive: Focus on social behaviour and roles or interpersonal losses. Some, but little focus on early life (e.g., Klerman et al. 1984).
Family	Therapeutic relationships supportive but not prominent. Focus on current family interactions and roles enacted, style of who puts whom down, issues of power. Some, but little focus on individual or historical data (e.g., Beach et al. 1990).
Archetype	Therapeutic relationship supportive. Guided discovery (e.g. focus on dreams, paintings, fantasies). Historical data if it comes up but not necessarily probed for. Understanding nature of internal archetypal life and developmental responsibilities (e.g., Jung, 1964, Samuels, 1985).
Themes	Therapeutic relationship supportive, similar to Kohut. Identify main recurring (often related to biosocial goal) themes in behaviour and fantasy. As in cognitive based models guided discovery central rather than interpretation. Also like cognitive therapy reducing self-downing, experimenting, increasing explorative behaviour. Focus on splitting (conflicting themes) as in affect therapy, need to be in touch with affect of the theme (e.g., Gilbert, 1989, this volume). May use any of the "techniques" of therapy from other approaches but with a clear focus on the theme that is being reworked or challenged.

> In some instances, a distorted viewpoint that has been targeted for change is isolated, recorded, monitored, logically analyzed, and ultimately brought under the patient's control with the teaching and support of the therapist. This process brings about salutary change, overt symptom relief, and/or prophylactic effects that endure beyond the acute episode and can be applied to subsequent recurrences. In other cases, the sociocultural context may be crucial because of specific environmental stresses. In yet other cases, where the effects of these approaches are at best temporary and changes in depressogenic thinking or environmental management do alter chronic conflicts or profound fears of loss of love, a deeper approach may be necessary to tap the unconscious memories, or schemata, beneath the surface thereby requiring greater efforts towards structural modification.
> Psychotherapy may thus be used not only by default, that is, to increase compliance with medication or as an alternative for patients who cannot or will not respond to pharmacotherapy, but in itself as an independent intervention. Cognitive therapy can be used to change depressogenic attitudes and ingrained thinking patterns. Interpersonal therapy emphasizes teaching specific communication and social skills to counter deficits or disputes involving a spouse or significant others in one's personal or work life; these deficits can be causes or consequences of depression. Psychodynamic therapy addresses the individual's intrapsychic conflictual personality structure so that the underlying demoralization of the damaged self, which dominates the clinical core of depression, can be understood and thus altered.

Hence Karasu (1990) clearly indicates that therapists must have a number of skills. Basically, to treat depression you can't be "a one-club golfer".

CULTURE

Over and above the study of the individual and their relationships, is culture. We have presented the view that humans have an evolved archetypal life, or a life that is set to follow certain general aims (biosocial goals). Our affective life tends to track social success (see Chapter 5). Yet at the same time this inner life must engage the social world and make sense of it, come to know and understand the rules of relationships, and so forth. Our minds, above all else, evolved for social living and not rationality. Our minds are extraordinarily sensitive to social information and working out one's sense of social place, rank, ingroup–outgroup, allies, and belonging. The meaning-creating systems of mind require a social, relational life that constantly feeds back and shapes the inner experience and biological state of self.

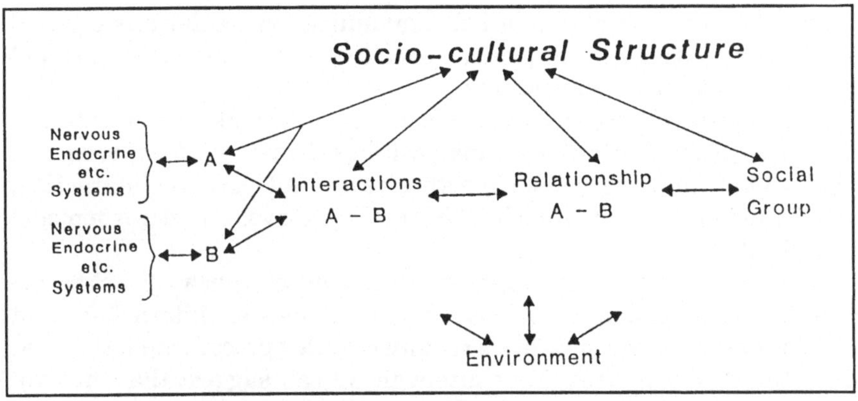

FIG. 16.2. The dialectics between successive levels of social complexity. From: Hinde 1987, reprinted with kind permission Cambridge University Press.

In my view one of the best models for outlining these complex interactions has been put forward by Hinde (1987). This is given in Fig. 16.2.

What this model outlines is the complex dialectal interactions between an individual's biological state, the nature of the relationships they seek, the type of relationships they elicit and how all these are embedded in a socially prescribed set of cultural patterns and values. These values are also the rules for gaining or losing SAHP.

Only slowly are we beginning to recognise how power has been a prime mover in evolution and how it has shifted up into cultural forms. Philosophers and sociologists have long been aware of this but psychologists less so, and psychopathologists hardly at all. Although attachment theory helped us to understand how we come to internalise our sense of power, it cannot address the issues at a cultural level. Cultures are riddled with power, as exercised by social-economic systems, religions, traditions, and families. As I have tried to show, if we want to understand psychopathology, and depression in particular, then we must recognise how power over children, power over outgroups and individualistic greed and envy produce many casualties. Behind the human veneer are archetypal processes and potential self-organisational patterns that will render one vulnerable to suffering.

In Chapters 5–8 we explored the similarities between depressive phenomenology and animals who are in involuntary subordinate positions. Both the depressed and the involuntary subordinate share the following: various biological changes (e.g. in cortisol, and monoamine functioning), inhibition of assertive behaviour, inhibition of explorative behaviour, patterns of nonverbal communication, social anxiety and sensitivity to social threat, raised sensitivity to attachment loss and raised sensitivity to helplessness.

In this work, *the theory* of depression relates to rank and the internal inhibition of involuntary low rank positions. However, *the approach* is biopsychosocial. Thus, we can hypothesize multiple levels of interaction, which are in tune with Hinde's (1987) outline above. These are depicted in table 16.3

In the biopsychosocial approach the issue of causality arises for complex interactions of various levels. Moreover interaction and feedback between various levels require complex process models rather than simple linear ones. Thus although we can suggest that internal inhibition and involuntary subordinate behaviour plays a major role in depression this begs other questions of why this particular individual at this particular time suffers from it. It is our readiness to engage this complexity, to move from culture to biology, that will have an impact on strategies of prevention.

PREVENTION

Unless one is going to slip lithium into the water supply we must recognise that drug and disease orientations are quite inadequate to instigate preventive programmes. You can only give a drug once

TABLE 16.3
Levels of Interaction in the Biopsychosocial Approach

CULTURE	At this level are role possibilities and values that are part of the culture and are transmitted from generation to generation (e.g. designated roles for masculinity, femininity and parenting styles, economic opportunities, religious behaviour, traditions, etc.).
FAMILY	At this level families operate within the values of their own culture and from their own earlier experiences. Their relationships may be supportive/loving or more towards dominating, downing and controlling other family members. These experienced styles become part of a personal history.
SOCIAL	At this level are the quality of current relationships that the individual experiences (family, friends, etc.). In depression significant relationships may be downing, controlling and devaluing of the individual.
PERSONAL	At this level is the person's internal judgements of self and others. Especially important are judgements of negative social comparison, ideals, aspirations and needs (basic personal themes and life scripts). In depression the judgements are often of inferiority, and being thwarted, trapped and hopeless.
BIOLOGICAL	At this level are the various measurable state factors, such as hormones and neurotransmitter integrity, and variations of brain functioning.
ORGAN	At this level are the specific biological targets of study, for example, synaptic control.

someone has become depressed. If we create a world that is so dehumanised and competitive (Lorenz, 1989), that has within it many forms of traps and cages, such that we need increasing levels of medication to survive, should we reclassify depression to allow such widespread use of drugs or should we look closely at how far we have deviated from our evolved hunter-gatherer patterns of life? Should we not begin to think of basic human needs in an effort to facilitate the creation of psychological environments that better fit humans, rather than economic systems or ideologies (Galbraith, 1987).

What is important is to recognise that theory and practice are closely intertwined. If you believe in diseases then this will affect your practice and research. However, perhaps the most significant changes in physical health have come from improvement in hygiene. Consider, for example, a disease theorist in the 15th century. There was excrement in the streets and goodness knows what else. We could study the diseases associated with poor hygiene and even find evidence for a genetic risk to some diseases and infant mortality no doubt (not everyone died or became seriously ill). But it was only with radical changes in our social living that prevention made a major impact. The plague was a clear biological disease but its destruction of vast numbers was because of living conditions.

I can put it no more strongly than to say that—in many of our child-rearing environments, our abuse of children and other humans, our turning of humans into objects of production, in our economic patterns that have emerged purely from the impetus of profit and efficiency—we are the creators of our own psychic bacteria. We infect each other. No one is to blame for this, for in a sense we are all victims to the culture we inherit. But as our knowledge base increases and we see the steady rise in rates of depression and suicide, maybe the time has come to start to think of economic systems as serving people rather than the other way around (Galbraith, 1987; Smail, 1987). It remains possible that in so far as a depression may run in families and be associated with increasing life events (Bebbington & McGuffin, 1989) we may be observing the effects of incompatible social environments interacting with evolved biological needs and social propensities (e.g., for secure attachments and small hunter-gatherer band life styles).

Although, as a psychologist I am deeply committed to the evolutionary and psychological understanding of depression, one has to admit that it will never be possible to treat or help the vast numbers of sufferers with individual therapy. Social solutions are essential. More serious perhaps is that whereas drugs are helpful for individuals they may be counterproductive at the cultural, societal level. In the first place they send implicit messages to the miserable that their affective experience is illness and that drugs provide solutions to problems—so keep taking the tablets. Second, they provide cheap answers to misery and one that any government will prefer to radical social policy of early detection of children at risk, better education policies for families, and more economic support. No government will accept that a deliberate policy of creating unemployment to deal with inflation will be a major factor in suicide for some, a major source of despair for others, and create a climate of such competitiveness where even our modicum of social coherence begins to fragment and break up—so again keeping taking the tablets.

And depression is only one problem. Other forms of psychopathology arise and crime increases when a culture can no longer offer a sense of belonging and coherent values. Unless one is going to argue for genetic differences in crime (which is an obvious nonsense) then the vastly higher rates of murder and other crimes in the USA compared to rural Britain lies clearly in the social fabric of life. So where are the disease theorists when it comes to early educational policies to protect and prevent and a call for radical changes in how we live our lives at work and home, if we are to protect the vast numbers from these serious sources of suffering?

Our social groups are now vastly larger than those we were evolved to fit. This is a major factor. To quote an old point: although in theory, every American is able to become President of the United States, judging by the number there has been in relation to the population size, the success rate has not been too high. We have to create a place for ourselves, it is not automatically given. We no longer see ourselves as mutually dependent on each other but rather are concerned with maintaining a self-identity that works, and works in the face of potential shamers and competitors. And this sense of self is something new (Baumeister, 1986). We are bombarded with pictures of people who are better, brighter, more wealthy, more beautiful. We are fed myths of the happy family (despite divorce rates being at 40% and a good number of other families being unhappy). People are beaten up in their homes, lose their jobs, and are socially marginalised. And when these individuals become casualties and come to believe that they are not so bright, that they are different and inferior to others, that among the masses they are treated as subordinates, that they cannot live in the minds of others as an agent of value because there are so many competitors for that role, we explicitly tell them they are suffering from a disease called depression, or implicitly tell them: "It's your fault you are too pessimistic."

It is not that our theories are wrong. People can be unrealistically pessimistic, self-devaluing and so on. But the point is one of prevention.

How on earth have we got into the state where there are so many who are depressed and ashamed of themselves? How come so many, in the lands of plenty, feel so trapped? A colleague who has recently returned from Spain informed me that there is a real problem of depression in the older population. With the growing cities, the young have moved out of the villages, leaving parents "de-roled" and lonely.

All of us will have our own solutions and mine are likely to be no better than anyone else's. Many have advocated rather sensible ideas like more self-help programmes, a greater push on our part for education and use of mass communication channels, acting against our "its all wonderful (marriage, babies, school, and work) myths", greater involvement in schools and in political debate, pointing out the possible mental health consequences of various social policies and political ideologies (see for example the *American Psychologist*, Feb. 1989). I would also suggest we should be more aware of the shamer (punisher) that lives in our own hearts and seeks to control others by threat.

But let me assure those who are dubious about evolutionary theory and the re-biologising of mind. This does not lead to reductionism (Gilbert, 1989; Nesse, 1990); far from it. It leads to a recognition of human needs and the problems of creating environments that are not psychologically toxic. The mind is not a machine—that is a most unfortunate metaphor. The mind is a goal-searching, meaning-making, self-organising organ that comes into the world predisposed to find meaning in the social fabric of its life. Within it are the mentalities/archetypes that evolved over millions of years and are orientated to social success, but the social environment is required to function and live out these possibilites in a relatively optimistic way. If humans have failed it is because we no longer act like humans (Lorenz, 1989) and have forgotten our human needs for love, respect, and compassion. For far too many, the roles that are played out are those of inferiority and tragedy and the socially unsuccessful.

Depression and other forms of mental suffering are not therefore only a problem of individuals, but also of groups and societies. There is no question that suffering involves biology, or that there are individual variations and thresholds for becoming depressed, or that some depressions are sadly genetically loaded. However, what this book has tried to articulate is that depression is associated with roles and relationships; with self-organisation and self-value. In my clinics one constantly observes the effects of poor relational style that are sometimes the consequences of economic stress, past and present abuse, the rendering of people into objects of gratification, early life histories of affectionless parenting, and so forth. In this book I have formulated the problem, as others have also, in terms of power and belonging and related these in turn to evolved needs for social success (see Chapter 5) and various brain mechanisms (e.g., subordinate inhibition and defeat). This is but one approach among others, but one I personally believe has potential as an integrating multidisciplinary paradigm.

> Without peace and social justice, without enough food and water, without education and decent housing, and *without providing each and all of us with a useful role in society* and an adequate income, there can be no health for the people, no growth and no social development.
> (World Health Organization, 1985. *Targets for health for all*, p.13, [italics added])

NOTE

1. Females, like males have the full repertoire of submissive responses and are often subject to both male and female aggression (Kevles, 1986). Their social lives are often dominated by males who sometimes directly or indirectly try to control them by putting them down. Welner et al. (1979) found that in female physicians depression ran at about 31%. Evidence is coming through that female children receive less attention than males both in the home and at school (perhaps because males are more active and restless and may elicit more attention). Infanticide is more directed at females than males. The sociobiologists argue that it is in the parents' own reproductive interest to attend to boys more because they can sire more offspring. Whatever the reason females are rarely regarded as the dominant group.

References

Abraham, K. (1911). Notes on the psycho-analytic investigation and treatment of manic depressive insanity and allied conditions. In K. Abraham (Ed.), *Selected Papers on Psycho-analysis.* London: Hogarth Press.
Abrams, D., Cochrane, S., Hogg, M.A., & Turner, J.C. (1990). Knowing what to think by knowing who you are: Self categorization and the nature of norm formation, conformity and group polarization. *British Journal of Social Psychology, 29*, 97-119.
Abramson, L.Y., & Alloy, L.B. (1990). Search for the "negative cognition" subtype of depression. In C.D. McCann & N. Endler (Eds.), *Depression: New Directions in Theory, Research and Practice.* Toronto: Wall & Emerson.
Abramson, L.Y., Metalsky, G.I., & Alloy, L.B. (1989). Hopelessness: A theory-based subtype of depression. *Psychological Review, 96*, 358-372.
Abramson, L.Y., Seligman, M.E.P., & Teasdale, J.D. (1978). Learned helplessness in humans: Critique and reformulation. *Journal of Abnormal Psychology, 87*, 49-74.
Ainsworth, M.D.S., Biehar, M.C., Waters, E., & Wall, S. (1978). *Patterns of attachment: A Psychological Study of the Strange Situation.* Hillsdale, N.J.: Lawrence Erlbaum Associates Inc.
Akiskal, H.S. (1979). A bio-behavioral approach to depression. In R.A. Depue (Ed.), *The Psychobiology of the Depressive Disorders: Implications for the Effects of Stress.* New York: Academic Press.
Akiskal, H.S. (1988). Personality as a mediating variable in the pathogenesis of mood disorders: Implications for theory, research, and prevention. In T. Helgason & D.J. Daly (Eds.), *Depressive Illness: Prediction of Course and Outcome.* New York: Springer-Verlag.
Akiskal, H.S. (1990). Towards a definition of dysthymia: boundaries with

personality and mood disorders. In S.W. Burton & H.S Akiskal (Eds.), *Dysthymic Disorder.* London: Gaskell: Royal College of Psychiatrists.
Akiskal, H.S., Bitar, A.H., Puzantian, V.R., Rosenthal, T.L., & Walker, P.W. (1978). The nosological status of neurotic depression: A prospective three-to-four year follow-up examination in the light of the primary–secondary and unipolar–bipolar dichotomies. *Archives of General Psychiatry, 35,* 756-766.
Akiskal, H.S., Hirschfeld, R.M.A., & Yerevanian, B.I. (1983). The relationship of personality to affective disorders. *Archives of General Psychiatry, 40,* 801-810.
Akiskal, H.S., & McKinney, W.T. (1973a). Psychiatry and pseudopsychiatry. *Archives of General Psychiatry, 28,* 367-373.
Akiskal, H.S., & McKinney, W.T. (1973b). Depressive disorders: Toward a unified hypothesis. *Science, 182,* 20-29.
Akiskal, H.S., & McKinney, W.T. (1975). Overview of recent research in depression: Integration of ten conceptual models into a comprehensive frame. *Archives of General Psychiatry, 32,* 285-305.
Akiskal, H.S., Rosenthal, T.L., Haykal, R.F. Lemmi, H., Rosenthal, R.H., & Scott-Strauss. (1980). Characterological depressions. *Archives of General Psychiatry, 37,* 777-783.
Alder, G. (1986). Psychotherapy of the narcissistic personality disorder patient. *American Journal of Psychiatry, 143,* 430-436.
Alloy, L.B. (1988) (Ed.). *Cognitive Processes in Depression.* New York: Guilford Press.
Alloy, B., Abramson, L.Y., Metalsky, G.I., & Hartledge, S. (1988). The hopelessness theory of depression: Attributional aspects. *British Journal of Clinical Psychology, 27,* 5-12.
Alter-Reid, K., Gibbs, M.S., Lachenmeyer, J.R., Sigal, J., & Massoth, N.A. (1986). Sexual abuse of children: A review of empirical findings. *Clinical Psychology Review, 6,* 246-266.
Ambelas, A. (1987). Life events and mania: A special relationship? *British Journal of Psychiatry, 150,* 235-240.
Amenson, C.S., & Lewinsohn, P.M. (1981). An investigation into the observed sex differences in the prevalence of unipolar depression. *Journal of Abnormal Psychology, 90,* 1-13.
American Psychiatric Association. (1987). *The Diagnostic and Statistical Manual for the DSM-111-R.*
Amies, P.L., Gelder, M.G., & Shaw, P.M. (1983). Social phobia: A comparative study. *British Journal of Psychiatry, 142,* 174-179.
Ammerman, R.T., Cassi, J.E., Hersen, M., & Van Hassett, V.B. (1986). Consequences of physical abuse and neglect in children. *Clinical Psychology Review, 6,* 291-310.
Amsel, A. (1958). The role of frustrative non-reward in non-continuous reward situations. *Psychological Bulletin, 55,* 102-119.
Amsel, A. (1962). The frustrative non-reward in partial reinforcement and discrimination learning: Some recent history and theoretical extensions. *Psychological Review, 69,* 306-328.
Andreasen, N.C. (1989). Some reflections on the concept of endogenous depression. In K. Davison & A. Kerr (Eds.), *Contemporary Themes in Psychiatry.* London: Gaskell: The Royal College of Psychiatrists.
Andreasen, N.C., Schefter, W., Reich, T., Hirschfeld, R.M.A., Endicott, J., & Keller,

M.B. (1986). The validation of the concept of depression: A family study approach. *Archives of General Psychiatry, 43,* 246-251.

Andrews, B., & Brewin, C.R. (1990). Attributions of blame for marital violence: A study of antecedents and consequences. *Journal of Family and Marriage, 52,* 757-767.

Andrews, G., Tennant, C., Hewson, D. M., & Vaillant, G. E. (1978). Life event stress, social support, coping style and risk of psychological impairment. *Journal of Nervous and Mental Disease, 166,* 307-316.

Andrews, G., Stewart, G., Morris-Yates, A., Holt, P., & Henderson, S. (1990). Evidence for a general neurotic syndrome. *British Journal of Psychiatry, 157,* 6-12.

Andrews, J.D.W. (1989). Integrating visions of reality: Interpersonal diagnosis and the existential vision. *American Psychologist, 44,* 803-817.

Angst, J. (1988). Clinical course of affective disorders. In T. Helgason & R.J. Daly (Eds.), *Depressive Illness: Prediction of Course and Outcome.* New York: Springer-Verlag.

Anisman, H. (1978). Neurochemical changes elicited by stress: Behavioral correlates. In H. Anisman & G. Bignami (Eds.), *Psychopharmacology of Aversively Motivated Behavior.* New York: Plenum Press.

Anisman, H., Pizzino, A., & Sklar, L.S. (1980b) Coping with stress, norepinephrine depletion and escape performance. *Brain Research, 191,* 583-588.

Anisman, H., & Sklar, L.S. (1979). Catecholamine depletion in mice upon re-exposure to stress: Mediation of the escape deficits produced by inescapable shock. *Journal of Comparative and Physiological Psychology, 93,* 610-625.

Anisman, H., Suissa, A., & Sklar, L.S. (1980a). Escape deficits induced by uncontrollable stress: Antagonism by dopamine and norepinephrine agonists. *Behavioural and Neural Biology, 28,* 34-47.

Anisman, H., & Zacharko, R,M. (1982) Depression: The predisposing influence of stress (plus commentary). *Behavioral and Brain Sciences, 5,* 89-137.

Anthony, E. J., & Benedek, T. (1975) (Eds.). *Depression and Human Existence.* Boston: Little Brown.

Arana, G.W., Baldessarini, R.J., & Ornsteen, M. (1985). The dexamethasone suppression test for diagnosis of and prognosis in psychiatry. *Archives of General Psychiatry, 42,* 1193-1204.

Archer, J. (1988). *The Behavioural Biology of Aggression.* Cambridge: Cambridge University Press.

Argyle, M. (1984). *The Psychology of Interpersonal Behaviour* (4th edition). Harmondsworth: Penguin Books.

Argyle, M. (1987). *The Psychology of Happiness.* London: Methuen & Co.

Arieti, S. (1977). Psychotherapy of severe depression. *American Journal of Psychiatry, 134,* 864-868.

Arieti, S. (1978). A psychotherapeutic approach to severely depressed patients. *American Journal of Psychotherapy, 32,* 33-47.

Arieti, S., & Bemporad, J. (1980a). The psychological organization of depression. *American Journal of Psychiatry, 137,* 1360-1365.

Arieti, S., & Bemporad, J. (1980b). *Severe and Mild Depression: The Psychotherapeutic Approach.* London: Tavistock.

Aronson, T.A. (1989). A critical review of psychotherapeutic treatments of the borderline personality: Historical trends and future directions. *Journal of*

Nervous and Mental Disease, 177, 511-528.

Arrindell, W.A., Sanderman, R., Van der Molen, H., Van der Ende, J., & Mersch, P.P. (1988). The structure of assertiveness: A confirmatory approach. *Behaviour Research and Therapy, 26,* 337-339.

Asch, S. (1956). Studies of independence and conformity: 1. A minority of one against an unanimous majority. *Psychological Monographs, 70,* 1-70.

Atkinson, J.W. (1964). *An Introduction to Motivation.* Princeton, N.J.: Van Nostrand.

Averill, J.R. (1968). Grief: Its nature and significance. *Psychological Bulletin, 70,* 721-748.

Bagshaw, V.E. (1977). A replication study of Foulds' and Bedford's hierarchical model of depression. *British Journal of Psychiatry, 131,* 53-55.

Bailey, K. (1987). *Human Paleopsychology. Applications to Aggression and Pathological Processes.* Hillsdale, N.J.: Lawrence Erlbaum Associates Inc.

Baker, H.S., & Baker, M.N. (1987). Heinz Kohut's self psychology. *American Journal of Psychiatry, 144,* 1-9.

Baker, H.S., & Baker, M.N. (1988). Arthur Miller's *Death of a Salesman*: Lessons for the self psychologist. In A. Goldberg (Ed.), *Progress in Self Psychology, Vol. 4.* Hillsdale, N.J.: The Analytic Press.

Bandura, A. (1977). *Social Learning Theory.* Englewood Cliffs, N.J.: Prentice-Hall.

Barash, D.P. (1977). *Sociobiology and Behavior.* London: Heineman.

Barkow, J.H. (1975). Prestige and culture: A biosocial interpretation (plus peer review). *Current Anthropology, 16,* 533-572

Barkow, J.H. (1980). Prestige and self-esteem: A biosocial interpretation. In D.R. Omark, D.R Strayer & J. Freedman (Eds.), *Dominance relations: An ethological view of social conflict and social interaction.* New York: Garland STPM Press.

Barlow, D.H. (1991). Disorders of emotion (plus peer commentary). *Psychological Inquiry, 2,* 51-105.

Barlow, D.H., Di Nardo, P.A., Vermilyea, B.B., Vermilyea, J.A., & Blanchard, E.B. (1986). Co-Morbidity and depression among anxiety disorders. *Journal of Nervous and Mental Disease, 174,* 63-72.

Barnard, P.J., & Teasdale, J.D. (1991). Interacting cognitive subsystems: A systematic approach to cognitive-affective interaction and change. *Cognition and Emotion, 5(1),* 1-39.

Basch, M.F. (1975). That encompasses depression: A revision of existing causal hypotheses in psychoanalysis. In E.J. Anthony & T. Benedek (Eds.), *Depression and Human Existence.* Boston: Little Brown.

Basch, M.F. (1984). Selfobject theory of motivation and the history of psychoanalysis. In P.E. Stepansky & A. Goldberg (Eds.), *Kohut's Legacy: Contributions to Self Psychology.* Hillsdale, N.J.: The Analytic Press.

Baumeister R.F. (1982). A self-presentational view of social phenomena. *Psychological Bulletin, 91,* 3-26.

Baumeister, R.F. (1986). How the self became a problem: A psychological review of historical research. *Journal of Personality and Social Psychology, 52,* 163-176.

Beach, S.R.H., Sandeen, E.E., & O'Leary, K.D. (1990). *Depression in Marriage.* New York: Guilford Press.

Bebbington, P. (1980). Causal models and logical inference in epidemiological psychiatry. *British Journal of Psychiatry, 136,* 317-325.

Bebbington, P., Hurry, J., Tennant, C., Sturt, E., & Wing, J.K. (1981). Epidemiology of mental disorders in Camberwell. *Psychological Medicine, 11,* 561-580.

Bebbington, P., Katz, R., McGuffin, P., Sturt, E., & Wing, J.K. (1989). The risk of minor depression before age 65: Results from a community survey. *Psychological Medicine, 19,* 393-400.

Bebbington, P.E., & McGuffin P. (1989). The integrative models of depression: The evidence. In K. Herbst & E. Paykel (Eds.), *Depression: An interactive Approach.* Oxford: Heinemann Medical Books.

Beck, A.T. (1963). Thinking and depression: 1. Idiosyncratic content and cognitive distortions. *Archives of General Psychiatry, 9,* 324-333.

Beck, A.T. (1967). *Depression: Clinical, Experimental and Theoretical Aspects.* New York: Harper & Row.

Beck, A.T. (1970). Cognitive therapy: Nature and relationship to behavior therapy. *Behavior Therapy, 1,* 184-200.

Beck, A.T. (1973). *The Diagnosis and Management of Depression.* Philadelphia: University of Pennsylvania Press.

Beck, A.T. (1974a). The development of depression. In R.J. Friedman & M.M. Katz (Eds.), *The Psychology of Depression: Contemporary Theory and Research.* New York: Winston-Wiley.

Beck, A.T. (1974b). Cognition, affect and psychopathology. In H. London & R.E. Nisbett (Eds.), *Thought and Feeling.* Chicago: Aldine Publishing Company.

Beck, A.T. (1976). *Cognitive Therapy and the Emotional Disorders.* New York: International Universities Press.

Beck, A.T. (1983). Cognitive therapy of depression: New perspectives. In. P.J. Clayton & J.E. Barrett (Eds.), *Treatment of Depression: Old Controversies and New Approaches.* New York: Raven Press.

Beck, A.T. (1987). Cognitive models of depression. *Journal of Cognitive Psychotherapy: An International Quarterly, 1,* 5-38.

Beck. A.T. (1989). *Love is Never Enough.* London: Harper and Row.

Beck, A.T., Emery, G., & Greenberg, R.L. (1985). *Anxiety Disorders and Phobias: A Cognitive Approach.* New York: Basic Books.

Beck, A.T., Epstein, N., Harrison, R.P., & Emery, G. (1983). *Development of the sociotropy-autonomy scale: A measure of personality factors in depression.* University of Pennsylvania: Philadelphia.

Beck, A.T., Freeman, A., & Associates. (1990). *Cognitive Therapy of Personality Disorders.* New York: Guilford Press.

Beck, A.T., Rush, A.J., Shaw, B.F., & Emery, G. (1979). *Cognitive Therapy of Depression.* New York: J. Wiley & Sons.

Beck, A.T., Steer, R.A., & Garbin, M.G. (1988). Psychometric properties of the Beck Depression Inventory: Twenty five years of evaluation. *Clinical Psychology Review. 8,* 77-100.

Beck, A.T., Ward, C.H., Mendelson, M., Mock, J., & Erbaugh, J. (1961). An inventory for measuring depression. *Archives of General Psychiatry, 4,* 561-571.

Beck, A.T., Weissman, A., Lester, D., & Trexler, L. (1974). The measurement of pessimism: The hopelessness scale. *Journal of Consulting and Clinical Psychology, 42,* 861-865.

Becker, J. (1960). Achievement related characteristics of manic-depressives. *Journal of Abnormal and Social Psychology, 60,* 334-339.

Becker, J. (1974). *Depression: Theory and Research.* New York: Winston-Wiley.

Becker, J. (1977). *Affective Disorders.* New Jersey: General Learning Press.
Becker, J. (1979). Vulnerable self-esteem as a predisposing factor in depressive disorders. In R.A. Depue (Ed.), *The Psychobiology of the Depressive Disorders: Implications for the Effects of Stress.* New York: Academic Press.
Beckham, E.E. (1990). Psychotherapy of depression research at a crossroads: Directions for the 1990s. *Clinical Psychology Review, 10,* 207-228.
Belsher, G., & Costello, C.G. (1988). Relapse after recovery from unipolar depression: A Critical Review. *Psychological Bulletin, 104,* 84-86.
Bergner, R.M. (1988). Status dynamic psychotherapy with depressed patients. *Psychotherapy, 25,* 266-272.
Berke, J.E. (1987). Shame and Envy. In D.L. Nathanson (Ed.), *The Many Faces of Shame.* New York: Guilford Press.
Berndt, D.J. (1990). Inventories and scales. In B.B. Wolman & G. Stricker (Eds.), *Depressive Disorders: Facts, Theories and Treatment Methods,* New York: J. Wiley & Sons Inc.
Bibring, E. (1953). The mechanism of depression. In P. Greenacre (Ed.), *Affective Disorders.* New York: International Universities Press.
Biglan, A., Hops, H., Sherman, L., Friedman, L.S., Authur, J., & Osteen, V. (1985). Problem-solving interactions of depressed women and their husbands. *Behavior Therapy, 16,* 431-451.
Bird, W.H., Martin, P.A., & Schulman, A. (1983). The marriage of the "collapsible" man of prominence. *American Journal of Psychiatry, 140,* 290-295.
Birney, R.C., Burdick, H., & Teevan, R.C. (1969). *Fear of Failure.* New York: Van Nostrand-Reinhold.
Birtchnell, J. (1988a). Defining dependence. *British Journal of Medical Psychology, 61,* 111-124.
Birtchnell, J. (1988b). Depression and family relationships: A study of young, married women on a London housing estate. *British Journal of Psychiatry, 153,* 758-769.
Birtchnell, J. (1990). Interpersonal theory: Criticism, modification and elaboration. *Human Relations,* 43, 1183-1201.
Blackburn, I.M. (1974). The pattern of hostility in affective illness. *British Journal of Psychiatry, 125,* 141-145.
Blackburn, I.M. (1989). Severely depressed in-patients. In J. Scot, J.M.G. Williams, & A.T. Beck (Eds.), *Cognitive Therapy in Clinical Practice.* London: Routledge.
Blackburn, I.M., Bishop, S., Glen, A.I.M., Walley, L.J., & Christie, J.E. (1981). The efficacy of cognitive therapy in depression: A treatment trial using cognitive therapy and pharmacotherapy, each alone and in combination. *British Journal of Psychiatry, 139,* 181-189.
Blackburn, I.M., & Davidson, K. (1990). *Cognitive Therapy for Depression and Anxiety.* London: Blackwell.
Blackburn, I.M., & Eunson, K.M. (1989). A content analysis of thoughts and emotions elicited from depressed patients during cognitive therapy. *British Journal of Medical Psychology, 62,* 23-35.
Blackburn, I.M., Jones, S., & Lewis, R.J.P. (1986). Cognitive style in depression. *British Journal of Clinical Psychology, 25,* 241-251.
Blackburn, I.M., Roxborough, H.M., Muir, W.J., Glabus, M., & Blackwood, D.H.R. (1990). Perceptual and physiological dysfunction in depression. *Psychological Medicine, 20,* 95-103.

Blackburn, R. (1988). On moral judgements and personality disorders: The myth of psychopathic personality revisited. *British Journal of Psychiatry, 153,* 505-512.

Blackwood, D.H.R. (1988). The biological determinants of personality. In R.E. Kendell & A.K. Zeally (Eds.), *Companion to Psychiatric Studies* (4th edition). Edinburgh: Churchill Livingstone.

Blakely, A.A., Howard, R.C., Sosich, R.M., Murdoch, J.C., Menkes, D.B., & Spears, G.F.S. (1991). Psychiatric symptoms, personality and ways of coping in chronic fatigue syndrome. *Psychological Medicine, 21,* 347-362.

Blaney, P.H. (1977). Contemporary theories of depression: Critique and comparison. *Journal of Abnormal Psychology, 86,* 203-223.

Blaney, P.H. (1986). Affect and memory: A review. *Psychological Bulletin, 99,* 229-246.

Blatt, S.J. (1974). Levels of object representation in anaclitic and introjective depression. *Psychoanalytic Study of the Child, 29,* 107-157.

Blatt, S.J., Quinlan, D.M., Chevron, E.S., McDonald, C., & Zuroff, D. (1982). Dependency and self criticism: psychological dimensions of depression. *Journal of Consulting and Clincal Psychology, 50,* 113-124.

Blatt, S.J., Wein, S.J., Chevron, E.S., & Quinlan, D.M. (1979). Parental representations and depression in normal young adults. *Journal of Abnormal Psychology, 88,* 388-397.

Blumenthal, M.D. (1971). Heterogeneity and research on depressive disorders. *Archives of General Psychiatry, 24,* 524-531.

Boesch, C. (1990). First hunters of the forest. *New Scientist,* May 19th, No 1717, 38-41.

Bonhoeffer, K. (1909). Exogenous psychoses. In S.R. Hirsch & M. Shepherd (Eds.), *Themes and Variations in European Psychiatry.* Bristol: J. Wright.

Bonhoeffer, K. (1911). How far should all psychogenic illness be regarded as hysterical? In S.R. Hirsch & M. Shepherd (Eds.), *Themes and Variations in European Psychiatry.* Bristol: J. Wright.

Boulton, M.G. (1983). *On Being a Mother.* London: Tavistock.

Bowlby, J. (1969). *Attachment. Attachment and Loss, Vol. 1.* London: Hogarth Press.

Bowlby, J. (1973). *Separation, Anxiety and Anger. Attachment and Loss, Vol. 2.* London: Hogarth Press.

Bowlby, J. (1977a). The making and breaking of affectional bonds: I. Aetiology and psychopathology in the light of attachment theory. *British Journal of Psychiatry, 130,* 201-210.

Bowlby, J. (1977b). The making and breaking of affectional bonds: 11. Some principles of psychotherapy. *British Journal of Psychiatry, 130,* 421-431.

Bowlby, J. (1980). *Loss: Sadness and Depression. Attachment and Loss, Vol. 3.* London: Hogarth Press.

Bowlby, J. (1988). Developmental psychiatry comes of age. *American Journal of Psychiatry, 145,* 1-10.

Bowman, L.A., Dilley, S.R., & Keverne, E.B. (1978). Suppression of oestrogen-induced LH surges by social subordination in talapoin monkeys. *Nature, 275,* 56-58.

Boyd, J.H., & Weissman, M.M. (1981). Epidemiology of affective disorders. *Archives of General Psychiatry, 38,* 1039-1046.

Braddock, L. (1986). The dexamethasone suppression test: fact or artefact. *British Journal of Psychiatry. 148,* 363-374.
Braden, W., & Ho, C.K. (1981). Racing thoughts in psychiatric inpatients. *Archives of General Psychiatry, 38,* 71-75.
Bradford, D.T. (1990). Early christian martyrdom and the psychology of depression, suicide and bodily mutilation. *Psychotherapy, 27,* 30-41.
Bradley, V.A., & Power, R. (1988). Aspects of the relationship between cognitive theories and therapies of depression. *British Journal of Medical Psychology, 61,* 329-338.
Breier, A., Albus, M., Pickar, D., Zahn, T.P., Wolkowitz, O.M., & Pauls, S.M. (1987). Controllable and uncontrollable stress in humans: Alterations in mood and neuroendocrine and psychophysiological functioning. *American Journal of Psychiatry, 144,* 1419-11425.
Brewin, C.R. (1985). Depression and causal attributions. What is their relation? *Psychological Bulletin, 98,* 297-309.
Brewin, C.R. (1988). *Cognitive Foundations of Clinical Psychology.* London: Lawrence Erlbaum Associates Ltd.
Brewin, C.R. (1989). Cognitive change processes in psychotherapy. *Psychological Review, 96,* 379-394.
Brewin, C.R. (1990). *The role of early memories in depression.* Paper presented at the Morton Trust Conference on depression. September. Sheffield, England.
Brewin, C.R., & Furnham, A. (1986). Attributional and pre-attributional variables in self-esteem and depression: A comparison and test of learned helplessness theory. *Journal of Personality and Social Psychology, 50,* 1013-1020.
Brewin, C.R., MacCarthy, B., & Furnham, A. (1989). Social support in the face of adversity: The role of cognitive appraisal. *Journal of Research in Personality, 23,* 354-372.
Brown, B.B., & Lohr, M.J. (1987). Peer-group affiliation and adolescent self-esteem: An integration of ego-identity and symbolic-interaction theories. *Journal of Personality and Social Psychology, 52,* 47-55.
Brown, G.W. (1979a). The social etiology of depression—London studies. In R.A. Depue (Ed.), *The Psychobiology of the Depressive Disorders: Implications for the Effects of Stress.* New York: Academic Press.
Brown, G.W. (1979b). Depression—a sociologist's view. *Trends in the Neurosciences, 2,* 253-256.
Brown, G.W. (1989). Depression: A Radical Social Perspective. In K. Herbst & E. Paykel (Eds.), *Depression: An interactive Approach.* Oxford: Heinemann Medical Books.
Brown, G.W., (1991). Epidemiological studies of depression: Definition and case findings. In J. Becker & A. Kleinman (Eds.), *Psychosocial Aspects of Depression.* Hillsdale, N.J.: Lawrence Erlbaum Associates Inc.
Brown, G.W., Adler, W.Z., & Bifulco, A. (1988). Life events, difficulties and recovery from chronic depression. *British Journal of Psychiatry, 152,* 487-498.
Brown, G.W., Bifulco, A., Harris, T.O., & Bridge, L. (1986). Social support, self-esteem and depression. *Psychological Medicine, 16,* 813-831.
Brown, G.W., Bifulco, A., & Harris, T.O. (1987). Life events, vulnerability and onset of depression: Some refinements. *British Journal of Psychiatry, 150,* 30-42.
Brown, G.W., & Harris, T.O. (1978a). *The Social Origins of Depression.* London: Tavistock.

Brown, G.W., & Harris, T. (1978b). Social origins of depression: A reply. *Psychological Medicine, 8,* 577-588.

Brown, G.W., & Harris, T. (1980). Further comments on the vulnerability model. *British Journal of Psychiatry, 137,* 584-585.

Brown, R. (1986). *Social Psychology: The Second Edition.* New York: Macmillan.

Brugha, T. S., Bebbington, P.E., MacCarthy, B., Potter, J., Sturt, E., & Wykes, T. (1987). Social networks, social support and the type of illness. *Acta Psychiatrica Scandinavia, 76,* 664-673.

Brugha, T.S., Bebbington, P.E., MacCarthy, B., Sturt, E., Wykes, E., & Potter, J. (1990). Gender, social support and recovery from depressive disorders: A prospective study. *Psychological Medicine, 20,* 147-156.

Brugha, T.S., & Conroy, R. (1985). Categories of depression: Reported life events in a controlled design. *British Journal of Psychiatry, 147,* 641-646.

Bucholz, K.K., & Dinwiddie, S.H. (1989). Influence of nondepressive psychiatric symptoms on whether patients tell a doctor about depression. *American Journal of Psychiatry, 146,* 640-644.

Burns, D.D. (1980). *Feeling Good: The New Mood Therapy.* New York: Morrow.

Burton, S.W., & Akiskal, H.S. (1990) (Eds.). *Dysthymic Disorder.* London: Gaskell: Royal College of Psychiatrists.

Buss, A.H. (1988). *Personality: Evolutionary Heritage and Human Distinctiveness.* Hillsdale, N.J.: Lawrence Erlbaum Associates Inc.

Buss, D.M. (1989). Sex differences in human mate preference: Evolutionary hypotheses tested in 37 cultures. *Brain and Behavioral Sciences, 12,* 1-49.

Buss, D.M. (1991). Evolutionary personality psychology. *Annual Review of Psychology, 42,* 459-491.

Buss, D.M., & Craik, K.H. (1986). Acts, dispositions and clinical assessment: The psychopathology of everyday conduct. *Clinical Psychology Review, 6,* 387-406.

Buss, D.M., Gomes, M., Higgins, D.S., & Lauterbach, K. (1987). Tactics of manipulation. *Journal of Personality and Social Psychology, 52,* 1219-1229.

Calloway, S.P. (1989). Thyroid function in depression. In J.G. Howells (Ed.), *Modern Perspectives in the Psychiatry of the Affective Disorders. Modern perspective in Psychiatry, Vol. 13.* New York: Brunner-Mazel.

Campos, J.J., Barrett, K.C., Lamb, M.E., Goldsmith, H.H., & Steinberg, C. (1983). Socioemotional development. In M.M. Haith & J.J. Campos (Eds.), *Handbook of Child Psychology, Vol. 2: Infancy and Psychobiology.* New York: J. Wiley.

Carmin, C.N., & Dowd, E.T. (1988). Paradigms in cognitive psychotherapy. In W. Dyden & P. Trower (Eds.), *Developments in Cognitive Psychotherapy.* London: Sage.

Carney, M.W.P. (1989). The differential diagnosis of depression and the prediction of response to ECT: A continuing odyssey. In K. Davison & A. Kerr (Eds.), *Contemporary Themes in Psychiatry.* London: Gaskell: The Royal College of Psychiatrists.

Carney, M.W.P., Roth, M., & Garside, R.F. (1965). The diagnosis of depressive syndromes and the prediction of E.C.T. response. *British Journal of Psychiatry, 111,* 659-674

Carroll, B.L., Feinberg, M., & Smouse, P. (1981). The Carroll rating scale for depression: 1 Development, reliability, and validation. *British Journal of Psychiatry, 138,* 194-200.

Carroll, B.J., Feinberg, M., Greden, J.F., Takika, J., Albala, A.A., Haskett, R.F.,

James, N.M., Kronfol, Z., Lohr, N., Steiner, M., Vigne, J.P.D., & Young, E. (1981). A specific laboratory test for the diagnosis of melancholia. *Archives of General Psychiatry, 38,* 15-22.

Carson, H. (1969). *Interaction Concepts in Personality.* London: Allen and Unwin.

Chamberlain, D.B. (1987). The cognitive newborn: A scientific update. *British Journal of Psychotherapy, 4,* 30-71

Champion, L. (1990). The relationship between social vulnerability and the occurence of severely threatening life events. *Psychological Medicine, 20,* 157-161

Chance, M.R.A. (1980). An ethological approach assessment of emotion. In R. Plutchik & H. Kellerman (Eds.), *Emotion: Theory Research and Experience, Vol. 1.* New York: Academic Press.

Chance M.R.A. (1984). Biological systems synthesis of mentality and the nature of the two modes of mental operation: Hedonic and agonic. *Man-Environment Systems, 14,* 143-157.

Chance, M.R.A. (1988a). Introduction. In M.R.A. Chance (Ed.), *Social Fabrics of the Mind.* Hove: Lawrence Erlbaum Associates Ltd.

Chance, M.R.A. (1988b) (Ed.). *Social Fabrics of the Mind.* Hove: Lawrence Erlbaum Associates Ltd.

Chance, M.R.A., & Jolly, C. (1970). *Social Groups of Monkeys, Apes and Men.* London: J. Cape.

Charlesworth, W.R. (1988). Resources and resource acquisition during ontogeny. In K.M. MacDonald (Ed.), *Sociobiological Perspectives on Human Development.* New York: Springer Verlag.

Chenery, D., Seyfarth, R., & Smuts, B. (1986). Social relationships and social cognition in nonhuman primates. *Science, 234,* 1361-1365.

Chisholm, J.S. (1988). Toward a developmental evolutionary ecology of humans. In K.M. MacDonald (Ed.), *Sociobiological Perspectives on Human Development.* New York: Springer-Verlag.

Chodoff, P. (1972). The depressive personality. *Archives of General Psychiatry, 27,* 666-673.

Claridge, G. (1985). *Origins of Mental Illness.* Oxford: Blackwell.

Claridge, G. (1987). The schizophrenias as nervous types revisited. *British Journal of Psychiatry, 151,* 735-743.

Clark, C. (1990). Emotions and micropolitics in everyday life: Some patterns and paradoxes of "place". In T.D. Kemper (Ed.), *Research Agendas in the Sociology of Emotions.* New York: State University of New York Press.

Clark, D.A., & Beck, A.T. (1989). Cognitive theory and therapy of anxiety and depression. In P.C. Kendall & D. Watson (Eds.), *Anxiety and Depression: Distinctive and Overlapping Features.* New York: Academic Press.

Clark, D.A., & Hemsley, D.R. (1985). Individual differences in the experience of depressive and anxious, intrusive thoughts. *Behaviour Research and Therapy, 23,* 625-633.

Clark, L.A., & Watson, D. (1991). Theoretical and empirical issues in differentiating depression from anxiety. In J. Becker & A. Kleinman (Eds.), *Psychosocial Aspects of Depression.* Hillsdale, N.J.: Lawrence Erlbaum Associates Inc.

Clarke, A.M., & Clarke, A.D.B. (1976). *Early Experience: Myth and Evidence.* London: Open Books.

Clarkin, J.F., Haas, G.L., & Glick, I.D. (1988). *Affective Disorders and the Family: Assessment and Treatment.* New York: Guilford Press.

Cochrane, N., & Neilson, M. (1977). Depressive illness: The role of aggressiveness further considered. *Psychological Medicine, 7,* 282-288.

Coe, C.L., Weiner, S.G., Rosenberg, L.T., & Levine, S. (1985). Endocrine and immune responses to separation and maternal loss in nonhuman primates. In M. Reite & T. Field (Eds.), *The Psychobiology of Attachment and Separation.* New York: Academic Press.

Cogill, S.R., Caplan, H.L., Alexandra, H., Robson, K.M., & Kumar, K.M. (1986). Impact of maternal postnatal depression on cognitive development of young children, *British Medical Journal, 292,* 1165-1167.

Cohen, M.B., Baker, G., Cohen, R.A., Fromm-Reichman, F., & Weigert, E.V. (1954). An intensive study of twelve cases of manic depressive psychosis. *Psychiatry, 17,* 103-137.

Cohen, R.M., Weingartner, H., Smallberg, S.A., Pickar, D., & Murphy, D L. (1982). Effort and cognition in depression. *Archives of General Psychiatry, 39,* 593-597.

Cohen, S., & Dunner, D. (1989). Bipolar affective disorder: Review and Update. In J.G. Howells (Ed.), *Modern Perspectives in the Psychiatry of the Affective Disorders: Modern Perspectives in Psychiatry, Vol. 13.* New York: Brunner/Mazel Inc.

Collins, N.L., & Read, S.J. (1990). Adult attachment, working models, and relationship quality in dating couples. *Journal of Personality and Social Psychology, 58,* 644-663.

Cook, B.L., & Winokur, G. (1989). Nosology of affective disorders. In J.G. Howells (Ed.), *Modern perspectives in the Psychiatry of the Affective Disorders: Modern Perspectives in Psychiatry, Vol. 13.* New York: Brunner/Mazel Inc.

Cooke, D.J. (1980a). The structure of depression found in the general population. *Psychological Medicine, 10,* 455-463.

Cooke, D.J. (1980b). Causal modelling with contingency tables. *British Journal of Psychiatry, 137,* 582-584.

Cooper, J.E. (1988). The structure and presentation of contemporary psychiatric classifications with special reference to ICD-9 and 10. *British Journal of Psychiatry, 152* (Suppl. 1), 21-28.

Coopersmith, S. (1967). *The Antecedents of Self Esteem.* San Francisco: W.H. Freeman.

Cosmides, L. (1989). The logic of social exchange: Has natural selection shaped how humans reason? Studies with the Wason selection task. *Cognition, 31,* 187-276.

Costello, C.G. (1972). Depression: Loss of reinforcers or loss of reinforcer effectiveness. *Behaviour Therapy, 3,* 240-247.

Costello, C.G. (1978). A critical review of Seligman's laboratory experiments on learned helplessness and depression in humans. *Journal of Abnormal Psychology, 87,* 21-31.

Cox, J.L. (1988). The life event of child birth: Sociocultural aspects of postnatal depression. In R. Kumar & I.F. Brockington (Eds.), *Motherhood and Mental Illness. Vol. 2: Causes and Consequences.* London: Wright.

Cox, J.L., Connor, Y., & Kendell, R.E. (1982). Prospective study of the psychiatric disorders in childbirth. *British Journal of Psychiatry, 140,* 11-117.

Cox, J.L., Holden, J.M., & Sagovsky, R. (1987). Detection of postnatal depression:

Development of the 10-item Edinburgh postnatal depression scale. *British Journal of Psychiatry, 150,* 782-786.

Cox, J.L., Rooney, A., Thomas, P.F., & Wrate, R.W. (1984). How accurately do depressed mothers recall postnatal depression: Further data from a three year follow-up study. *Journal of Psychosomatic Obstetrics and Gynaecology, 3,* 185-189.

Coyne, J.C. (1976a). Depression and response to others. *Journal of Abnormal Psychology, 85,* 186-193.

Coyne, J.C. (1976b). Towards an interactional description of depression. *Psychiatry, 39,* 28-40.

Coyne, J.C. (1982). A critique of cognitions as causal entities with particular reference to depression. Cognitive *Therapy and Research, 6,* 3-13.

Coyne, J.C. (1988). Strategic Therapy. In J.F. Clarkin, G.L. Haas, & I.D. Glick. *Affective Disorders and the Family: Assessment and Treatment.* New York: Guilford Press.

Coyne, J.C. (1989). Thinking postcognitively about depression. In A. Freeman, K.M. Simon, L.E. Beutler, & H. Arkowitz (Eds.), *Comprehensive Handbook of Cognitive Therapy.* New York: Plenum.

Coyne, J.C., Aldwin, C., & Lazarus, R. S. (1981). Depression and coping in stressful episodes. *Journal of Abnormal Psychology, 90,* 439-447.

Coyne, J.C., Kahn, J., & Gotlib, I.H. (1987). Depression. In T. Jacob (Ed.), *Family Interaction and Psychotherapy.* New York: Plenum Press.

Crammer, D. (1990). Self-esteem and close relationships: A statistical refinement. *British Journal of Social Psychology, 29,* 189-191.

Crombie, I.K. (1990). Suicide in England and Wales and in Scotland: An examination of recent trends. *British Journal of Psychiatry, 157,* 529-532.

Crook, J.H. (1980). *The Evolution of Human Consciousness.* Oxford: Oxford University Press.

Crook, J.H. (1986). The evolution of leadership: A preliminary skirmish. In C.F. Graumann & S. Moscovici (Eds.), *Changing Concepts of Leadership.* New York: Springer Verlag.

Dalgleish, T., & Watts, F.N.(1990). Biases of attention and memory in disorders of anxiety and depression. *Clinical Psychology Review, 10,* 589-604.

Dalton, K. (1985). Progesterone prophylaxis used successfully in postnatal depression. *Practitioner,* June, 507-508.

Davidson, J., Turnball, C., Strickland, R., & Belyea, M. (1984). Comparative diagnostic criteria for melancholia and endogenous depression. *Archives of General Psychiatry. 41,* 506-511.

Davidson, J., Zisook, S., Giller, E., & Helms, M. (1989). Symptoms of interpersonal sensitivity in depression. *Comprehensive Psychiatry, 30,* 357-368.

Davis, K.L., Hollister, L.E., Overall, J., Johnson, A., & Train, K. (1976). Physostigmine: Effects on cognition and affect in normal subjects. *Psychopharmacology, 51,* 23-27.

Dawkins, R. (1976). *The Selfish Gene.* Oxford: Oxford University Press.

Day, S. (1990). Genes that control genes. *New Scientist, 1741:* special supplement -inside science, No 40, 1-4.

Debus, J.R., & Rush, A.J. (1990). Sleep EEG findings in depression. In C.D McCann & N.S. Endler (Eds.), *Depression: New Directions in Theory, Research and Practice.* Toronto: Wall & Emerson.

de Catanzaro, D. (1980). Human suicide: A biological perspective. *Behavioral and Brain Sciences, 3,* 265-290.

de Coverley Veale, D.M.W. (1987). Exercise and mental health. *Acta Psychiatrica Scandinavia, 76,* 113-120.

Deitz, J. (1988). Self-psychological interventions for major depression. *American Journal of Psychotherapy, XLII,* 597-609.

Deitz, J. (1989). The evolution of the self-psychology approach to depression. *American Journal of Psychotherapy, XLIII,* 494-505.

Depue, R.A., & Monroe, S.M. (1978a). Learned helplessness in the perspective of the depressive disorders: Conceptual and definitional issues. *Journal of Abnormal Psychology,* 87, 3-20.

Depue, R.A., & Monroe, S.M. (1978b). The unipolar-bipolar distinction in the depressive disorders. *Psychological Bulletin, 85,* 1001-1029.

Depue, R.A., & Monroe, S.M. (1979). The unipolar-bipolar distinction in the depressive disorders: Implications for stress-onset interactions. In R.A. Depue (Ed.), *The Psychobiology of the Depressive Disorders. Implications for the Effects of Stress.* New York: Academic Press.

de Waal, F.M.B (1988). The reconciled hierarchy. In M.R.A. Chance (Ed.), *Social Fabrics of the Mind.* Hove: Lawrence Erlbaum Associates Ltd.

Dixon, N.F., & Henley, S.H.A. (1980). Without awareness. In M. Jeeves (Ed.), *Psychology Survey No. 3.* London: Allen & Unwin.

Dixon, T., & Lucas, K. (1982). *The Human Race.* London: Thames-Methuen.

Dobzhansky, T. (1950). Evolution and man's self-image. In V. Goodall, (Ed.), *The Search for Man.* London: Phaidon Press.

Douglas, D., & Anisman, H. (1975). Helplessness or expectation incongruency: Effects of aversive stimulation on subsequent performance. *Journal of Experimental Psychology: Human Perception and Performance, 1,* 411-417.

Dowd, E.T., & Pace, T.M. (1989). The relativity of reality: Second order change in psychotherapy. In A. Freeman, K.M. Simon, L.E. Beutler, & H. Arkowitz (Eds.), *Comprehensive Handbook of Cognitive Therapy.* New York: Plenum.

Driscoll, R. (1988). Self-condemnation: A conceptual framework for assessment and treatment. *Psychotherapy, 26,* 104-111.

Dryden, W. (1984) (Ed.). *Individual Therapy in Britain.* London: Harper & Row.

Dryden, W. (1989). The use of chaining in rational-emotive therapy. *Journal of Rational-Emotive Therapy, 7,* 59-66.

Dryden, W. (1990) (Ed.). *Individual Therapy: A Handbook.* Milton Keynes: Open University Press.

Dryden, W., & Golden, W. (1986) (Eds.). *Cognitive Behavioural Approaches to Psychotherapy.* London: Harper & Row.

Duke, M.P., & Nowicki, S.J. (1982). A social learning analysis of interactional concepts and a multi-dimensional model of human interaction constellations. In J.C. Anakin & D.J. Kiesler (Eds.), *Handbook of Interpersonal Psychotherapy.* New York: Pergamon.

Dunbar, R.I.M. (1988). *Primate Social Systems.* London: Croom Helm.

Dunn, J. (1988). Sibling influences on childhood development. *Journal of Child Psychology and Psychiatry, 29,* 119-127.

Dweck, C.S. (1975). The role of expectations and attributions in the alleviation of learned helplessness. *Journal of Personality and Social Psychology, 31,* 674-685.

D'Zurilla, T.J., & Goldfried, M.R. (1971). Problem solving and behavior modification. *Journal of Abnormal Psychology, 78,* 107-126.

Eagle, M. (1987). Theoretical and clinical shifts in psychoanalysis. *American Journal of Orthopsychiatry, 57,* 175-185.

Eastwood, M.R., Whitton, J.L., Krammer, P.A., & Peter, A.M. (1985). Infradian rhythms: A comparison of affective disorders and normal persons. *Archives of General Psychiatry, 42,* 295-299.

Efron, A. (1985). The sexual body: An interdisciplinary perspective. *Journal of Mind and Behavior, Vol. 6* (1 & 2), 1-314 (special issue).

Eibl-Eibesfeldt, I. (1989). *Human Ethology.* New York: Aldine de Gruyter.

Eisenberg, L. (1986). Mindlessness and brainlessness in psychiatry. *British Journal of Psychiatry, 148,* 497-508.

Eisenberg, N. (1986). *Altruism, Emotion, Cognition and Behavior.* Hillsdale, N.J.: Lawrence Erlbaum Associates Inc.

Eisenberg, N., & Mussen, P.N. (1989). *The Roots of Prosocial Behavior in Children.* New York: Cambridge University Press.

Elkin, I., Shea, T.M., Watkins J.T., Imner, S.T., Sotsky, S.M., Collins, J.F., Fiester, S.J., & Parloff, M.B. (1989). National institute of mental health treatment of depression collaborative research program. *Archives of General Psychiatry, 46,* 971-982.

Ellenberger, H.F. (1970). *The Discovery of the Unconscious. The History and Evolution of Dynamic Psychiatry.* New York: Basic Books.

Ellgring, H. (1989). *Nonverbal communication in depression.* Cambridge: Cambridge University Press.

Ellicott, A., Hammen, C., Gitlin, M., Brown, G., & Jamison, K. (1990). Life events and the course of bipolar disorder. *American Journal of Psychiatry. 147,* 1194-1198.

Ellis, A. (1977a). Psychotherapy and the value of a human being. In A. Ellis & R. Grieger (Eds.), *Handbook of Rational Emotive Therapy.* New York: Springer.

Ellis, A. (1977b). Characteristics of psychotic and borderline psychotic individuals. In A. Ellis & R. Grieger (Eds.), *Handbook of Rational Emotive Therapy.* New York: Springer.

Ellis, A . (1977c). A rational approach to interpretation. In A. Ellis & R. Grieger (Eds.), *Handbook of Rational Emotive Therapy.* New York: Springer.

Ellis, A., & Whiteley, J.M. (1979) (Eds.). *Theoretical and Empirical Foundations of Rational Emotive Therapy.* California: Brooks-Cole.

Emmons, R.A. (1984). Factor analysis and construct validity of the narcissistic personality inventory. *Journal of Personality Assessment, 48,* 291-300.

Emmons, R.A. (1987). Narcissism: Theory and measurement. *Journal of Personality and Social Psychology, 52,* 11-17.

Emmons, R.A., & Diener, E. (1986). Influence of impulsivity and sociability on subjective well-being. *Journal of Personality and Social Psychology, 50,* 1211-1215.

Endicott, J., & Spitzer, R.L. (1978). A diagnostic interview—the schedule for affective disorders and schizophrenia. *Archives of General Psychiatry, 35,* 837-844.

Endler, N.S. (1990). Sociopolitical factors and stigma in depression. In C.D. McCann & N.S. Endler (Eds.), *Depression: New Directions in Theory, Research and Practice.* Toronto: Wall & Emerson Inc.

Engle, G.L. (1977). The need for a new medical model: A challenge for biomedicine. *Science, 196,* 129-136.

Erdelyi, M.H. (1985). *Psychoanalysis: Freud's Cognitive Psychology.* New York: Freeman & Co.

Ewen, R.B. (1988). *An Introduction to Theories of Personality.* Hillsdale, N.J.: Lawrence Erlbaum Associates Inc.

Eysenck, H.J. (1967). *The Biological Basis of Personality.* Springfield: C Thomas.

Eysenck, H.J. (1970). The classification of depressive illness. *British Journal of Psychiatry, 117,* 241-250.

Eysenck, H.J. (1979). The conditioning model of neurosis. *Behavioral and Brain Sciences, 2,* 155-199.

Eysenck, H.J., & Eysenck, S.B.G. (1975). *Manual of the Eysenck Personality Questionnaire.* London: Hodder & Stoughton.

Eysenck, M.W. (1988). Trait anxiety and stress. In S. Fisher & J. Reason (Eds.), *Handbook of Life Stress, Cognition and Health.* Chichester: J. Wiley & Sons.

Falloon, I.R.H. (1988). Expressed emotion: Current status. *Psychological Medicine, 18,* 269-274.

Farmer, A.M., & McGuffin, P. (1989). The classification of the depressions: Contemporary confusion revisited. *British Journal of Psychiatry, 155,* 437-443.

Farmer, R., & Nelson-Gray, R.O. (1990). Personality disorders and depression: Hypothetical relations, empirical findings, and methodological considerations. *Clinical Psychology Review, 10,* 453-476.

Farrant, J., & Perez, M. (1989). Immunity and depression. In J.G. Howells (Ed.), *Modern perspectives in the Psychiatry of the Affective Disorders: Modern Perspectives in Psychiatry. Vol. 13.* New York: Brunner/Mazel Inc.

Fava, G.A., Kellner, R., Lisansky, J., Park, S., Perini, G.I., & Zielenzny, K. (1986). Hostility and recovery from melancholia. *Journal of Nervous and Mental Disease, 174,* 414-417.

Fava, M., Anderson, K., & Rosenbaum, J.F. (1990). "Anger attacks": Possible variants of panic in major depressive disorders. *American Journal of Psychiatry, 147,* 867-870.

Feighner, J.P., Robins, E., Guze, S.B., Woodruff, R.W., Winkour, G., & Munoz, R. (1972). Diagnostic criteria for use in psychiatric research. *Archives of General Psychiatry, 26,* 57-63.

Fennell, M.J.V. (1989). Depression. In, K. Hawton, P.M. Salkovskis, J. Kirk, & D.M. Clark, (Eds.), *Cognitive Behaviour Therapy for Psychiatric Problems.* Oxford: Oxford University Press.

Ferguson, B., & Tyrer, P. (1989). Rating instruments in psychiatric research. In C. Freeman & P. Tyrer (Eds.), *Research Methods in Psychiatry: A Beginner's Guide.* London: Gaskell: The Royal College of Psychiatrists.

Ferster, C.B. (1973). A functional analysis of depression. *American Psychologist, 28,* 857-870.

Ferster, C.B. (1974). Behavioral approaches to depression. In R.J. Friedman & M.M. Katz (Eds.), *The Psychology of Depression: Contemporary Theory and Research.* New York: Winston-Wiley.

Festinger, L. (1954). A theory of social comparison processes. *Human Relations, 7,* 117-140.

Finch, Jr, A.J., Lipovsky, J.A., & Casat, C.D. (1989). Anxiety and depression in children and adolescents: Negative affectivity or separate constructs? In P.C.

Kendall & D. Watson (Eds.), *Anxiety and Depression: Distinct and Overlapping Features.* New York: Academic Press.

Fink, M. (1989). Convulsive therapy: A reappraisal. In J.G. Howells (Ed.), *Modern Perspectives in the Psychiatry of the Affective Disorders: Modern Perspectives in Psychiatry, Vol.13.* New York: Brunner/Mazel Inc.

Firestone, R.W. (1986). The "inner" voice of suicide. *Psychotherapy, 23,* 439-444.

Fish, M. (1974). *Fish's Clinical Psychopathology: Signs and Symptoms in Psychiatry* (Ed. Hamilton, M.). Bristol: J. Wright.

Fisher, J.D., Nadler, A., & Whitcher-Alagna, S. (1982). Recipient reactions to aid. *Psychological Bulletin, 91,* 27-54.

Fitzgibbons, R.B. (1986). The cognitive and emotive uses of forgiveness in the treatment of anger. *Psychotherapy, 23,* 629-633.

Fodor, J.A. (1985). Précis of the modularity of mind (plus peer commentary). *Behavioral and Brain Sciences, 8,* 1-42.

Fogel, A., Melson, G.F., & Mistry, J. (1986). Conceptualising the determinants of nurturance: A reassessment of sex differences. In A. Fogel & G.F. Melson (Eds.), *Origins of Nurturance: Developmental, Biological and Cultural Perspectives on Caregiving.* Hillsdale, N.J.: Lawrence Erlbaum Associates Inc.

Forrest, M.S., & Hokanson, J.E. (1975). Depression and autonomic arousal reduction accompanying self-punitive behavior. *Journal of Abnormal Psychology, 84,* 346-357.

Foulds, G.A. (1973). The relationship between the depressive illnesses. *British Journal of Psychiatry, 123,* 531-533.

Foulds, G.A., & Bedford, A. (1975). Hierarchy of classes of personal illness. *Psychological Medicine, 5,* 181-192.

Foulds, G.A., & Bedford, A. (1976). Classification of depressive illness: A re-evaluation. *Psychological Medicine, 6,* 15-19.

Fowles, D.C., & Gersh, F.S. (1979a). Neurotic depression: The endogenous-neurotic distinction. In R.A. Depue (Ed.), *The Psychobiology of the Depressive Disorders: Implications for the Effects of Stress.* New York: Academic Press.

Fowles, D.C., & Gersh, F.S. (1979b). Neurotic depression: The concept of anxious depression. In R.A. Depue (Ed.), *The Psychobiology of the Depressive Disorders: Implications for the Effects of Stress.* New York: Academic Press.

Fox. R. (1986). Fitness by any other name. *Behavioral and Brain Sciences, 9,* 192-193.

Frank, E., Kupfer, D.J., Jacob, M., & Jarrett, D. (1987). Personality features and response to acute treatment in recurrent depression. *Journal of Personality Disorders, 1,* 14-26.

Frank, E., Kupfer, D.J., & Perel, J.M. (1989). Early recurrence in unipolar depression. *Archives of General Psychiatry. 46,* 397-400.

Frank, J.D. (1982). Therapeutic components shared by psychotherapies. In J.H. Harvey & M.M. Parkes (Eds.), *Psychotherapy Research and Behavior Change, Vol. 1.* Washington D.C. American Psychological Association.

Free, M.L., & Oei, T.P.S. (1989). Biological and Psychological processes in the treatment and maintenance of depression. *Clinical Psychology Review, 9,* 653-688.

Freeman, A. Simon, K.M., Beutler, L.E., & Arkowitz, H. (1989) (Eds.). *Comprehensive Handbook of Cognitive Therapy.* New York: Plenum.

Freeman, C., & Tyrer, P. (1989) (Eds.). *Research Methods in Psychiatry: A Beginner's Guide.* London: Gaskell: The Royal College of Psychiatrists.
Freud, S. (1917). Mourning and Melancholia. In *Completed Psychological Works, Vol. 14.* (standard ed.). Translated and edited by J. Strachey. London: Hogarth Press.
Frost R. (1963). *Selected Poems of Robert Frost.* New York: Holt, Rinehart & Winston.
Fuchs, C. Z., & Rehm, L. P. (1977). A self-control behavior therapy program for depression. *Journal of Consulting and Clinical Psychology, 45,* 206-215.
Galanter, M. (1990). Cults and zealous self-help movements: A psychiatric perspective. *American Journal of Psychiatry, 147,* 543-551.
Galbraith, J.K. (1987). *The Affluent Society.* 4th edition. Harmondsworth: Penguin Books.
Ganzini, L., McFarland, B.H., & Cutler, D. (1990). Prevalence of mental disorder after a catastrophic financial loss. *Journal of Nervous and Mental Disease, 178,* 680-685.
Garber, J., & Hollon, S.D. (1980). Universal versus personal helplessness in depression: Belief in uncontrollability or incompetence. *Journal of Abnormal Psychology, 89,* 56-66.
Gardner, H. (1985). *Frames of Mind.* London: Palidain.
Gardner, R. (1982). Mechanisms of manic-depressive disorder: An evolutionary model. *Archives of General Psychiatry, 39,* 1436-1441.
Gardner, R. (1988). Psychiatric infrastructures for intraspecific communication. In M.R.A. Chance (Ed.), *Social Fabrics of the Mind.* Hove: Lawrence Erlbaum Associates Ltd.
Gazzaniga, M.S. (1989). Organization of the human brain. *Science, 245,* 947-952.
Gelfand, D.M., & Teti, D.M. (1990). The effects of maternal depression on children. *Clinical Psychology Review, 10,* 329-354.
Gerlsma, C, Emmelkamp, P.M.G., & Arrindell, W.A. (1990). Anxiety, depression, and the perception of early parenting: A meta-analysis. *Clinical Psychology Review, 10,* 251-277.
Gilbert, P. (1980). *An investigation of cognitive factors in depression.* Unpublished PhD Thesis, University of Edinburgh.
Gilbert, P. (1984). *Depression: From Psychology to Brain State.* London: Lawrence Erlbaum Associates Ltd.
Gilbert, P. (1988a). Psychobiological interaction in depression. In S. Fisher & J. Reason (Eds.), *Handbook of Life Stress, Cognition and Health.* Chichester: J. Wiley & Sons.
Gilbert, P. (1988b). Emotional disorders, brain state and psychosocial evolution. In W. Dyden & P. Trower (Eds.), *Developments in Cognitive Psychotherapy.* London: Sage.
Gilbert, P. (1989). *Human Nature and Suffering.* Hove: Lawrence Erlbaum Associates Ltd.
Gilbert, P. (1990). Changes: Rank, status and mood. In S. Fisher & C.L. Cooper (Eds.), *On the Move: The Psychology of Change and Transition.* Chichester: J. Wiley & Sons.
Gilbert, P., Hughes, W., & Dryden, W. (1989). The therapist as the crucial variable in psychotherapy. In W. Dryden & L. Spurling (Eds.), *On Becoming a Psychotherapist.* London: Routledge.

Gilbert, P., & Reynolds, S. (1990). The relationship between the Eysenck personality questionnaire and Beck's concepts of sociotropy and autonomy. *British Journal of Clinical Psychology, 29,* 319-325.

Gilbert, P., & Trent, D. (submitted for publication). Depression in relation to submission and other rank related attributes. *British Journal of Medical Psychology*

Gilbert, P., & Trower P. (1990). The evolution and manifestation of social anxiety. In W.R. Crozier (Ed.), *Shyness and Embarrassment: Perspectives from Social Psychology.* Cambridge: Cambridge University Press.

Gilboa, S., Levav, I., Gilboa, L., & Ruiz, F. (1990). The epidemiology of demoralization in a kibbutz. *Acta Psychiatrica Scandinavia, 82,* 60-64.

Giles, D.E., Jarret, R.B., Roffwarg, H.P., & Rush, A.J. (1987). Reduced REM latency: A predictor of recurrence in depression. *Neuropsychopharmacology, 1,* 33-39.

Gilmore, D. (1981). Internal responses to environmental stimuli. In D. Gilmore & B. Cook (Eds.), *Environmental factors in mammal reproduction.* London : Macmillan.

Glantz, K., & Pearce, J.K. (1989). *Exiles from Eden: Psychotherapy From an Evolutionary Perspective.* New York: W.W. Norton & Co.

Glass, R.M., Uhlenhuth, E.H., Hartel, F.W., Matuzas, W., & Fischman, M.D. (1981). Cognitive dysfunction and imipramine in outpatients. *Archives of General Psychiatry, 38,* 1048-1051.

Gleick, J (1987). *Chaos.* Harmondsworth: Penguin Books.

Glen, A.I.M., Johnson, A.L., & Shepherd, M. (1984). Continuation therapy with lithium and amitriptyline in unipolar depressive illness: A randomized, double-blind, controlled trial. *Psychological Medicine, 14,* 37-50.

Goffman, E. (1968). *Stigma: Notes on the management of a spoiled identity.* Harmondsworth: Penguin Books.

Gold, J.R. (1990). Levels of depression. In B.B. Wolman & G. Stricker (Eds.), *Depressive Disorders: Facts, Theories and Treatment Methods.* New York: J. Wiley & Sons Inc.

Goldberg, A.I. (1975). The evolution of psychoanalytic concepts of depression. In E.J. Anthony & J. Benedek (Eds.), *Depression and Human Existence.* Boston: Little Brown.

Goldberg, D.P., Bridges, K., Duncan-Jones, P., & Grayson, D. (1987). Dimensions of neurosis seen in primary-care settings. *Psychological Medicine, 17,* 461-470.

Goldberg, D.P., & Bridges, K.W. (1990). Epidemiological observations on the concept of dysthymic disorder. In S.W. Burton & H.S. Akiskal (Eds.), *Dysthymic Disorder.* London: Gaskell: Royal College of Psychiatrists.

Goldberg, J.O., & Shaw, B.F., (1989). The measurement of cognition in psychopathology. In A.Freeman, K.M. Simon, L.E. Beutler, & H. Arkowitz (Eds.), *Comprehensive Handbook of Cognitive Therapy.* New York: Plenum.

Goldstein, W.N., & Anthony, R.N. (1989). DSM-111 and depression. In J.G. Howells (Ed.), *Modern perspectives in the Psychiatry of the Affective Disorders: Modern Perspectives in Psychiatry, Vol. 13.* New York: Brunner/Mazel Inc.

Goodall, J. (1973). The behavior of chimpanzees in their natural habitat. *American Journal of Psychiatry, 130,* 1-12.

Goodall, J. (1975). The chimpanzee. In V. Goodall (Ed.), *The Quest for Man.* London: Phaidon Press.

Goodyer, I.M., Wright, C., & Altham, P.M.E. (1989). Recent friendships in anxious and depressed school age children. *Psychological Medicine, 19,* 165-174.

Gordon, D., Burge, D., Hammen, C., Adrian, C., Jaenicke, C., & Hiroto, D. (1989). Observations of interactions of depressed women with their children. *American Journal of Psychiatry, 146,* 50-55.

Gotlib, I.H., & Cane, D.B. (1989). Self-report assessment of depression and anxiety. In P.C. Kendall & D. Watson (Eds.), *Anxiety and Depression: Distinctive and Overlapping Features.* New York: Academic Press.

Gotlib, I.H., & Colby, C.A. (1987). *Treatment of Depression: An Interpersonal Systems Approach.* New York: Pergamon Press.

Gotlib, I.H., & Lee, C.M. (1990). Children of depressed parents: A review and directions for future research. In C.D. McCann & N.S. Endler (Eds.), *Depression: New Directions in Theory, Research and Practice.* Toronto: Wall & Emerson Inc.

Gotlib, I.H., Mount, J.H., Cordby, N.I., & Whiffen, V.E. (1988). Depression and perceptions of early parenting: A longitudinal Investigation. *British Journal of Psychiatry, 152,* 24-27.

Gottschalk, L.A. (1988). Narcissism: Its normal evolution and development and the treatment of its disorders. *American Journal of Psychotherapy, XLII,* 4-27.

Gray, J.A. (1971). *The Psychology of Fear and Stress.* London: Weidenfeld & Nicolson.

Gray, J.A. (1979). *Pavlov.* London: Fontana (Modern Masters).

Gray, J.A. (1982) *The Neuropsychology of Anxiety.* Oxford: Oxford University Press.

Greenberg, J.R., & Mitchell, S.A. (1983). *Object Relations in Psychoanalytic Theory.* Cambridge, Mass.: Harvard University Press.

Greenberg, L.S. (1979). Resolving splits: Use of the two-chair technique. *Psychotherapy, Theory, Research and Practice, 16,* 316-324.

Greenberg, L.S., Elliott, R.K., & Foerster, F.S (1990). Experiential Processes in the psychotherapeutic treatment of depression. In C.D. McCann & N.S. Endler (Eds.), *Depression: New Directions in Theory, Research and Practice.* Toronto: Wall & Emerson Inc.

Greenberg, L.S., & Safran, J.D. (1987). *Emotion in Psychotherapy.* New York: Guilford Press.

Grove, W.M., Andreasen, N.C., Young, M.A., Endicott, J., Keller, M.B., & Hirschfeld, R.M.A. (1987). Isolation and characterization of a nuclear depressive syndrome. *Psychological Medicine, 17,* 471-484.

Guidano, V.F., & Liotti, G. (1983). *Cognitive Processes and Emotional Disorders.* New York: Guilford Press.

Gunderson, J.G., & Elliott, G.L. (1985). The interface between borderline personality disorder and affective disorder. *American Journal of Psychiatry, 142,* 277-288.

Gunderson, J.G., & Phillips, K.A. (1991). A current view of the interface between borderline personality disorder and depression. *American Journal of Psychiatry, 148,* 967-975.

Gut, E. (1989). *Productive and Unproductive Depression: Success or Failure of a Vital Process.* London: Routledge & Kegan Paul.

Haldipur, C.V. (1989) Psychiatric nosology and taxonomy in ancient India. *Acta Psychiatrica Scandinavia, 80,* 148-150

Hall, C.S. (1979). *A Primer of Freudian Psychology.* New York: Mentor Books.
Hall, C.S., & Nordby, V. J. (1973). *A Primer of Jungian Psychology.* New York: Mentor.
Hamilton, M. (1960). A rating scale for depression. *Journal of Neurology, Neurosurgery and Psychiatry, 32,* 50-55.
Hamilton, N.G. (1989). A critical review of object relations theory. *American Journal of Psychiatry, 146,* 1552-1560.
Hammen, C. (1988). Depression and cognitions about personal stressful life events. In L.B. Alloy (Ed.), *Cognitive Processes in Depression.* New York: Guilford Press.
Hammen, C., Adrian, C, & Hiroto, D. (1988). A longitudinal test of the attributional vulnerability model in children at risk for depression. *British Journal of Clinical Psychology, 27,* 37-46.
Hammen, C., & Peters, S.D. (1978). Interpersonal consequences of depression: Responses to men and women enacting a depressed role. *Journal of Abnormal Psychology, 87,* 322-332.
Hampden-Turner, C. (1970). *Radical Man.* London: Duckworth.
Harlow, H.F., & Mears, C. (1979). *The Human Model: Primate Perspectives.* New York: Winston & Sons.
Harre, R. (1980). The notion of causality. *British Journal of Psychiatry, 137,* 578-579.
Harris, T.O., Surtees, P., & Bancroft, J. (1991). Is sex necessarily a risk factor to depression? *British Journal of Psychiatry, 158,* 708-712.
Harrow, M., Colbert, J., Detre, T., & Bakeman, R. (1966). Symptomatology and subjective experiences in current depressive states. *Archives of General Psychiatry, 14,* 203-212.
Hartung, J. (1988). Deceiving down: Conjectures on the management of subordinate status. In J.S. Lockard & D.L. Paulus (Eds.), *Self-Deception: An Adaptive Mechanism.* Englewood Cliffs, N.J.: Prentice Hall Inc.
Hartup, W. (1989). Social relationships and their developmental significance. *American Psychologist, 44,* 120-126.
Haviland, W.A. (1990). *Cultural Anthropology* (6th edition). New York: Holt, Rinehart & Winston.
Hawton, K. (1987). Assessment of suicide risk. *British Journal of Psychiatry, 150,* 145-153.
Hawton, K., & Catalan, J. (1987). Attempted Suicide: A practical Guide to its nature and management (2nd edition). Oxford: Oxford Univerity Press.
Hawton, K., Salkovskis, P.M., Kirk, J., & Clark, D.M. (1989) (Eds). *Cognitive Behaviour Therapy for Psychiatric Problems.* Oxford: Oxford University Press.
Hay, D.P., & Hay, L.K (1990). The role of ECT in the treatment of depression. In C.D McCann & N.S. Endler (Eds.), *Depression: new directions in Theory, Research and Practice.* Toronto: Wall & Emerson.
Haynes, R. (1984). Suicide in Fiji: A preliminary study. *British Journal of Psychiatry, 145,* 433-438.
Hazan, C., & Shaver, P. (1987). Romantic love conceptualised as an attachment process. *Journal of Personality and Social Psychology, 52,* 511-524.
Healy, D., & Paykel, E.S. (1989). Neurochemistry of depression. In J.G. Howells (Ed.), *Modern Perspectives in the Psychiatry of the Affective Disorders. Modern perspectives in Psychiatry, Vol. 13.* New York: Brunner-Mazel.

Healy, D., & Williams, J.M.G. (1988). Dysrhythmia, dysphoria, and depression: The interaction of learned helplessness and circadian dysrhythmia in the pathogenesis of depression. *Psychological Bulletin, 103,* 163-178.
Heard, D.H., & Lake, B. (1986). The attachment dynamic in adult life. *British Journal of Psychiatry, 149,* 430-438.
Henderson, S. (1974). Care-eliciting behavior in man. *Journal of Nervous and Mental Disease, 159,* 172-181.
Henry, G.M., Weingartner, H., & Murphy, D. L. (1973). Influence of affective states and psychoactive drugs on verbal learning and memory. *American Journal of Psychiatry, 130,* 966-971.
Henry, J.P. (1982). The relation of social to biological process in disease. *Social Science Medicine, 16,* 369-380.
Henry, J.P., & Stephens, P.M. (1977). *Stress, Health and the Social Environment: A Sociobiologic Approach to Medicine.* New York: Springer Verlag.
Hesse H. (1971). *A child's heart* (short story). London: Cape.
Hickie, I., Parker, G., Wilhelm, K., & Tennant, C. (1991). Perceived interpersonal risk factors of non-endogenous depression. *Psychological Medicine, 21,* 399-412.
Hill, C.A. (1987). Affiliation motivation: People who need people...but for different reasons. *Journal of Personality and Social Psychology, 52,* 1008-1018.
Hill, D. (1968). Depression: Disease, reaction or posture? *American Journal of Psychiatry, 125,* 445-457.
Hill, E. (1981). Mechanisms of the mind: A psychiatrists's perspective. *British Journal of Medical Psychology, 54,* 1- 13.
Hill, J. (1984). Human altruism and sociocultural fitness. *Journal of Social and Biological Structures, 7,* 17-35.
Hill, K., & Hurtado, A.M. (1989). Hunter-gatherers of the new world. *American Scientist, 77,* 437-443.
Hinde, R.A. (1982). *Ethology.* Fontana Paperbacks.
Hinde, R.S. (1987). *Individuals, Relationships and Culture. Links Between Ethology and the Social Sciences.* Cambridge: Cambridge University Press.
Hinde, R.S. (1989). Relations between levels of complexity in behavioral sciences. *Journal of Nervous and Mental Disease, 177,* 655-667.
Hippocrates (460-367 BC). As quoted in Zilboorg & Henry (1941).
Hiroto, D.S., & Seligman, M.E.P. (1975). Generality of learned helplessness in man. *Journal of Personality and Social Psychology, 31,* 311-327.
Hirsch, S.R., & Shepherd, M. (1974) (Eds.). *Themes and Variations in European Psychiatry.* Bristol: John Wright.
Hirschfeld, R.M.A. (1982). Situational depression: Validity of the concept. *British Journal of Psychiatry, 139,* 297-305.
Hirschfeld, R.M.A., Klerman, G.L., Clayton, P.L., Clayton, P.J., Keller, M.B., McDonald-Scott, M.A., & Larkin, B.H. (1983a). Assessing personality: Effects of the depressive state on trait measurement. *American Journal of Psychiatry, 140,* 695-699.
Hirschfeld, R.M.A., Klerman, G.L., Clayton, P.L., & Keller, M.B. (1983b). Personality and depression: Empirical findings. *Archives of General Psychiatry, 40,* 993-998.
Hirschfeld, R.M.A., Klerman, G.L., Lavori, P., Keller, M.B., Griffith, P., & Coryell, W. (1989). Premorbid personality assessments of first onset of major

depression. *Archives of General Psychiatry, 46,* 345-350.

Hirschowitz, J., Casper, R., Garver, D. L., & Chang, S. (1980). Lithium response in good prognosis schizophrenia. *American Journal of Psychiatry, 137,* 916-920.

Hobfoll, S.E. (1989). Conservation of resources: A new attempt at conceptualising stress. *American Psychologist, 44,* 513-524.

Hoblitzelle, W. (1987). Differentiating shame and guilt: The relationship between shame and depression. In H.B. Lewis (Ed.), *The Role of Shame in Symptom Formation.* Hillsdale, N.J.: Lawrence Erlbaum Associates Inc.

Hofer, M.A. (1981). *The Roots of Human Behavior.* San Fransico: W.H. Freeman.

Hofer, M.A. (1984). Relationships as regulators: A psychobiologic perspective on bereavement. *Psychosomatic Medicine, 46,* 183-197.

Hojat, M., & Crandall, R. (1989) (Eds.). *Loneliness: Theory, Research, and Applications.* London: Sage.

Hojat, M., & Vogel, W.H. (1989). Socioemotional bonds and neurochmistry. In M. Hojat & R. Crandall (Eds.), *Loneliness: Theory, Research, and Applications.* London: Sage.

Hold-Cavell, B.C.L., & Borsutzky, D. (1986). Strategies to obtain high regard: A longitudinal study of a group of preschool children. *Ethology and Sociobiology, 7,* 39-56.

Hollon, S.D., & Kriss, M.R (1984). Cognitive factors in clinical research and practice. *Clinical Psychology Review, 4,* 35-76.

Hollon, S.D., & Najavits, L. (1988). Review of empirical studies on cognitive therapy. In A.J. Frances & R.E. Moles (Eds.), *Review of Psychiatry, Vol. 7.* Washington DC: American Psychiatric Press.

Hollon, S., Shelton, R.C., & Loosen, P.T. (1991). Cognitive therapy and pharmacotherapy for depression. *Journal of Consulting and Clinical Psychology, 59,* 88-99.

Holmes, D.S. (1978). Projection as a defense mechanism. *Psychological Bulletin, 85,* 677-688.

Holmes, D.S. (1981). Existence of classical projection and the stress-reducing function of attributive projection: A reply to Sherwood. *Psychological Bulletin, 90,* 460-466.

Holt, J. (1969). *How Children Fail.* Harmondsworth: Penguin Books.

Hong, M.K., Wirt, R.D., Yellin, A.M., & Hopwood, J. (1979). Psychological attributes: Patterns of life change and illness susceptibility. *Journal of Nervous and Mental Disease, 167,* 275-281.

Hooley, T.M., & Teasdale, J.D. (1989). Predictors of relapse in unipolar depressives: Expressed emotion, marital distress and perceived criticism. *Journal of Abnormal Psychology, 98,* 229-235.

Horner, A. (1989). *The Wish for Power and the Fear of Having It.* Northdale: Jason Aronson.

Horowitz, L.M., & Vitkus, J. (1986). The interpersonal basis of psychiatric symptoms. *Clinical Psychology Review, 6,* 443-470.

Horowitz, M.J. (1988) Formulation of states of mind. *American Journal of Psychotherapy, XLII,* 514-520.

Horowitz, M.J., & Wilner, N. (1976). Stress films, emotion and cognitive response. *Archives of General Psychiatry, 33,* 1339-1344.

Horowitz, M.J., Wilner, N., Marmar, C., & Krupnick, J. (1980a). Pathological grief and the activation of latent self-images. *American Journal of Psychiatry, 137,* 1157-1162 .

Horowitz, M.J., Wilner, N., Kaltreider, N., & Alvarez, W. (1980b). Signs and symptoms of posttraumatic stress disorder. *Archives of General Psychiatry, 37,* 85-92.

Horowitz, M.J., & Zilberg, N. (1983). Regressive alterations of the self concept. *American Journal of Psychiatry, 140,* 284-289.

Horrobin, D.F., & Manku, M.S. (1980). Possible role of prostaglandin E in the affective disorders and in alcoholism. *British Medical Journal, 280,* 1363-1366.

Hudson, J.I., & Pope, H.G. (1990). Affective spectrum disorder: Does antidepressant response identify a family of disorders with a common pathophysiology? *American Journal of Psychiatry, 147,* 552-564.

Hyman, S., & Arana, G.W. (1989). Suicide and affective disorders. In D. Jacobs & H.N. Brown (Eds.), *Suicide: Understanding and responding: Harvard Medical School Perspectives.* Connecticut: International Universities Press.

Imber, S.D., Pilkonis, P.A., Sotsky, S.M., Elkin, I., Watkins, J.T., Collins, J.F., Shea, M.T., & Leber, W.R. (1990). Mode-specific effects among three treatments for depression. *Journal of Consulting and Clinical Psychology, 58,* 352-359.

Iran-Nejad, A., & Ontony, A. (1984). A biofunctional model of disturbed mental content, mental structures, awareness and attention. *Journal of Mind and Behavior, 5,* 171-210.

Isen, A.M. (1990). The influence of positive and negative affect on cognitive organisation: Some implications for development. In N.L. Stein, B. Levanthal, & T. Trabasco (Eds.), *Psychological and Biological Approaches to Emotion.* Hillsdale, N.J.: Lawrence Erlbaum Associates Inc.

Isen, A.M., Daubman, K.A., & Nowicki, G.P. (1987). Positive affect facilitates creative problem solving. *Journal of Personality and Social Psychology, 52,* 1122-1131.

Itzkoff, S.W. (1990). *The Making of the Civilized Mind.* New York: Peter Lang.

Izard, C.E., & Blumberg, S.H. (1985). Emotion Theory and the role of emotions in anxiety in children and adults. In A.H. Tuma & J.D. Maser (Eds.), *Anxiety and Anxiety Disorders.* Hillsdale, N.J.: Lawrence Erlbaum Associates Inc.

Jackson, S.W. (1986). *Melancholia & Depression: From Hippocratic Times to Modern Times.* New Haven: Yale University Press.

Jacobi. J (1968). *The Psychology of Jung* (seventh edition). London: Routledge & Kegan Paul.

Jacobs, W.J., & Nadel, L. (1985). State-induced recovery of fears and phobias. *Psychological Review, 92,* 512-531.

Jacoby, M. (1989). Reflections on Heinz Kohut's concept of narcissism. In A. Sammuels (Ed.), *Psychopathology: Contemporary Jungian Perspectives.* London: Routledge & Kegan Paul.

Janoff-Bulman, R. (1979). Characterological versus behavioral self-blame: Inquiries into depression and rape. *Journal of Personality and Social Psychology, 37,* 1798-1809.

Janoff-Bulman, R., & Hecker, B. (1988). Depression, vulnerability, and world assumptions. In L.B. Alloy (Ed.), *Cognitive Processes in Depression.* New York: Guilford Press.

Jantsch, E. (1980). *The Self-Organising Universe: Scientific and Human Implications of the Emerging Paradigm of Evolution.* Oxford: Pergamon Press.

Jehu, D. (1988). *Beyond Childhood Abuse: Therapy for Women who were Childhood Victims.* Chichester: John Wiley.

Jehu, D. (1989). Mood disturbances among women clients abused in childhood: Prevalence, etiology and treatment. *Journal of Interpersonal Violence, 4,* 164-184.

Jenkins, J.H., Kleinman, A., & Good, B.J. (1991). Cross-cultural studies of depression. In J. Becker & A. Kleinman (Eds.), *Psychosocial Aspects of Depression.* Hillsdale, N.J.: Lawrence Erlbaum Associates Inc.

Joffe, W.W. (1969). A critical review of the status of envy. *International Journal of Psychoanalysis, 50,* 533-545.

Johnson, R.C., Danko, G.P., Huang, Y.H., Park, J.Y., Johnson, S.B., & Nagoshi, C.T. (1987). Guilt, shame and adjustment in three cultures. *Personality and Individual Differences, 8,* 357-364.

Jung, C.G. (1933). *Modern Man in Search of a Soul.* London: Routledge & Kegan Paul.

Jung, C.G. (1940). *The Integration of the Personality.* London: Routledge & Kegan Paul.

Jung, C.G. (1963). *Memories, Dreams, Reflections.* London: Collins/Fount Paperbacks.

Jung, C.G. (1964) (ed.). *Man and his Symbols.* London: Aldus-Jupiter Books.

Jung, C.G. (1972). *Four Archetypes.* London: Routledge & Kegan Paul.

Kagan, J. (1984). *The Nature of the Child.* New York: Basic Books.

Kahn, E. (1985). Heinz Kohut and Carl Rogers: A timely comparison. *American Psychologist, 40,* 893-904.

Kahn, E. (1989). Heinz Kohut and Carl Rogers: Towards a constructive collaboration. *Psychotherapy, 26,* 555-563.

Kalma, A. (1991). Hierarchisation and dominance assessment at first glance. *European Journal of Social Psychology, 21,* 165-181.

Karasu, T.B. (1990). Toward a clinical model of the psychotherapy for depression, II: An integrative and selective treatment approach. *American Journal of Psychiatry, 147,* 269-278.

Kasper, S., & Rosenthal, N.E (1989). Anxiety and depression in seasonal affective disorder. In P.C. Kendall & D.Watson (Eds.), *Anxiety and Depression: Distinctive and Overlapping Features.* New York: Academic Press.

Katakis, C.D. (1989). Stages of psychotherapy: Progressive reconceptualisation as a self-organizing process. *Psychotherapy, 26,* 484-493.

Katkin, E.S., Sasmor, D.B., & Tan, R. (1966). Conformity and achievement-related characteristics of depressed patients. *Journal of Abnormal Psychology, 71,* 407-412.

Katona, C.L.E. (1989). Biological markers and the diagnostic status of schizo-affective disorder. In K. Davison & A. Kerr (Eds.), *Contemporary Themes in Psychiatry.* London: Gaskell: The Royal College of Psychiatrists.

Katschnig, H., & Nutzinger, D.O. (1988). Psychosocial aspects of course and outcome in depressive illness. In T. Helgason & R.J. Daly (Eds.), *Depressive Illness: Prediction of Course and Outcome.* New York: Springer-Verlag.

Kaufman, J., & Zigler, E. (1987). Do abused children become abusive parents? *American Journal of Orthopsychiatry, 57,* 186-192.

Kegan, R. (1982). *The Evolving Self: Problem and Process in Human Development.* Cambridge, Mass.: Harvard University Press.

Keitner, G.I., & Miller, I.W. (1990). Family functioning and major depression: An overview. *American Journal of Psychiatry, 147,* 1128-1137.

Kelleher, M.J., & Daly, M. (1990). Suicide in Cork and Ireland. *British Journal of Psychiatry, 157,* 533-538.

Keller, M.B ., & Shapiro, R.W. (1982). "Double depression" superimposition of acute depressive episodes on chronic depressive disorders. *American Journal of Psychiatry, 139,* 438-442.

Keller, M.B., Klerman, G.L., Lavori, P.W., Coryell, W., Endicott, J., & Taylor, J. (1984). Long-term outcome of episodes of major depression: Clinical and public health significance. *Journal of the American Medical Association, 252,* 788-792.

Keller, M.B., Lavori, P.W., Klerman, G.L., Rice, J., Coryell, W., & Hirschfeld, R.M.A. (1986). The persistent risk of chronicity in recurrent episodes of non-bipolar major depressive disorder: A prospective follow-up. *American Journal of Psychiatry, 143,* 24-28.

Kellner, R. (1990). Somatization: Theories and research. *Journal of Nervous and Mental Disease, 178,* 150-160.

Kelly, G. (1955). *The Psychology of Personal Constructs.* New York: Norton & Co.

Kemper, T.D. (1988). The two dimensions of sociality. In M.R.A. Chance (Ed.), *Social Fabrics of the Mind.* Hove: Lawrence Erlbaum Associates Ltd.

Kemper, T.D. (1990a). Social relations and emotions: A structural approach. In T.D. Kemper (Ed.), *Research Agendas in the Sociology of the Emotions.* New York: State University of New York Press.

Kemper, T.D. (1990b). *Social Structure and Testosterone: Explorations of the Socio-Bio-Social Chain.* New Brunswick: Rutgers University Press.

Kemper, T.D., & Collins, R. (1990). Dimensions of microinteraction. *American Journal of Sociology, 96,* 32-68.

Kendall P.C., Hollon S.D., Beck, A.T., Hammen, C.L., & Ingram, R.E. (1987). Issues and recommendations regarding use of the Beck Depression Inventory. *Cognitive Therapy and Research, 11,* 298-299.

Kendall, P.C., & Watson, D. (1989) (Eds.). *Anxiety and Depression: Distinctive and Overlapping Features.* New York: Academic Press.

Kendell, R.E. (1968). The problem of classification. In A. Coppen & A. Walker (Eds.), Recent Developments in Affective Disorders: A Symposium. *British Journal of Psychiatry, Special Publication, No. 2.*

Kendell, R.E. (1974). The stability of psychiatric diagnoses. *British Journal of Psychiatry, 124,* 352-356.

Kendell, R.E. (1975). *The Role of Diagnosis in Psychiatry.* London: Blackwell Scientific Publications.

Kendell, R.E. (1976). The classification of depression: A review of contemporary confusion. *British Journal of Psychiatry, 129,* 15-28.

Kendell, R.E. (1988). What is a case? Food for thought for epidemiologists. *Archives of General Psychiatry, 45,* 374-376.

Kendell, R.E., & Brockington, I.F. (1980). The identification of disease entities and the relationship between schizophrenic and affective psychoses. *British Journal of Psychiatry, 137,* 324-331.

Kendell, R.E., MacKenzie, W.E., West, C., McGuire, J., & Cox, J.L. (1984). Day-to-day mood changes after childbirth: Further data. *British Journal of Psychiatry, 145,* 620-625.

Kendler, K.S., Kessler, R.C., Heath, A.C., Neale, M.C., & Eavas, L.J. (1991).

Coping: A genetic epidemiological investigation. *Psychological Medicine, 21,* 337-346.

Kennedy, H.G. (1988). Fatigue and fatigability. *British Journal of Psychiatry, 153,* 1-5.

Kennedy, J.L., & McKenzie, K.R. (1986). Dominance hierarchies in psychotherapy groups. *British Journal of Psychiatry, 148,* 625-631.

Kernberg, O.F. (1989) (Eds.). Narcissistic Personality Disorder. *The American Psychiatric Clinics of North America, 12,* 505-776.

Kevles, B. (1986). *Females of the Species: Sex and Survival in the Animal Kingdom.* Cambridge, Mass.: Harvard University Press.

Kiesler, D.J. (1983). The 1982 interpersonal circle: A taxonomy for complementarity in human transactions. *Psychological Review, 90,* 185-214.

Kiloh, L.G., & Garside, R.F. (1963). The independence of neurotic depression and endogenous depression. *British Journal of Psychiatry, 109,* 451-463.

Kiloh, L.G., Andrews, G., & Neilson, M. (1988). The long-term outcome of depressive illness. *British Journal of Psychiatry, 153,* 752-757.

King, R., Rases, J.D., & Barchas, J.D. (1981). Catastrophe theory of dopaminergic transmission: A revised dopamine hypothesis of schizophrenia. *Journal of Theoretical Biology, 92,* 373-400.

Klein, D.C., Fencil-Morse, E., & Seligman, M.E.P. (1976) Learned helplessness, depression and the attribution of failure. *Journal of Personality and Social Psychology, 33,* 508-516.

Klein, D.C., & Seligman, M.E.P. (1976). Reversal of performance deficits and perceptual deficits in learned helplessness and depression. *Journal of Abnormal Psychology, 85,* 11-25.

Klein, D.F. (1974). Endogenomorphic depression: A conceptual and terminological revision. *Archives of General Psychiatry, 31,* 447-454.

Klein, M. (1957/1975a). *Envy and Gratitude and Other Works (1946-1963).* London: Hogarth Press.

Klein, M. (1957/1975b). Envy and gratitude. In *Envy and Gratitude and Other Works (1946-1963).* London: Hogarth Press.

Klerman, G.L. (1988). The current age of youthful melancholia: Evidence for increase in depression among adolescents and young adults. *British Journal of Psychiatry, 152,* 4-14.

Klerman, G.L., Weissman, M.M., Rounsaville, B.J., & Chevron, E.S. (1984). *Interpersonal Psychotherapy of Depression.* New York: Basic Books.

Klinger, E. (1975). Consequences and commitment to aid disengagement from incentives. *Psychological Review, 82,* 1-24.

Klinger, E. (1977). *Meaning and Void.* Minneapolis: University of Minnesota Press.

Kohut, H. (1971). *The Analysis of the Self.* New York International Universities Press.

Kohut, H. (1977). *The Restoration of the Self.* New York: International Universities Press.

Kohut, H. (1982). Introspection, empathy, and the semi circle of mental health. *International Journal of Psychoanalysis, 63,* 395-407.

Kovacs, M. (1989). Depression in children and adolescents. *American Psychologist, 44,* 209-215.

Kraemer, G.W. (1985). Effects in early social experiences on primate neurobiological-behavioral development. In M. Reite & T. Field (Eds.), *The Psychobiology of Attachment and Separation.* New York: Academic Press.

Kraepelin, E. (1855-1926). As quoted in Zilboorg & Henry (1941).

Kräupl Taylor, F. (1980). The concepts of disease. *Psychological Medicine, 10,* 419-424.

Krebs, D., Denton, K., & Higgins, N.C. (1988). On the evolution of self-knowledge and self-deception. In K.M. MacDonald (Ed.), *Sociobiological Perspectives on Human Development.* New York: Springer Verlag.

Kripke, D.F., Risch, C.S., & Janowsky, D.S. (1983a). Lighting up depression. *Psychopharmacological Bulletin, 19,* 526-530.

Kripke, D.F., Risch, C.S., & Janowsky, D.S. (1983b). Bright light alleviates depression. *Psychiatry Research, 10,* 105-112.

Kuiper, N.A., & Olinger, L.J. (1986). Dysfunctional attitudes and a self-worth contingency model of depression. In P.C. Kendall (Ed.), *Advances in Cognitive-Behavioral Research and Therapy.* New York: Academic Press.

Kuiper, N.A., Olinger, L.J., & MacDonald, M.R. (1988). Vulnerability and episodic cognitions in a self-worth contingency model of depression. In L.B. Alloy (Ed.), *Cognitive Processes in Depression.* New York: Guilford Press.

Kuiper, N.A., Olinger, L.J., & Martin, R.A. (1990). Are cognitive approaches to depression useful? In C.D. McCann & N.S. Endler (Eds.), *Depression: New Directions in Theory, Research and Practice.* Toronto: Wall & Emerson Inc.

Kumar, R., & Brockington, I.F. (1988) (Eds.). *Motherhood and Mental Illness. Vol. 2: Causes and Consequences.* London: Wright.

Kumar, R., & Robson, K.M. (1984). A prospective study of emotional disorders in childbearing women. *British Journal of Psychiatry, 144,* 35-47.

Lader, M.M. (1975). *The Psychophysiology of Mental Illness.* London: Routledge & Kegan Paul.

Lamb, M.E., Thompson, R.A., Gardner, W.P., Chanon, K.L., & Estes, D. (1984). Security of infantile attachment as assessed in the strange situation: Its study and biological interpretation (plus peer review). *Behavioral and Brain Sciences, 7,* 127-162.

Lane, R.D., & Schwartz, G.E. (1987). Levels of emotional awareness: A cognitive-developmental theory and its application to psychopathology. *American Journal of Psychiatry, 144,* 133-143.

Lasch, C. (1985). *The Minimal Self: Psyche Troubles in Troubled Times.* London: Picador.

Lazarus, R.S. (1966). *Psychological Stress and the Coping Processes.* New York: McGraw Hill.

Lazarus, R.S. (1982). Thoughts on the relationship between emotion and cognition. *American Psychologist, 37,* 1019-1024.

Leary, M.R. (1983). A brief version of the fear of negative evaluation scale. *Personality and Social Psychology Bulletin, 9,* 371-375.

Leary, T. (1957). *The Interpersonal Diagnosis of Personality.* New York: Ronald Press.

Lee, A.S., & Murray, R.M. (1988). The long-term outcome of Maudsley depressives. *British Journal of Psychiatry, 153,* 741-750.

Leff, J.P. (1978). Social and psychological causes of the acute attack. In J.K. Wing (Ed.), *Schizophrenia: Towards a New Synthesis.* London: Academic Press.

Leonhard, K. (1959). Aufteilung der endogenen Psychosen. As quoted in Becker,

1974: *Depression: Theory and Research.* New York: Winston Wiley.
Leshner, A.I (1978). *An Introduction to Behavioral Endocrinology.* New York: Oxford University Press.
Leventhal, H., & Scherer, K. (1987). The relationship of emotion to cognition. *Cognition and Emotion, 1,* 3-28.
Lewinsohn, P.M. (1974). A behavioral approach to depression In R.J. Friedman & M.M. Katz (Eds.), *The Psychology of Depression: Contemporary Theory and Research.* New York: Winston-Wiley.
Lewinsohn, P.M. (1975). The behavioral study and treatment of depression. In M. Hersen, R.M. Eisler, & P.M. Miller (Eds.), *Progress in Behavior Modification, Vol. 1.* New York: Academic Press.
Lewinsohn, P.M., Mischel, W., Chaplin, W., & Barton, R. (1980). Social competence and depression: The role of illusory self-perceptions. *Journal of Abnormal Psychology, 89,* 203-212.
Lewinsohn, P.M., & Rosenbaum, M. (1987). Recall of parental behavior by acute depressives, remitted depressives, and non depressives. *Journal of Personality and Social Psychology, 52,* 611-619.
Lewinsohn, P.M., Steinmetz, J.L., Larson, D.W., & Franklin, J. (1981). Depression related cognitions: Antecedent or consequence? *Journal of Abnormal Psychology, 90,* 213-219.
Lewinsohn, P.M., Youngren, M.A., & Grosscup. S.J. (1979). Reinforcement and depression. In R.A. Depue (Ed.), *The Psychobiology of Depressive Disorders: Implications for the Effects of Stress.* New York: Academic Press.
Lewis, A. (1967). *Inquiries in Psychiatry: Clinical and Social Investigations.* London: Routledge & Kegan Paul.
Lewis, A. (1971). "Endogenous" and "exogenous". A useful dichotomy? *Psychological Medicine, 1,* 191-196.
Lewis, G., & Appleby, L. (1988). Personality disorder: The patients psychiatrists dislike. *British Journal of Psychiatry, 153,* 44-49.
Lewis, H.B. (1986). The role of shame in depression. In M. Rutter, C.E. Izard, & P.B. Read (Eds.), *Depression in Young People: Developmental and Clinical Perspectives.* New York: Guilford Press.
Lewis, H.B. (1987a). Introduction: Shame-the "sleeper" in psychopathology. In H.B. Lewis (Ed.), *The Role of Shame in Symptom Formation.* Hillsdale, N.J.: Lawrence Erlbaum Associates Inc.
Lewis, H.B. (1987b). The role of shame in depression over the life span. In H.B. Lewis (Ed.), *The Role of Shame in Symptom Formation.* Hillsdale, N.J.: Lawrence Erlbaum Associates Inc.
Lewis, H.B. (1987) (Ed.). *The Role of Shame in Symptom Formation.* Hillsdale, N.J.: Lawrence Erlbaum Associates Inc.
Lewy, A.J., Nurnberger, J.I., Wehr, T.A., Pack, D., Becker, L.E., Powell, R.L., & Newsome, D.A. (1985). Super-sensitivity to light: Possible trait marker for manic-depressive illness. *American Journal of Psychiatry, 142,* 725-727.
Liebert, R.M., & Spielger, M.D. (1990). *Personality: Strategies and Issues.* Belmont: Brooks/Cole.
Linville, P.W. (1985). Self-complexity and affective extremity: Don't put all your eggs in one basket. *Social Cognition, 3,* 94-120.
Liotti, G. (1988). Attachment and cognition: A guide for the reconstruction of early pathogenic experiences in cognitive therapy. In C. Perris, I.M. Blackburn, &

H. Perris (Eds.), *Handbook of Cognitive Psychotherapy.* New York: Springer.
Liotti, G. (in press). Egocentricism and cognitive psychotherapy of personality disorders. *Journal of Cognitive Psychotherapy: An International Quarterly.*
Littlewood, R. (1990). From categories to contexts: A decade of the 'new cross-cultural psychiatry'. *British Journal of Psychiatry, 156,* 308-327.
Lockard, J.S., & Paulhus, D.L. (1988) (Eds.). *Self deception: Adaptive mechanism.* Englewood Cliffs, N.J.: Prentice Hall.
Loftus, E.F., & Loftus, G.R. (1980). On the permanence of stored information in the human brain. *American Psychologist, 35,* 409-420.
Lorenz, K. (1981). *The Foundations of Ethology.* New York: Springer Verlag.
Lorenz, K. (1989). *The Waning of Humaneness.* Unwin Paperbacks.
Lyketsos, G.C., Blackburn, I.M., & Tsiantis, J. (1978). The movement of hostility during recovery from depression. *Psychological Medicine, 8,* 145-149.
Lyons, J.S., Rosen, A.J., & Dysken, M.W. (1985). Behavioral effects of tricyclic drugs in depressed in-patients. *Journal of Consulting and Clinical Psychology, 53,* 17-24.
McAllister, T.W., & Price, T.R.P. (1990). Psychopharmacology and depression. In C.N. McCann & N.S. Endler (Eds.), *Depression: New Directions in Theory, Research and Practice.* Toronto: Wall & Emerson Inc.
McCarley, R.W., & Hobson, A.J. (1977). The neurobiological origins of psychoanalytic dream theory. *American Journal of Psychiatry, 134,* 1211-1221.
McCarley, R.W. (1982) REM sleep and depression: Common neurobiologic control mechanisms. *American Journal of Psychiatry, 139,* 565-570.
McC.Miller, P., & Ingham, J.G. (1976). Friends, confidants and symptoms. *Social Psychiatry, 11,* 51-58.
McClelland, D.C. (1985). *Human Motivation.* Dallas: Scott, Foresman & Co.
McClelland, D.C., Atkinson, J.W., Clark, R.H., & Lowell, E.L. (1953). *The Achievement Motive.* New York: Appleton-Century-Crofts.
McCraine, E.W., & Buss, J.D. (1984). Childhood family antecedents of dependency and self-criticism. *Journal of Abnormal Psychology, 93,* 3-8.
McCrea, R.R. (1987). Creativity, divergent thinking, and openness to experience. *Journal of Personality and Social Psychology, 52,* 1258-1265.
Macdiarmid, D. (1989). Self-cathexis and other-cathexis: Vicissitudes in the history of an observation. *British Journal of Psychiatry, 154,* 844-852.
MacDonald, K.B. (1988). *Social and Personality Development: An Evolutionary Synthesis.* New York: Plenum Press.
MacDonald, K.B. (1988) (Ed.). *Sociobiological Perspectives on Human Development.* New York: Springer-Verlag.
McGuffin, P., & Katz, R. (1989). The genetics of depression and manic-depressive disorder. *British Journal of Psychiatry, 155,* 294-304.
McGuffin, P., Katz, R., & Rutherford, J. (1991). Nature, nurture and depression: A twin study. *Psychological Medicine, 21,* 329-338.
McGuire, M.T. (1988). On the possibility of ethological explanations of psychiatric disorders. *Acta Psychiatrica Scandinavia,* (suppl. 341, Van den Hoofdakker (Ed.)) *77,* 7-22.
McGuire, M.T. (1990). *Proximate cognitive mechanisms in depression.* Paper presented at the American Psychiatric Association, New York.
McGuire, M.T., & Troisi, A. (1987). Physiological regulation-deregulation and psychiatric disorders. *Ethology and Sociobiology, 8,* 9-25.

MacKie, A.J. (1982). Attachment theory: Its relevance to the therapeutic alliance. *British Journal of Medical Psychology, 54,* 203-212.

Mackintosh, N.J. (1974). *The Psychology of Animal Learning.* London: Academic Press.

Mackintosh, N.J. (1978). Conditioning. In B.M. Foss (Ed.), *Psychology Survey, No. 1.* London: G. Allen & Unwin.

MacLean, P. (1977). The triune brain in conflict. *Psychotherapy and Psychosomatics, 28,* 207-220.

MacLean, P. (1985). Brain evolution relating to family, play and the separation call. *Archives of General Psychiatry, 42,* 405-417.

MacVane, J.R., Lange, J.D., Brown, W.A., & Zayat, M. (1978). Psychological functioning of bipolar manic-depressives in remission. *Archives of General Psychiatry, 35,* 1351-1354.

Mahoney, M.J. (1974). *Cognition and Behavior Modification.* Cambridge, Mass.: Ballinger.

Mahoney, M.J., & Arnkoff, D.B. (1978). Cognitive and self-control therapies. In S.L. Garfield & J.W. Bergin (Eds.), *Handbook of Psychotherapy and Change, 2nd edition.* New York: Wiley & Sons.

Mahoney, M.J., & Gabriel, T.J. (1987). Psychotherapy and cognitive science. *Journal of Cognitive Psychotherapy: An International Quarterly, 1,* 39-60.

Mandell, A.J. (1979). On the mechanism of mood and personality changes of adult and later life: A Psychobiological hypothesis. *Journal of Nervous and Mental Disease, 167,* 457-466.

Mandler, G. (1975). *Mind and Emotion.* New York: John Wiley.

Marce, L. (1858). *Traité de la Folie des Femmes Enceintes, des Nouvelles Accouchées et des Nourrices.* Paris: Baillier.

Marks, I.M. (1987). *Fears, Phobias, and Rituals: Panic, Anxiety and their Disorders.* Oxford: Oxford University Press.

Markus, H., & Nurius, A. (1986). Possible selves. *American Psychologist, 41,* 945-969.

Marsella, A.J. (1980). Depressive experience and disorder across cultures. In H.C. Triandis & J.G Draguns (Eds.), *Handbook of Cross-Cultural Psychology. Vol. 6. Psychopathology.* Boston: Allyn & Bacon Inc.

Marzillier, J.S. (1980). Cognitive therapy and behavioural practice. *Behaviour Therapy and Research, 18,* 249-258.

Matson, S.T., & Zeiss, R.A. (1979). The buddy system: A method of generalised reduction of inappropriate interpersonal behaviour of retarded psychiatric patients. *British Journal of Social and Clinical Psychology, 18,* 401-405.

Matussek, P., & Feil, W.B. (1983). Personality attributes of depressive patients. *Archives of General Psychiatry, 40,* 783-790.

Maynard Smith, J. (1982). *Evolution and the Theory of Games.* Cambridge: Cambridge University Press.

Mazure, C., Nelson, C., & Price, L. (1986). Reliability and validity of the symptoms of major depression. *Archives of General Psychiatry, 43,* 451-456.

Melges, F.T., & Bowlby, J. (1969). Types of hopelessness in psychopathological processes. *Archives of General Psychiatry, 20,* 690-699.

Melges, F.T., & Swartz, M.S. (1989). Oscillations of attachment in borderline personality disorder. *American Journal of Psychiatry, 146,* 1115-1120.

Melhuish, E.C., Gambles, C., & Kumar, R. (1988). Maternal mental illness and the mother-infant relationship. In R. Kumar & I.F. Brockington (Eds.), *Motherhood and Mental Illness. Vol. 2: Causes and Consequences.* London: Wright.

Mendels, J., & Cochrane, C. (1968). The nosology of depression: The endogenous-reactive concept. *American Journal of Psychiatry, 124,* 1-11.

Mendels, J., & Frazer, A. (1974). Brain biogenic amine depletion and mood. *Archives of General Psychiatry, 30,* 447-451.

Menninger, K. (1963). *The Vital Balance: The Life Processes in Mental Health and Illness.* New York: Viking Press.

Merikangas, K.R., Spence, A.M., & Kupfer, D.J. (1989). Linkage studies of bipolar disorder: Methodologic and analytic issues. *Archives of General Psychiatry, 46,* 1137-1141.

Meyersburg, H.A., & Post, R.M. (1979). A holistic developmental view of neural and psychobiological processes: A neurobiologic-psychoanalytic integration. *British Journal of Psychiatry, 135,* 139-155.

Mezzich, J.E. (1988). On developing a psychiatric multiaxial schema for ICD-10. *British Journal of Psychiatry, 152 (suppl. 1),* 38-43.

Milgram, S. (1974). *Obedience to Authority.* New York: Harper and Row.

Miller, A. (1983). *For Your Own Good: The Roots of Violence in Child-rearing.* London: Virago.

Miller, I.W., Norman, W.H., & Keitner, G.I. (1989). Cognitive behavioral treatment of depressed inpatients: Six- and twelve-month follow-up. *American Journal of Psychiatry, 146,* 1274-1279.

Miller, N.E., & Weiss, J.M. (1969). Effects of somatic or visceral responses to punishment. In B.A. Campbell & R.M. Church (Eds.), *Punishment and Aversive Behavior.* New York: Appleton-Century-Crofts.

Miller, W.R. (1975). Psychological deficit in depression. *Psychological Bulletin, 82,* 238-260.

Miller, W.R., & Seligman, M.E.P. (1973). Depression and the perception of reinforcement. *Journal of Abnormal Psychology, 82,* 62-73.

Miller, W.R., & Seligman, M.E.P. (1975). Depression and learned helplessness in man. *Journal of Abnormal Psychology, 84,* 228- 238.

Millon, T. (1986). Theoretical derivations of pathological personalities. In T. Millon & G.L. Klerman (Eds.), *Contemporary Directions in Psychopathology: Toward the DSM-1V.* New York: Guilford Press.

Millon, T., & Klerman, G.L. (1986) (Eds.). *Contemporary Directions in Psychopathology: Toward the DSM-1V.* New York: Guilford Press.

Mineka, S., & Suomi, S.J. (1978). Social separation in monkeys. *Psychological Bulletin, 85,* 1376-1400.

Minkoff, K., Bergman, E., Beck, A.T., & Beck, R. (1973). Hopelessness, depression and attempted suicide. *American Journal of Psychiatry, 130,* 455-459.

Mischel, W., Ebbesen, E.B., & Zeiss, A.R. (1973). Selective attention to the self: Situational and dispositional determinants. *Journal of Personality and Social Psychology, 27,* 129-142.

Mischel, W., Ebbesen, E.B., & Zeiss, A.R. (1976). Determinants of selective memory about the self. *Journal of Consulting and Clinical Psychology, 44,* 92-103.

Mitchell, G., & Maple, T.L. (1985). Dominance in nonhuman primates. In S.L. Ellyson & J.F. Dovidio (Eds.), Power, Dominance and Nonverbal Behavior.

New York: Springer-Verlag.
Mollon, P. (1984). Shame in relation to narcissistic disturbance. *British Journal of Medical Psychology, 57,* 207-214.
Mollon, P., & Parry, G. (1984). The fragile self: Narcissistic disturbance and the protective function of depression. *British Journal of Medical Psychology, 57,* 137-145.
Montagu, A. (1986). *Touching: The Human Significance of the Skin* (third edition). New York: Harper and Row.
Moore, R.G., Watts, F.N., & Williams, J.M.G (1988). The specificity of personal memories in depression. *British Journal of Clinical Psychology, 27,* 275-276.
Moore, R.G., & Blackburn, I.M. (in preparation). Sociotropy, autonomy and personal memories in depression. University of Edinburgh.
Moretti, M.M., Higgins, E.T., & Feldman, L.A. (1990). The self-system in depression: Conceptualization and treatment. In C.D. McCann & N.S. Endler (Eds.), *Depression: New Directions in Theory, Research and Practice.* Toronto: Wall & Emerson Inc.
Morey, L.C. (1985). A comparative validation of the Foulds and Bedford hierarchy of psychiatric symptomatology. *British Journal of Psychiatry, 146,* 424-428.
Morey, L.C. (1988). Personality disorders in DSM-111 and DSM-111-R: Convergence, coverage, and internal consistency. *American Journal of Psychiatry, 145,* 573-577.
Morris, D. (1978). *Manwatching.* London: Triad/Granada.
Morris, L.W. (1979). *Extraversion and Introversion: An Interactional Perspective.* New York: J Wiley & Sons.
Morrison, A.P. (1984). Shame and the psychology of the self. In P.E. Stepansky & A. Goldberg (Eds.), *Kohut's Legacy: Contributions to Self Psychology.* The Analytic Press, (Distributed by Lawrence Erlbaum Associates: Hillsdale, N.J.)
Morrison, N. (1987). The role of shame in schizophrenia. In H.B. Lewis (Ed.), *The Role of Shame in Symptom Formation.* Hillsdale, N.J.: Lawrence Erlbaum Associates Inc.
Mowrer, O.H., & Viek, P. (1948). An experimental analogue of fear from a sense of helplessness. *Journal of Abnormal Psychology, 43,* 193-200.
Mullaney, J.A. (1989). The measurement and classification of affective disorders. In K. Davison & A. Kerr (Eds.), *Contemporary Themes in Psychiatry.* London: Gaskell: The Royal College of Psychiatrists.
Murphy, H.B.M. (1978). The advent of guilt feelings as a common depressive symptom: A historical comparison on two continents. *Psychiatry, 41,* 229-242.
Murray, L. (1988). Effects of postnatal depression on infant development: Direct studies of early mother-infant interactions. In R. Kumar, & I.F. Brockington (Eds.), *Motherhood and Mental Illness, Vol. 2: Causes and Consequences.* London: Wright.
Murray, L.G., & Blackburn, I.M. (1974). Personality differences in patients with depressive illness and anxiety neurosis. *Acta Psychiatrica Scandinavia, 50,* 183-191.
Musson, R.F., & Alloy, L.B. (1988). Depression and self-directed attention. In L.B. Alloy (Ed.), *Cognitive Processes in Depression.* New York: Guilford Press.
Nathanson, D.L. (1987) (Ed.). *The Many Faces of Shame.* New York: Guilford Press.
Nelson, J.C., & Charney, D.S. (1981). The symptoms of major depressive illness.

American Journal of Psychiatry, 138, 1-13.

Nesse, R.M. (1990). Evolutionary explanations of emotions. *Human Nature, 1,* 261-289.

Nietzel, M.T., & Harris, M.J. (1990). Relationship of dependency and achievement/autonomy to depression. *Clinical Psychology Review, 10,* 279-297.

Nisbitt, R.E., & Wilson, T.D. (1977). Telling more than we can know: Verbal reports on mental processes. *Psychological Review, 84,* 231-259.

Nolen-Hoeksema, S. (1987). Sex differences in unipolar depression: Evidence and theory. *Psychological Bulletin, 101,* 259-282.

Oatley, K. (1988). Life events, social cognition and depression. In S. Fisher, & J. Reason (Eds.), *Handbook of Life Stress, Cognition and Health.* Chichester: J. Wiley & Sons.

Oatley, K., & Boulton, W. (1985). A social theory of depression in reaction to life events. *Psychological Review, 92,* 372-388.

Ogata, S.N., Silk, K.R., Goodrich, S., Lohr, N.E., Westen, D., & Hill, E.M. (1990). Childhood sexual and physical abuse in adult patients with borderline personality disorder. *American Journal of Psychiatry, 147,* 1008-1013.

O'Hara, M.W. (1986). Social support, life events and depression during pregnancy and the puerperium. *Archives of General Psychiatry, 43,* 569-573.

O'Hara, M.W., & Zekoski, E.M. (1988). Postpartum depression: A comprehensive review. In R. Kumar & I.F. Brockington (Eds.), *Motherhood and Mental Illness, Vol. 2: Causes and Consequences.* London: Wright.

Oliver, J.M., & Simmons, M.E. (1985). Affective disorders and depression as measured by the Diagnostic Interview Schedule and the Beck Depression Inventory in an unselected adult population. *Journal of Clinical Psychology, 41,* 469-477.

Ollendick, T.H., & Yule, W. (1990). Depression in British and American children and its relation to anxiety and fear. *Journal of Consulting and Clinical Psychology, 58,* 126-129.

Orford, J. (1986). The rules of complementarity: Does hostility beget hostility and dominance, submission. *Psychological Review, 93,* 365-377.

Ornstein, R. (1986). *Multimind: A new way of looking at human beings.* London: Macmillan.

Overall, J.E., & Zisook, S. (1980). Diagnosis and the phenomenology of depressive disorders. *Journal of Consulting and Clinical Psychology, 48,* 626-634.

Overmier, J.B., & Seligman, M.E.P. (1967). Effects of inescapable shock upon subsequent escape and avoidance learning. *Journal of Comparative and Physiological Psychology, 63,* 28-33.

Parker, G.A. (1974). Assessment strategy and the evolution of fighting behaviour. *Journal of Theoretical Biology, 47,* 223-243.

Parker, G.A. (1984). Evolutionary strategies. In J.R. Krebs & N.B. Davies (Eds.), *Behavioral Ecology: An Evolutionary Approach.* Oxford: Blackwell.

Parker, G.A., Blignault, I., & Manicavasagar, V. (1988). Neurotic depression: Delineation of symptom profiles and their relation to outcome. *British Journal of Psychiatry, 152,* 15-23.

Parkes, C.M. (1972). *Bereavement: Studies of Grief in Adult Life.* London: Tavistock.

Parry, G., & Brewin, C.R. (1988). Cognitive style and depression: Symptom-related, event-related or independent provoking factor? *British*

Journal of Clinical Psychology, 27, 23-35.

Parry-Jones, W.L. (1989). Depression in adolescence. In K. Herbst & E. Paykel (Eds.), *Depression: An Integrative Approach.* Oxford: Heinemann Medical Books.

Pascal, B. (1670). *Pensées: Notes on Religion and Other Subjects.* Edited by L. Lafuma. Translation by J. Warrington. London: Dent.

Paulhus, D.L., & Martin. C.L. (1987). The structure of personal capabilities. *Journal of Personality and Social Psychology, 52,* 354-365.

Paykel, E.S. (1971). Classification of depressed patients: A cluster analysis derived grouping. *British Journal of Psychiatry, 118,* 275-288.

Paykel, E.S. (1978). Contribution of life events to causation of psychiatric illness. *Psychological Medicine, 8,* 245-253.

Paykel, E.S. (1979). Recent life events in the development of the depressive disorders. In R.A. Depue (Ed.), *The Psychobiology of the Depressive Disorders: Implications for the Effects of Stress.* New York: Academic Press.

Paykel, E.S. (1989). The background: Extent and nature of the disorder. In K. Herbst & E.S. Paykel (Eds.), *Depression: An Integrative Approach.* Oxford: Heinemann Medical Books.

Paykel, E.S., & Dowlatshahi, D. (1988). Life events and mental illness. In S. Fisher & J. Reason (Eds.), *Handbook of Life Stress, Cognition and Health.* Chichester: J. Wiley & Sons.

Paykel, E.S., & Henderson, A.J. (1977). Application of cluster analysis in the classification of depression: a replication study. *Neuropsychobiology, 3,* 111-119.

Paykel, E.S., & Tanner, J. (1976). Life events, depressive relapse and maintenance treatment. *Psychological Medicine, 6,* 481-485.

Paykel, E.S., Weissman, M.M., & Prusoff, B.A. (1978). Social maladjustment and severity of depression. *Comprehensive Psychiatry, 19,* 121-128.

Pedder, J.R. (1982). Failure to mourn and melancholia. *British Journal of Psychiatry, 141,* 329-337.

Pedersen, J., Schelde, J.T.M., Hannibal. E., Benke, K., Neilsen, B.M., & Hertz, M. (1988). An ethological description of depression. *Acta Psychiatrica Scandinavia, 78,* 320-330.

Pehl, J. (1990). *An investigation of the relation between shame proneness and fear of negative evaluation.* Unpublished Manuscript: University of Leicester.

Pennebaker, J.M. (1988). Confiding traumatic experiences and health. In S. Fisher & J. Reason (Eds.), *Handbook of Life Stress, Cognition and Health.* Chichester: J. Wiley & Sons.

Pennebaker, J.W., & Becall, S.K. (1986). Confronting a traumatic event: Toward an understanding of inhibition and disease. *Journal of Abnormal Psychology, 95,* 274-287.

Pennebaker, J.W., & O'Heeron, R.C. (1984). Confiding in others and illness rates among spouses of suicide and accident-death victims. *Journal of Abnormal Psychology, 93,* 473-476.

Perris, C. (1966). A study of bipolar (manic depressive) and unipolar (recurrent depressive) psychoses. *Acta Psychiatrica Scandinavia, 42 (Suppl. 194),* 1-189.

Perris, C., Arrindell, W.A., & Perris, H., Eisemann, M., Van der Ende, J., & von Knorring, L. (1986). Perceived depriving parental rearing and depression. *British Journal of Psychiatry, 148,* 170-175.

Persons, J.B., Burns, D.D., & Perloff, J.M. (1988). Predictors of dropout and outcome in cognitive therapy for depression in a private practice setting. *Cognitive Therapy and Research, 12,* 557-576.

Peselow, E.D., Robins, C.J., Block, P., Barouche, F.M., & Fieve, R.R. (1990). Dysfunctional attitudes in depressed patients before and after clinical treatment and normal control subjects. *American Journal of Psychiatry, 147,* 439-444.

Pfeffer, C. (1989). Suicidal episodes and risk factors in children. In J.G. Howells (Ed.), *Modern Perspectives in the Psychiatry of the Affective Disorders. Modern perspective in Psychiatry, Vol. 13.* New York: Brunner-Mazel.

Phillips, K.A., Gunderson, J. G., Hirschfeld, R., & Smith, L.E. (1990). A review of depressive personality. *American Journal of Psychiatry, 147,* 830-837.

Pilkonis, P.A., & Frank, E. (1988). Personality pathology in recurrent depression: Nature, prevalence, and relationship to treatment response. *American Journal of Psychiatry, 145,* 435-441.

Pilowsky, I., & Spence, N.D. (1975). Hostility and depressive illness. *Archives of General Psychiatry, 32,* 1154-1157.

Pitt, B. (1968). 'Atypical' depression following childbirth. *British Journal of Psychiatry, 114,* 1325-1335.

Plato (427-347 BC). As quoted in Zilboorg & Henry (1941).

Platz, C., & Kendell, R.E. (1988). A matched-control follow-up and family study of 'puerperal psychoses'. *British Journal of Psychiatry, 153,* 90-94.

Plotkin, H.C., & Odling-Smee, F.J. (1981). A multiple-level model of evolution and its implications for sociobiology. *Behavioral and Brain Sciences, 4,* 225-268.

Popper, K.A., & Eccles, J.C. (1977). *The Self and Its Brain.* London: Springer-Verlag.

Postle, D. (1980). *Catastrophe Theory: Predict and Avoid Personal Disasters.* London: Fontana.

Power, M.D. (1988). The cohesive foragers: Human and Chimpanzee. In M.R.A. Chance (Ed.), *Social Fabrics of the Mind.* Hove: Lawrence Erlbaum Associates Ltd.

Power, M.J., & Brewin, C.R. (in press). From Freud to cognitive science: A contemporary account of the unconscious. *British Journal of Clinical Psychology.*

Price, J.A. (in press). Change or Homeostasis? A systems theory approach to depression. *British Journal of Medical Psychology.*

Price, J.S. (1972). Genetic and phylogenetic aspects of mood variations. *International Journal of Mental Health, 1,* 124-144.

Price, J.S. (1988). Alternative channels for negotiating asymmentry in social relationships. In M.R.A. Chance (Ed.), *Social Fabrics of the Mind.* Hove: Lawrence Erlbaum Associates Ltd.

Price, J.S. (1989). The effects of social stress on the behaviour and physiology of monkeys. In K. Davison & A. Kerr (Eds.), *Contemporary Themes in Psychiatry.* London: Gaskell: Royal College of Psychiatrists.

Price, J.S., & Sloman, L. (1987). Depression as yielding behavior: An animal model based on Schjelderup-Ebbe's pecking order. *Ethology and Sociobiology, 8,* 85-98.

Price, V.A. (1982). *Type A Behavior Pattern: A Model for Research and Practice.* New York: Academic Press.

Prusoff, B., & Klerman, G. L. (1974). Differentiating depressed from anxious neurotic outpatients. *Archives of General Psychiatry, 30,* 302-309.

Pyszczynski, T., & Greenberg, J. (1987). Self-regulatory perseveration and the depressive self focusing style: A self-awareness theory of reactive depression. *Psychological Bulletin, 102,* 122-138.

Rachman, S. (1978). *Fear and Courage.* San Francisco: Freeman.

Rachman, S. (1981). The primacy of affect: Some theoretical implications. *Behaviour Research and Therapy, 19,* 279-290.

Rahe, R.H., & Arthur, R.J. (1978). Life change and illness studies: Past history and future directions. *Journal of Human Stress, 3,* 3-15.

Raleigh, M.J., McQuire, M.T., Brammer, G.L., & Yuwieler, A. (1984). Social and environmental influences on blood serotonin concentrations in monkeys. *Archives of General Psychiatry, 41,* 405-410.

Rao, R.V.A., & Coppen, A. (1979). Classification of depression and response to amitriptyline therapy. *Psychological Medicine, 9,* 321-325.

Raphael-Leff, J. (1986). Facilitators and regulators: Conscious and unconscious processes in pregnancy and motherhood. *British Journal of Medical Psychology, 59,* 43-56.

Raskin, A., & Crook, T.H. (1976). The endogenous-neurotic distinction as a predictor of response to antidepressant drugs. *Psychological Medicine, 6,* 59-70.

Raskin, A., Schulterbrandt, J.G., Raetig, N., & McKeon, J.J. (1970). Differential response to chlorpromazine, imipramine and placebo: A study of sub-groups of hospitalized depressed patients. *Archives of General Psychiatry, 23,* 164-173.

Rasmussen, K.L.R., & Reite, M. (1982). Loss-induced depression in an adult Macaque monkey. *American Journal of Psychiatry, 139,* 679-681.

Rehm, L.P. (1977). A self-control model of depression. *Behavior Therapy, 8,* 787-804.

Rehm, L.P. (1981) (Ed.). *Behavior Therapy for Depression.* New York: Academic Press.

Rehm, L.P. (1988). Self-management and cognitive processes in depression. In L.B. Alloy (Ed.), *Cognitive Processes in Depression.* New York: Guilford.

Rehm, L.P. (1989). Behavioral models of anxiety and depression. In P.C. Kendall & D. Watson (Eds.), *Anxiety and Depression: Distinctive and Overlapping Features.* New York: Academic Press.

Rehm, L.P., Fuchs, C.Z., Roth, D.M., Kornblith, S.J., & Romano, J. M. (1979). A comparison of self-control and assertion skills treatments of depression. *Behavior Therapy, 10,* 429-442.

Reich, J., Noyes, R., Hirschfeld, R.M.A., Coryell, W.H., & O'Gorman, T. (1987). State and personality in depressed and panic patients. *American Journal of Psychiatry, 144,* 181-187.

Reiss, D., Plomin, R., & Hetherington, E.M. (1991). Genetics and psychiatry: An unheralded window on the environment. *American Journal of Psychiatry,* 283-291.

Reite, M., & Field, T. (1985) (Eds.). *The Psychobiology of Attachment and Separation.* New York: Academic Press.

Reite, M., Short, R., Seiler, C., & Pauley, J.D. (1981). Attachment, loss and depression. *Journal of Child Psychology and Psychiatry, 22,* 141-169.

Rescorla, R.A. (1988). Pavlovian Conditioning: It's not what you think it is. *American Psychologist, 43,* 151-160.

Reus, V.I., Weingartner, H., & Post, R.M. (1979a). Clinical implications of state-dependent learning. *American Journal of Psychiatry, 136,* 927-931.

Reus, V.I., Silberman, E., Post, R.M., & Weingartner, H. (1979b). H-amphetamine: Effects on memory in a depressed population. *Biological Psychiatry, 14,* 345-356.

Reynolds, S., & Gilbert, P. (1991). Psychological impact of unemployment: Interacting effects of individual vulnerability and protective factors. *Journal of Counselling Psychology, 38,* 76-84.

Richards, G. (1987). *Human Evolution: An Introduction for the Behavioural Sciences.* London: Routledge & Kegan Paul.

Riley, W.T., Treiber, F.A., & Woods, M.G. (1989). Anger and hostility in depression. *Journal of Nervous and Mental Disease, 177,* 668-674.

Rippere, V. (1981). Depression, common sense, and psychosocial evolution. *British Journal of Medical Psychology, 54,* 379-387.

Rippere, V. (1984). Depression: Investigation. In S. Lindsay & G. Powell (Eds.), *A Handbook of Clinical Adult Psychology.* Aldershot: Gower.

Robins, C.J., & Block, P. (1988). Personal vulnerability, life events and depressive symptoms: A test of a specific interactional model. *Journal of Personality and Social Psychology, 54,* 846-852.

Robins, C.J., Block, P., & Peselow, E.D. (1989). Relations of sociotropic and autonomous personality characteristics to specific symptoms in depressed patients. *Journal of Abnormal Psychology, 98,* 86-88.

Robins, C.J., & Luten, A. (1991). Personality characteristics and clinical features of depression. *Journal of Abnormal Psychology, 100,* 74-77.

Robins, E., Munoz, R. A., Martin, S., & Gentry, K.A. (1972). Primary and secondary affective disorders. In J. Zubin & F.A. Freyhan (Eds.), *Disorders of Mood.* Baltimore: John Hopkins University Press.

Robson, P.J. (1988). Self-esteem: A psychiatrists view. *British Journal of Psychiatry, 153,* 6-15.

Rohner, R.P. (1986). *The Warmth Dimension: Foundations of Parental Acceptance-rejection Theory.* Beverly Hills: Sage.

Rook, K.S. (1987). Social support versus companionship: Effects on life stress, loneliness and evaluations of others. *Journal of Personality and Social Psychology, 52,* 1132-1147.

Rose, S., Lewontin, R.C., & Kamin, L.K. (1984). *Not All in Our Genes.* Pelican Books.

Rosen, H. (1989). Piagetian theory and cognitive therapy. In A. Freeman, K.M. Simon, L.E. Beutler, & H. Arkowitz (Eds.), *Comprehensive Handbook of Cognitive Therapy.* New York: Plenum.

Rosenbaum, A.H. (1989). Advances in lithium therapy. In J.G. Howells (Ed.), *Modern perspectives in the Psychiatry of the Affective Disorders: Modern Perspectives in Psychiatry, Vol. 13.* New York: Brunner/Mazel Inc.

Rosenhan, D.L., & Seligman, M.E.P. (1984). *Abnormal Psychology* (Chapter 16, Personality Disorders). New York: W.W. Norton & Co.

Rosenthal, N.E., Sack, D.A., Gillian, C.J., Lewy, A.T., Goodwin, F.K., Davenport, Y., Mueller, P.S., Newsome, D.A., & Wehr, T.A. (1984). Seasonal affective disorder: A description of the syndrome and preliminary findings with light therapy. *Archives of General Psychiatry, 41,* 72-79.

Rossi, E.L. (1989). Consciousness, emotional complexes, and the mind-gene connection. In M.D. Yapko (Ed.), *Brief Approaches to treating Anxiety and*

Depression. New York: Brunner/Mazel.

Roth, S., & Kubal, L. (1975). Effects of noncontingent reinforcement on tasks of different importance: Facilitation and learned helplessness. *Journal of Personality and Social Psychology, 32,* 680-691.

Rotter, J.B. (1966). *Generalized expectancies for internal versus external control of reinforcement.* Psychological Monographs (Whole No. 609).

Rotter, J.B., Seeman, M., & Liverant, S. (1962). Internal versus external control of reinforcement: A major variable in behavior theory. In N.F. Washburne (Ed.), *Decisions, Values and Groups, Vol. 2.* Oxford: Pergamon Press.

Rush, A.J., Erman, M.K., Giles, D.E., Schlesser, M.A., Carpenter, G., Vasavada, N., & Roffwarg, H.P. (1986). Polysomnographic findings in drug-free and clinically remitted depressed patients. *Archives of General Psychiatry, 43,* 878-884.

Russell, G.A. (1985). Narcissism and narcissistic personality disorder; A comparison of the theories of Kernberg and Kohut. *British Journal of Medical Psychology, 58,* 137-148.

Rutter, M. (1975). *Helping Troubled Children.* Harmondsworth: Penguin Books.

Rutter, M. (1981). *Maternal Deprivation Reassessed* (2nd edition). Harmondsworth: Penguin Books.

Rutter, M. (1987a). Temperament, personality and personality disorder. *British Journal of Psychiatry, 150,* 443-458.

Rutter, M. (1987b). The role of cognition in child development. *British Journal of Medical Psychology, 60,* 1-18.

Ryle, A. (1982). *Psychotherapy. A Cognitive Integration of Theory and Practice.* London: Academic Press.

Sabini, J., & Silver, M. (1982). *The Moralities of Everyday Life.* New York: Oxford University Press.

Sadd, S., Lenauer, M., Shaver, P., & Dunivant, N. (1978). Objective measurement of fear of success and fear of failure: A factor analytic approach. *Journal of Consulting and Clinical Psychology, 46,* 405-416.

Safran, J.D., & Segal, Z.V. (1990). *Interpersonal Process in Cognitive Therapy.* New York: Basic Books.

Samuels, A. (1985). *Jung and the Post Jungians.* London: Routledge & Kegan Paul.

Sanderson, W.C., Beck, A.T., & Beck, J. (1990). Syndrome comorbidity in patients with major depression and dysthymia: Prevalence and temporal relationships. *American Journal of Psychiatry, 147,* 1025-1028.

Sapolsky, R.M. (1989). Hypercortisolism among socially subordinate wild baboons originates at the CNS level. *Archives of General Psychiatry, 46,* 1047-1051.

Sartorius, N., Jablensky, A., Gulbinat, W., & Ernberg, G. (1980). WHO collaborative study: Assessment of depressive disorders. *Psychological Medicine, 10,* 743-749.

Sartorius, N., Davidian, H., & Ernberg, G. (1983). *Depressive disorders in different cultures: Report on the WHO collaborative study on standardized assessment of depressive disorders.* Geneva: World Health Organization.

Savin-Williams, R.C. (1979). Dominance hierarchies in groups of early adolescents. *Child Development, 50,* 923-935.

Scadding, J. (1980). The concepts of disease: A response. *Psychological Medicine, 10,* 415-427.

Scheff, T.J. (1988). Shame and conformity. The deference-emotion system. *American Review of Sociology, 53,* 395-406.

Schjerlderup-Ebbe T. (1935). Social behaviour in birds. In C. Murchison (Ed.), *Handbook of Social Psychology.* Worster: Clark University Press.

Schlenker, B.R. (1987). Threats to identity: Self-identification and social stress. In C.R. Snyder & C.E. Ford (Eds.), *Coping with Life Events: Clinical and Social Perspectives.* New York: Plenum Press.

Schless, A.P., Schwartz, L., Goetz, C., & Mendels, J. (1974). How depressives view the significance of life events. *British Journal of Psychiatry, 125,* 406-410.

Schwab, J.J. (1970). Coming in the 70s: An epidemic of depression. *Attitude, 1,* 2-6.

Schwab, J.J. (1989). The epidemiology of the affective disorders. In Howells, J.G. (Ed.), *Modern perspectives in the psychiatry of the affective disorders. Modern Perspectives in Psychiatry Number 13.* New York: Brunner/Marzel.

Schwartz, B. (1986). *The Battle for Human Nature: Science, Morality and Modern Life.* New York: W.W. Norton & Co.

Schwartz, R.M., & Gottman, J.M. (1976). Toward a task analysis of assertive behavior. *Journal of Consulting and Clinical Psychology, 44,* 910-920.

Scott, J. (1988). Chronic depression. *British Journal of Psychiatry, 153,* 287-297.

Scott, J., Williams, J.M.G., & Beck, A.T. (1989). *Cognitive Therapy in Clinical Practice.* London: Routledge.

Sedler, M.J. (1983). Falret's discovery: The origin of the concept of bipolar affective illness. *American Journal of Psychiatry, 140,* 1127-1133.

Segal, H. (1975). *Introduction to the Work of Melanie Klein.* London: Hogarth Press.

Segal, J. (1985). *Phantasy in Everyday Life: A Psychological Approach to Understanding Ourselves.* New York: Pelican Books.

Seligman, M.E.P. (1971). Phobias and preparedness. *Behavior Therapy, 2,* 307-320.

Seligman, M.E.P. (1975). *Helplessness: On Depression Development and Death.* San Francisco: Freeman & Co.

Seligman, M.E.P (1989). Explanatory style: Predicting depression, achievement and health. In M.D. Yapko (Ed.), *Brief Approaches to Treating Anxiety and Depression.* New York: Brunner/Mazel.

Seligman, M.E.P., Abramson, L.Y., Semmel, A., & Baeyer, C.V. (1979). Depressive attributional style. *Journal of Abnormal Psychology, 88,* 242-247.

Seligman, M.E.P., & Maier, S.F. (1967). Failure to escape traumatic shock. *Journal of Experimental Psychology, 74,* 1-9.

Serney, G. (1990). The sins of the fathers. *The Sunday Times Colour Magazine, September 23,* 22-36.

Shapiro, M.B. (1989). A phenomenon-orientated strategy in depression research. *British Journal of Clinical Psychology, 28,* 298-306.

Shaw, B.F., Steer, R.A., Beck, A.T., & Schut, J. (1979). The structure of depression in heroin addicts. *British Journal of Addiction, 74,* 295-303.

Sheldon, A.E., & West, M. (1989). The functional discrimination of attachment and affiliation: Theory and empirical demonstration. *British Journal of Psychiatry, 155,* 18-23.

Sherwood, G.G. (1982). Consciousness and stress reduction in defensive projection: A reply to Holmes. *Psychological Bulletin, 91,* 372-375.

Shevrin, H., & Dickman, S. (1980). The psychological unconscious: A necessary assumption for all psychological theory? *American Psychologist, 35,* 421-434.
Shively, C. (1985). The evolution of dominance hierarchies in nonhuman primates. In S.L. Ellyson & J.F. Dovidio (Eds.), *Power, Dominance and Nonverbal Behavior.* New York: Springer-Verlag.
Shneidman, E.S. (1989). Overview: A multidimensional approach to suicide. In D. Jacobs & H.N. Brown (Eds.), *Suicide: Understanding and responding.* Harvard Medical School Perspectives: Connecticut: International Universities Press.
Sholomskas, D.E. (1990). Interviewing Methods. In B.B. Wolman & G. Stricker (Eds.), *Depressive Disorders: Facts, Theories and Treatment Methods.* New York: J. Wiley & Sons Inc.
Silberman, E.K., Reus, V.I., Jimerson, D.C., Lynott, A.M., & Post, R.M. (1981). Heterogeneity of amphetamine response in depressed patients. *American Journal of Psychiatry, 138,* 1302-1307.
Silberstein, L.R., Striegel-Moore, R., & Rodin, J. (1987). Feeling fat: A woman's shame. In H.B. Lewis (Ed.), *The Role of Shame in Symptom Formation.* Hillsdale, N.J.: Lawrence Erlbaum Associates Inc.
Simon, D.I. (1987). On change, catastrophe and therapy. *Journal of Family Therapy, 8,* 59-73.
Simons, A.D., McGrowan, C.R., & Epstein, L.H. (1985). Exercise as a treatment for depression: An update. *Clinical Psychology Review, 5,* 553-568.
Sitaram, N., Nurnberger, J.I., Gershon, E.S., & Gillin, C.J. (1982). Cholinergic regulations of mood and REM sleep: Potential model and marker of vulnerability to affective disorder. *American Journal of Psychiatry, 139,* 571-576.
Slater, J., & Depue, R.A. (1981). The contribution of environmental events and social support to serious suicide attempts in primary depressive disorder. *Journal of Abnormal Psychology, 90,* 275-285.
Smail, D. (1987). *Taking Care: An Alternative to Therapy.* London: J. Dent & Sons.
Smith, T.W., & Allred, K.D. (1989). Major life events in anxiety and depression. In P.C. Kendall & D. Watson (Eds.), *Anxiety and Depression: Distinctive and Overlapping Features.* New York: Academic Press.
Solomon, R.L. (1980). The opponent-process theory of acquired motivation: The cost of pleasure and the benefits of pain. *American Psychologist, 35,* 691-712.
Sommers, S. (1981). Emotionality reconsidered: The role of cognition in emotional responsiveness. *Journal of Personality and Social Psychology, 41,* 553- 561.
Spielman, L.A., & Bargh, J.A (1990). Does the depressive self schema really exist? In C.N. McCann & N.S. Endler (Eds.), *Depression: New Directions in Theory, Research and Practice.* Toronto: Wall & Emerson Inc.
Spitzer, R., Endicott, J., & Robins, E. (1975). *Research Diagnostic Criteria.* New York: State Psychiatric Institute.
Spitzer, R., Endicott, J., & Robins, E. (1978). Research Diagnostic Criteria: Rational and reliability. *Archives of General Psychiatry, 35,* 773-782.
Sroufe, A.L., & Fleeson, J. (1986). Attachment and the construction of relationships. In W.W. Hartup, & Z. Rubin (Eds.), *Relationships and Development.* Hillsdale, N.J.: Lawrence Erlbaum Associates Inc.
Sroufe, A.L., & Rutter, M. (1984). The domain of developmental psychopathology. *Child Development, 55,* 17-29.
Staats, A.W., & Eifert, G.H. (1990). The paradigmatic behaviorism theory of

emotion: Basis for unification. *Clinical Psychology Review, 10,* 539-566.

Staude, J.R. (1981). *The Adult Development of C.G. Jung.* Boston: Routledge & Kegan Paul.

Stevens, A. (1982). *Archetype: A Natural History of the Self.* London: Routledge & Kegan Paul.

Stewart, J.M., McGrath, P.J., Quitkin, F.M., Harrison, W., Markowitz, J., Wager, S., & Leibowitz, M.R. (1989). Relevance of DSM-111 depressive subtype and the chronicity of antidepressant efficacy in atypical depression. *Archives of General Psychiatry, 46,* 1080-1087.

Stigler, J.W., Shweder, R.A., & Herdt, G. (1990) (Eds.). *Cultural Psychology: Essays on Comparative Human Development.* Cambridge: Cambridge University Press.

Stokes, J.P., & McKirnan, D.J. (1989). Affect and the social environment: The role of social support in depression and anxiety. In P.C. Kendall & D. Watson (Eds.), *Anxiety and Depression: Distinctive and Overlapping Features.* New York: Academic Press.

Stone, M.H. (1989). Long term follow-up of narcissistic/borderline patients. *The Psychiatric Clinics of North America, 12,* 621-641.

Storr, A. (1973). *Jung.* London: Fontana.

Storr, A. (1989). *Solitude.* London: Flamingo.

Suls, J., & Wills, T.A. (1991). *Social Comparison: Contemporary Theory and Research.* Hillsdale, N.J.: Lawrence Erlbaum Associates Inc.

Surtees, P.G., & Kendell, R.E. (1979). The hierarchy model of psychiatric symptomatology: An investigation based on present state examination ratings. *British Journal of Psychiatry, 135,* 438-443.

Swallow S.R., & Kuiper, N.A. (1988). Social comparison and negative self evaluation: An application to depression. *Clinical Psychology Review, 8,* 55-76.

Szasz, T. (1974). *Ideology and Insanity.* New York: Penguin.

Tarnopolsky, A., & Berelowitz, M. (1987). Borderline personality: A review of recent research. *British Journal of Psychiatry, 151,* 724-734.

Tarrier, N., Vaughn, C., Lader, M.H., & Leff, J.P. (1979). Bodily reactions to people and events in schizophrenics. *Archives of General Psychiatry, 36,* 311-315.

Taylor, S.E., & Brown, J.D. (1988). Illusion and well begin: A social psychological perspective on mental health. *Psychological Bulletin, 103,* 193-210.

Teasdale, J.D. (1988). Cognitive Vulnerability to persistent depression. *Cognition and Emotion, 2,* 247-274.

Teasdale, J. D., & Dent, J. (1987). Cognitive vulnerability to depression: An investigation of two hypotheses. *British Journal of Clinical Psychology, 26,* 113-126.

Tellegen, A., Lykken, D.T., Bouchard., T.J., Wilcox, K.J., & Rich, S. (1988). Personality similarity in twins reared apart and together. *Journal of Personality and Social Psychology, 54,* 1031-1039.

Tennant, C., & Andrews, G. (1978). The pathogenic quality of life stress in neurotic impairment. *Archives of General Psychiatry, 35,* 859-863.

Tennant, C., & Bebbington, P. (1978). The social causation of depression: A critique of the work of Brown and his colleagues. *Psychological Medicine, 8,* 565-575.

Tennant, C., Bebbington, P., & Hurry, J. (1981a). The short-term outcome of neurotic disorders in the community: The relation of remission to clinical factors and to 'neutralizing' life events. *British Journal of Psychiatry, 139,*

213-220.
Tennant, C., Bebbington, P., & Hurry, J. (1981b). The role of life events in depressive illness: Is there a substantial causal relation? *Psychological Medicine, 11,* 379-389.
Tennant, C., Smith, A., Bebbington, P., & Hurry, J. (1979). The contextual threat of life events: The concept and its reliability. *Psychological Medicine, 9,* 525-528.
Tennant, N., & Thompson, I.E. (1980). Causal models and logical inference. *British Journal of Psychiatry, 137,* 579-582.
Tennen, H., & Eller, S.J. (1977). Attributional components of learned helplessness and facilitation. *Journal of Personality and Social Psychology, 35,* 265-271.
Thompson, P.J., & Trimble, M.R. (1982). Non-MAOI antidepressant drugs and cognitive functions: A review. *Psychological Medicine, 12,* 539-548.
Thornton, J.W., & Jacobs, P.D. (1971). Learned helplessness in human subjects. *Journal of Experimental Psychology, 87,* 367-372.
Tinbergen, N. (1963). On the aims and methods of ethology. *Zeitschrift für Tierpsychologie, 20,* 410-433.
Torgersen, S. (1990). Comorbidity of major depression and anxiety disorders in twin pairs. *American Journal of Psychiatry, 147,* 1199-1202.
Trivers, R. (1971). The evolution of reciprocal altruism. *Quarterly Review of Biology, 46,* 35-57.
Trivers, R. (1985). *Social Evolution.* California: Benjamin/Cummings.
Tronick, E.Z. (1989). Emotions and emotional communication in infants. *American Psychologist, 44,* 112-119.
Tronick, E.Z., Winn, S., & Morelli, G.A. (1985). Multiple caretaking in the context of human evolution: Why don't the Efe know the western prescription for child care? In M. Reite & T. Field (Eds.), *The Psychobiology of Attachment and Separation.* New York: Academic Press.
Trower, P., & Gilbert, P. (1989). New theoretical conceptions of social anxiety and social phobia. *Clinical Psychology Review (special issue; social phobia), 9,* 19-35.
Trower, P. Gilbert, P., & Sherling, G. (1990). Social anxiety, evolution and self-presentation. An inter-disciplinary perspective. In H. Leitenberg (Ed.), *Handbook of Social Anxiety.* New York, Plenum Press.
Tucker, D.M. (1981). Lateral brain function, emotion and conceptualisation. *Psychological Bulletin, 89,* 19-46.
Tucker, D.M., Stenslie, C.E., Roth, R.S., & Shearer, S.L. (1981). Right frontal lobe activation and right hemisphere performance: Decrement during depressed mood. *Archives of General Psychiatry, 38,* 169-174.
Turner, B.S. (1987). *Medical Power and Social Knowledge.* London: Sage.
Tyson, R.L. (1986). The roots of psychopathology and our theories of development. *Journal of the American Academy of Child Psychiatry, 25,* 12-22.
van der Post, L. (1976). *Jung and the Story of our Time.* Harmondsworth: Penguin Books.
Vasile, R.G., Samson, J.A., Bemporad, J., Bloomingdale, K.L., Creasey, D., Fenton, B.T., Gudeman, J.E., & Schildkraut, J.J. (1987). A biopsychosocial approach to treating patients with affective disorders. *American Journal of Psychiatry, 144,* 341-344.
Vaughn, C.E., & Leff, J.P. (1976). The influence of family and social factors on the

course of psychiatric illness: A comparison of schizophrenic and depressed neurotic patients. *British Journal of Psychiatry, 129,* 125-137.

Vaughn, C.E., & Leff, J. (1985). *Expressed Emotion in Families: Its Significance for Mental Illness.* New York: Guilford Press.

Vining, D.R. Jr, (1986). Social success versus reproductive success: The central theoretical problem for sociobiology (plus peer commentary). *Behavioral and Brain Sciences, 9,* 167-216.

Volkan, V. (1985) (Ed.). *Depressive States and Their Treatment.* Northvale, N.J.: Jason Aronson.

Wachtel, P.L. (1977). *Psychoanalysis and Behavior Therapy: Toward an Integration.* New York: Basic Books.

Warburton, D.M. (1979). Physiological aspects of information processing and stress. In V. Hamilton & D.M. Warburton (Eds.), *Human Stress and Cognition: An Information Processing Approach.* Chichester: J.Wiley.

Warheit, G.J. (1979). Life events, coping, stress and depressive symptomatology. *American Journal of Psychiatry, 136,* 502-507.

Watson, D., & Clark, L.A. (1984). Negative affectivity: The disposition to experience aversive emotional states. *Psychological Bulletin, 96,* 465-490.

Watson, D., & Clark, L.A. (1988). Positive and negative affectivity and their relation to anxiety and depressive disorders. *Journal of Abnormal Psychology, 97,* 346-353.

Wehr, T.A., Sack, D.A., Parry, B.L., & Rosenthal, N.E. (1985). Treatment of seasonal affective disorder with light in the evening. *British Journal of Psychiatry, 147,* 424-428.

Wehr, T.A., Jacobson, F.M., Sack, D.A., Arendt, J., Tamarkin, L., & Rosenthal, N.E. (1986). Phototherapy of seasonal affective disorder. *Archives of General Psychiatry, 43,* 870-875.

Weiner, B. (1972). *Theories of Motivation: From Mechanism to Cognition.* Chicago: Rand McNally.

Weiner, B. (1974) (Ed.). *Achievement, Motivation and Attribution Theory.* Morristown, N.J.: General Learning Press.

Weiner, B., Heckhausen, H., Meyer, W.U., & Cook, R.E. (1972). Causal ascriptions and achievement motivation. *Journal of Personality and Social Psychology, 21,* 239-248.

Weiner, B., Nierenberg, R., & Goldstein, M. (1976). Social learning (locus of control) versus attributional (causal stability) interpretations of expectancy of success. *Journal of Personality, 44,* 52-68.

Weiner, B., Russell, D., & Lerman, D. (1978). Affective consequences of causal ascriptions. In J.H. Harvey, W.J. Ickes, & R.F. Kidd (Eds.), *New Directions in Attribution Research, Vol. 2.* Hillsdale, N.J.: Lawrence Erlbaum Associates Inc.

Weiner, B. Russel, D., & Lerman, D. (1979). The cognition-emotion process in achievement related contexts. *Journal of Personality and Social Psychology, 37,* 1211-1220.

Weingartner, H., Cohen, R.M., Murphy, D.L., Martello, J., & Gerdt, C. (1981). Cognitive processes in depression. *Archives of General Psychiatry, 38,* 42-47.

Weingartner, H., Miller, H., & Murphy, D.L. (1977). Mood- state-dependent retrieval of verbal associations. *Journal of Abnormal Psychology, 86,* 276-284.

Weisner, T.S. (1986). Implementing new relationship styles in American families. In W.W. Hartup & Z. Rubin (Eds.), *Relationships and Development.* Hillsdale,

N.J.: Lawrence Erlbaum Associates Inc.

Weiss, J.M., Glazer, H.I., & Pohorecky, L.A. (1976). Coping behavior and neurochemical changes. An alternative explanation for the original 'learned helplessness' experiments. In G. Serban & A. Kling (Eds.), *Animal Models in Human Psychobiology.* New York: Plenum Press.

Weiss, J.M., Glazer, H.I., Pohorecky, L.A., Bailey, W.H., & Schneider, L.H. (1979). Coping behavior and stress-induced behavioral depression: Studies of the role of brain catecholamines. In R.A. Depue (Ed.), *The Psychobiology of the Depressive Disorders.* New York: Academic Press.

Weiss, J.M., & Simson, P.G. (1985). Neurochemical mechanisms underlying stress-induced depression. In T.M. Field, P.M. McCabe, & N. Schneiderman (Eds.), *Stress and Coping.* London: Lawrence Erlbaum Associates Ltd.

Weiss, R.S. (1986). Continuities and transformation in social relationships from childhood to adulthood. In W.W. Hartup & Z. Rubin (Eds.), *Relationships and Development.* Hillsdale, N.J.: Lawrence Erlbaum Associates Inc.

Weissman, M.M. (1979). The psychological treatment of depression. *Archives of General Psychiatry, 36,* 1261-1269.

Weissman, M.M. (1985). The epidemiology of anxiety disorders: Rates, risks and familial patterns. In A.H. Tuma & J.D. Maser (Eds.), *Anxiety and Anxiety Disorders.* Hillsdale, N.J.: Lawrence Erlbaum Associates Inc.

Weissman, M.M., & Klerman, G. L. (1977a). Sex differences and the epidemiology of depression. *Archives of General Psychiatry, 34,* 98-111.

Weissman, M.M., & Klerman, G.L. (1977b). The chronic depressive in the community: Unrecognized and poorly treated. *Comprehensive Psychiatry, 18,* 523-532.

Weissman, M.M., Klerman, G.L., & Paykel, E.S. (1971). Clinical evaluation of hostility in depression. *American Journal of Psychiatry, 128,* 261-266.

Weissman, M.M., Merikangas, K.R., Wickramaratne, P., Kidd, K.K., Prusoff, B.A., Leckman, J.F., & Pauls, D.L. (1986). Understanding the clinical heterogeneity of major depression using family data. *Archives of General Psychiatry, 43,* 430-434.

Welner, A., Marten, S., Wochnick, E., Davis, M.A., Fishman, R., & Clayton, P.J. (1979). Psychiatric disorders among professional women. *Archives of General Psychiatry, 36,* 169-173.

Wender, P., Kety, H., Rosenthal, D., Schulsinger, F., Orthmann, J., & Lunde, I. (1986). Psychiatric disturbance in the biological and adoptive families of adopted individuals with affective disorder. *Archives of General Psychiatry, 43,* 923-929.

Wenegrat, B. (1984). *Sociobiology and mental disorder: A New View.* California: Addison-Wesley.

Westen, D. (1988). Transference and information processing. *Clinical Psychology Review, 8,* 161-180.

Wetzel, R.D. (1976). Hopelessness, depression and suicide intent. *Archives of General Psychiatry, 33,* 1069-1073.

Whitlock, F.A., & Siskind, M. (1979). Depression and cancer: A follow-up study. *Psychological Medicine, 9,* 747-752.

Whybrow, P.C., Akiskal, H.S., & Mckinney. W.T. (1984). *Mood Disorders: Towards a New Psychobiology.* New York: Plenum Press.

Wicker, F.W., Payne, G.C., & Morgan, R.D. (1983). Participant descriptions of guilt and shame. *Motivation and Emotion, 7,* 25-39.

Wilhelm, K., & Parker, G. (1989). Is sex necessarily a risk factor to depression? *Psychological Medicine, 19,* 401-413.

Williams, C.L., & Poling, J. (1989). An epidemiological perspective on the anxiety and depressive disorders. In P.C. Kendall & D. Watson (Eds.), *Anxiety and Depression: Distinctive and Overlapping Features.* New York: Academic Press.

Williams, J,M.G. (1986). Social skills training and depression. In C.R. Hollin & P. Trower (Eds.), *Handbook of Social Skills Training: Applications and New Directions.* Oxford: Pergamon.

Williams, J.M.G. (1989). Cognitive treatment for depression. In K. Herbst & E. Paykel (Eds.), *Depression: An Integrative Approach.* Oxford: Heinemann Medical Books.

Williams, J.M.G., & Scott, J. (1988). Autobiographical memory in depression. *Psychological Medicine, 18,* 689-695.

Willner, P. (1984). Cognitive functioning in depression: A review of theory and research. *Psychological Medicine, 14,* 807-823.

Willner, P. (1985). *Depression: A Psychobiological Synthesis.* Chichester: J.Wiley & Sons.

Wilson, E.O. (1975). *Sociobiology.* Cambridge, Mass.: Harvard University Press.

Wilson, J. (1989). The role of self-help groups in the management of depression. In K. Herbst & E.S. Paykel (Eds.), *Depression: An Intergative Approach.* Oxford: Heinemann Medical Books.

Wing, J.K., Cooper, J.E., & Sartorius, N. (1974). *Measurement and Classification of Psychiatric Symptoms: An Introduction Manual for the PSE and Catego Program.* London: Cambridge University Press.

Winokur, G. (1973). Diagnostic and genetic aspects of affective illness. *Psychiatric Annals, 3,* 6-15.

Winokur, G. (1984). Psychosis in bipolar and unipolar affective illness with special reference to schizo-affective disorder. *British Journal of Psychiatry, 145,* 236-242.

Wolf, E.S. (1988). *Treating the Self.* New York: Guilford Press.

Wolfe, B. (1989). Heinz Kohut's self psychology: A conceptual framework. *Psychotherapy, 26,* 545-554.

Wolff, S. (1988). Personality development. In R.E. Kendell & A.K. Zeally (Eds.), *Companion to Psychiatric Studies* (4th edition). Edinburgh: Churchhill Livingstone.

Wollheim, R. (1971). *Freud.* London: Fontana.

Wolpe, J. (1971). Neurotic depression: Experimental analogue, clinical syndromes and treatment. *American Journal of Psychotherapy, 25,* 362-368.

Wolpe, J. (1979). The experimental model and treatment of neurotic depression. *Behaviour Research and Therapy, 17,* 555-565.

Wolpe, J. (1981a). The dichotomy between classically conditioned and cognitively learned anxiety. *Journal of Behavior Therapy and Experimental Psychiatry, 12,* 35-42.

Wolpe, J. (1981b). Commentary on the report of the behavior therapy conference. *Journal of Consulting and Clinical Psychology, 49,* 604-605.

Wood, J.V. (1989). Theory and research concerning social comparisons of personal attributes. *Psychological Bulletin, 106,* 231-248.

World Health Organization (1978). *Mental Disorders: Glossary and Guide to their*

Classification in Accordance with the Ninth Revision of the International Classification of Diseases. Geneva: WHO.

Wrate, R.M., Rooney, A.C., Thomas, P.F., & Cox, J.L. (1985). Postnatal depression and child development: A three year follow-up study. *British Journal of Psychiatry, 146,* 622-627.

Wright, J.C., Giammarino, M., & Parad, H.W. (1986). Social status in small groups: Individual-group similarity and social "misfit". *Journal of Personality and Social Psychology, 50,* 523-536.

Yalom. I.D (1980). *Existential Psychotherapy.* New York: Basic Books.

Young, J.E. (1988, June). *Schema-focused therapy,* presented at the World Conference in Cognitive Therapy, Oxford.

Young, M.A., Sheftner, W.A., Klerman, G.L., Andreasen, N.C., & Hirschfeld, R.M.A. (1986). The endogenous subtype of depression: A Study of its internal construct validity. *British Journal of Psychiatry, 148,* 257-267.

Youngren, M.A., & Lewinsohn, P.M. (1980). The functional relation between depression and problematic interpersonal behavior. *Journal of Abnormal Psychology, 89,* 333-341.

Zajonc, R.B. (1980). Feeling and thinking: Preferences need no inferences. *American Psychologist, 35,* 151-175.

Zajonc, R.B (1984). On the primacy of affect. *American Psychologist, 39,* 117-123.

Zilboorg, G., & Henry, G.W. (1941). *History of Medical Psychology.* New York: W.W. Norton & Co.

Zimmerman, M., & Coryell, W. (1989). DSM-111 Personality disorder diagnoses in a nonpatient sample: Demographic correlates and comorbidity. *Archives of General Psychiatry, 46,* 682-689.

Zimmerman, M., Coryell, W.H., & Black, D.W. (1990). Variability in the application of contemporary diagnostic criteria: Endogenous depression as an example. *American Journal of Psychiatry, 147,* 1173-1179.

Zimmerman, M., Coryell, W., Pfohl, B., & Stangl, D. (1986). The validity of four definitions of endogenous depression: 11. Clinical, demographic, familial and psychosocial correlates. *Archives of General Psychiatry, 43,* 234-244.

Zimmerman, M., Pfohl, M.D., Coryell, W., Stangl, D., & Corenthal, C. (1988). Diagnosing personality disorder in depressed patients: A comparison of patient and informant interviews. *Archives of General Psychiatry, 45,* 733-737.

Zimmerman, M., & Spitzer, R.L. (1989). Melancholia: From DSM-111 to DSM-111-R. *American Journal of Psychiatry, 146,* 20-28.

Zuckerman, M. (1989). Personality in the third dimension: a psychobiological approach. *Personality and Individual Differences, 10,* 391-418.

Zung, W.W.K. (1965). A self-rating depression scale. *Archives of General Psychiatry, 13,* 508-516,

Zuroff, D.C., & Mongrain, M. (1987). Dependency and self criticism: Vulnerability factors for depressive affective states. *Journal of Abnormal Psychology, 96,* 14-22.

Author Index

Subject Index

APPENDIX A: MEASUREMENT OF DEPRESSION

There are three main issues in the measurement/assessment of depression: 1) self-rating versus clinical or objective rating; 2) severity versus diagnosis of type and 3) the use family or other external sources of information. Assessment can have various functions: to indicate a form of treatment (e.g. ECT, drug, or psychosocial therapy); to plot change from day to day, week to week, or the course of change during treatment; and/or for research of syndromes. According to the purpose of the assessment the clinician may utilise different instruments. Mazure, Nelson and Price (1986) discuss the issues involved in differences between patient-reported symptoms and clinical evaluation. Other issues relate to the use of external sources of information such as family members or ward staff. As we have mentioned, while a patient may complain of their depression their family may complain of their aggression and irritability. Observers may note different behaviours to those reported by the patient. Sometimes if a patient is challenged with the idea that they do seem to enjoy things, (e.g. laughing with other patients) they may say, "yes but it's only an act." So the question of whether one places more weight on observed behaviour or on self-reports is a complex issue.

There are no self-rating scales of depression that are regarded as reliable diagnostic instruments and most are used as measures of severity. There are a variety of self-rating instruments available (Ferguson & Tyrer, 1989; Berndt, 1990). The two most well known are the Beck Depression Inventory BDI (Beck et al., 1961) and the Zung self-rating depression scale (Zung, 1965). The BDI was restandardised in 1979 (Beck et al., 1979) and researchers and clinicians should now use this form which is included on pages 550 and 551.

Kendall, Hollon, Beck, Hammen, and Ingram (1987) have outlined the guidelines for use. They suggest 0–9 = non-depressed, 10-15 and meeting no diagnostic criteria = dysphoric, 16 and above and meeting diagnostic criteria for affective disorder = depressed. Whether these cut-off scores have cross cultural validity is unknown since in other cultures depression is often shifted in the somatic direction (Marsella, 1980; Jenkins et al., 1991). Oliver and Simmons (1985) found that there may be cultural variation on the scoring of the BDI. Also more research is needed to look at personality disorder (e.g. borderline) since these patients can score very highly on the BDI. Shaw, Steer, Beck, and Schut (1979) found that the factor structure of the BDI for heroin addicts did not differ from a depressed population. Hence the BDI like all others that rate for severity of mood disturbance is not a diagnostic instrument.

Objective assessment of depression is achieved by various means. The Hamilton rating scale (HRSD) for depression was originally a 21-item scale but has since been shortened to 17 items (Ferguson & Tyrer, 1989). This requires training in its use and involves the clinician rating severity of various symptoms. The HRSD was put into a self-rating format by Carroll et al., (1981). The HRSD is also a severity rating scale and not a diagnostic scale. Together the BDI and HRSD are common instruments used by researchers.

Diagnosis depends on objective criteria and we met some of these in Chapter 2. Systematic methods of assessment for diagnosis are based on semi-structure or structured interviews. Here the most important are the Schedule for Affective Disorders and Schizophrenia (SADS) designed by Endicott and Spitzer (1978) and the Present State Examination developed by Wing, Cooper, and Sartorius (1974). There are three forms of the SADS, training is necessary, and it takes about 2 hours to complete. The PSE also requires training to use. The data is then classified by a CATEGO computer program. Diagnosis takes note of the time over which mood has been disturbed, its form and previous history (e.g. bipolar-unipolar). Self-rating scales do not address these issues. Sholomskas (1990) has given a clear and very helpful overview of various types of interview methods for depression and their validity.

Relationship of measures

Beck, Steer, and Garbin (1988) have given a major review of the psychometric properties of the BDI. In ten studies the BDI correlated with the HRSD between 0.41 and 0.86, giving a mean of 0.73 for clinical populations and 0.74 for non-clinical. Correlations with clinical ratings of severity and BDI in 14 studies range from 0.96-0.55, yielding a mean correlation of 0.72 for clinical populations and 0.60 for non-clinical populations. Hence the relationship between observer rating and subjective rating is fairly good. The BDI also has good correlations with other subjective rating, e.g. the Zung and the MMPI-D scales. Beck et al. (1988) also report on various factor analysis of the BDI. In general these studies suggest three main factors: negative attitudes towards the self; performance impairment; and somatic disturbance.

There have been various reviews of findings from research that have compared different scales. For example, Rippere (1987) found that the Zung and the BDI correlate between 0.52 and 0.70 across studies. Zung and HRSD correlate at 0.57. (Rippere also reports on one study that gave a very low correlation but this seems atypical). She also found that BDI and HRSD correlated 0.55–0.82. across studies, and BDI with psychiatrist global assessment of severity the correlation are 0.62 and

0.77 for two studies. An excellent review of various self-report and other scales is given by Berndt (1990). If you wish to explore scales relating to both depression and anxiety then Gotlib and Cane (1989) is also excellent. If you wish to research in this area then I recommend both the chapters by Berndt (1990) and Gotlib and Cane (1989).

Change

Mood rating scales like the BDI and the HRSD can be used to measure change and this can be very useful for clinical practice as well as research. Clinicians are encouraged to use some recognised rating of change rather than rely on vague subjective reports given by the patient or others (e.g. nurses). This vague impressionistic assessment of depression is sadly all too common at present. Standardised rating allows clinicians to see which symptoms are changing and which are not.

In the cognitive therapy literature, the BDI is a prominent instrument. However, the level by which recovery might be defined (normally less than 9 or 10) is controversial. For example, there may be important individual differences. For a person who before onset would have a typical score of (say) 7 then less than nine is a return to premorbid levels. However, a score of say 7–8 for someone who before becoming depressed would have scored 0, then the person may still be mildly depressed and not fully recovered (see Belsher & Costello 1988 and Chapters 3 & 4, this volume).

The BDI can be used not only as a measure of depression but also to alert the clinician to various patterns of symptoms that might need to be followed up e.g., a combination of hopelessness and desire to kill self should be explored further. High scores on the feelings of being punished should also be explored. The therapist may also wish to use the BDI to help start discussion if a patient is difficult to engage; e.g. "I note that you are feeling particularly guilty, could you tell me more about that?" or, "could we look at that?"

For those interested in this area of research and for a general overview of measuring instruments the reader is referred to the Freeman and Tyrer's edited volume (1989), and chapters by Brendt (1990), Gotlib & Cane (1989) and Sholomskas (1990). Brown's (1991) chapter is more slanted to issues of epidemiology but includes much discussion on measurement. It addresses some of the issues in assessment not considered by the others and is therefore also recommended.

APPENDIX B: THE THEORY AND STYLES OF PERSONAL ADJUSTMENT

From Leary's (1957) work it is possible to derive eight sets of possible styles for eliciting and maintaining a particular interpersonal style between sender and respondent. The sender chooses a particular style because of possible advantages. Different psychopathologies tend to be associated with different positions on the circumplex model. Leary calls these preferences for adjustment. This is because an individual has come to adjust their self to the social world (dealing with its threats, fears and reinforcers) by adopting and amplifying particular aspects of a interpersonal styles. In other words, they represent forms of social coping strategies to deal with or avoid social conflict(s), or to promote positive (reinforcing) interactions. In my view the interpersonal model provides an excellent, but as yet largely untapped source for research on personality and affective disorder. It was these ideas that lead me to consider interpersonal themes (see chapter 11).

Adjustment Through Rebellion: The Distrustful Personality

These individuals compulsively eschew closeness with others; they are traumatised and threatened by positive feelings (Leary 1957, p.269). They seem to evaluate interpersonal closeness as potentially reducing highly valued autonomy, freedom and individuality through closeness, nurturing and cooperation. In their extreme activation they actually provoke the distrust and rejection they feel themselves. This leads to a vicious circle of more distrust and rejection in both sender and respondent. Not only do they distrust the nurturing and cooperative behaviour of others, they are prone to distrust the same feelings in themselves. It is likely that they are poor empathisers (as indeed all those on the hostile dimension may be). They can be cynical, wary, uncompromising and, in the extreme, paranoid and prone to schizophrenia and psychosomatic complaints.

Adjustment Through Self-Effacement: The Masochistic Personality

These individuals have more developed submissive tendencies. They respond to interpersonal difficulties and dilemmas with submissive gestures: I am a weak, inferior person. These individuals ward off anxiety of interpersonal threat by submission and are depression prone. There is experimental evidence that this may indeed be so (Forrest & Hokanson, 1975). There seems to be a fear or taboo on assertive responses; hence, submission is the solution to avoid interpersonal threats, injuries and losses (much as ethological models suggest). These behavioural styles tend to provoke arrogant, punitive and leadership behaviours in others. This style is highly represented in depressive conditions and is marked by low assertiveness with a tendency to suppress the open expression of anger/rage, and a harbouring of secret grievances.

Adjustment Through Docility: The Dependent Personality

This style is also submissive but less hostile, and there is generally a more open and affiliative component. They give out responses such as: I am a meek, admiring person in need of your help. Hence, nurturance-seeking rather than the avoidance of interpersonal attack is more of a central concern here. Autonomy and competitive competency may be inhibited because of self-doubt and the fear that a demonstration (display) of autonomy would threaten help provision from others. These individuals believe that a degree of self humility and admiration of the other is required to secure help. Whereas when the masochist tends to get depressed there is a good deal of self-castigation, the dependent personality is more tearful, pleading, and reassurance-seeking. He does not endear himself to personalities on the more hostile dimension but may provoke caring, helpful, nurturing responses from those on the more friendly side of the dimension. Carson (1969, p.109) suggests: The extreme of this form of behaviour is a clinging, ingratiating dependency that may become very sticky indeed for the person towards whom it is directed. According to Leary, these individuals are more prone to diffuse anxieties, phobias and obsessions. As with other submissive postures there is a tendency to inhibit competitive assertiveness.

Adjustment Through Cooperation: The Over-conventional Personality

This style for solving interpersonal dilemmas and conflicts is primarily one of cooperation. In the extreme, these individuals are inappropriately and excessively agreeable, striving to maintain harmony in their interpersonal domains. They are easily influenced by others but are uncomfortable in the presence of hostile, unhappy, or power-oriented feelings in both themselves and others and avoid these if possible. They tend to be self-sacrificing. Brotherly love is preferred together with the avoidance of aggression. They tend to provoke friendliness and openness in others since they pose no competitive threat, nor threaten to become dependent on or needy of others. Anxiety is aroused by situations which call for assertive, non cooperative responses. They run the risk of being seen as kind but bland and unforceful people. In some cases they can activate aggressive responses in people who are looking for some definite viewpoint or positive reaction from them. Although they cooperate they may have difficulty in cooperating with others when there is an intra-group aggressive dispute. They may not like to take sides.

Adjustment Through Responsibility: The Hypernormal Personality
Of these, Leary (1957, p.315) says: "Here we deal with the individual who attempts to present himself with a 'normal' persona. He presents himself as strong, but his power and self-confident independence are used in an affiliative way. He strives to be close to others to help, counsel, support and sympathise. He wants to be tender with his intimates, reasonable and responsible with his acquaintances." These behaviours tend to invite others to lean on him and foster dependency. In the extreme this may manifest as inappropriate over-protectiveness. They may need to be needed to fend off their own anxieties and helplessness or fears of loss of importance. In Leary's view the majority of these individuals do not self-refer but are referred by physicians for psychosomatic complaints. These patients may repress and deny a good deal of inner conflict in their efforts to maintain the hypernormal persona.

Adjustment Through Power: The Autocratic Personality
These are individuals are rank orientated; they use status, respect and prestige to secure and maintain self-esteem. In today's arena some of these may fall into the category of people labelled Type A. These individuals in the extreme are prone to be energetic, compulsive, perfectionist, and prone to mania. There is an avoidance of anxiety (related to inferiority, weakness, and helplessness) via striving. Like the masochist, their interpersonal activity tends to be basically one of social competition but unlike the masochist who surrenders quickly, the autocrat challenges and pushes for success. They can be overly controlling and demanding of respect from others and attribute weakness or incompetence to subordinates, usually in the emotional domain. That is they may see in others what they fear in themselves. These individuals may be poor therapy clients in the normal course of events, manifesting distress through psychosomatic difficulties and overactive autonomic systems. They have a tendency to abandon therapeutic methods quickly. It may also be noted that these individuals, in so far as they relate to Type A personalities, are prone to defeat depression and cardiac disorder.

Adjustment Through Competition: The Narcissistic Personality
These individuals are also status seekers but, as the model suggests, are rather more hostile, arrogant, and smug. They may be boastful in words rather than deeds although also inappropriately exhibitionist. They are prone to focus on their outward appearance, dress, physical beauty or superior talents. These individuals feel most secure when they are independent of other people or feel they are triumphing over them (Leary, 1957, p.332). There is a greater tendency than with the

autocratic personality to use people for selfish ends (boost self-esteem) and a significant lack of empathy. They tend to be envious and disdainful of others, instilling resentment. They tend to provoke in others more passive, hostile, and negative submissive responses. They are prone to break down with anxiety about weakness, shame, and humiliation. They describe their parents as sadistic.

Adjustment Through Aggression: The Sadistic Personality
These individuals are the most destructive of all the personality types so far considered. Self-security is based on the wielding of power through threat and physical and verbal abuse. Leary includes all those who maintain dominance through the humiliation of others. Although the narcissist uses other people primarily for his own ends, the purpose is not to humiliate but to acquire independence, admiration, and prestige. To strike humiliation, fear or guilt is not the primary purpose of the narcissistic type but is so of the sadistic personality. Leary (1957, p.342) says: "We think here, for example, of the stern unforgiving father, the bad-tempered wife, the moralistic guilt-provoking mother, the sharp-tongued mocking husband, the grim-faced punitive official, the truculent fiery-natured colleague, the disciplinarian. We include all those law-abiding, often pious and self-righteous individuals who maintain a role for potential insult, degradation or punishment." As Leary points out, these styles are by no means confined to the delinquent few but can be found to various degrees in the ruling classes of many societies and subgroups. These individuals do not, interestingly, come to the clinics for phobic anxieties or depressive problems but primarily for marital and interpersonal difficulties. Delinquency, bed-wetting and phobias often appear in the offspring of these patients (p.347). As with the distrusting personality that we met earlier, these individuals fear intimate, loving, and nurturing responses in themselves. Sometimes they are in states of vengeful retaliation to cruel early parental experiences. Again, there is a lack of empathy.

APPENDIX C: ENDOGENOUS AND NEUROTIC DEPRESSION

One way to consider differences between types of depression, such as endogenous-neurotic and unipolar-bipolar, is by the strategies of ranking.

Consider the following:

1. Are there biological and symptom differences in depression in individuals who are highly up-rank motivated, with autocratic and achievement-focused personalities (high on trait dominance, Buss,

1988) compared to those who are more affiliative and less autocratic? Personality studies have found that endogenous depressives and bipolar patients are more ambitious and competitive than neurotics (Chapter 4). Is the endogenous depression similar to Type A depression (called vital exhaustion, Price, 1982), which arises when these individuals feel they haven't been successful or are trapped or thwarted in their competitive behaviour?

2. In marriage, is the endogenous patient the one who falls from being dominant, while the neurotic becomes (or is pushed) into a more subordinate position? (see Price, in press). These issues of dominance may relate particularly to males. Men may do less well with family therapy (Keitner & Miller, 1990), perhaps because therapy does not sanction their autocratic control. Also depressed men are more likely to kill themselves by violent means.

3. Consider the evidence on nonverbal behaviour (Chapter 6). Is it possible that endogenous depression is more akin to a primitive defeat and yielding response whereas the neurotic is more akin to a highly subordinate response? Can one shade into the other? Is yielding and defeat controlled via a different psychobiological process than those of heightened submissiveness?

4. One key issue that may also separate neurotic from endogenous depression might be coping behaviour (or response rules) and their attitudes to seeking help and expressing emotion. The endogenous depressive might be more prone to hiding distress and social withdrawal (and social withdrawal itself has biological effects) and expressing somatic symptoms, whereas the neurotic is more orientated to eliciting support and expressing distress. Hence, the neurotic will show high levels of subordinate appeasement behaviour and reassurance seeking.

5. I am intrigued by the possibility that the trait of dominance has three aspects 1) aggression 2) competing for attention and 3) initiative taking (Buss, 1988). Is it possible that hypomania and mania reflect instability in the SAHP ranking system? Hypomanic individuals rarely show increased aggressive dominance behaviour (although they can be easily frustrated). In the early stages their good moods make them attractive to others and they like to be the 'centre of attention'. Indeed it is hard not to be impressed by their need for attention. Thus perhaps, as we have evolved from an agonic to a hedonic type of species, genetic changes have occurred in the brain that have had major implications for the control of internal inhibition. If this is so then bipolar disorder is of late phylogenetic origin. In other words bipolar disorders are essentially disorders of the SAHP system.

There are more questions than answers, but if ranking theory proves useful, then the nature of the differences between the old reptilian yielding responses and the newer mammalian submissive responses may offer a useful research paradigm. Also since the tactics of ranking have changed over evolutionary time then we may need to be more precise as to what aspect of ranking has been effected in depression (e.g. desires for attractiveness or desires for aggressive power). At this point we must wait for our questions to be clearly formulated and researched. At present there is little research that has attempted to test ranking theory directly and most evidence is indirect.

APPENDIX D: CULTURE AND CHANGE

Culture proliferated with the shift from social rank and asymmetry derived from aggression and intimidation to rank and asymmetry derived from attractiveness. With the emergence of SAHP as a way to gain access to resources, find acceptance in a group and even leadership roles, a host of changes took place.

1. There had to be changes (reductions) in internal (agonic) processes of inhibition such that many individuals rather than just the strongest felt free and motivated to explore their social worlds, display talents, skills and problem-solving abilities to others. Hence the reassuring/relaxing/calming qualities of gaining SAHP were profoundly important. Furthermore, very inhibited individuals would find it hard to display and be 'noticed' or to explore enough to develop helpful networks. Hence the reduction of internal inhibition was crucial for hedonic social life.

2. Communication and empathy become vital to discover what others feel about oneself (how to impress them) and also to learn from others (copy) skills and values that will gain SAHP.

3. These changes meant that copying behaviour and intelligence would now be positively selected for. This is because intelligent individuals would learn quickly from others and be able to demonstrate to others various behaviours that would be seen to offer advantage (i.e. give advantage to the 'select/accept me' signal). Thus we have a kind of 'value added' situation which allows for the accumulation of knowledge and skill.

4. New threats also evolved however, such as: loss of SAHP in the form of shame, and new tactics to undermine others' SAHP by envious attacks (e.g. running others down behind their back), and the fear of eliciting envy, emerge; there is no equivalent of spoiling-envious behaviour in non-human primates. Hence in some contexts too much evidence of positive difference is threatening and may make one an envied individual (see Chapter 8 and Gilbert, 1989). Sharing and reducing discrepancies in resources may lower this fear and so altruism may play a role in reducing envy and gain SAHP.

5. If SAHP becomes a primary strategy for gaining access to resources and security, then we may assume that this would have exerted great selective pressure on the brain, facilitating algorithms that could evaluate how to be attractive to others on the one hand, and biologic possibilities to be calmed or encouraged with others' approval/ acceptance on the other. Hence the algorithm might go like this "if you value me then you will wish to be with me and be an ally; you will not attack me, nor drive me from your group nor ignore me. You will share your resources with me. However if you do not value me and send signals of SAHP then none of these things can be relied upon and the social world is far more threatening." Without SAHP the best strategy might be to become aggressive and take what one can or be submissive and seek out others on whose coat-tails one can ride. Thus signals of SAHP are crucial for the safety system. Some individuals can be charming to others provided they are eliciting SAHP but become aggressive if these signals fall below a certain level.

6. At this level and only at this level, group selection (not species selection) occurs, for those groups that do indeed bestow status on the talented will gain over those that do not. This is true especially if 'tribes are warlike' (Itzkoff, 1990) or if the environment changes and requires intelligence to compensate (e.g. the discovery of fire). It is, in a way, the path to the rise of the meritocracy.

7. Individuals and groups will now come to differentiate themselves on the dimension of values and ideas. Competition arises from the battle "to win hearts and minds", to win people over to one's point of view and way of doing things. But the scale is a problem here for we evolved in small hunter-gather bands. Thus there is a tendency to form ingroups out of larger groups (e.g. the religious leaders who may set up their own sects). This has remarkable similarities to animals who breakaway when a group gets too large but still surround themselves with other defectors who become dutiful subordinates. The arousal of paranoid fears of outsiders might be just the thing to help bind a group together and to a particular leader.

8. There is another new problem with SAHP which, in a way, is paradoxical. It can increase aggression between groups. Followers, for example, may use aggression to win favour or approval (gain SAHP) from some higher ranker, be this a God, an Archbishop, a Mafia leader or the group in general. Usually it is requested as a demonstration of loyalty. For example, in competitive sportsthose teams that show aggressive determination to win often gain increased SAHP from supporters. Thus demonstration of aggression to outsiders can increase the attractiveness of the 'select me and I will be useful to you', signal especially for an ingroup that has fear of outsiders (the Rambo character).

Thus the most serious forms of aggression to humans are not from the individual but from groups or nations. Few of us wish to believe that our aggression is outright selfishness, paranoia, envy, or need for revenge. So we wrap it up in SAHP terms and appeal to the virtue of the fight (e.g. the crusades, and so forth). Once SAHP is involved everyone wants to prove themselves to the group—that they too are willing to fight and are therefore virtuous and deserving of a place. The virtuous war is often the most savage and Hitler relied on ideas of the appeal to virtue. Even economic policies that maybe harmful to many are accepted because we need to strengthen our competitive edge, we become paranoid about losing our place and those that are not up to it can be seen as different from ourselves. Here one does not have to see oneself as aggressive but as moral and pursuing a moral cause—we tell ourselves 'it has to be done'. The need to belong and prove ourselves has therefore a shadow side. It is wise to remember this when we focus on the positive side of our belongingness as a protection against depression.

9. The SAHP system does not replace the RHP system and various individuals in power (or attempting to get it) can use coercion to control others or bestow power on kin rather than the talented. The serious consequences of agonic fear-based social systems are evident in various societies today. The events that have unfolded with the collapse of agonic societies in Eastern Europe has, for me, raised the issue of depressive societies and social structures. How we move from biology to culture remains complex but possible (e.g. Kemper, 1990b). When we are able to move freely through these different levels of discourse then biopsychosocial models of health will have moved forward.